W9-BKV-233

DATE DUE

NOV 5 2003			

If this book should get lost, will the finder please call or notify nearest address at once, and the owner will call for same. May I thank you very much for this courtesy.

STUDENT'S NAME	
STREET ADDRESS	
CITY	STATE
TELEPHONE NUMBER	
NAME OF SCHOOL	
ADDRESS OF SCHOOL	
CITY	STATE
TELEPHONE NUMBER	

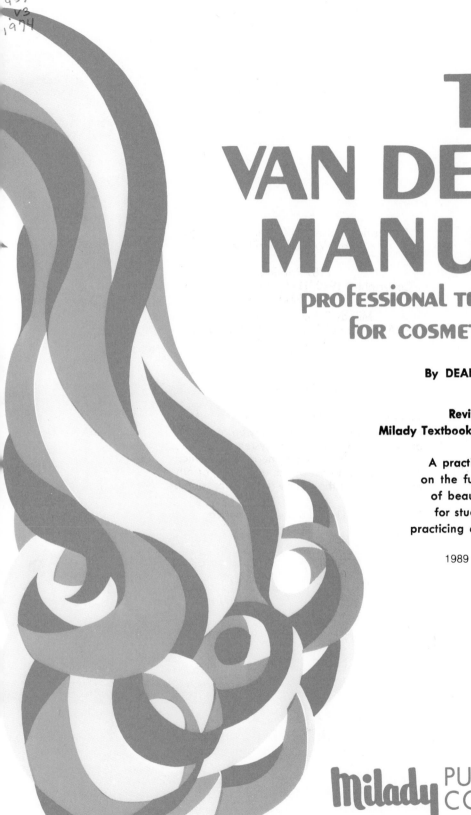

THE VAN DEAN MANUAL

professional techniques for cosmetologists

By DEAN BARRETT

Revised by
Milady Textbook Educational Board

A practical course
on the fundamentals
of beauty culture
for students and
practicing cosmetologists

1989 Printing

Milady PUBLISHING
COMPANY

(A Division of Delmar Publishers, Inc.)
2839 WHITE PLAINS ROAD
BRONX, NEW YORK 10467

Illustrations based on Original Drawings
by WARREN MEEK

1989 Printing
Copyright © 1940, 1945, 1948, 1951, 1957,
1962, 1974, 1976
Milady Publishing Company
(A Division of Delmar Publishing, Inc.)
Bronx, N.Y.

ISBN 0-87350-368-6

PREFACE

The Van Dean Manual has been redesigned to provide students and teachers with an up-to-date learning tool. It offers a step-by-step, practical development of the subject matter that unfolds the complete cosmetology course in easily understood segments. Further, the material contained herein reflects the most current information and procedures available.

A new format was devised in which headings and sub-headings have been placed in the margin, providing teachers with an outline of each chapter and thus facilitating the presentation of the material. Students can use the side headings to locate and identify subject matter more readily, and to isolate specific subjects for concentrated study.

The information contained in this text offers a great measure of flexibility, whereby teachers and students can adapt the material to whichever routine they find comfortable. No attempt has been made to present the "one and only" method for the practice of cosmetology. In fact, no such method exists. 'But what has been stressed is that a correct approach to cosmetology can lead to the development of other correct approaches, and in the process provide cosmetology educators with an impetus to be flexible, modern, and alert to change and improvements.

With the greater demand by the general public for more knowledgeable cosmetologists, it became necessary to de-emphasize certain theory subjects and to include more detailed information on hair structure and chemistry. This text will help lay the foundation for a better understanding of the nature of hair and skin as protein substances and the products used in professional beauty culture work.

Graduating students who enter the job market will be better qualified to keep pace with the new techniques which are developed and to understand the new products with which they will be working.

To those outstanding educators, State Board members, teachers and school administrators, whose contributions have greatly enhanced the value of the new Van Dean Manual, we offer our sincere appreciation.

Milady Textbook Educational Board

CONTENTS

continued

8   SCALP AND HAIR CARE   51

9   HAIR SHAPING   59

10   FINGER WAVING   75

11   HAIRSTYLING   81

continued

31   SALON MANAGEMENT   447

Welcome to Cosmetology and its Opportunities

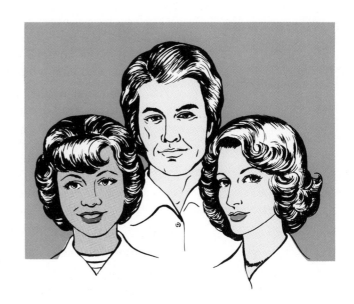

CONGRATULATIONS

. . . for making the decision to study beauty culture. By enrolling in this school, you have taken the first step toward a most glamorous and interesting profession. Beauty culture offers the opportunity for a lifetime career in one of the country's largest and most profitable industries. Within a comparatively short training time, you can be ready to embark upon a career offering a good income for the balance of your working life.

For A Young Woman

Beauty culture is a vocation that can be tailored to fit into the pattern of your private life. When you are ready to raise a family, you can leave and then return and pick up where you left off. You can live a normal married family life and work at your own convenience.

For A Young Man

The opportunities available are greater in the cosmetology field than in any other field comparable in preparation time and expense. Beauty culture offers a lucrative, exciting and growth filled future if you are an ambitious young man.

The practice of beauty culture also offers the opportunity for a great deal of personal satisfaction. It appeals to the artistic and esthetic needs of the cosmetologist. It encourages the free exercise of one's abilities. And it combines job satisfaction with financial stability.

Welcome

We extend a most sincere welcome to you. We know that you will be pleased with your choice of this fascinating career.

How well you succeed will depend to a great degree on your own ambitions. The field and the opportunities are unlimited. You have opened the door to a new world . . . now enter.

OPPORTUNITIES

Unlimited opportunities are available to young men and women who complete their training and acquire a license to practice cosmetology.

The doors to over 45 fascinating and exciting careers are thrown open to the trained cosmetologist. Passing through any one of these doors presents an opportunity for a lifetime career in some facet of the dynamic and glamorous field of beauty culture.

An examination of the following chart will give you some idea of the many areas available to the licensed cosmetologist.

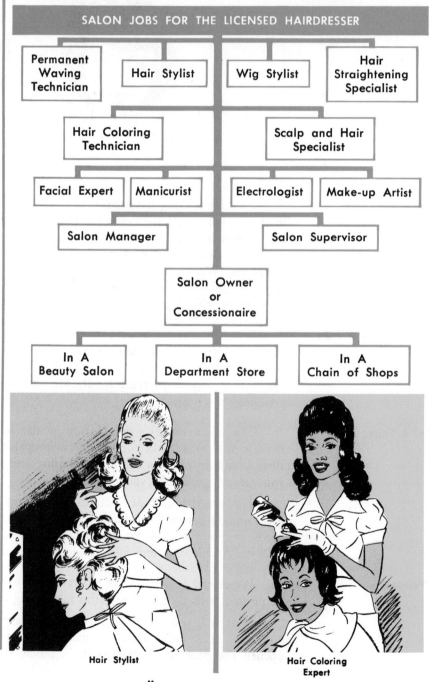

SALON JOBS FOR THE LICENSED HAIRDRESSER

- Permanent Waving Technician
- Hair Stylist
- Wig Stylist
- Hair Straightening Specialist
- Hair Coloring Technician
- Scalp and Hair Specialist
- Facial Expert
- Manicurist
- Electrologist
- Make-up Artist
- Salon Manager
- Salon Supervisor
- Salon Owner or Concessionaire
- In A Beauty Salon
- In A Department Store
- In A Chain of Shops

Hair Stylist

Hair Coloring Expert

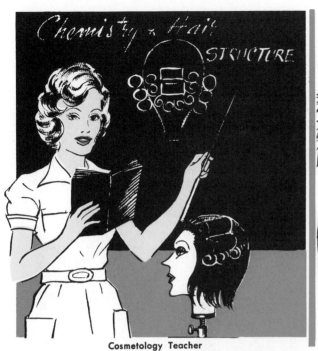

Cosmetology Teacher

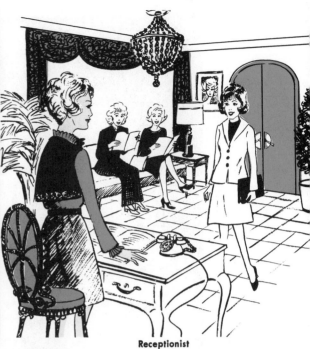

Receptionist

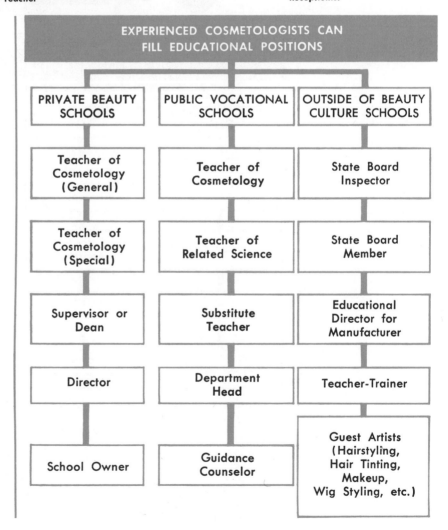

EXPERIENCED COSMETOLOGISTS CAN FILL EDUCATIONAL POSITIONS		
PRIVATE BEAUTY SCHOOLS	PUBLIC VOCATIONAL SCHOOLS	OUTSIDE OF BEAUTY CULTURE SCHOOLS
Teacher of Cosmetology (General)	Teacher of Cosmetology	State Board Inspector
Teacher of Cosmetology (Special)	Teacher of Related Science	State Board Member
Supervisor or Dean	Substitute Teacher	Educational Director for Manufacturer
Director	Department Head	Teacher-Trainer
School Owner	Guidance Counselor	Guest Artists (Hairstyling, Hair Tinting, Makeup, Wig Styling, etc.)

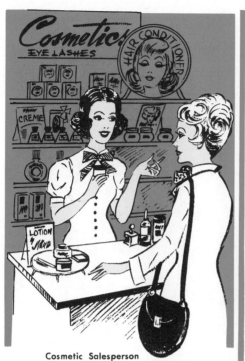

Cosmetic Salesperson

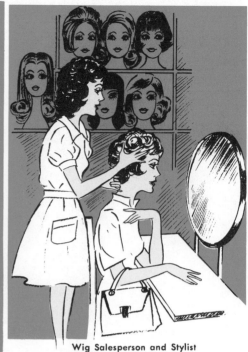

Wig Salesperson and Stylist

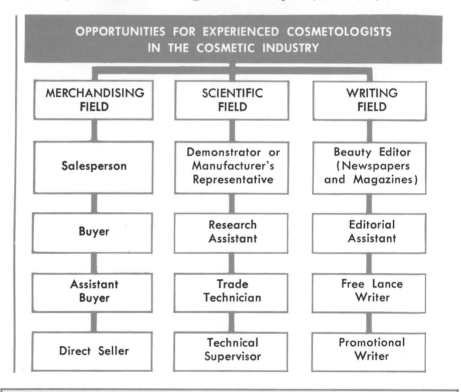

OPPORTUNITIES FOR EXPERIENCED COSMETOLOGISTS IN THE COSMETIC INDUSTRY		
MERCHANDISING FIELD	**SCIENTIFIC FIELD**	**WRITING FIELD**
Salesperson	Demonstrator or Manufacturer's Representative	Beauty Editor (Newspapers and Magazines)
Buyer	Research Assistant	Editorial Assistant
Assistant Buyer	Trade Technician	Free Lance Writer
Direct Seller	Technical Supervisor	Promotional Writer

SUMMARY

Cosmetology is as exciting as it is profitable, and represents to many men and women a profession that will bring happiness and financial independence.

CHAPTER 1

HYGIENE AND GOOD GROOMING

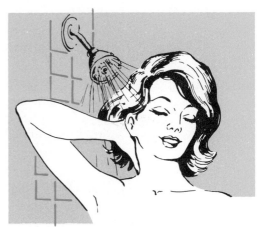

Daily shower

INTRODUCTION

Good health is required for the successful practice of cosmetology. Without it, one can neither work efficiently nor enjoy the pleasures of life. With it, the greatest constructive work and happiness are made possible.

In keeping with his/her profession, the cosmetologist should be a living example of health and be able to advise patrons on how to attain it by hygienic living. In this way, she will increase her value to herself, to her employer and to the community.

HYGIENE

Hygiene is a branch of applied science which deals with healthful living. It includes both personal and public hygiene.

Personal Hygiene

Personal hygiene concerns the intelligent care given by the individual to preserve health through following the rules of healthful living, especially as they relate to such aspects as:

1. Cleanliness
2. Oral hygiene
3. Posture
4. Exercise
5. Relaxation
6. Adequate sleep
7. Balanced diet
8. Wholesome thoughts

Public Hygiene

Public hygiene or **sanitation** refers to the steps which should be taken by the government to promote public health. In order for the government to carry out its responsibilities to protect the health, safety and welfare of its citizens, steps should be taken to assure:

1. Pure air
2. Pure food
3. Pure water
4. Adequate sewerage
5. Control of disease
6. Adequate medical facilities

Public Safety

To protect public health, any person suffering from an infectious or contagious disease must not be allowed to attend school or work in a beauty salon. The public **must never** be served by one having an infectious or contagious disease.

HYGIENIC RULES OF LIVING

Beauty Problems

Beauty problems are also **health problems.** Good health reflects itself in a clear complexion, a fine-textured skin, sparkling eyes and luxuriant hair. The complexion is the outward expression of inner health. A dull, sallow complexion is indicative of:

1. A sluggish circulation
2. Lack of fresh air
3. Irregular elimination
4. Improper diet

Balanced Meals

Eating well-balanced meals at regular intervals and drinking a sufficient amount of water will keep the digestive system functioning properly. However, one of the basic causes of poor health is a **faulty diet.** It is essential to avoid such poor eating habits as:

1. **Not eating enough** of the **right kinds** of food, which may lead to loss of weight, lower resistance, or nutritional diseases
2. **Over-eating,** which taxes the digestive system and organs of elimination

Exercise And Recreation

Exercise and recreation in the form of walking, dancing, sports and gym activities develop muscles and help keep the body fit. A few of the benefits resulting from regular and non-strenuous exercises are:

1. An improvement in nutrition
2. An improvement in blood circulation
3. A larger supply of life-giving oxygen to the body, due to the increased action of the lungs

Sunshine. Any form of recreation in the sunshine adds vigor as well as helps to supply the body with essential vitamin "D."

Fatigue

Fatigue or **tiredness,** resulting from work, exercise, mental effort or the strain caused by hurry and worry, should always be followed by a period of rest or relaxation. Over-exertion and lack of rest tend to drain the body of its vitality. Therefore, an adequate amount of sleep, not less than seven hours, is necessary. This allows the body to recover from the fatigue of the day's activities and replenish itself with renewed energy.

Healthy Thoughts

The mind and body operate as a unit. A well-balanced condition of body and mind results in good health. This enables them to perform all their functions normally. Healthy thoughts can be cultivated by self-control. In place of worry and fear, the health-giving qualities of cheerfulness, courage and hope should be encouraged. Outside interests and recreation relieve the strain of monotony and hard work.

Thoughts and **emotions** influence body activities. A thought may cause the face to turn red and increase the heart action. A thought may either stimulate or depress the functions of the body. Strong emotions, such as worry and fear, have a harmful effect on the heart, arteries and glands. Mental depression weakens the functions of the organs, thereby lowering the resistance of the body to disease.

REMINDER

Observing the rules of hygienic living and cultivating healthy thoughts will help you become a successful cosmetologist.

A WELL-GROOMED FEMALE COSMETOLOGIST

The cosmetologist's care of her personal appearance sets a good example and is the best advertisement of the benefits of cosmetology.

To keep your appearance at its best, give daily attention to all the important details which make for a clean, neat and charming personality.

Daily Bath And Deodorant

Keep the body fresh and pleasant by taking a daily shower or bath and by using an underarm deodorant.

Teeth And Breath (Oral Hygiene)

Clean and brush the teeth regularly. Use mouth wash to eliminate unpleasant breath odor.

Hairstyle

Keep the hair clean and lustrous. Wear an attractive and practical hairstyle at all times.

Clothes

Wear a uniform that is spotlessly clean, neat and properly fitted. Keep slip out of sight and wear fresh underclothes.

Facial Makeup

Use the correct cosmetics to match your skin tones. Have a fresh, flawless complexion, sparkling eyes, well-shaped eyebrows and lips.

Hands And Nails

Keep your hands clean and smooth and your nails well-manicured.

Jewelry

Avoid gaudy jewelry. A wristwatch is permissible.

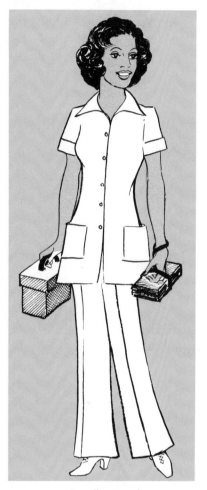

A well-groomed cosmetologist

Shoes And Stockings

Wear low-heeled shoes that are well-fitted and sensibly styled. Keep the shoes shined and the heels straight. Wear clean hose. Watch out for stocking runs, wrinkles and crooked seams.

Appearance And Personality

Beauty salon owners consider appearance and personality to be almost as important to the cosmetologist as technical knowledge and manual skills.

TO BE SUCCESSFUL. In addition to being well-groomed and proficient in your work, you must learn to do the little things that will make patrons like you. Have you done a **good** deed today? If not, try **tomorrow.**

A WELL-GROOMED MALE COSMETOLOGIST

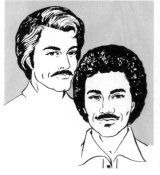

CHECK LIST
(Personal Cleanliness)

Proper grooming is equally important to male cosmetologists. They must give careful attention to cleanliness of uniform, skin, hair, hands, teeth, to the daily shower or bath, and use an underarm deodorant, if needed. Shave each day. Mustache or beard must be trimmed and styled. Trim hair from nostrils.

Personal cleanliness is an important hygienic habit. The cosmetologist must observe cleanliness in the following ways:

1. Keep the body clean by taking a daily bath or shower.
2. Avoid body odor by using a deodorant, when necessary.
3. Keep teeth and gums in good condition. Brush teeth at least twice daily with a good dentifrice.
4. Have a dental examination every six months.
5. Avoid bad breath by rinsing mouth with a good antiseptic.
6. Never wear shoes without clean hose or peds.
7. Keep shoes clean and neat.
8. Wear clean undergarments and a clean uniform each day.
9. Keep hair well-groomed.
10. Keep hands and fingernails in good condition.
11. Wash hands before and after serving each patron, and after visiting the toilet.
12. Avoid the common use of towels, drinking cups, cosmetics, hairbrushes and combs.

Maintaining Good Health

In order to maintain good health, observe the following rules:

1. Breathe clean and fresh air.
2. Drink sufficient water each day.
3. Follow a balanced diet. Do not over-eat.
4. Have regular and daily elimination.
5. Stand, sit and walk with good posture.
6. Get adequate sleep.
7. Get recreation and outdoor exercise.
8. Have regular physical examinations.

REVIEW QUESTIONS

Hygiene And Good Grooming

1. Define hygiene.
2. Define personal hygiene.
3. Define public hygiene.
4. List eight basic requirements for good personal hygiene.
5. List six basic requirements for good public health under the supervision of the government.
6. Which three mental qualities promote good health?
7. Which two emotions can injure health?
8. A daily bath or shower keeps the body ....
9. Avoid body odors by using a ....
10. Avoid bad breath by rinsing mouth with a good ....
11. The public must never be served by a cosmetologist having an infectious or .... disease.
12. How would you define oral hygiene?

CHAPTER 2

VISUAL POISE

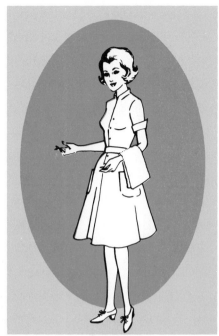

Correct stance

INTRODUCTION

Correct posture is very important to your body because it helps to prevent fatigue, improves your personal appearance and permits graceful movements in relation to your everyday work as a cosmetologist.

Good posture is an important part of personal care. Its continued **practice** assists in the **prevention** of many physical disturbances. In addition, it is a self-disciplinary factor which contributes to the development of other good habits. These are determining elements of a gracious and pleasing personality. When present, they indicate a **poised,** well-ordered individual.

Beauty salon owners consider appearance, visual poise and personality to be almost as important to the cosmetologist as technical knowledge and manual skills.

CORRECT STANCE

Regular exercise keeps the muscles of the body in good condition and assists in forming the habit of **good posture.** Practice will train the muscles to hold the body correctly. Good posture is a matter of habit. Avoid slouching, humped shoulders, and spinal curvature while working.

To **walk and stand** correctly and to attain good body balance, the body weight must be properly distributed.

For the basic stance or standing position:
1. Turn left foot out at a forty-five degree angle.
2. Point right foot straight ahead on a straight line.
3. Bend right knee slightly over line of the left knee.
4. Flex left knee slightly.

This basic stance will give body balance and be graceful to the eye.

POSTURE

Good Posture

GOOD POSTURE
  Head up.
  Chin level with floor.
  Chest up.
  Shoulders relaxed.
  Lower abdomen flat.

CENTER LINE
  Extends from center of head,
  through neck, shoulders, hips,
  knees and arches of feet.

BODY WEIGHT
  Body weight is balanced along
  this center line and supported
  by the weight-bearing arches
  of the feet.

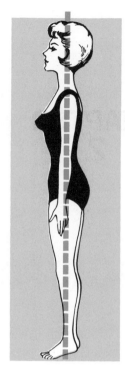

Good posture

FIVE DEFECTIVE BODY POSTURES

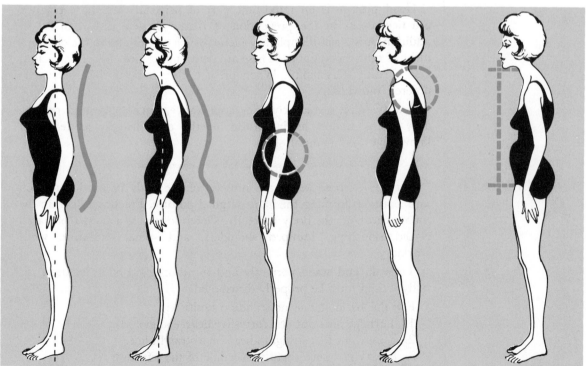

Stiff-rigid
Poor posture

Slumped-humped
Poor posture

Sway-back or
lordosis (lor-dō'sis)

Drooped shoulders
kyphosis (kī-fō'sis)

Sway-back and
drooped shoulders
scoliosis (skō-lē-ō'sis)

Back Strain

TO AVOID BACK STRAIN,
MAINTAIN GOOD POSTURE

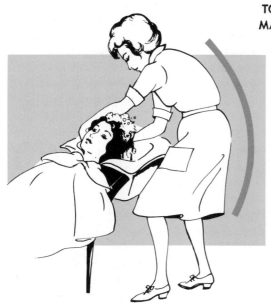

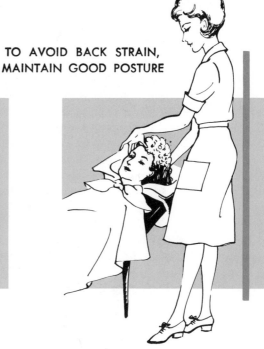

Poor posture

Good posture

COMFORT FOR PATRON AND COSMETOLOGIST

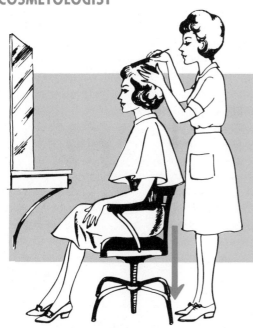

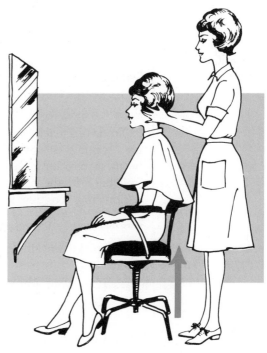

Short cosmetologist, tall patron —
lower the chair

Short patron, tall cosmetologist —
raise the chair

CORRECT SITTING POSITION

Never fall into a chair. Glide gracefully into a sitting position. When sliding to the back of the chair, place both hands on the front edge of the chair at either side of the hips, raise the body slightly, and then slide back. Do not wiggle back.

Rules For Correct Sitting

1. Keep the feet close together.
2. Keep the knees together.
3. Place the feet out slightly farther than the knees.
4. Never push your feet under the chair.
5. Keep the soles of your shoes on the floor.

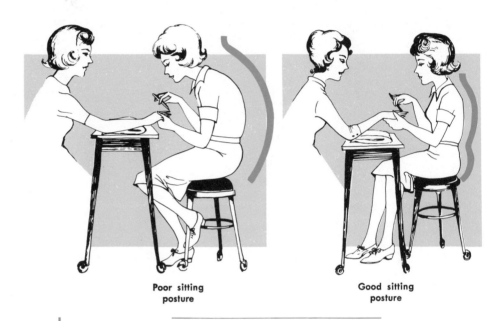

Poor sitting posture   Good sitting posture

Manicure Sitting Position

The correct sitting position is important in order to avoid general fatigue and back strain. Sit with the lower back against the chair, leaning slightly forward while giving a manicure. If a stool is used, sit on the entire stool. Keep chest up. Body weight should rest upon the full length of the thighs.

To avoid back strain while reading, writing or studying, whether it be in school, business or at home, sit well back in the chair. Do not sit in a slouching position at any time.

STOOPING POSITION

To pick up an article from the floor:

1. Place your feet close together.
2. Keep the back perpendicular as the knees bend.
3. Lift with the muscles of your legs and buttocks, not with the back.

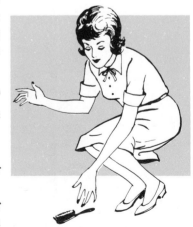

CARE OF FEET

High heels are often responsible for poor posture, malformed feet and aching backs. The weight of the body is thrown forward, exerting an extra strain on the feet and back.

Low, broad heels give the body support and balance which help to maintain good posture. Wearing low-heeled shoes contributes to greater comfort and tends to offset fatigue resulting from prolonged standing.

The cosmetologist should give her feet daily care, as follows:

1. After bathing, apply cream or oil and massage each foot for five minutes.
2. Remove cream and apply an antiseptic foot lotion.
3. Keep the toenails filed smooth.
4. Corns, bunions or ingrown nails should receive care from a chiropodist.

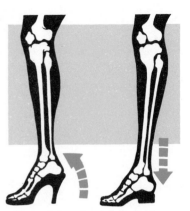

For comfort and to help maintain good posture, wear well-fitted, low-heeled shoes.

Wearing well-fitted, low-heeled shoes and giving the feet a few minutes daily care are essential to good posture and to good health. Healthy feet help to produce a radiant smile and a pleasing personality.

NORMAL AND WEAK ARCHES

A **normal footprint** is narrow in the middle and wide at the heel and at the toes. Good arches are characteristic of the normal footprint.

A **weak foot** is caused by a weak arch. Its footprint is wider in the middle than a normal footprint.

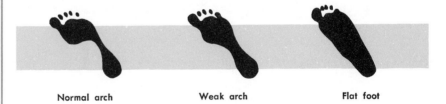

Normal arch   Weak arch   Flat foot

Fallen arches or flat feet is a common foot ailment. The flat foot leaves a footprint that is almost the same width throughout its entire length.

Weak and flat feet may be eased by means of massage, exercise, or the wearing of arch supports and proper shoes. These remedial measures should be taken only after consultation with a foot specialist.

10

Visual Poise

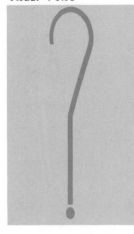

1. What are three benefits of correct posture?
2. In a basic stance or standing position, place the left foot at a .... degree angle and point the right foot straight ahead.
3. For a good standing posture, keep the head ....; chin level with ....; chest ....; shoulders relaxed and lower abdomen ....
4. For a good sitting posture, keep the feet and knees close ....
5. For a comfortable sitting posture, keep the soles of the feet on the ....
6. When giving a manicure, sit with the lower back against the ....
7. The cosmetologist who stands for long periods of time should wear well-fitted, ... shoes.
8. How does regular exercise assist in forming the habit of good posture?
9. Why should the cosmetologist wear low, broad-heeled shoes?
10. Why should the cosmetologist give his/her feet daily care?
11. Why is a correct sitting position important?
12. How should one sit to avoid back strain?

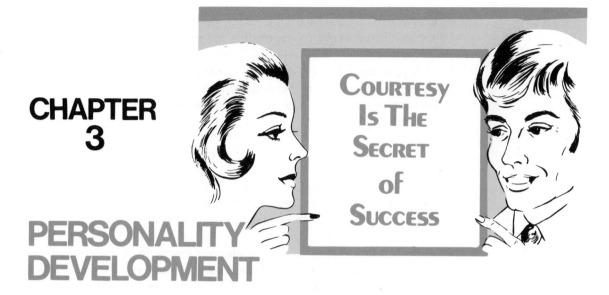

COURTESY IS THE SECRET of SUCCESS

CHAPTER 3

PERSONALITY DEVELOPMENT

INTRODUCTION

Your personality is the key to a successful career in the "world of work." You can build a personality that helps to open doors to a life full of happy experiences.

Only you **can draft the pattern** of the "ideal you," who can step through these doors. No one can make you over — **no one but yourself.**

Without a pleasing personality, a student's fine workmanship or attractive appearance will be overlooked. People develop their personalities according to the way they meet their everyday problems. Both the good and the adverse conditions that affect their lives can be used to develop better personalities.

DESIRABLE QUALITIES TO CULTIVATE

Attitude

Attitude has a great deal to do with personality. It influences your likes and dislikes and your response to people, events and things. People who meet difficult situations with calmness and who are cheerful, pleasant and easy to get along with are said to have a **healthy attitude toward life.**

Behavior

Control your temper. Once you have spoken, you cannot recall a single word. One person with his/her controls off balance can throw others into a state of confusion. Everything you say or do starts a chain of reactions which, be they good or bad, will have a continuing and lasting effect. When you have begun to be master of your own behavior you will be free to choose the course your behavior will take —to **cultivate** those characteristics which are **desirable** and to **discard** those which are **unwanted.**

Vocabulary

Thinking should be a part of your personality. If you want people to listen when you speak, think clearly and then communicate your thoughts as interestingly as you can. Increase your word power by building a vocabulary. This can be done by reading good literature and incorporating new words into your vocabulary. Use the dictionary.

Learn new words each day. Look up the unfamiliar ones you encounter in conversation or reading so you can use them correctly.

Pleasant Voice

A pleasant voice is needed, for words alone do not project a friendly feeling. If speech is to be both fluent and pleasing, a tone of voice properly pitched must be used. **A monotone** voice is both dull and uninteresting.

Emotional Stability

Realize what a great beautifier serenity is, and strive for emotional balance. If you want to be admired, develop the qualities of character that command respect, chief among them being emotional stability. **Learn to suppress the signs that betray unpleasant emotions, such as facial grimaces or gestures of anger, impatience, envy or greed.**

Graciousness

Be gracious. Learn to display pleasant emotions. A smile of greeting and a word of welcome, the willingness to assume the responsibilities of friendship, the ability to fit into new situations and to meet new people with charm and grace, **all are parts of graciousness.** Especially important is a sincere smile. It sets the mood for a warm friendly meeting.

Politeness

The root of politeness is thoughtfulness of others. Politeness should be easy to practice for it includes all the little things, such as saying "Thank you," "Please," and treating people with respect, exercising care of other people's property, being tolerant and understanding of other people's efforts and being considerate of those with whom you work. Let your heart choose your words and you will never be rude.

Good Grooming And Posture

Be well-groomed. When you meet a stranger, you make an instinctive appraisal and, of course, have a similar appraisal made of you. This is also true of patrons you meet each day.

To meet good grooming requirements, your hair should be clean and styled to make a pleasing frame for your face. Your grooming goes hand-in-hand with good posture, whether standing, walking or sitting. Your clothing should be immaculately clean; your hands smooth and your nails properly cared for.

Sense Of Humor

Cultivate your sense of humor. Take yourself less seriously. When you can laugh at yourself, you have gained the ability to evaluate realistically your relative personal importance.

Remember, a pleasant personality is the key to success. Be sure to **develop yours to the utmost.**

VOICE AND CONVERSATION

Voice and conversation, plus good English = **success.** The use of good English and intelligent conversation will serve you well as a professional cosmetologist.

Success is not made within the beauty salon alone but depends also on personal contacts, associations, and active participation in many social and cosmetology functions.

The necessity for using proper English, for cultivating a pleasant voice and for developing an interesting conversational manner is not limited to contacts with salon patrons. To make progress within the cosmetology profession, these essentials must be relied upon during association meetings, trade shows, conventions, workshops and social gatherings where you come in contact with the people who create, develop and direct cosmetology activities.

Your Voice Is You

A satisfactory speaking voice should be complementary to the physical self. Speech should convey the real you, since it communicates to everyone what you really are. Separation cannot take place between "what you say" and "what you are." The voice should convey:
1. **Sincerity**—honesty of mind or intention
2. **Intelligence**—the act of understanding
3. **Friendliness**—friendly behavior
4. **Vitality**—vigor and liveliness
5. **Flexibility**—pliable, not rigid in voice tones
6. **Expressiveness**—the expression of one's individuality

Tone Of Voice

The **tone of voice** expresses a living comment on personality and individual effectiveness. It betrays the emotions: anger, joy, hate, love, jealousy, friendliness and envy. The voice cannot conceal an emotion you feel.

The voice should be **clear** and **understandable** and have the quality of softness. If the spoken words cannot be understood, a good voice tone is useless.

To be successful, a pleasing voice is needed:
1. To greet the patron
2. For professional and social conversation
3. To sell yourself
4. To sell services and products
5. To help build business   6. To talk on the telephone

Conversation

Conversation includes the use of voice, speech, intelligence, charm and personality.

The use of good speech is vital to the art of conversation. The most serious violations of good English are the use of slang, vulgarisms and poor grammar.

Topics of conversation should be as non-controversial as possible. Friendly relations are easily achieved through pleasant conversations.

Topics To Discuss

Topics to discuss in conversation:
1. Patron's interest in herself, her personal grooming and cosmetic needs
2. Patron's own activities
3. Fashions
4. Literature
5. Art
6. Music
7. Education
8. Travel
9. Civic affairs
10. Vacations

Try to understand the patron's state of mind and the kind of person she is. Your conversation should be directed toward her interests. Fit your conversation to the patron's mood and temperament.

Conversational Charm

To acquire conversational charm:
1. Guide the conversation.
2. Do not be argumentative.
3. Be a good listener.
4. Do not monopolize the conversation.
5. Do not become personal by prying into personal affairs.
6. Talk about ideas rather than people
7. Use simple language that all can understand
8. Never gossip. (This is small talk used by uninteresting people.)
9. Be pleasant.
10. Use good English.

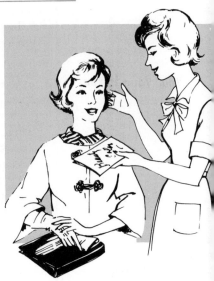

Ability to carry on a conversation is an asset to the cosmetologist.

Topics Not To Discuss

Never discuss the following topics:
1. Your own personal problems
2. Religion
3. Other patrons' poor behavior
4. Your love affairs
5. Your own financial status
6. Poor workmanship of fellow workers
7. Your own health problems
8. Information given you in confidence.

Traits To Avoid

Unpopular persons annoy or irritate others. To become popular, develop a desirable personality by adhering to the following rules:
1. Do not be bossy.
2. Do not be sarcastic.
3. Do not ridicule people.
4. Do not lose your temper.
5. Do not be rude to others.
6. Do not start an argument.
7. Do not talk continually.
8. Do not spread gossip.
9. Do not use profanity, slang or poor grammar.
10. Do not monopolize the conversation.

YOUR PERSONALITY CHART

Personality is your **greatest** asset in life. It is the inner charm revealed in your speech, appearance, behavior and manners. What you think and how you feel are expressed by your speech. How you behave in school, business or social life can either add to or take away from your personality.

Try to make the personality chart a true picture of your inner and outer self. Study yourself first. If your rating is low, consult your teacher, friends or doctor, to find out what can be done to enrich and improve it. Check your progress by analyzing your personality every three months to find out what progress you are making.

PERSONALITY QUIZ

Check the proper box in this Personality Quiz to find out if you have the personality qualities listed below:

1. **Girl.** Do you give careful attention to personal grooming, such as clothes, hair, makeup, hose and shoes?
☐ Always ☐ Sometimes ☐ Never
Young man. Do you give careful attention to personal grooming, such as clothes, hair, shave, mustache, beard, hair in nose?
☐ Always ☐ Sometimes ☐ Never
2. Do you check your posture, sitting, standing and walking erect?
☐ Always ☐ Sometimes ☐ Never
3. Do you change undergarments regularly and avoid halitosis and body odor (B.O.) at all times?
☐ Always ☐ Sometimes ☐ Never
4. Are you loyal to others? ☐ Always ☐ Sometimes ☐ Never
5. Are you friendly and courteous to others?
☐ Always ☐ Sometimes ☐ Never
6. Are you truthful in dealing with others?
☐ Always ☐ Sometimes ☐ Never
7. Can you get along and work with others?
☐ Always ☐ Sometimes ☐ Never
8. Can you accept responsibility?
☐ Always ☐ Sometimes ☐ Never
9. Do you have confidence in your knowledge and ability?
☐ Always ☐ Sometimes ☐ Never
10. Do you have a good tone of voice and choice of words and do you smile sincerely? ☐ Always ☐ Sometimes ☐ Never

RATING YOUR PERSONALITY

Give yourself 10 points for **Always**; 5 points for **Sometimes**; and zero (0) for **Never.** Compare the final rating with the following standards:

Excellent Personality 85-100%
Good Personality 75- 85%
Fair Personality 60- 75%
Poor Personality .... 59% or less

REMINDER

About two-thirds of all job dismissals are due to bad manners, poor personality and inability to get along with people. It would be to your advantage, therefore, to do all you can to improve your personality.

16

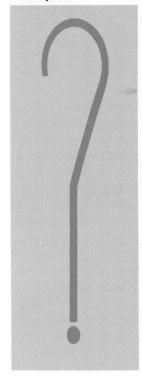

1. Define personality.
2. How are personalities developed?
3. How does the use of good English affect a personality?
4. Why should the student develop a pleasing personality?
5. Why is it necessary to analyze our own personalities?
6. List some "enemies" of a pleasing personality.
7. What is the foundation of politeness?
8. What are two personality characteristics that reflect graciousness?
9. Your personality is the key to ....
10. Voice and conversation, plus good English, equal ....
11. Vitality in a speaking voice means vigor and ....
12. The most serious errors of good English are slang, vulgarisms and poor ....
13. To acquire conversational charm, talk about .... rather than people.
14. Which of the following topics can be pleasantly discussed in conversation?
    Fashions
    Health problems
    Personal grooming
    Love affairs
    Religion
    Education
    Literature
15. Personality is revealed in your speech, appearance, behavior and ....

CHAPTER 4

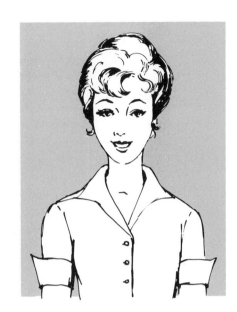

PROFESSIONAL ETHICS

INTRODUCTION

Cosmetology as a professional career offers many opportunities and rewards to young men and women who have received a thorough training, have developed a pleasing personality, have an attractive appearance and who observe professional ethics in their actions.

ETHICS

Ethics deal with the accepted professional standards of conduct and business practices that are followed by cosmetologists in their relations with patrons and co-workers.

Simply stated, living by standards of **good ethics** will assure your doing what is right, whether at work or at play. In the practice of cosmetology, the employment of a set of high moral principles and values is a prerequisite for building confidence and developing increased patronage.

Good Ethics

Financial and professional success is based upon the following rules and professional standards:

1. Be friendly and give courteous services to all patrons. Always maintain your dignity.
2. Treat all patrons honestly and fairly; do not show favoritism.
3. Be polite and courteous and respect the feelings and rights of others.
4. Let people know that you are dependable, by keeping your word and fulfilling your obligations.
5. Set an example of good conduct and professional behavior. Cherish your reputation.
6. Be loyal to your employer, manager, school and associates.
7. Cooperate with school and salon personnel, and fellow students and employees.

8. Comply with the rules established by the State Board, your school and your salon.
9. Practice the highest standards of sanitation at all times.
10. Keep faith with your profession. Do your best at all times. (Always strive for perfection.)

Poor Ethics

Poor ethics. Questionable practices, extravagant claims and unfulfilled promises violate the rules of good ethical conduct. They cast an unfavorable light on cosmetology in general and on the individual student, cosmetologist and beauty salon in particular.

A PROFESSIONAL ATTITUDE TOWARD PATRONS

Greet the patron by name, with a pleasing tone of welcome in your voice. See that her personal belongings are cared for. Help the patron to be seated. Study her mood. Often, the patron will prefer quiet and relaxation. Confine your own conversation to her cosmetic needs. If she wishes to talk, be a good listener. Never repeat a tidbit of gossip to her as she may lose confidence in you. **Never gossip about anyone.**

Off-color stories are distasteful to most women and have no place in a beauty salon.

CHECK LIST

Good habits and practices, acquired during your school training, will lay the foundation for a successful career in cosmetology. To become successful, the cosmetologist should:

1. Follow the rules of good ethics.
2. Make a good impression on others.

3. Be punctual. Get to work on time and you will not miss any patrons. Tardiness never pays.

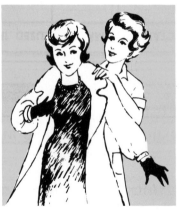

4. Be courteous. Have a sunny disposition and everyone will like you. Discourtesy is inexcusable.

5. Cultivate charm, confidence and a pleasing personality.
6. Pay attention to the minor details which will make patrons like you.
7. Adopt a cordial manner in greeting patrons in person and over the telephone.

8. Address patrons by their name . . . Miss or Mrs. Smith. Never use terms, such as "Honey" or "Dearie," when addressing patrons.

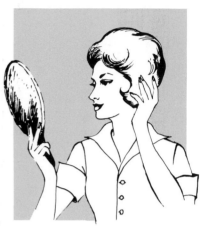

9. Be neat, clean and attractive. Be good to look at, and patrons will admire you.

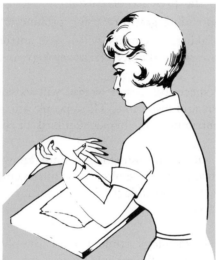

10. Handle patrons with tact. Be gentle when giving treatments, and they will return time and again. Harsh treatment will lose them as patrons.

11. Set a good example of what you are selling. Your personal appearance is the best advertisement.

12. Develop business and sales abilities along with common sense. Use tact when suggesting additional services to patrons.

13. Plan each day's schedule. Avoid long waiting periods.

14. Be prompt and judicious in adjusting patrons' complaints and grievances.

15. Listen attentively when others speak.

16. Learn to talk intelligently about your work.

17. Develop a pleasing and cultured voice.

Make People Like You

The first requirement for success is the ability to make people like you. If they like you, they will look forward to being with you. You should expend every effort in this direction, because your status as a successful cosmetologist depends to a great extent upon being liked by patrons.

TO BE AVOIDED

The successful cosmetologist must avoid:

1. Bad breath and body odor.
2. Chewing gum and smoking in the presence of patrons.
3. Speaking in a loud or harsh voice.
4. Criticizing the services of fellow cosmetologists.
5. Discussing personal problems with patrons.
6. Lounging on the arms of chairs, table tops or in the reception room.
7. Poor posture when working, and shuffling the feet when walking.
8. Playing the television or radio loudly in the presence of patrons.
9. Spreading gossip or using profane or sarcastic language.
10. Making statements which are untrue or unduly critical. (This lowers the dignity of cosmetology as a profession.)

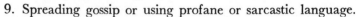

Do not gossip or criticize.

State Board Members And Inspectors

The successful cosmetologist will extend **courtesy** to State Board members and inspectors. These people are acting in the line of duty and they contribute to the higher standards of cosmetology.

Laws, Rules And Regulations

The successful cosmetologist must know the laws, rules and regulations governing cosmetology, and must comply with them. By such compliance, the cosmetologist is contributing to the public health, welfare and safety.

School Rules And Regulations

The cosmetology student must comply with all rules of conduct promulgated by the school. By so doing, students develop the habits of good citizenship and self-discipline which are essential for success in the practice of cosmetology.

REVIEW QUESTIONS

Ethics

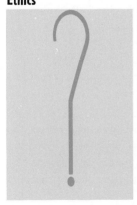

1. Define ethics.
2. Check which ones you consider as ethical practices.
   - [ ] Courtesy
   - [ ] Honesty
   - [ ] Extravagant claims
   - [ ] Unfulfilled promises
   - [ ] Obeying the cosmetology law
   - [ ] Keeping your word
3. Why should the cosmetologist avoid bad breath and body odor?
4. Why should the cosmetologist never repeat gossip to patrons or co-workers?
5. Why should the cosmetologist avoid the use of profane language?
6. Why should the cosmetologist extend courtesy to State Board members?
7. Why should the cosmetologist comply with the cosmetology laws?
8. Why should the student in training follow and obey the rules and regulations set by the school?

CHAPTER 5

BACTERIOLOGY

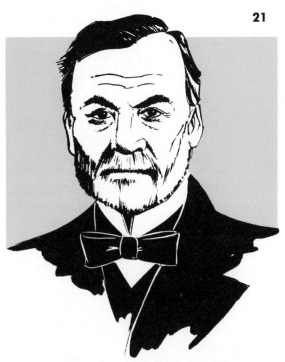

LOUIS PASTEUR (1822-1895), French chemist and biologist, devised the method of treating liquids known as pasteurization.

INTRODUCTION

Cosmetologists should first study bacteriology in order to understand the importance of sanitation and sterilization.

Bacteriology (bak-tē-r̄e-ol′ō-jē) is the science that deals with the study of micro-organisms (mi′kro-or′gan-izms) called **bacteria**.

Cosmetologists must understand how the spread of disease can be prevented and become familiar with the precautions that must be taken to protect their own as well as their patrons' health. They must understand the **relation** of bacteria to the **principles** of school and salon cleanliness and sanitation. The State Board of Cosmetology and the Health Department require the application of sanitary measures while serving the public. Contagious diseases, skin infections and blood poisoning are caused either by the conveyance of infectious material from one individual to another, or by unsanitary implements (such as combs, brushes, hairpins, clippies, rollers) that have been used first on an infected person and then on another person. Other sources of contagion are dirty hands and fingernails.

BACTERIA

Bacteria (bak-tē′re-āh) are minute, one-celled vegetable micro-organisms found nearly everywhere, and are especially numerous in dust, dirt, refuse and diseased tissues. Bacteria are also known as **germs** or **microbes** (mī′krōbs).

Bacteria exist almost everywhere, particularly on the skin of the body, in water, air, decayed matter, the secretion of body openings, on the clothing and under the free edge of the nails.

Ordinarily, bacteria are not visible except with the aid of a **microscope** (mī′krō-skōp). Fifteen hundred rod-shaped bacteria will barely reach across a pinhead.

Types Of Bacteria

While there are hundreds of different kinds of bacteria, they are classified generally into two types, depending on whether they are **beneficial** (harmless) or **harmful** (disease producing):

1. **Non-pathogenic** (non-path-ō-jen′ik) **organisms** (beneficial or harmless type) constitute the majority of all bacteria. They perform many useful functions, such as decomposing refuse and improving the fertility of the soil. To this group belong the **saprophytes** (sap′rō-fīts), which live on dead matter but do not produce disease.

2. **Pathogenic** (path-ō-jen′ik) **organisms (microbes or germs)** (harmful type), although in the minority, cause considerable damage when they invade plant or animal tissues. Pathogenic bacteria are harmful because they produce disease. To this group belong the **parasites** (par′ah-sīts), which require living matter for their growth.

It is because of pathogenic bacteria that the practice of cleanliness and sanitation is especially necessary in a beauty school or salon.

Classification Of Pathogenic Bacteria

Bacteria show distinct forms or shapes which aid in their identification. However, we are concerned with pathogenic bacteria, classified as follows:

1. **Cocci** (singular, **coccus**) are round-shaped organisms which appear singly or in groups as follows:

   a) **Staphylococci** (singular, **staphylococcus**) are pus-forming organisms which grow in bunches or clusters. They are present in abscesses, pustules and boils.

   b) **Streptococci** (singular, **streptococcus**) are pus-forming organisms which grow in chains. They are found in blood poisoning.

   c) **Diplococci** (singular, **diplococcus**) grow in pairs. They cause pneumonia.

2. **Bacilli** (singular, **bacillus**) are rod-shaped organisms which present either a short, thin or thick structure. They are the most common and produce such diseases as tetanus (lockjaw), influenza, typhoid fever, tuberculosis and diphtheria. Many bacilli are **spore** producers.

3. **Spirilla** (singular, **spirillum**) are curved or corkscrew-shaped organisms. They are subdivided into several groups, of chief importance being the treponema pallida, the causative agent of syphilis.

Pronunciation Of Terms Relating To Pathogenic Bacteria

Singular	Plural
coccus (kok′us)	cocci (kok′sī)
bacillus (bah-sil′us)	bacilli (bah-sil′ī)
spirillum (spī-ril′um)	spirilla (spī-ril′ah)
staphylococcus (staf-i-lō-kok′us)	staphylococci (staf-i-lō-kok′sī)
streptococcus (strep-tō-kok′us)	streptococci (strep-tō-kok′sī)
diplococcus (dip-lō-kok′us)	diplococci (dip-lō-kok′sī)
treponema pallida (trep-ō-nē′mah pal′i-dah)	syphilis (sif′i-lis)

THREE GENERAL FORMS OF BACTERIA

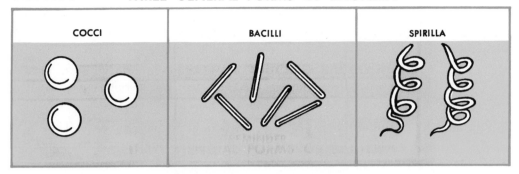

| COCCI | BACILLI | SPIRILLA |

GROUPINGS OF BACTERIA

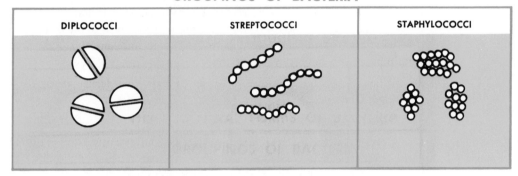

| DIPLOCOCCI | STREPTOCOCCI | STAPHYLOCOCCI |

SIX DISEASE PRODUCING BACTERIA

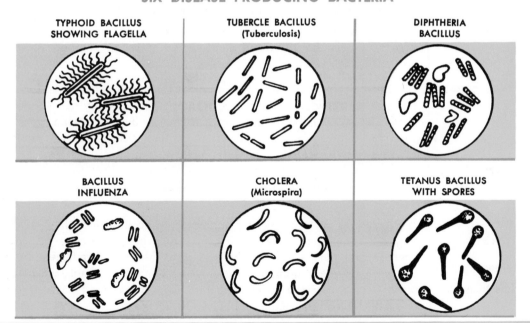

| TYPHOID BACILLUS SHOWING FLAGELLA | TUBERCLE BACILLUS (Tuberculosis) | DIPHTHERIA BACILLUS |
| BACILLUS INFLUENZA | CHOLERA (Microspira) | TETANUS BACILLUS WITH SPORES |

REMINDER

Although bacteria cannot be seen with the naked eye, it is very important to practice cleanliness and sanitation at all times, to prevent the spread of contagious disease.

BACTERIAL GROWTH AND REPRODUCTION

Bacteria generally consist of an outer cell wall and internal protoplasm. They manufacture their own food from the surrounding environment, give off waste products and grow and reproduce.

Bacteria may exhibit two distinct phases in their life cycle: the active (or **vegetative**) stage, and the **inactive** (or **spore-forming**) stage.

Active Or Vegetative Bacteria

During the active stage, bacteria grow and reproduce. These microorganisms multiply best in warm, dark, damp and dirty places where sufficient food is present.

When conditions are favorable, bacteria reproduce very fast. As food is absorbed, the bacterial cell grows in size. When the limit of growth is reached, the bacterial cell divides crosswise into halves, thereby forming two daughter cells. From one bacterium, as many as sixteen million germs may develop in half-a-day.

When favorable conditions cease to exist, bacteria either die or become inactive.

Inactive Or Spore-Forming Bacteria

Certain bacteria (such as the anthrax and tetanus bacilli), during their inactive stage and in order to withstand periods of famine, dryness and unsuitable temperature, form **spherical spores** having tough outer coverings. In this stage, spores can be blown about in the dust and are not harmed by disinfectants, heat or cold.

When favorable conditions are restored, the spores **change** into the **active** or **vegetative** form and then start to grow and reproduce.

Movement Of Bacteria

The ability to move about is limited to the bacilli and spirilla, for the cocci rarely show active mobility. Wherever any mobility of bacteria is shown, there are hairlike projections, known as **flagella** or **cilia**, extending from the sides, or sides and end, of certain bacilli. A whiplike motion of these hairs propels the bacteria about in liquid.

BACTERIAL INFECTIONS

Local Infections
General Infections

Pathogenic bacteria become a menace to health when they invade the body. An **infection** occurs if the body is unable to cope with the bacteria and their harmful toxins. A **local infection** is indicated by a boil or a pimple containing pus. A **general infection** results when the blood stream carries the bacteria and their toxins to all parts of the body, as in blood poisoning.

The presence of **pus** is a sign of infection. **Staphylococci** are the most common pus-forming bacteria. Found in pus are bacteria, waste matter, decayed tissue, body cells and blood cells, both living and dead.

Contagious Disease

An infectious disease becomes **contagious** or **communicable** when it spreads from one person to another by contact. Some of the more common contagious diseases which would prevent a cosmetologist from working are tuberculosis, ringworm, scabies, lice and virus infections.

Source Of Infection

The chief sources of infection are: unclean hands, unclean implements, open sores and pus, mouth and nose discharges, and the common use of drinking cups and towels. Uncovered coughing or sneezing,
and spitting in public also spread germs.

Through personal hygiene and public sanitation, infections can be
prevented and controlled.

Bacteria Enter Body

There can be no infection without the presence of a **pathogenic** agent.
Pathogenic bacteria may enter the body by way of:
1. A break in the skin, such as a cut, pimple or scratch
2. Breathing or by swallowing (air, water or food)
3. The nose (air)
4. The eyes or ears (dirt)

Body Fights Infection

The **body fights infection** by means of its defensive forces:
1. The unbroken skin, which is the body's first line of defense
2. Body secretions, such as perspiration and digestive juices
3. White blood cells, within the blood, to destroy bacteria
4. Antitoxins to counteract the toxins produced by bacteria

OTHER INFECTIOUS AGENTS

Filterable viruses (fil'ter-ah-bl vī'ru-sez) are living organisms so small
that they will pass through the pores of a porcelain filter. They cause
the common cold and other **respiratory** (re-spīr'ah-tō-rē) and **gastro-
intestinal** (gas'tro-in-tes'te-nal) infections.

Parasites are plants or animals which live upon another living
organism without giving anything in return.

Plant parasites or **fungi** (fun'jī), such as molds, mildews and yeasts,
can produce such contagious diseases as ringworm and favus.

Animal parasites, such as certain insects, are responsible for such
contagious diseases as scabies, due to the itch mite, and **pediculosis**
(pe-dik-ū-lō'sis), caused by lice.

Contagious diseases caused by parasites should never be treated in a
beauty school or salon. Patrons should be referred to their physicians.

IMMUNITY

Immunity (i-mū'ni-tē) is the ability of the body to resist invasion
and destroy bacteria once they have gained entrance. Immunity against
disease is a sign of good health. It may be natural or acquired. **Natural
immunity** means natural resistance to disease, being partly inherited
and partly developed by hygienic living. **Acquired immunity** is secured
after the body has by itself overcome certain diseases, or when it has
received certain kinds of vaccinations.

HUMAN DISEASE CARRIER

Human disease carrier is a person immune to a disease, yet harbors
germs that can infect other people. **Typhoid** (tī'foid) **fever** and **diphtheria** (dif-thē'rē-ah) may be transmitted in this manner.

DESTRUCTION OF BACTERIA

The destruction of bacteria may be accomplished by disinfectants,
intense heat, such as boiling, steaming, baking, or burning, and ultra-
violet rays. This subject is covered in the next chapter.

PRECAUTION

**To avoid the spread of disease keep yourself clean. Keep your
surroundings clean. Keep everything you come in contact with
clean. See that everything you use is clean.**

Bacteriology

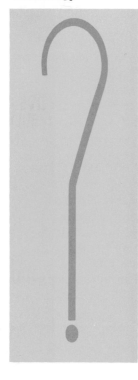

1. Define bacteriology.
2. Why should the student and cosmetologist practice strict sanitary rules?
3. What are bacteria?
4. By what other terms are bacteria known?
5. Why are bacteria not visible to the naked eye?
6. Name and briefly describe two types of bacteria.
7. What are: a) parasites; b) saprophytes?
8. Name three general forms of bacteria and the shape of each.
9. Which bacteria grow in: a) clusters; b) chains?
10. How do bacteria multiply?
11. What is the difference between local infection and general infection?
12. What causes an infection?
13. Name two common pus-forming bacteria.
14. Name four common contagious diseases that prevent a cosmetologist from working.
15. a) Briefly describe spore-forming bacteria. b) Name two.
16. What is a contagious or communicable disease?
17. How can infection be prevented in the beauty salon?
18. Name four principal routes through which bacteria may enter the body.
19. In which four ways does the body resist infection?
20. What is immunity?
21. Differentiate between natural and acquired immunity.
22. What is a human disease carrier? Give two examples.
23. What will destroy bacteria?

CHAPTER 6

STERILIZATION AND SANITATION

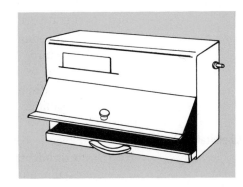

INTRODUCTION

Sterilization (ster-i-li-zā′shun) is the process of making an object germ-free by the destruction of all kinds of bacteria, whether beneficial or harmful.

Sterilization is of practical importance to the cosmetologist because it deals with methods used to prevent the growth of germs or destroy them entirely, particularly those that are responsible for infections and communicable (ko-mū′ni-kah-bl) diseases.

METHODS OF STERILIZATION AND SANITATION

Physical Agents

There are five well-known methods of sterilization and sanitation. These may be grouped under two main headings:

1. **Physical agents:**

   a) **Moist heat.**

   Boiling water at 212° Fahrenheit (far′en-hĭt) for twenty minutes. (This method is no longer used in beauty salons.)

   Steaming—requires a steam pressure sterilizer. It is used in the medical field to kill bacteria and spores.

   b) **Dry heat** (baking) is used in hospitals to sterilize sheets, towels, gauze, cotton and similar materials.

   c) **Ultra-violet rays** in an electrical sanitizer are used in beauty salons to keep sanitized implements sanitary.

Health Departments and other governmental agencies recognize that it is impossible to completely sterilize implements and equipment in the beauty school or beauty salon. Therefore, it is generally recognized that implements and equipment are SANITIZED and not sterilized.

Throughout the entire text the term SANITIZE will be used to indicate all forms of sanitation.

Chemical Agents

2. **Chemical agents:**
   a) **Antiseptics** and **disinfectants** are presently used in beauty salons.
   b) **Vapors** (fumigants) in a cabinet sanitizer are used to keep sanitized implements sanitary.

Chemicals are the most effective sanitizing agents that may be used in beauty salons for destroying or checking bacteria. The chemical agents used for sanitizing purposes are antiseptics and disinfectants.

1. An **antiseptic** (an-ti-sep'tik) is a substance which may kill or retard the growth of bacteria without killing them. Antiseptics can as a general rule be used with safety on the skin.
2. A **disinfectant** (dis-in-fek'tant) destroys bacteria and is used to sanitize implements.

Chemicals Classified

Several chemicals may be classified as either a **strong solution**, used as a disinfectant, or a **weak solution**, used as an antiseptic. (Example: Formalin, alcohol or "quats.")

Requirements Of Good Disinfectant

Requirements of a good disinfectant:
1. Convenient to prepare   4. Non-corrosive
2. Quick acting   5. Economical
3. Preferably odorless   6. Non-irritating to skin

There are many chemical disinfectant agents on the market prepared ready for use. If these are used, select the ones that have been approved by the Board of Health or the State Board of Cosmetology. Chemicals commonly used in the beauty salon are:

1. Quaternary ammonium compounds ("quats") — to sanitize implements
2. Formaldehyde—to sanitize implements
3. Alcohol—to sanitize sharp cutting instruments and electrodes
4. Prepared products—to clean floors, sinks and toilet bowls

SANITIZERS

Wet Sanitizer

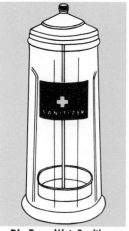

Dip-Type Wet Sanitizer

A **wet sanitizer** is any receptacle large enough to hold a disinfectant solution in which the objects to be sanitized are completely immersed. A cover is provided to prevent contamination of the solution. Wet sanitizers come in various sizes and shapes.

Before immersing objects in a wet sanitizer containing a disinfectant solution, be sure to:
1. Remove hair from combs and brushes.
2. Wash thoroughly with hot water and soap.
3. Rinse thoroughly.

This procedure prevents contamination of the solution. Besides, soap and hot water remove most of the bacteria.

After the implements are removed from the disinfectant solution, they should be rinsed in clean water, wiped dry with a clean towel and stored in a dry cabinet sanitizer until ready to be used.

**Dry Or Cabinet
Sanitizer**

Dry or cabinet sanitizer is an airtight cabinet containing an active fumigant. The sanitized implements are kept clean by placing them in the cabinet until ready for use.

How fumigant is prepared. Place one tablespoonful of borax and one tablespoonful of Formalin on a small tray on the bottom of the cabinet. This will form formaldehyde vapors. Replace chemicals periodically, as they lose their strength, depending on how often the cabinet door is opened and closed.

Formalin is also available in tablet form. Follow manufacturer's directions.

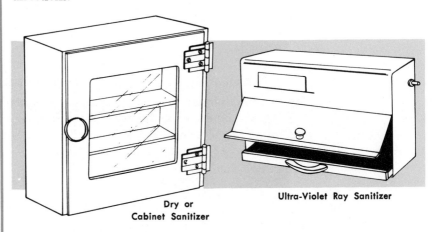

Dry or
Cabinet Sanitizer

Ultra-Violet Ray Sanitizer

**ULTRA-VIOLET RAY
SANITIZERS**

Ultra-violet ray electrical sanitizers are effective for keeping combs, brushes or implements clean until ready for use. These materials must be sanitized before they are placed in the ultra-violet sanitizer. Follow manufacturer's directions for proper use.

**CHEMICAL
SANITIZING
AGENT "QUATS"**

Quaternary ammonium compounds ("**Quats**") is pronounced kwa-ter′nah-rē ah-mō′nē-um kom′pounds—kwats.

This group of compounds is effective as disinfectants. These disinfectants are available under different trade and chemical names, and in liquid and tablet form.

The **advantages** claimed are: short disinfection time, odorless and colorless, non-toxic and stable. A 1:1000 solution is commonly used to sanitize implements. **Immersion time** ranges from 1 to 5 minutes, depending upon the strength of the solution used.

CAUTION. Before using any "quat," read and follow manufacturer's directions on label and accompanying literature. Find out if product can be used in naturally soft or hard water or water that has been softened. Inquire whether it contains a rust inhibitor (in-hib′i-tor). Should the product lack a rust inhibitor, the addition of ½% of sodium nitrite (sō′dē-um nī′trīt) to the solution prevents the rusting of metallic implements.

How to Prepare a 1:1000 Strength Solution of a Quaternary Ammonium Compound

If the product contains:

10% active ingredient, add 1¼ oz. "quat" solution to 1 gallon of water.

12½% active ingredient, add 1 oz. "quat" solution to 1 gallon of water.

15% active ingredient, add ¾ oz. "quat" solution to 1 gallon of water.

FORMALIN

Formalin (fōr′ma-lin) is a safe and effective sanitizing agent which can be used either as an antiseptic or disinfectant, depending on its percentage strength. As purchased, Formalin is composed of approximately 37% to 40% of formaldehyde (fōr-mal′dĕ-hĭd) gas in water.

Formalin is used in various strengths, as follows:

25% solution (equivalent to 10% formaldehyde gas)—used to sanitize implements. Immerse them in the solution for at least 10 minutes. (Preparation: 2 parts Formalin, 5 parts water, 1 part glycerine — glycerine keeps implements from rusting.)

10% solution (equivalent to 4% formaldehyde gas)—used to sanitize combs and brushes. Immerse them for at least 20 minutes. (Preparation: 1 part Formalin, 9 parts water.)

5% solution (equivalent to 2% formaldehyde gas)—used to cleanse the hands after they have been in contact with wounds, skin eruptions, and other sources of bacteria. Also used to sanitize shampoo bowls and chairs. (Preparation: 1 part Formalin, 19 parts water.)

SANITIZING METHODS
With Chemicals

1. Wash implements thoroughly with soap and hot water.
2. Use plain water rinse to remove all traces of soap.
3. Immerse implements in a wet sanitizer (containing approved disinfectant) for the required time.*
4. Remove implements from wet sanitizer, rinse in water and wipe dry with clean towel.
5. Store sanitized implements in individually wrapped cellophane envelopes in cabinet sanitizer or in ultra-violet ray cabinet until ready to be used.

SANITIZING WITH ALCOHOL

To sanitize **electrodes** and **implements**, immerse them in 70% alcohol. *70% alcohol refers to ethyl or grain alcohol.*
99% isopropyl alcohol is the same strength as 70% ethyl alcohol.

Implements having a fine cutting edge are best sanitized by rubbing the surface with a cotton pad dampened with 70% alcohol. This application prevents the cutting edges from becoming dull.

Electrodes (ē-lek′trōds) may be safely sanitized by gently rubbing the exposed surface with a cotton pad dampened with 70% alcohol.

Then place the articles into a dry sanitizer until ready for use.

---

* *Consult your State Board of Cosmetology or Health Department for list of approved disinfectants to be used in beauty salons.*

SANITIZING FLOORS, SINKS, TOILET BOWLS

The disinfection of floors, sinks and toilet bowls in the beauty salon calls for the use of such commercial products as Lysol, pine needle oil or similar disinfectants. **Deodorizers** are also useful to offset offensive smells and for imparting a refreshing odor.

Whatever disinfectant is being used, make sure that it is properly diluted as suggested by manufacturer.

> IT IS ALWAYS A PLEASURE FOR PATRONS TO RECEIVE SERVICES IN A BEAUTY SALON THAT IS SPOTLESS. GET INTO THE HABIT NOW. KEEP EVERYTHING CLEAN AND IN ORDER.

DISINFECTANTS

DISINFECTANTS COMMONLY USED IN BEAUTY SALONS

Name	Form	Strength	Uses
Quaternary Ammonium Compounds ("Quats")	Liquid or tablet	1:1000 solution	Immerse implements into solution for 1 to 5 minutes. minutes.
Formalin	Liquid	25% solution	Immerse implements into solution for 10 minutes.
Formalin	Liquid	10% solution	Immerse implements into solution for 20 minutes.
Ethyl or Grain Alcohol	Liquid	70% solution	Sanitize sharp cutting implements and electrodes.
Cresol (Lysol)	Liquid	10% soap solution	Cleanse floors, sinks and toilets.

ANTISEPTICS

ANTISEPTICS COMMONLY USED IN BEAUTY SALONS

Name	Form	Strength	Uses
Boric Acid	White crystals	2-5% solution	Cleanse the eyes.
Tincture of Iodine	Liquid	2% solution	Cleanse cuts and wounds.
Hydrogen Peroxide	Liquid	3% solution	Cleanse skin and minor cuts.
Ethyl or Grain Alcohol	Liquid	60% solution	Cleanse hands and skin. Not to be used if irritation is present.
Formalin	Liquid	5% solution	Cleanse hands, shampoo bowl, cabinet, etc.
Chloramine-T (Chlorazene; Chlorozol)	White crystals	½% solution	Cleanse skin and hands and for general use.
Sodium Hypochlorite (Javelle water; Zonite)	White crystals	½% solution	Rinse the hands.

Other approved disinfectants and antiseptics are being used in beauty salons. Consult the State Board of Cosmetology or the Health Department.

SAFETY PRECAUTIONS

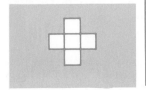

In order to prevent mistakes and accidents in the use of sanitizing chemical agents, follow these safety rules:

1. Purchase chemicals in small quantities and store them in a cool, dry place; otherwise, they deteriorate due to contact with air, light and heat.
2. Weigh and measure chemicals carefully.
3. Keep all containers labeled, covered and under lock and key.

4. Do not smell chemicals or solutions, as some of them have pungent odors.
5. Avoid spilling when diluting chemicals.
6. Keep a complete first aid kit on hand.

SANITATION DEFINITIONS

1. **Sterilize** (ster'i-līz)—to render sterile; to make free from all bacteria (harmful or beneficial) by the act of sterilizing.
2. **Sterile** (ster'il)—free from all germs.
3. **Antiseptic** (an-ti-sep'tic)—a chemical agent which may kill or retard the growth of bacteria.
4. **Disinfect** (dis-in-fekt')—to destroy bacteria on any object.
5. **Disinfectant** (dis-in-fek'tant)—a chemical agent having the power to destroy bacteria (germs or microbes).
6. **Bactericide** (bak-tē'ri-sīd)—a chemical agent having the power to destroy bacteria (germs or microbes).
7. **Germicide** (jer'mi-sīd)—a chemical agent having the power to destroy germs (bacteria or microbes).
8. **Asepsis** (ah-sep'sis)—freedom from disease germs.
9. **Sepsis** (sep'sis)—poisoning due to pathogenic bacteria.
10. **Fumigant** (fū'mi-gant)—vapor used to keep clean objects sanitary.
11. **Sanitize** (san'i-tīz)—to render objects clean and sanitary.

SANITIZING RULES

1. **Chemical solutions** in sanitizers should be changed when necessary.
2. **Manicuring implements** must be kept in a disinfectant solution (70% alcohol) during the process of giving a manicure.
3. **All manicuring implements** must be sanitized after each use on a patron.
4. **All articles** must be clean and free from hair before being sanitized.
5. **Combs and brushes** must be sanitized after each patron has been served.
6. **Shampoo bowls** must be sanitized after each use.
7. **Sanitize electrical appliances** by rubbing surface with a cotton pad dampened with 70% alcohol.
8. **Finger bowls** or **similar objects** must be sanitized prior to being used for another patron.

Note—The immersing of implements in a chemical solution should conform to State Board of Cosmetology regulations issued by your state.

SANITATION

Sanitation is the application of measures to promote public health and prevent the spread of infectious diseases.

Importance Of Sanitation

The importance of sanitation cannot be overemphasized. Cosmetic services bring the cosmetologist in direct contact with the patron's skin, scalp, hair and nails. Understanding sanitary measures contributes to the **protection** of the patron's health.

Precautions

Various governmental agencies protect community health by providing for a wholesome food and water supply and the quick disposal of refuse. These steps are only a few of the ways in which the public health is safeguarded.

Water for drinking purposes should be odorless, colorless and free from any foreign matter. Crystal clear water may still be unsanitary because of the presence of **pathogenic bacteria** which cannot be seen with the naked eye.

The **air within a beauty salon** should be neither dry nor stagnant, nor have a stale, musty odor. Room temperature should be about 70 degrees Fahrenheit.

The beauty salon can also be ventilated with the aid of an exhaust fan or an air conditioning unit. Air conditioning has the advantage of permitting changes in the quality and quantity of air brought into the beauty salon. The temperature and moisture content of the air can also be regulated by means of air conditioning.

A person with an infectious disease is a source of contagion to others. Hence, cosmetologists who have colds or any communicable disease must not be permitted to serve patrons. Likewise, patrons obviously suffering from an infectious disease must not be accommodated in a beauty salon. In this way, the best interests of other patrons will be served.

The public has learned the importance of sanitation and is now demanding that every possible sanitary measure be used in the beauty salon for the promotion of public health.

The **State Board of Cosmetology** and **Board of Health** in each state or locality have formulated sanitary regulations governing beauty salons. Every cosmetologist must be familiar with these regulations in order to obey them.

SANITARY RULES

Adherence to the following sanitary rules will result in cleaner and better service to the public:

1. Every beauty salon **must** be well-lighted, heated or cooled, as the case may be, and properly ventilated, and **must** be kept in a clean and sanitary condition.
2. The walls, curtains and floor or floor coverings in a beauty salon **must** be washable and kept clean.
3. All beauty establishments must be supplied with continuous running hot and cold water. Drinking facilities (individual cups, and water-cooler and/or fountain) should be provided.
4. All plumbing fixtures should be properly installed.
5. The premises should be kept free from rodents, vermin, flies or similar insects.
6. The beauty salon is **not to be used** for cooking, sleeping or living quarters.
7. All hair, cotton or other waste material **must be removed** from the floor without delay, and deposited in closed containers. Remove them from the premises at frequent intervals.
8. Rest rooms **must be kept** in a sanitary condition, and provided with hot and cold running water, liquid soap, paper towels and toilet tissues.
9. Each cosmetologist **must wear** a clean washable uniform while working on patrons.

10. The cosmetologist **must cleanse** her hands thoroughly **before** and **after** serving a patron and **after** using the **toilet.**

11. A freshly laundered towel **must be used** for each patron. Towels that are ready for use must be stored in a clean, closed cabinet. Soiled towels and linens must be placed **immediately** in containers used for this purpose. Keep dirty towels away from clean towels.

12. Headrest coverings and neck strips **must be changed** for each patron.

13. **Do not permit** the shampoo cape to come in contact with the patron's skin.

14. The **common use** of powder puffs, lipstick, rouge, solid soap, sponges or styptic pencils, by more than one person, is **prohibited.**

15. Lotions, ointments, creams and powders **must be kept** in clean, closed containers. Use clean spatula to remove creams or ointments from jars. Use sterile cotton pledgets to apply lotions and powders. Re-cover cosmetic containers after each use.

16. When manicuring, provide sanitized finger bowl or finger bowl with an individual paper cup for each patron.

17. **Discard** emery boards after use on a patron.

18. Soiled combs, brushes, towels or other used material **must be removed** from tops of work stations **immediately** after use.

19. Clippies, hairpins or bobby pins **must not** be placed in the mouth.

20. Combs or implements **must not** be carried in pockets of the uniform.

21. Hair nets **must not** be carried in pockets or cuffs of the uniform.

22. Hair nets **must be washed** after each use.

23. Clipper blades, curlers, bobby pins and hairpins **must be sanitized** after each use.

24. All implements and articles used **must first be sanitized** and then placed in a dustproof or airtight container or a cabinet sanitizer.

25. Objects dropped on the floor **are not to be used** until sanitized.

26. Dogs, cats, birds or other pets **shall not be permitted** in a beauty school or salon.

REMINDERS

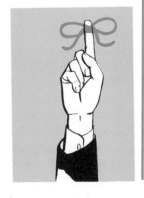

The responsibility for sanitation rests with **each student** in the beauty school and **each cosmetologist** in the beauty salon. The manager must provide the necessities for school and salon sanitation.

The cosmetologist **must** obey the rules on sanitation issued by the Health Department and the State Board of Cosmetology regarding acceptable methods of sanitation.

Use clean, fresh linen. Wash your hands before and after working on patron. Never pick up a comb or brush dropped on the floor and use it until it has been sanitized. Never place an implement in your mouth or uniform pocket or combs in your own hair. Hair dryers should not be placed so close as to touch the hair.

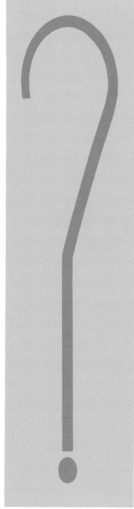

REVIEW QUESTIONS

Sterilization

1. What is sterilization?
2. Physical and .... agents are used in sanitation.
3. Name two methods of keeping objects clean after they have been sanitized.
4. What type of bacteria makes necessary the practice of sanitation in the beauty salon?
5. What are the dangers of using unsanitary implements and linens on patrons?
6. Distinguish between asepsis, sterile and sepsis.
7. What is the chemical sanitizing agent quaternary ammonium compound commonly called?
8. Formaldehyde is the active gas found in ....
9. What is an antiseptic?
10. What is a disinfectant?
11. What is a fumigant?
12. About how long does it take to sanitize implements when using: a) "quats"; b) 25% Formalin; c) 10% Formalin?
13. What is a wet sanitizer; how is it best used?
14. When using a disinfectant, how are objects sanitized?
15. List four requirements of a good disinfectant.
16. What should be done with implements after they are sanitized in a disinfectant solution?
17. How should combs and brushes be kept after they are sanitized?
18. What is a dry or cabinet sanitizer?
19. What is the proper way to produce formaldehyde vapors in a cabinet sanitizer?
20. What is the composition of Formalin?
21. What is the best way to sanitize sharp implements and prevent their dulling?
22. What is a safe way to sanitize electrodes?
23. Effective sanitation prevents the spread of .... in the beauty salon.
24. What strength Formalin solution is recommended to sanitize implements?
25. What are four advantages of using "quats" as a disinfectant?
26. In what strength is "quats" commonly used?
27. List six safety precautions when using chemical agents.
28. Is there a difference in the action of a disinfectant, germicide, or bactericide? Give reason for your answer.

Sanitation

1. Define sanitation.
2. Which two governmental agencies formulate sanitary regulations for beauty schools and salons?
3. On whom does the responsibility for sanitation rest within the beauty school?
4. Which do you consider the two most important of the sanitary rules and regulations?
5. How should loose hair and other waste material be disposed of?
6. How often should the cosmetologist cleanse her hands?
7. Why is it important to have a pure water supply?
8. What is the objection to the use of the common towel?
9. What is a sanitary way to remove cosmetic creams from their container?
10. How are face powders kept, and how are they applied?
11. **List items required in the beauty school or salon to keep it sanitary.**
12. What is the regulation governing the sanitizing of all towels used in a beauty salon?
13. If a towel or an implement is accidentally dropped on the floor, how should it be treated?

THE
PRACTICE
OF
COSMETOLOGY

"Practice Makes Perfect"

New products and developments in beauty culture bring about changes in the practice of cosmetology. This text contains acceptable procedures which reflect current trends. The procedures outlined herein can be modified to conform to your instructor's requirements, as their techniques are equally correct.

BE GUIDED BY THE INSTRUCTIONS OF YOUR COSMETOLOGY TEACHER.

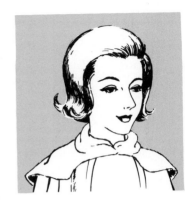

DRAPING
For Wet Or Dry Hair Work

INTRODUCTION

Correctly draping a patron for the various services given in the beauty salon is an important aspect of a cosmetologist's service to a patron. It protects the patron's skin and clothing from stains. In addition, a patron feels more comfortable when she knows care has been taken with her personal needs.

PREPARATION

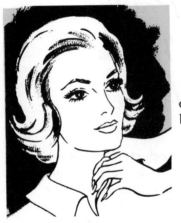

Before draping a patron for any type of hair service, the following steps should be followed:

1. Seat patron comfortably.
2. Select and arrange required materials.
3. Wash and sanitize hands.
4. Smooth dress or blouse collar under the garment and adjust cape over the neck strip or towel.
5. Place neck strip or towel around patron's neck.
6. Remove all hair pins and combs from the hair.
7. Ask patron to remove necklace, ear jewelry and glasses, and to put them into her purse.
8. Proceed with the desired hair treatment.

> **Reminder.** The instructor may have developed her own methods for draping; they are equally correct.

DRAPING FOR
DRY HAIR WORK

The following procedure is for **draping for dry hair shaping, or any service where hair is dry, and for brushing the hair.**

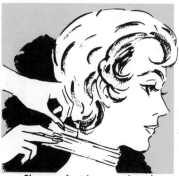

The neck strip is used for sanitary as well as protective purposes. At no time should the protective cape come in direct contact with the patron's skin.

Place neck strip around neck; fold ends over and tuck in.

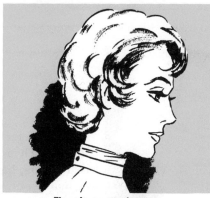

Tie, pin or attach cape over neck strip.

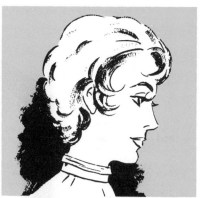

Fold neck strip down over cape neckband. Cape should not touch patron's skin.

DRAPING FOR
COMB-OUT

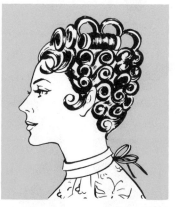

Draping for comb-out is the same as for dry hair shaping, with the exception that a short cape is used.

Courtesy is the Secret of Success. In addition to being well-groomed and proficient in your work, you must learn to do the little things that will make patrons like you. It is when you are draping the patron that you can make her relax and comfortable so that she may enjoy the treatment or service you are about to give her.

DRAPING FOR
WET HAIR WORK

Method 1

When draping for hair services, such as shampoo and set, wet hair shaping, or scalp treatment, place a small towel around patron's neck and then drape the patron the same as for dry hair shaping. Then, place a towel over the shoulders and fasten it in front with a clamp.

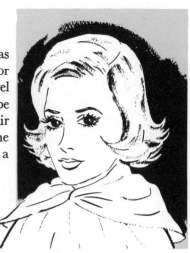

Method 2

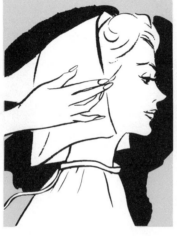

The second method of draping patrons, such as for permanent waving, hair relaxing, hair coloring and all other wet hair work.

Place cape in front of patron loosely.

Slide towel down and fold around neck.

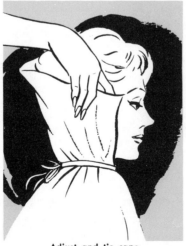

Adjust and tie cape
over towel.

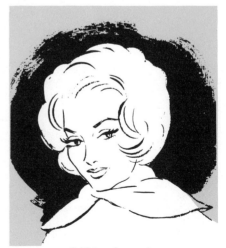

Fold towel over in
cape effect.

CHAPTER 7

SHAMPOOING AND RINSING

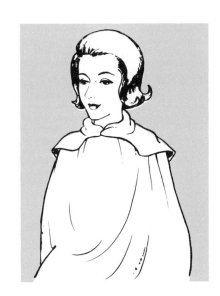

SHAMPOOING

INTRODUCTION

Shampooing the hair is not only an important preliminary step for various hair treatments, but is also the **first impression** a patron has of how professionally a cosmetologist practices her art. In this respect, a shampoo can be considered to be a valuable selling aid, because a patron who is pleased with the way her hair has been shampooed is more likely to look favorably upon any recommendation of additional services made by the cosmetologist. Therefore, the cosmetologist who can give a professional quality shampoo becomes a valuable asset to a salon.

Importance Of Shampoo

While shampoos are primarily given to clean the hair and scalp, they perform another important function: they initiate the "relaxing experience" to which the patron has been looking forward with pleasant anticipation. If the cosmetologist can make this expected pleasurable experience a reality, the patron is likely to make her visits to this salon a regular habit.

Purpose Of Shampoo

A shampoo, to be effective, must remove all dirt, oils, cosmetics and skin debris from the scalp and hair shaft, without adversely affecting either the scalp or hair. **Shampoos which are strongly alkaline should not be used because they are liable to make the hair dry and brittle.**

Unless the scalp and hair are cleansed regularly, the accumulation of oils and perspiration, which mixes with natural scales and dirt, offers a breeding place for disease-producing bacteria. This condition can lead to scalp disorders.

Frequency Of Shampooing

Hair should be shampooed as often as necessary, depending on how quickly the scalp and hair become soiled. As a general rule, **oily hair should be shampooed more often than normal or dry hair.**

WATER

Soft Water

Hard Water

Water is composed of hydrogen and oxygen. The cosmetologist should know whether the water she is using is soft or hard.

Soft water. Rain water, or water that has been chemically softened, contains very small amounts of minerals and lathers freely. For this reason, it is preferred for soap shampooing.

Hard water contains certain minerals and soap shampoo does not readily lather in this water. Depending on the kind of hard water available in your community, it can be softened by a chemical process and made suitable for shampooing.

PRE-STEPS IN SHAMPOOING

Selecting The Correct Shampoo

To make an intelligent choice of shampoo, the cosmetologist should know the composition and action of the shampoo and whether it will do an effective job. To obtain this information, carefully read the label and accompanying literature.

Select the shampoo according to the hair's condition. Hair is not considered normal if it has been:

1. Lightened
2. Toned or tinted
3. Permanently waved
4. Chemically relaxed
5. Sun bleached
6. Abused by the use of harsh shampoos
7. Damaged by improper care
8. Damaged by exposure to the elements

Required Materials And Implements

Before giving a shampoo, gather all necessary materials and implements. There is nothing more annoying to the patron than to have the cosmetologist wet her hair and leave her stranded, while she dashes out to get shampoo or other necessities. Required materials and implements are:

1. Neck strip
2. Towels
3. Shampoo cape
4. Comb and hair brush
5. Shampoo
6. Hair rinse

Draping Patron For Shampoo

Draping a patron for a shampoo is a very important step. It is of the utmost importance that the patron's clothing be fully protected. *For draping consult pages* 38 to 40.

Hair Brushing

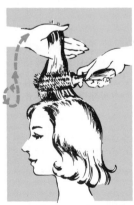

Brushing procedure with natural bristle brush

Brushing should always be a part of both shampoo and scalp treatments, with the following **exceptions:**

1. Do not brush before giving a lightening treatment.
2. Do not brush before the application of a tint or toner.
3. Do not brush before giving a permanent wave.
4. Do not brush before applying a chemical hair relaxer.
5. Do not brush if the scalp is irritated.

Brushing stimulates the scalp, helps to remove dust and dirt from the hair, and gives it added sheen. Stimulation of the scalp by brushing helps to normalize the oil glands. Therefore, the hair should receive thorough brushing, whether the scalp and hair is in a **dry or oily condition.** The comb **should not** be used to loosen scales from the scalp.

To brush the hair, first part it through the center, from **front to** nape. Part a section from about one-half inch off the center **parting,** to the crown of the head. Holding this strand of hair in the left **hand,** between the thumb and fingers, place the brush (held in the **right** hand) with the bristles near the scalp; sweep the bristles the full length of the hair, turning the wrist slightly in doing so, and continuing to the ends of the hair. Repeat three times. Then part the hair again one-half inch from the first parting, and continue until the entire head has been brushed.

PLAIN SHAMPOO

This is the shampoo most often given in the salon. The procedure described here is one way of giving a shampoo. In all instances, follow your instructor's recommendations.

**Preparation For
A Shampoo**

1. Seat patron comfortably.
2. Select and arrange required materials.
3. Wash and sanitize hands.
4. Drape patron.
5. Ask patron to remove neck jewelry, ear jewelry and glasses, and to put them into her purse.
6. Remove all hair pins and combs from the hair.
7. Examine condition of patron's hair and scalp.
8. Brush the hair thoroughly.
9. Cover neck of shampoo bowl with a folded towel.
10. Adjust shampoo cape over back of shampoo chair.
11. Adjust volume and temperature of water spray.

Procedure

The cosmetologist should be able to use both hands with equal ease and to work from either side of the patron.

Unless there is a reason to use cool or cold water, use water as warm as the patron can comfortably stand. Her preference should always be considered.

Test the temperature of the water by spraying it on your wrist.

Turn the spray on and curl the fingers over the edge of it, so that any sudden change in the water temperature will be detected. Proceed as follows:

1. **Wet the hair thoroughly** with warm water, holding spray off the head. Lift the hair and work it with the free hand to be sure it is saturated right to the scalp. Shift hand to protect patron's face and ears from the spray when working around the hairline, as in Figs. 1 and 2.

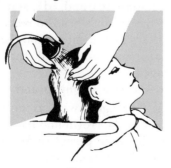 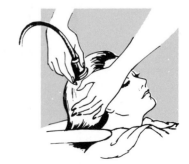

Fig. 1   Fig. 2

2. **Apply shampoo** over the hair a little at a time.
   a) Starting at the crown, apply a small amount to scalp, working shampoo in well with the free hand as it is being applied.
   b) Apply in like manner at the sides, front hairline, and back of the head. It is important to work the shampoo as it is being applied so that complete coverage is achieved and its loss down the drain is prevented.

MANIPULATIONS — CAUTION

Do not use vigorous scalp massage movements if scalp is sensitive or irritated, or if patron requests less pressure. Give light manipulations if the shampoo is to be followed by a permanent wave, hair coloring or hair relaxing.

3. **Give manipulations.**
   a) Starting at the hairline in front of the ears (using both hands) work in a back-and-forth movement until the top of the head is reached. Use the cushions or balls of the fingers. Do not use fingertips. See Fig. 3.
   b) Shifting the fingers back one inch at a time, continue in this manner to the back of the head.
   c) Lift the patron's head and brace her neck against the shampoo bowl, as in Fig. 4, with the left hand controlling the movement of her head. With the right hand, start at the top of the right ear; using the same movement, work to back of the head.

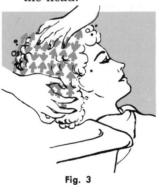 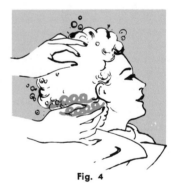

Fig. 3   Fig. 4

   d) Drop the fingers down one inch, and repeat until right side of the head is covered.
   e) Repeat steps (c) and (d), starting at the left ear.
   f) Allow the patron's head to relax, and work with your thumbs in a rotary movement around the hairline.
   g) Repeat movements until the scalp has been thoroughly massaged.
   h) Remove excess shampoo and foam by squeezing the hair.
4. **Rinse hair thoroughly** with strong spray, as in Figs. 1 and 2.
   a) Lift hair at the crown and back of the head with the fingers of the left hand, to permit spray to rinse the hair thoroughly.
   b) Cup left hand along nape line and pat the hair, forcing the spray of water against the base of the scalp area.

5. **Apply shampoo again.**

Place the cushions or balls of the fingers of both hands at the hairline, just behind the ears. With a continuous rotary movement, proceed up and along the edge of the hairline to the temples, and then up to the center of the forehead. With large rotary movements, cover the sides of the head, the crown, the back, the nape hairline and work back to the original starting position. Repeat these movements until the scalp and hair have been thoroughly cleansed.

6. **Rinse the hair thoroughly** with strong spray in the manner outlined in Step 4.

   (*For after-shampoo rinses for various hair conditions, consult "Rinses" section of this chapter.*)

7. **Partially towel dry.**
   a) Remove excess moisture from the hair at the shampoo bowl.
   b) Wipe excess moisture from around the face and ears with ends of towel.
   c) Lift towel over back of patron's head and drape head with towel.
   d) Massage the scalp with the palms and fingers of both hands, through the towel, using a circular motion, until the hair is partially dry.

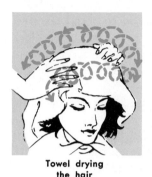

Towel drying
the hair

Completion

1. Comb the hair, starting with hair ends at nape of neck.
2. If no other service is to be given, set the hair to the desired style.
3. Remove shampoo cape, towel or neck strip.
4. Dry and comb out hair to appropriate hairstyle.

Clean-up

1. Discard used materials and place unused supplies in their proper place.
2. Remove hair from combs and brushes; wash combs and brushes with hot, soapy water; rinse and place them in wet sanitizer for required time.
3. Place used towels into towel hamper.
4. Clean and sanitize shampoo bowl.
5. Wash and sanitize hands.

SAFETY MEASURES FOR SHAMPOOING

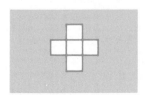

1. Do not permit shampoo to get into patron's eyes.
2. Protect patron's ears with pieces of clean cotton, if she is sensitive to water in the ears.
3. Test the water temperature before applying to patron's head.
4. Do not permit the fingernails to scratch the patron's scalp.
5. Always towel blot excess moisture from patron's hair before she leaves the shampoo bowl.
6. Do not turn the dryer to "hot" if the patron is subject to high blood pressure.
7. Do not permit the shampoo cape to come in contact with patron's skin.

8. Do not permit water to remain on the floor around the shampoo bowl.
9. Use sanitized combs, brushes, towels and other implements for each patron.
10. Clean shampoo bowl and sanitize the neck of the bowl after each use.

SHAMPOOING LIGHTENED HAIR

Since lightened hair is likely to mat and tangle when wet, it must be handled with great care. The shampoo used should be mild or **low in alkalinity**.

Use lukewarm or tepid water. Pour shampoo on hair very slowly to avoid matting. Always work with the hands **underneath the hair**—not on the top. Never, under any circumstances, bring the ends of the hair to the top of the head. Rinse hair thoroughly with clear water. Apply a special rinse for lightened hair, for easier combing. Carefully towel dry hair. Comb the hair gently. Do not force the comb through tangles.

Hair that has been tinted or damaged should receive the same consideration in shampooing.

TYPES OF SHAMPOOS

There are many types of shampoos available to the professional cosmetologists. They learn through experience which type gives them the results they require. The student should follow the instructor's recommendation at all times.

Plain Shampoos

Plain shampoos are usually clear and transparent. They contain no added ingredients, such as **medication** or **oily compounds.** They may have a natural amber shade, or a greenish yellow color.

A plain shampoo may be used on **virgin** hair which is in good condition. A plain shampoo should never be used on **lightened, toned, tinted, damaged** or **permanently waved** hair. It will strip or fade the color and may further damage the hair.

Soap

A plain shampoo may be of the **soap** type. It contains an oil or fat and an alkali. A soap shampoo should be used with soft water.

Soapless

A plain shampoo may be of the **soapless** type and be a **detergent-based** product. It is made from synthetic detergents mainly derived from petroleum by-products, or from natural fats that have been chemically treated. Detergent shampoos can be used with either soft or hard water.

Shampoos for **oily** and **normal** hair can be either the soap or soapless type plain shampoos. Shampoos for oily hair usually contain a higher concentrate of soap or detergent.

Liquid Cream Shampoos

Liquid cream shampoos are usually used for **dry** hair. As a rule, they are detergent-based products in which soap, or sometimes soap jelly, is used as a thickening agent. **Magnesium stearate** is also used as a whitening agent. Cream shampoos are mostly emulsions. They often contain oily compounds to make the hair feel silky and softer. Use **this** type of shampoo as directed by your instructor, or by the product's manufacturer.

Cream Or Paste Shampoos

Cream or paste shampoos are essentially the same as the liquid cream shampoos, except that more detergent material and more soap are used with less water. Some contain oily compounds to make the hair feel softer. Be guided by your **instructor,** or the product's manufacturer.

Acid Balanced Shampoos (Non-Strip)

Acid balanced shampoos are formulated to prevent the stripping of **tints** or **toners** from the hair. They are mild in action, contain conditioners, and are low in alkaline content. They are also recommended for **brittle, dry** or **damaged hair.** Follow manufacturer's directions concerning their use.

Anti-Dandruff Shampoos

Anti-dandruff shampoos are used to control a dandruff condition of the scalp. They are made by adding a germicide to a plain shampoo. The appropriate anti-dandruff shampoo should be selected for either a dry or oily scalp condition. It is important that the manufacturer's directions be followed when using this type of shampoo.

Liquid Dry Shampoos

Liquid dry shampoos are cosmetic products used for cleansing the scalp and hair when the patron is prevented by illness from having a regular shampoo.

CAUTION. Make sure that the room is well ventilated when using a liquid dry shampoo.

Procedure

1. Brush hair thoroughly—comb lightly.
2. Part hair in one-inch sections from forehead to crown and from crown to nape of neck.
3. Saturate a piece of cotton with the cleaning liquid; squeeze liquid out lightly, then rub briskly along each part. Follow by rubbing vigorously with a towel along the part. Repeat over the entire head in this manner. Then apply liquid down length of hair strands with cotton pledget.
4. Rub the hair strands with the towel to remove soil.
5. Re-moisten hair lightly with liquid and set hair.

A dry shampoo will freshen the hair and tone the scalp without endangering the patron. (When using any type of shampoo, read instructions carefully, and follow manufacturer's directions.)

SHAMPOO FOR DAMAGED HAIR

Shampoo for damaged hair. For dry, brittle, over-lightened or tinted hair, the cosmetologist can use either of the following:

Egg Shampoo

1. **Egg shampoo**—a one or two whole egg mixture which is applied to the hair and scalp in the same way as for a regular shampoo. Only tepid water is used, as hot water will congeal the egg on the hair.

Commercial Egg Shampoo

2. **A commercial egg shampoo,** containing a small amount of egg. Apply it as directed by manufacturer.
3. Other commercial shampoos (such as a non-strip shampoo). They contain ingredients which are helpful to damaged hair.

Highlighting Shampoo

Consult chapter on **Hair Coloring.**

METHODS OF DISSOLVING SOAP CURDS

Minerals are present in all kinds of water; the more minerals, the harder the water. In soaps, there are fatty acids. Minerals and fatty acids combine to form a soap scum which dulls the hair and makes it difficult to comb.

It is impossible to remove all the soap curds from the hair with ordinary water. Vinegar, lemon or acid rinses are effective in removing soap residue from the hair. They separate hair and make it easier to comb.

Special rinses now on the market actually remove soap curds from the hair, thus making combing easier, and at the same time, adding brilliance to the hair. Follow manufacturer's directions.

HAIR RINSES

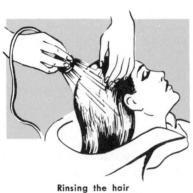

Rinsing the hair

A hair rinse consists of water, or a mixture of water with a mild acid, coloring agent, or special ingredients.

Hair rinses are given for the following purposes:

1. To add temporary color to the hair
2. To dissolve soap curds from the hair, and to make hair more manageable
3. To give hair a soft, lustrous appearance
4. To neutralize the yellow tinge of white or gray hair
5. To seal in tint or toner after a color treatment

Vinegar (Acid) Rinse

A vinegar (acetic) rinse is used to separate the hair, dissolve soap curds, give hair brightness, and make it soft and pliable.

A vinegar rinse may also be used to counteract the alkalinity of hair after a lightening, tint or a cold wave treatment.

Formula: Two tablespoons of white vinegar to one pint of tepid water. Use as a last rinse after a shampoo. After using the vinegar rinse, run water quickly over the hair to remove the odor.

Lemon (Acid) Rinse

A lemon rinse has a slight lightening quality. It separates the hair strands and is effective on lightened and blonde hair.

Formula: Use the strained juice of one or two lemons, or a few drops of concentrated lemon extract, and mix in one quart of warm water.

Rinse the hair with the lemon mixture several times. Finally, rinse the hair with clear warm water to remove all the lemon juice.

Citric Acid Rinse

A citric acid rinse is often used in place of a lemon rinse.

Formula: Place one tablespoon of citric acid crystals into a pint container and pour four ounces of boiling water over them. Fill the rest of the container with warm water, stirring while you add the water. Apply the same as you would the lemon rinse.

Cream Rinse

A cream rinse is a commercial product having a creamy appearance. It is used as a last rinse. It tends to soften the hair, add lustre, and make tangled hair easier to comb.

Cream rinses depend for their effectiveness on one or more chemicals having one property in common—that of being "substantive" to hair. Some substances will adhere to the hair shaft and refuse to be washed off by ordinary rinsing. This is so in the materials used in a cream rinse. The result is that the hair has a soft feel and is much easier to comb and handle.

A cream rinse does not have the same function as an acid rinse. Cream rinses are slightly acid in reaction, which is due to the nature of the ingredients used. However, the acidity is so low that in the dilutions used, **a cream rinse would have no effect as a soap film remover.**

CAUTION must be exercised in the use of a cream rinse immediately after a cold permanent wave. A cream rinse should not be used after a permanent which leaves only a shallow or body wave. The cream rinse could relax the hair to the point where the wave is entirely removed. In such a case, an acid rinse is recommended.

Acid Balanced Rinse (Non-Strip)

An acid balanced rinse is formulated to prevent the stripping of color after a toner or tint treatment. Most manufacturers design this type of rinse to be used in connection with their particular tint or toner product.

Reconditioning Rinse

A reconditioning rinse is used following a lightening or tint treatment. Follow manufacturer's directions.

Medicated Rinses

These are formulated with some medicinal properties to control minor conditions of dandruff. Follow the manufacturer's instructions.

Bluing Rinse

A prepared rinse containing a blue base color is used to give yellowish hair a silvery grey or white color tone. The porosity of the hair must be taken into consideration in order to avoid a two-toned effect on the porous ends. Follow the **manufacturer's directions** when mixing the type of rinse needed to achieve the desired silver or slate color tone.

Color Rinse

Color rinses are prepared rinses used to highlight, or add temporary color, to the hair. These rinses remain on the hair until the next shampoo. For additional information consult chapter on **Hair Coloring.**

REVIEW QUESTIONS

Shampooing

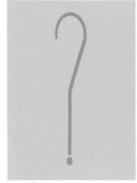

1. Define shampoos.
2. How often should the hair be shampooed?
3. Which important steps precede the shampoo?
4. What are the main steps in shampooing the hair?
5. What is done with the leftover supplies after the shampoo?
6. When does the cosmetologist wash and sanitize her hands?
7. Why is it necessary to cleanse the scalp and hair regularly?
8. List five conditions under which hair brushing is omitted before giving a shampoo.
9. Which type of shampoo will have a damaging effect on the hair?
10. When is a non-strip shampoo recommended?
11. When is a liquid dry shampoo recommended?

Rinsing

1. What are hair rinses?
2. List five purposes of hair rinses.
3. Give the purpose and effect of the following rinses:
   a) Lemon or citric acid
   b) Vinegar
4. What type of rinse is used to tone down a yellowish cast to grey or white hair?
5. How does a cream rinse act on the hair?
6. What is the purpose of color rinses?
7. How long do color rinses last?
8. When is a plain water rinse applied?
9. What is a non-strip rinse?
10. Which kind of rinse may be used to counteract the alkalinity of a lightener, tint or a cold wave lotion?

CHAPTER 8

SCALP AND HAIR CARE

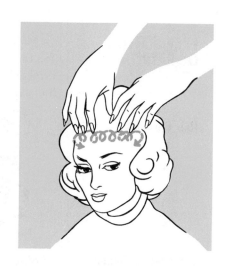

INTRODUCTION

The purpose of scalp treatments is to help preserve the health and beauty of the hair and scalp. Scalp treatments also assist in overcoming and combating disorders of the scalp, such as dandruff and loss of hair.

A basic requirement for a healthy scalp is constant cleanliness. The scalp and hair should be kept clean by frequent treatment and shampooing. A clean scalp will resist a wide variety of diseases.

Scalp manipulations stimulate the circulation of blood in the scalp, rest and soothe the nerves, stimulate the muscles and the activity of scalp glands, render a tight scalp more flexible, and promote the growth and health of the hair.

MAINTAINING A HEALTHY SCALP AND HAIR

Even the healthy person should have scalp treatments to preserve the natural health of the hair. While shampooing will keep the hair clean, it will not prevent the hair from becoming dry and brittle. The cosmetologist, therefore, should be careful to recommend the proper cosmetic applications to help counteract the danger of a dry and scaly scalp, or to administer the proper treatment in order to overcome an excessively oily condition of the scalp and hair.

Because the scalp and hair are vitally related, many scalp disorders need correction in order to keep the hair healthy. **A healthy scalp will usually produce healthy hair.** The cosmetologist may treat only common and minor conditions.

CAUTION: **Do not suggest a scalp treatment:**

1. If there are scalp abrasions or a scalp disease;
2. Or, if immediately prior to the application of a lightener, tint, toner, a permanent wave treatment, or a chemical hair relaxer treatment.

For serious or contagious scalp ailments, advise patrons to consult a physician. However, conditions caused by neglect, such as tight scalp muscles, overactive or inactive oil glands, and tense nerves, can often be corrected or alleviated by proper scalp treatments.

PREPARATION OF PATRON

As in any other treatment, first gather all the necessary equipment for the kind of scalp treatment you are about to give. Prepare patron as directed by your instructor. Be sure to remove all hairpins from the hair and comb out tangles.

Hair Brushing

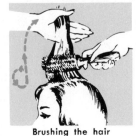

Brushing the hair should always be an essential part of a scalp treatment. Not only will proper brushing help to stimulate the scalp, but it will also help to remove dust and dirt from the hair and give it added luster and sheen. (For instructions on hair brushing, see chapter on **Shampooing and Rinsing.**)

Brushing the hair

Scalp Manipulations

Since the same manipulations are given with all scalp treatments, the cosmetologist should learn to give them with a continuous, even motion, which will have beneficial effects on the patron. Scalp massage is best applied as a series of treatments: once a week for normal scalps, and more frequently for scalp disorders, under the direction of a dermatologist.

Anatomy

Knowing the muscles, the location of blood vessels and the nerve points of the scalp and neck will help guide the cosmetologist to those areas in which massage movements are to be directed for most beneficial results.

OUTLINE OF SCALP MANIPULATION TECHNIQUE

Basic Technique in Scalp Manipulation

There are several ways in which scalp manipulations may be given. The following routine may be changed to meet your instructor's requirements.

With each movement described below, the hands are placed **under** the hair. Thus, the length of the fingers, the balls of the fingertips and the cushions of the palms stimulate the muscles, nerves and blood vessels in the scalp area.

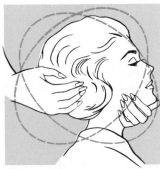

1. RELAXING MOVEMENT. Cupping chin in your left hand, place right hand at base of skull and rotate gently. Reverse positions of the hands and repeat.

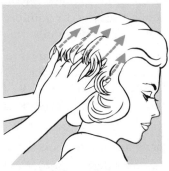

2. SLIDING MOVEMENT. Place fingertips on each side of head, slide firmly upward, spreading the fingertips until they meet at the top of head. Repeat four times.

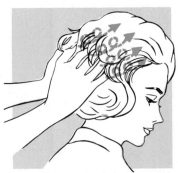

3. SLIDING AND ROTATING MOVEMENT. Same as movement No. 2, except that after sliding the fingertips one inch, rotate and move the scalp. Repeat four times.

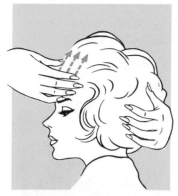

4. FOREHEAD MOVEMENT. Hold back of head with left hand. Place stretched thumb and fingers of right hand on forehead. Move hand slowly and firmly upward to one inch past hairline. Repeat four times.

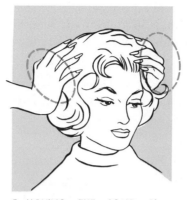

5. MOVING THE SCALP. Place palms of hands firmly against scalp. Lift scalp in a rotary movement: first, with hands placed above ears; second, with hands placed at front and back of head.

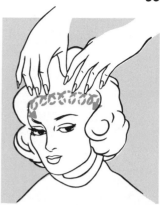

6. HAIRLINE MOVEMENT. Place fingers of both hands at forehead; massage around hairline by lifting and rotating.

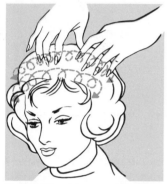

7. FRONT SCALP MOVEMENT. Dropping back one inch, repeat movement over entire front scalp.

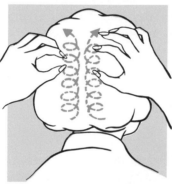

8. BACK SCALP MOVEMENT. Place fingers of each hand on sides of head; starting below ears, manipulate with thumbs upward to crown. Repeat four times. Repeat thumb manipulations, working towards center back of head.

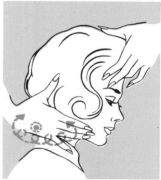

9. EAR-TO-EAR MOVEMENT. Place left hand on forehead; massage from right ear to left ear, along base of skull, with heel of hand, using rotary movement.

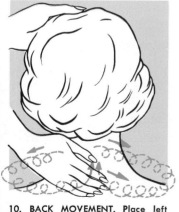

10. BACK MOVEMENT. Place left hand on forehead and stand at left of patron. Rotate with right hand from base of neck, along shoulder, and back across shoulder blade to spine. Slide up spine to base of neck. Repeat on opposite side.

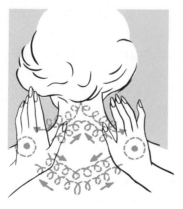

11. SHOULDER MOVEMENT. Place both palms together at base of neck. With rotary movement, catch muscles in the palms and massage along shoulder blades to point of shoulder and back again. Then massage from shoulders to spine and back again.

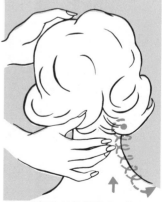

12. SPINE MOVEMENT. Massage with rotary movement from base of skull down the spine. Using a firm finger pressure, bring hand slowly to base of skull.

TREATMENT FOR NORMAL HAIR AND SCALP

The primary purpose of a general scalp treatment is to keep the scalp and hair in a clean and healthy condition. Regular scalp treatments are also beneficial in helping to prevent baldness.

Preparation

1. Assemble materials and supplies.
2. Help patron with dress or blouse.
3. Drape and prepare patron.

Procedure

1. Brush hair for about five minutes.
2. Apply scalp pomade or cream.
3. Apply infra-red lamp for about five minutes.
4. Give scalp manipulations for 10 to 20 minutes.
5. Shampoo the hair.
6. Towel dry the hair to remove excess moisture.
7. Apply suitable scalp lotion or tonic.
8. Style hair.
9. Clean up work station.

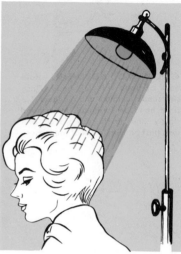

Apply heat with infra-red lamp.

DANDRUFF TREATMENT

The principal signs of dandruff are the appearance of white scales on the hair and scalp and the itching of the scalp. Dandruff may be associated with either a dry or oily condition of the scalp. The more common causes of dandruff are poor circulation of blood to the scalp, improper diet, lack of cleanliness, and infection. To help prevent the spread of dandruff in the beauty salon, the cosmetologist must sanitize all implements and avoid the use in common of combs, brushes and scalp applicators.

Procedure

1. Prepare patron as for normal scalp treatment.
2. Brush hair for five minutes.
3. Apply a scalp preparation according to scalp condition (dry or oily).
4. Apply infra-red lamp for about five minutes.
5. Give regular scalp manipulations using indirect high-frequency current.
6. Shampoo with corrective shampoo lotion.
7. Towel dry the hair.
8. Use direct high-frequency current with glass rake electrode for 3-5 minutes.
9. Apply scalp preparation suitable for the condition.
10. Style hair.
11. Clean up work station.

**DRY HAIR AND
SCALP TREATMENT**

This treatment should be used when there is a deficiency of natural oil on the scalp and hair. Select scalp preparations containing moisturizing and emollient materials. **Avoid** the use of strong soaps, cosmetics containing a mineral oil or sulfonated oil base, or greasy preparations and lotions with a high alcoholic content.

Procedure

1. Prepare patron as for normal scalp treatment.
2. Brush hair for about five minutes.
3. Apply the cosmetic preparation for this condition, as directed by your instructor or manufacturer.
4. Apply a steamer for 7-10 minutes, or apply some other form of moist heat for 7-10 minutes. Be guided by your instructor.
5. Give a mild shampoo.
6. Towel dry the hair, making sure that the scalp is thoroughly dry.

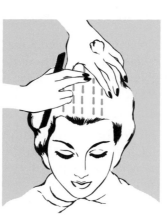

Applying scalp cream

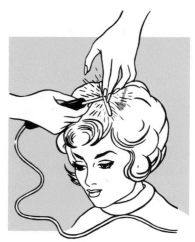

Applying high-frequency with
glass rake electrode

7. Apply moisturizing scalp cream sparingly with a rotary frictional motion.
8. Stimulate scalp with direct high-frequency current, using the glass rake electrode, for about five minutes.
9. Style hair.
10. Clean up work station.

**OILY SCALP
TREATMENT**

Excessive oiliness of the scalp is caused by the overactivity of the sebaceous (oil) glands. During manipulations, lift the scalp from the skull and knead it in the direction of the blood vessels and nerves. With the correct degree of pressing and squeezing, any hardened sebum in the pores of the scalp may be removed. To normalize the function of these glands, excess sebum should be flushed out with each treatment.

Procedure

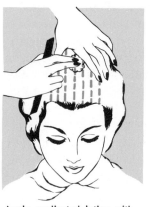

Apply medicated lotion with cotton pledget.

1. Prepare patron as for normal scalp treatment.
2. Brush hair for about five minutes. **Do not** irritate scalp with brush bristles.
3. Apply a medicated lotion to scalp only.
4. Apply infra-red lamp for about five minutes.
5. Give scalp manipulations.
6. Shampoo with a corrective shampoo.
7. Towel dry the hair.
8. Apply direct high-frequency current 3-5 minutes.
9. Apply a medicated scalp tonic containing an astringent base.
10. Style hair.
11. Clean up work station.

CAUTION. Creams or ointments may be applied **before** using high-frequency current. Hair tonics or lotions with alcoholic content may be applied only **after** the application of high-frequency current.

CORRECTIVE HAIR TREATMENT

Conditioning Agent

A corrective hair treatment deals with the **hair shaft,** not the scalp. Dry and damaged hair can be greatly improved by reconditioning agents. Hair treatments are especially beneficial and extremely important when given approximately a week or ten days before, and a week or ten days after, a permanent wave, tint, lightener, toner or chemical hair straightener treatment.

Dry hair may be softened quickly with a reconditioning preparation applied directly on the hair shaft. The product used for this purpose is usually an emulsion containing cholesterol and related compounds.

Some conditioners function more effectively when heat is applied to induce penetration into the cortex. The heat, applied directly to the hair, stimulates the opening of the imbrications of the cuticle and permits significantly more corrective agents to enter. This provides more conditioning and more lasting benefits.

(Heat may be supplied by a heating cap, a steamer, or a pre-heated hood dryer.)

Procedure

1. Prepare patron as for normal scalp treatment.
2. Brush hair for about five minutes.
3. Apply a mild shampoo.
4. Blot the hair with towel.
5. Apply reconditioning agent as directed by manufacturer.
6. Set the hair; dry with medium or cool dryer; style the hair.
7. Clean up work station.

TREATMENT FOR ALOPECIA

Alopecia refers to a condition of premature baldness or excessive hair loss. The chief causes responsible for alopecia are poor circulation, lack of proper stimulation, improper nourishment and certain infectious diseases, such as ringworm, or constitutional disorders. The treatment of alopecia is directed to stimulating the blood supply and reviving the hair papillae involved in hair growth.

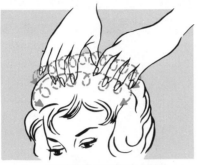

APPLYING INDIRECT HIGH-
FREQUENCY CURRENT
Cosmetologist manipulates scalp

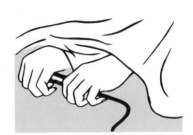

while patron holds
metal electrode.

Procedure

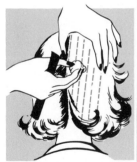

Apply medicated
scalp lotion.

1. Prepare patron as for normal scalp treatment.
2. Brush hair for about five minutes.
3. Apply a medicated scalp ointment as directed by a physician.
4. Apply infra-red rays for about five minutes.
5. Give scalp manipulations. You may use indirect high-frequency current.
6. Shampoo, using a mild shampoo.
7. Towel dry.
8. Apply direct high-frequency current for about five minutes.
9. Apply medicated scalp lotion.
10. Repeat scalp manipulations, including neck, shoulders and upper back.
11. Set hair; dry with warm or cool air, and style.
12. Clean up work station.

REMINDER

An abnormal scalp and hair condition requires very careful analysis in order to give the appropriate scalp and hair treatment.

Some scalp conditions may be infectious. Therefore, use only sanitized implements on patrons.

Procedure

Alopecia areata is a disease causing baldness in spots. This condition may be treated under the direction of a physician.

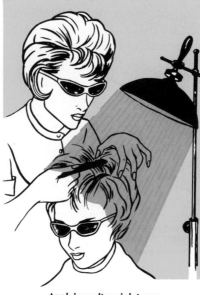

Applying ultra-violet rays

1. Prepare patron as for normal scalp treatment.
2. Give regular scalp manipulations.
3. Shampoo the hair according to the condition; if scalp is very tender, give a mild shampoo.
4. Dry the scalp and hair thoroughly.
5. Expose the scalp to ultra-violet rays for 5-10 minutes, especially the bald spots.
6. Apply ointment or lotion with light manipulations on the bald spots.
7. Apply high-frequency current for about five minutes. If an ointment is used, apply direct current; if a lotion is used, apply indirect current.
8. Style hair, using comb only.
9. Clean up work station.

REVIEW QUESTIONS

Scalp And Hair Treatments

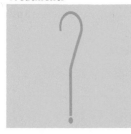

1. What is the purpose of giving scalp treatments?
2. What benefits are obtained from effective scalp manipulations?
3. What is the most effective method of stimulating the scalp?
4. What must be observed for a scalp and hair treatment?
5. How often should scalp massage be given?
6. What benefits are obtained from regular hair brushing?
7. Why does normal hair and scalp require scalp treatment?
8. Which scalp disorders are commonly treated in the beauty salon?
9. What are the common causes of dandruff?
10. List two reasons for not recommending a scalp treatment.
11. What precautions are required when using high-frequency current in connection with hair tonics or lotions?

CHAPTER 9

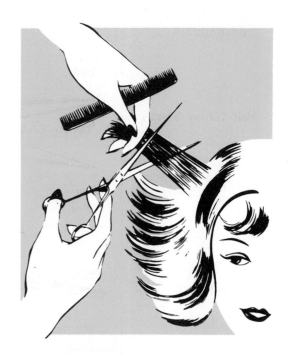

HAIR SHAPING

INTRODUCTION

The art of **hair shaping** must be mastered by the student of cosmetology before she can be qualified to work in the better salons. Thorough instruction is required in the proper way to shape the hair, using either regular scissors, thinning shears or razor. Instruction must be followed by practice under the guidance of the instructor. A good hair shaping serves as a foundation for beautiful coiffures. The cosmetologist's education is not complete until she has acquired the artistic skill and judgment necessary for successful hair shaping.

Modern Hairstyles

Modern hairstyles are designed to accentuate the patron's good points, while minimizing her poor features. The cosmetologist must be guided by the patron's wishes as well as by what is best for her personality. In selecting the proper hairstyle, the cosmetologist should take into consideration the patron's head shape, her facial contour, her neckline and hair texture.

HAIR SHAPING IMPLEMENTS

Implements used in hair shaping. A cosmetologist will find the quality of the implements she selects and uses in hair shaping to be important. To do her best work, the cosmetologist should buy and use only superior implements from a reliable manufacturer.

Improper use will quickly destroy the efficiency of any implement, however perfectly it might be made at the factory.

The following are the implements used in hair shaping:

1. Regular hair shaping scissors
2. Thinning shears
3. Straight razor
4. Razors with safety guards
5. Combs

HAIR SHAPING IMPLEMENTS

Hair Cutting Scissors

Thinning Shears

Straight Razor

Razors With Safety Guards

Popular Combs

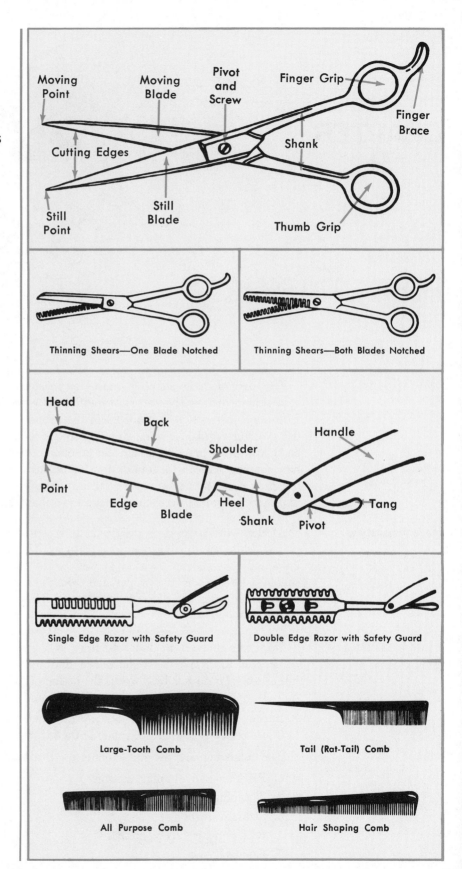

Moving Point — Moving Blade — Pivot and Screw — Finger Grip — Finger Brace — Cutting Edges — Shank — Still Point — Still Blade — Thumb Grip

Thinning Shears—One Blade Notched

Thinning Shears—Both Blades Notched

Head — Back — Shoulder — Handle — Point — Edge — Blade — Heel — Shank — Pivot — Tang

Single Edge Razor with Safety Guard

Double Edge Razor with Safety Guard

Large-Tooth Comb

Tail (Rat-Tail) Comb

All Purpose Comb

Hair Shaping Comb

SECTIONING FOR HAIR SHAPING

By following a step-by-step practical procedure, the student will soon learn how to give a professional hair shaping. The first step is to section the hair properly. The following illustrations cover the practical and accepted methods for dividing the hair, either into four or five sections. In any case, follow your instructor's methods, which are equally correct.

Partings—4 Sections

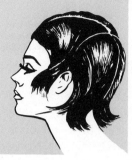 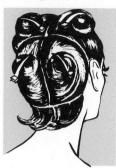

Part hair down the center from forehead to nape, and also across from ear to ear. Pin up the four sections and leave nape hair to use as a guide.

Partings—5 Sections

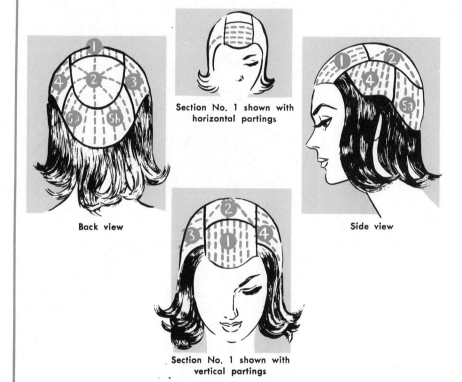

Back view

Section No. 1 shown with horizontal partings

Side view

Section No. 1 shown with vertical partings

Procedure

Five (5) section parting, with sub-parting panels. Section and pin up hair in the order shown in illustration. Leave nape and side hair loose to be used as a guide.

The back section (No. 5) may be divided into Sections No. 5a and No. 5b for easier handling.

Top section (No. 1) may be sub-parted in two ways, as shown in the above illustrations, with partings running in either a horizontal or vertical direction.

Alternate 5-Section Method

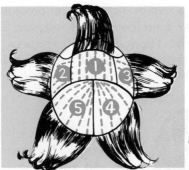

Another way to divide the hair into five sections is to part the hair from ear to ear; then subdivide the hair in the same order as shown in the illustration.

Hair divided into
5 sections with
center back parting

HOLDING HAIR-SHAPING IMPLEMENTS

Hair shaping scissors are correctly handled by inserting the third (ring) finger into the ring of the "still blade," and placing the little finger on the finger brace. The thumb is inserted into the ring of the "movable blade." The tip of the index finger is braced near the pivot of the scissors in order to have better control.

Scissors

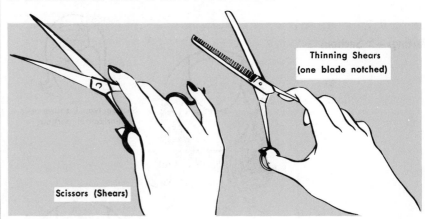

Thinning Shears
(one blade notched)

Scissors (Shears)

Thinning Shears

Excess bulk is removed from the hair by the use of **thinning shears**. As can be seen in the accompanying illustrations, they are quite similar to hair shaping scissors, except they have one or both blades notched, or serrated. Which one is used depends on the preference of the cosmetologist. The notches help the cosmetologist control the amount of hair that is removed. Both thinning shears and shaping scissors are held in the same way.

Holding Comb And Scissors

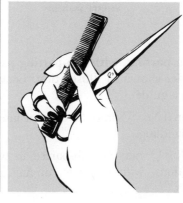

Whenever it is necessary to use the comb during hair shaping, close the blades of the scissors, remove thumb from the ring and rest scissors in the palm. The scissors are held securely with the ring finger. The thumb and index finger can be used to handle the comb.

HAIR THINNING

The purpose of thinning the hair is to remove the excess bulk without shortening its length. For best results, use the following suggestions:

1. When using a razor for thinning or shaping, you must dampen the hair first.
2. When using thinning shears or regular scissors, you may have the hair either dry or damp.

Hair Texture

Be guided by the **hair texture** when determining the point on the hair strand where thinning should start. As a rule, **fine hair** may be thinned **closer** to the scalp than coarse hair. The reason is that if coarse hair is thinned too close to the scalp, the short, stubby ends will protrude through the top layer. Fine hair, on the other hand, is softer and more pliable, and when cut very short will lay flat on the head.

How Much To Thin

How much to thin the hair depends on the particular hairstyle to be created. As a guide, start thinning different textures of hair as follows:

1. Fine hair—from $\frac{1}{2}$ to 1 inch from the scalp
2. Medium hair—from 1 to $1\frac{1}{2}$ inches from the scalp
3. Coarse hair—from $1\frac{1}{2}$ to 2 inches from the scalp

Thinning Areas

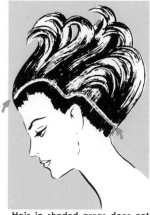

Hair in shaded areas does not require thinning.

There are several areas where it is not advisable to thin the hair. For instance, thinning the hair on the sides immediately above the ears or at the nape of the neck leaves the hair in the same shape as when you started, **only** with less hair to work with.

Areas where hair does not require thinning:

1. At nape of neck (ear to ear), as excess bulk is seldom found there.
2. At side of head, above ears.
3. $\frac{1}{4}$ inch around facial hairline. Usually hair is not heavy at hairline.
4. In the hair part. The cut ends would be seen in the finished hairstyle.

> **Never thin the hair near the ends of a strand; to do so will render the hair shapeless.**

THINNING WITH THINNING SHEARS

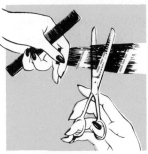

Holding hair between middle and index finger

When using the thinning shears, grip the hair firmly by overlapping the middle finger a little over the index finger, bracing the thumb against the index finger, as shown in the illustration.

Thinning the hair. Pick up a strand of hair from $\frac{1}{2}$ to 1 inch wide by 2 to 3 inches long, depending on the texture of the hair. Hold strand straight out between the middle and index fingers. Place thinning shears 1 or 2 inches from the scalp (depending on the hair texture) and cut into the hair as shown in illustration. Move out another $1\frac{1}{2}$ inches and cut again. **Caution.** It is advisable to avoid thinning the top layer of strand. The strand is cut by partly closing the thinning shears about $\frac{3}{4}$ through the strand. The top part is not cut.

Thinning Or Shaping With Shears

Slithering

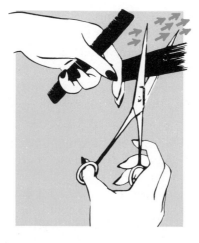

When using regular shears to thin the hair, pick up smaller sections of hair than you would when using thinning shears. The technique is also different. The process of thinning the hair with shears (scissors) is known as **slithering.**

Hold a strand of hair straight out between the middle and index fingers. Place the hair in the shears so that only the **underneath** hair will be cut. Slide the shears up and down the strand, closing them slightly each time the shears are moved toward the scalp. Repeat this procedure twice on each strand. **Alternate method** of holding the hair is with the thumb and index finger.

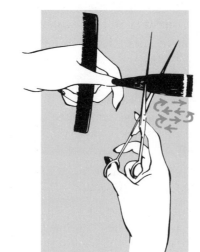

Holding the hair with thumb and index finger

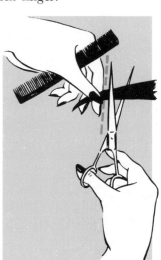

Blunt cutting

Back-Combing And Slithering

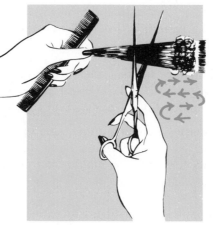

Slithering the hair after back-combing

Hold hair with thumb and index finger and back-comb the short hair; then slither as explained above.

Back-combing is also known as **matting, ratting, teasing,** or **French lacing.**

SCISSOR HAIR SHAPING

Scissor hair shaping may be done on either dry or wet hair.

1. **Dry shaping.** If the hair is shaped while dry, it is usually shampooed **after** the shaping is completed.

2. **Wet shaping.** The hair may be shaped immediately after it has been shampooed.

Preparation

1. Seat patron; adjust neck strip and plastic cape.
2. Examine head shape, facial features and hair texture.
3. Comb and brush hair free of tangles.
4. Shaping may be done dry or damp.

Procedure For Nape Section

1. Divide hair into five sections.
2. Determine the length of the nape guideline hair.
3. Blunt cut guideline strand of nape hair.
   a) Blunt cut strand on left side, using the earlobe as guide.
   b) Blunt cut strand on right side to match left side.

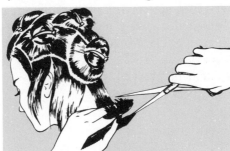

Blunt cutting strand at center
nape to desired length

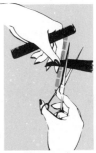

Blunt cutting

   c) Blunt cut from back center to left front.
   d) Blunt cut from back center to right front.

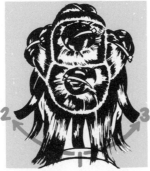

Following up by cutting all
remaining guideline hair

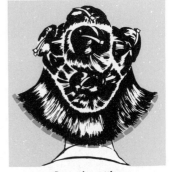

Properly cutting
guideline hair

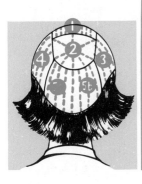

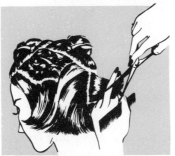

Blunt cutting section No. 5b

Let down section No. 5 and d¹
into two equal parts (No. 5a an⁷
5b). Match length with guidelⁱⁿ
Either left side or right side
done first.

Hold hair panels out frⁿe
while blunt cutting. Cⁿ
sections No. 3 and Nⁿ
manner.

Crown Section

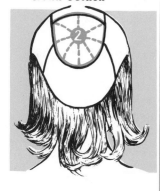

Top Section

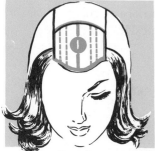

Top view.
Section No. 1 with
vertical partings.

Bangs

Reducing Bulk

Completion

Crown section No. 2. Hold pie-shaped strands out from the head; match length by picking up strands from section already cut. Continue around the head, matching length with sides and back hair.

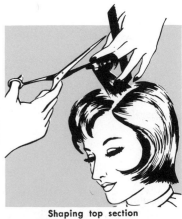

Shaping top section

Divide section No. 1 into two parts. Pick up hair from the middle of the section, using previously cut hair as a guide. Maintain the hand movement in a 45° arc. Proceed to cut both parts of section No. 1 in the prescribed manner.

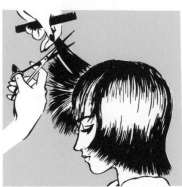

Shaping the top section

If **bangs** are to be cut, move from side to directly in front of patron for even cutting. Test hair for bounce (elasticity) then determine desired length. If bangs are to be short, use bridge of nose as a guide. If style is to be long, shape strands to blend into length of the sides.

Thinning. To complete the shaping of the hair, excess bulk should be removed by thinning with thinning shears or scissors. It is recommended that all hair be checked for proper length.

Remove neck strip and plastic cape. Thoroughly clean all hair clip-

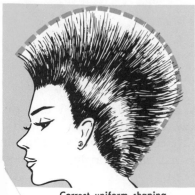

Correct uniform shaping

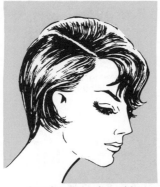

Completed shaping with
bang effect and/or
off-face style

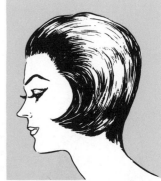

Hair shaping for straight
back styles

pings from cape, patron's clothing and from work area. You may then proceed with the next professional service desired by the patron.

SHINGLING

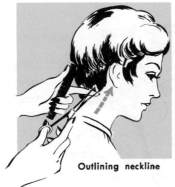

Outlining neckline

Shingling is cutting the hair close to the nape of the neck and gradually longer toward the crown, without showing a definite line.

Regardless of the prevailing hair fashion, there will always be a number of patrons who want their hair cut or molded short. To satisfy these patrons, you must know how to shingle the hair. The following illustrations show how shingling is accomplished using shears and comb.

Procedure

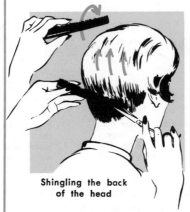

Shingling the back of the head

Shingling should be done at eye level. Starting at the nape line, shingle the hair upward in a graduated effect. After reaching the top of the section being shingled, turn the comb downward and comb the hair. Proceed, section by section, until the entire back of the head is shingled in a smooth, uniform manner.

Note—In shingling, the blades of the scissors are held parallel with the comb; only the top blade moves and does the cutting.

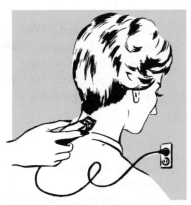

Cleaning neck with clippers

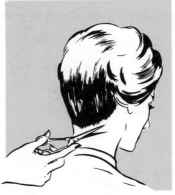

Cleaning neck with points of scissors

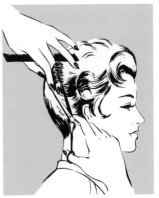

Clipping hair ends

USE OF CLIPPERS

There is a mistaken notion that the use of clippers to clean the neck line has a tendency to make the hair grow thicker at the neck. This is not true, as the amount of human hair can only be as great as the number of follicles in the area, and these do not increase in number with the use of the clippers, or any other implement.

SHAPING WITH RAZOR

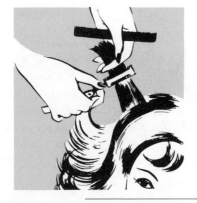

The successful cosmetologist must be able to handle all implements efficiently, including the straight razor.

How To Hold Razor

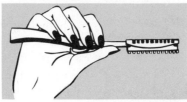

Finger Wrap Hold
Place the thumb in the groove part of the shank and fold the fingers over the handle of the razor. The guard faces the cosmetologist while working.

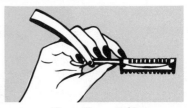

Three Finger Hold
Place three fingers over the shank, the thumb in the groove of the shank and the little finger in the hollow part of the tang.

When using the razor, keep the hair damp, in order to avoid pulling the hair and to prevent dulling the razor.

CHANGING BLADES

Removing Old Blade

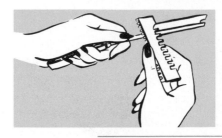

Remove guard. With left hand, hold shaper firmly above joint. Catching the blade in the teeth on upper part of guard, push blade out.

Inserting New Blade

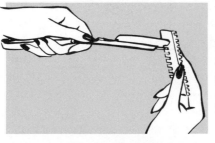

Slide blade into groove, pushing the end with your fingers. Place the tooth end of guard into the blade notch and slide the blade in until it clicks into position.

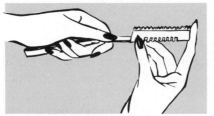

Slide the guard over blade, making sure free or open end is over cutting edge of blade.

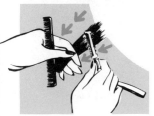

Thinning with razor

Hold a strand of wet hair straight out between the middle and index fingers. Place the razor flat, **not erect,** about 1 to 2 inches from the scalp (depending on the hair texture), use short, steady strokes toward the hair ends.

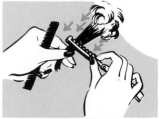

Tapering hair ends
after back-combing

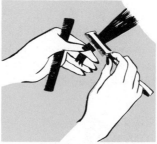

Blunt razor cutting

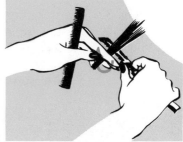

Razor undercutting with
upward stroke

**SHAPING
WITH RAZOR**

Preparation

1. Seat patron; adjust neck strip and plastic cape.
2. Examine head shape, facial features and hair texture.
3. Comb and brush hair free of tangles.
4. Shampoo or wet the hair.

**Procedure
Cutting Guideline**

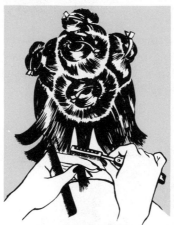

Blunt cutting a strand at
center nape for desired
hair length

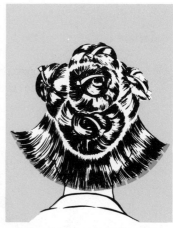

Completely cut guideline hair

1. Divide hair into five sections.
2. Determine the length of the nape guideline hair.
3. Blunt cut guideline strand of nape hair.
   a) Blunt cut strand on left side; use the earlobe as guide.
   b) Blunt cut strand on right side to match left side.
   c) Use guideline hair to cut from back center to left front.
   d) Blunt cut from back center to right front.

Shaping Back Section (5a, 5b)

Divide section No. 5 into two parts (Sections No. 5a and No. 5b). From center of section No. 5a, pick horizontal strands. Pick up guideline strand for length. When guideline hair falls away, cut hair — moving hands out and upward into a 45° arc.

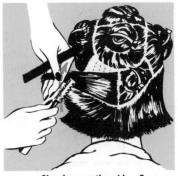

Shaping Section 4

Proceed to cut to the left into section No. 4 in the same manner.

Shaping Section 3

Return to section No. 5b and cut this section, moving to the right into section No. 3, always lifting hands in an upward 45° arc as the hair is cut. **Measure carefully with guideline.**

Shaping section No. 5a

Shaping Section 2

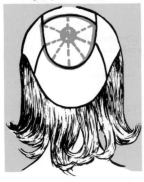

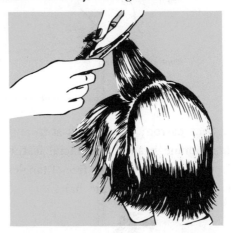

Next, proceed to cut section No. 2 (crown), using previously cut hair as a guide.

Shaping Section 1

Divide section No. 1 into two parts. Pick up hair from the middle of the section, using previously cut hair as a guide. Maintain the hand movement in a 45° arc. Proceed to cut both parts of section No. 1 in the prescribed manner.

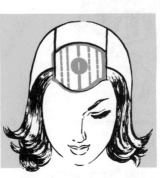

Section No. 1 shown with vertical parting

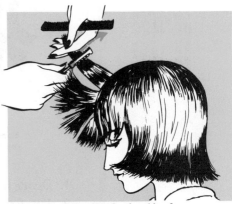

Shaping Section No. 1

Bangs

To cut **bangs** evenly, move your position from the side to directly in front of patron. Test hair for bounce (elasticity), then determine desired length. If bangs are to be short, use bridge of nose as a guide. If style is to be long, shape strands to blend into length of the sides.

Thinning

To complete the shaping of the hair, excess bulk should be removed by thinning with a razor, thinning shears or scissors. It is recommended that all hair be checked for proper length.

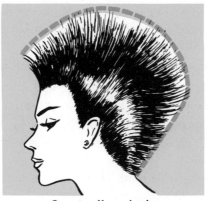
Correct uniform shaping

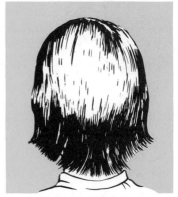
Back view—uniform shaping

Completion

Remove neck strip and plastic cape. Thoroughly clean all hair clippings from cape, patron's clothing and work area. You may then proceed with the next professional service desired by the patron.

> **Molding the hair properly with a razor serves as a foundation for a variety of beautiful hairstyles.**

LEARN HOW TO HANDLE CHILDREN

Special consideration should be given to children and teenagers. Hairstylists who know how to handle children will usually attract the mothers to the same salon for their own hairstyling.

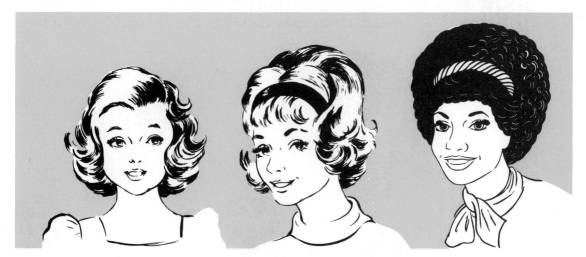
Popular hairstyles for youngsters

SHAPING OVER-CURLY HAIR

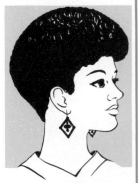

Medium length hair

Back view

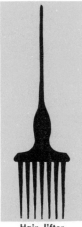

Hair lifter

Over-curly hair has its own particular characteristics, as have the other types of hair, which require special techniques for styling. Of prime importance to the cosmetologist is the ability to create a hairstyle that will enhance the appearance of the patron and to visualize how the finished hairstyle will look. Knowing the correct styling techniques and using common sense in their application are the marks of the trained cosmetologist.

The steps outlined below represent one method of styling over-curly hair. Where your instructor's methods differ, follow her techniques.

1. Drape patron in the usual manner for hair shaping.
2. Shampoo and dry hair thoroughly.
3. Apply an emollient product lightly to the scalp and hair to replace lost oil.
4. Using a wide-tooth comb, or a hair lifter, comb the hair upward and slightly forward, making the hair as long as possible. Start at the crown and continue until all hair has been combed out from the scalp and distributed evenly around the head. By combing in a circular pattern, splits are usually avoided.
5. Shape the hair. Visualize the style and length of hair desired. Start by tapering the sides, and cut in the direction hair will be combed.
6. Taper the back part of the head to blend with the sides.
7. Trim the extreme ends of the crown and top areas to desired length.
8. For an off-the-face hairstyle, comb hair up and backward. For forward movement, comb hair up and forward.
9. Blend side hair with the top, crown and back hair.
10. Outline the hairstyle at sides, around the ears and nape area, using either scissors or hairliner (special type clipper).
11. Give finishing touch. Fluff slightly with hair lifter, wherever needed. Lightly spray the hair to give it a natural, lustrous sheen.

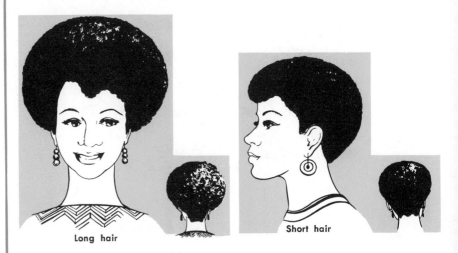

Long hair

Short hair

CORRECTING SPLIT HAIR ENDS

Trichoptilosis is the technical term for **split hair ends.** When the hair becomes dry and brittle, due to several causes, the hair ends frequently split. Temporary relief for this condition may be obtained by clipping the hair ends.

Procedure

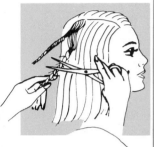

Clipping the protruding hair ends

The hair is combed thoroughly and divided into small, equal sections. Each section or strand is twisted tightly from the scalp to the ends.

The twisted strand is then held in the left hand while the extended fingers of the right hand ruff the strand upward toward the scalp.

The split hair ends are removed with regular shears. Beginning near the scalp, cut alongside of the strand all protruding hair ends, gradually moving downward to the end of the strand, where the remaining ends are cut. The hair is then brushed briskly to remove the short hair clippings.

DEFINITIONS

Hair Shaping

Hairstyling—the art of arranging the hair in various attractive shapes or styles. The contour of the face, shape of the head, and the current season's styles must all be considered in this phase of the work.

Hairstylist—one who has the artistic ability to suggest and create an attractive new hair fashion.

Hair shaping—the process of thinning, tapering and shortening the hair, using comb, scissors, thinning shears or razor, to mold the hair into a becoming shape. **Hair shaping** is now the commonly used term for **haircutting.**

Dry cutting—shaping the hair with scissors while it is in a dry condition.

Scissor cutting—shaping hair by means of scissors.

Basic hair shaping—shaping the hair to a length which is not too long, nor too short, in order that it properly fits many different hairstyles.

Guideline—a strand of hair at the nape or sides of the head that is cut to a precise length. This cut strand establishes a guide or line to be followed in shaping the balance of the head, and helps to establish the general shaping pattern.

Shingling—cutting the hair close to the nape of the neck, with the hair becoming gradually longer toward the crown, without showing a definite line.

Thinning—decreasing the thickness of the hair where it is too heavy.

Tapering—shortening the hair in a graduated effect. **Feathering** —another term for tapering.

Slithering—the process used in thinning the hair with scissors. **Effilating**—a French term for slithering.

Trimming or clipping—the removing of split hair ends, or cutting the extreme ends of the hair with the scissors is known as trimming, or clipping.

Blunt cutting—cutting the hair straight off, without tapering.

Layer cutting—tapering and thinning the hair by dividing it into many thin layers.

Razor cutting—the use of the razor in thinning or cutting wet hair.

Natural hairline—where no artificial hairline is created in short hairstyles, the hair at the nape of the neck is left in its natural hairline.

Feather edge—when the hair at the nape of the neck is shingled in a graceful upward effect, and the neck is cleansed with scissors, razor or clippers.

Back-combing—combing the short hairs of a strand towards the scalp. Other terms used for back-combing are **teasing, ratting, matting** and **French lacing.**

Neck trim—cutting and shaping the hair at the nape of the neck into a "V", oval, or round shape, or shingling the hair into a feather-edge effect.

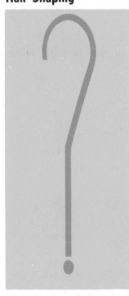

REVIEW QUESTIONS

Hair Shaping

1. Define hair shaping.
2. Name the main implements used in hair shaping.
3. Give four reasons for thinning, tapering and cutting the hair to the desired length.
4. What is meant by slithering the hair?
5. What is meant by back-combing?
6. Why is it not advisable to thin hair at the hairline, over the ears, or at the nape of the neck?
7. Why is it not advisable to thin hair in the hair part?
8. Why should you avoid removing too much hair during the thinning process?
9. About how close to the scalp should the following hair textures be thinned? a) Fine hair; b) Medium hair; c) Coarse hair
10. Why may thin hair be cut closer to the scalp than coarse hair?
11. Give a good reason for sectioning the hair prior to shaping.
12. Why should the hair be damp for razor shaping?
13. What causes a "stair-step" appearance at the back of the head in a shingle haircut?
14. What are three precautions which should be observed in giving a neck trim for tailored hairstyles?

CHAPTER 10

FINGER WAVING

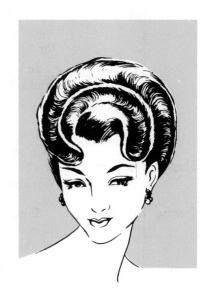

INTRODUCTION

Finger waving is the art of shaping the hair into waves with the aid of the fingers, comb, waving lotion, hairpins or clippies and a hair net. Proficiency in finger waving is important to the cosmetologist because it is the technique used to achieve many modern hairstyles.

Better results in producing soft, natural waves are obtained with hair that either has a natural wave or has been permanently waved, rather than with straight hair. A pleasing finger wave should harmonize with the shape of the patron's head, as well as with her features.

Finger Waving Lotion

A suitable waving lotion is an aid to better finger waving because it makes the hair pliable and keeps it in place.

The proper choice of waving lotion should be governed by the texture and condition of the patron's hair. A good waving lotion is harmless to the hair and should not flake upon drying.

Preparation

The cosmetologist washes his or her hands and has available all necessary sanitized implements and clean supplies. The cosmetologist prepares the patron in the same manner as for a shampoo.

The patron's hair is either shampooed or thoroughly saturated with water at the shampoo bowl. Her hair is towel blotted and she is seated comfortably before a dresserette.

Applying Lotion

The hair is parted, combed smooth and arranged to conform to the planned hairstyle. Waving lotion is applied to the hair with an applicator and distributed through the hair with a comb. The use of an excessive amount of waving lotion is avoided. **Note**—Lotion is applied on one side of the head at a time; this prevents it from drying and requiring an additional application.

Locating Natural Growth

To locate the natural hair growth, comb hair away from the face and push hair forward with the palm of your hand. (Consult Hairstyling chapter—"Finding the Natural Part.")

Parting Hair

The finger wave may be started on either side of the head. However, when the hair part is on the left side of the head, the work begins on the right or heavy side. (See illustrations below.)

In other words, in finger wave styling with a side part, the wave is usually started on the heavy side of the head.

HORIZONTAL FINGER WAVING

Shaping Top Area

Using the index finger of the left hand as a guide, shape the top hair with a comb, using a circular movement. Starting at the hairline, work towards the crown about one inch at a time until it has been reached. (Fig. 1.)

Forming First Ridge

Forming the first ridge. The index finger of the left hand is placed directly above the position planned for the first ridge. With the teeth of the comb pointing slightly upward, the comb is inserted directly under the index finger. The comb is drawn forward about one inch along the fingertip. (Fig. 2.)

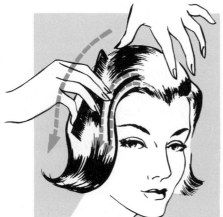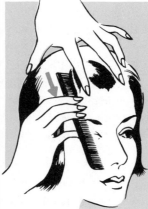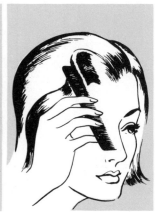

Fig. 1. Shaping top area   Fig. 2. Drawing hair about one inch   Fig. 3. Comb flattened against head

With the teeth still inserted in the ridge, the comb is flattened against the head in order to hold the ridge in place. (Fig. 3. The left hand is not shown so that you may see the ridge and position of the comb.)

The left hand is removed from the head, the middle finger is placed above the ridge, and the index finger is positioned on the teeth of the comb. The ridge is emphasized by closing the two fingers and applying pressure to the head. (Fig. 4.)

CAUTION. Do not try to increase the height of the ridge by pushing or lifting it up with the fingers. Such movement will distort the ridge formation and move it off its base.

Without removing the comb from the hair, turn the teeth downward and comb the hair in a right semi-circular direction to form a dip in the hollow part of the wave. (Fig. 5.)

This procedure is followed section by section until the crown has been reached, where the ridge phases out. (Fig. 6.)

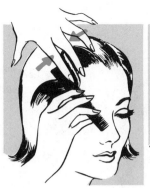

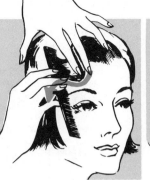

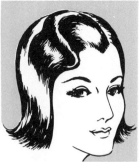

Fig. 4. Emphasizing ridge   Fig. 5. Combing hair in   Fig. 6. Completed first ridge
                                        semi-circular effect   at the crown

The ridge and wave of each section should match evenly without showing separations in the ridge and hollow part of the wave.

Forming Second Ridge

The formation of the second ridge is begun at the crown area. (Fig. 7.) The movements are the reverse of those followed in forming the first ridge. The comb is drawn from the tip towards the base of the index finger, thus directing the formation of the second ridge. All movements are followed in a reverse pattern (Fig. 8) until the hairline is reached, thus completing the second ridge. (Fig. 9.)

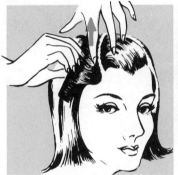

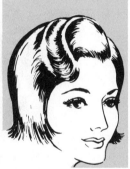

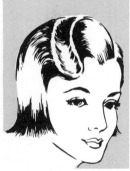

Fig. 7. Starting the second   Fig. 8. First section of   Fig. 9. Completed
          ridge.   second ridge   second ridge

Forming Third Ridge

Movements for the **third ridge** follow closely those used in creating the first ridge. The third ridge is formed starting from the hairline and extending back towards the back of the head. (Fig. 10.)

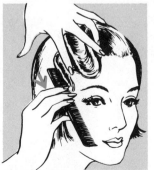

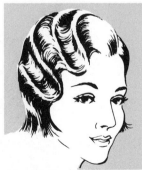

Fig. 10. Starting the third ridge   Fig. 11. Completed right side

Continue in alternating directions until the side of the head has been completed. (Fig. 11.)

Waving Left Side

Procedure

The same procedure is followed in finger waving the left (light) side of the head.

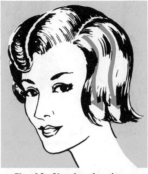

Fig. 12. Shaping for the left side.

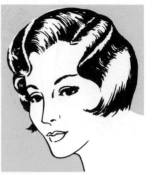

Fig. 13. First ridge starts at hairline.

1. The hair is first shaped as in Fig. 12.
2. The first ridge is made, starting at the hairline, section by section, until the second ridge of the opposite side is reached. (Fig. 13.)
3. Both the ridge and wave must blend and join with the ridge and wave from the right side of the head without splits or breaks. (Fig. 14.)

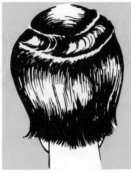

Fig. 14. Ridge and wave matched in the crown area.

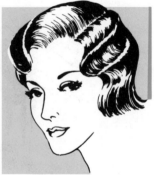

Fig. 15. Left side completed.

4. Start with the ridge and wave in the back of the head and proceed section by section towards the left side of the face.
5. Continue working back and forth until the entire side is completed. (Fig. 15.)

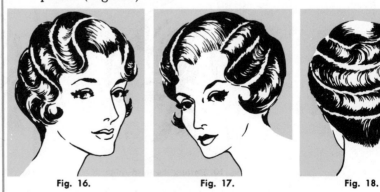

Fig. 16.   Fig. 17.   Fig. 18.

Figures 16, 17 and 18 illustrate the completed hairstyle.

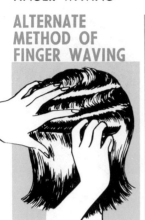

Fig. 19. Finger waving
around the head

Hair parted on left side. An alternate method in performing finger waving is done in the following manner:

1. Shape the top heavy right side.
2. The first ridge, front **right** side, phases out at the crown.
3. Start a ridge on the **left** front side and go all around the head; finish on the front **right** hairline.
4. Start another ridge on the front **right** hairline and finish on the **left** front side. Continue, left to right and right to left, until the entire head is completed.

This method eliminates the matching of ridges and waves at the back part of the head.

**VERTICAL
FINGER WAVING**

Vertical finger waving is different from horizontal finger waving in this respect: in vertical waving, the ridges and waves run up and down on the head, while the horizontal waves go parallel around the head.

Procedure for making ridges and waves is the same as for horizontal finger waving.

Make a side part extending from the forehead to the crown. Form shaping in a semi-circular effect. (Figs. 1 and 2.) Then make first section of ridge and wave. (Fig. 3.) Continue with additional sections until the part is reached.

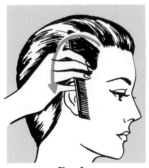

Fig. 1

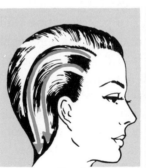

Fig. 2

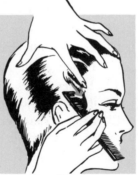

Fig. 3

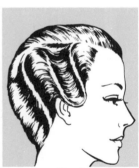

Fig. 4

Start the second ridge at the hair part. The third ridge is started at the hairline. Completed side is shown on Fig. 4.

COMPLETION

1. Place net over hair and safeguard patron's forehead and ears with cotton, gauze or paper protectors.
2. Adjust the dryer to medium heat and allow hair to dry thoroughly.
3. Remove patron from under dryer.
4. Remove hair net and clippies or pins from hair.
5. Comb out and reset waves into a soft coiffure.
6. Clean up booth.
7. Sanitize combs, hairpins, clippies and hair net after each use.

HAIRSTYLES IN FINGER WAVING

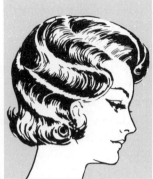
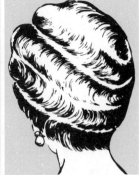
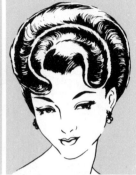

Side Part finger wave with fluff nape line

Swirl Back effect finger wave with tapered neck line

Horseshoe effect finger wave

REMINDER AND HINTS

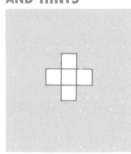

1. When preparing to give a finger wave, wash hands and have available sanitized implements and clean supplies.
2. Avoid the use of an excessive amount of waving lotion.
3. Use hard rubber combs that have both fine and coarse teeth.
4. Before waving, locate the natural or permanent wave in the hair.
5. To emphasize the ridges of a finger wave, press and close the fingers holding the ridge against the head.
6. To wave underneath hair, insert comb through the hair to scalp.
7. For a longer lasting wave, mold hair in direction of natural growth.
8. To safeguard the patron's forehead and ears from intense heat while under dryer, use cotton, gauze or paper protectors.
9. Place net over hair to protect setting while the hair is being dried.
10. Before combing out, dry the hair thoroughly.
11. Prolonged drying will dry the natural oils of the hair and scalp.
12. Finger waves will not remain in place if hair is combed out before it has been completely dried.
13. After a shampoo, lightened or tinted hair that tangles or snarls is easier to comb if a cream rinse is used.
14. Lightly spraying the hair with lacquer will hold the wave longer and give the hair a sheen.

REVIEW QUESTIONS

Finger Waving

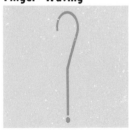

1. What is a finger wave?
2. How do you protect the patron's clothing?
3. How should the hair be protected while being dried?
4. Why is proficiency in finger waving important to the cosmetologist?
5. What types of hair are the easiest to finger wave?
6. Give two main points in judging a good finger-waved hairstyle?
7. Why are good waving lotions not harmful to the hair?
8. To what advantage is waving lotion used in giving a finger wave?
9. Why are cotton, gauze or paper protectors placed over the patron's ears and forehead?

CHAPTER 11

HAIRSTYLING

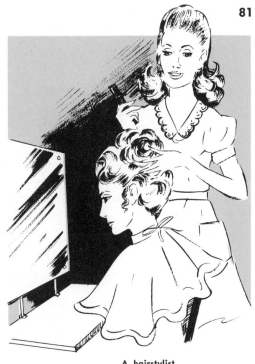

A hairstylist

INTRODUCTION

The cosmetologist must have a basic knowledge of hairstyling in order to keep up with the ever-changing fashions. The skilled and successful cosmetologist must be capable of giving a personal touch to each coiffure, making it appropriate and suitable to the individual.

It is always advisable to examine the patron's hair before starting the shampoo. This examination gives the cosmetologist the opportunity to perform a rough combing and to decide how the hair should be worn in order to produce the most becoming results.

Patrons realize that a good hairstyle is one which is not only becoming, but also can be handled easily and quickly between sets. They should be told that careful shaping is the secret of a well-groomed head.

Popular Combs

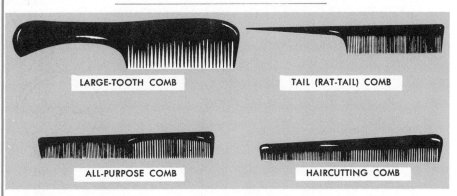

LARGE-TOOTH COMB

TAIL (RAT-TAIL) COMB

ALL-PURPOSE COMB

HAIRCUTTING COMB

The cosmetologist who hopes to become a proficient hairstylist must understand hair structure and the overall importance of hair shaping, permanent waving, hair straightening, thermal waving and curling, hair coloring, hair chemistry, and the action of hair conditioners.

For best results, the hair should be in good condition when being styled.

82

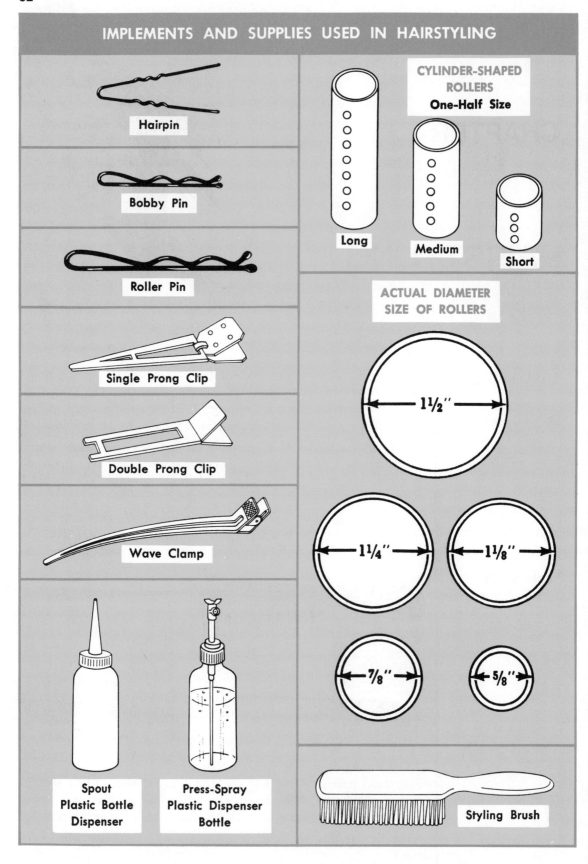

IMPLEMENTS AND SUPPLIES USED IN HAIRSTYLING

Hairpin

Bobby Pin

Roller Pin

Single Prong Clip

Double Prong Clip

Wave Clamp

Spout
Plastic Bottle
Dispenser

Press-Spray
Plastic Dispenser
Bottle

CYLINDER-SHAPED
ROLLERS
One-Half Size

Long

Medium

Short

ACTUAL DIAMETER
SIZE OF ROLLERS

$1\frac{1}{2}''$

$1\frac{1}{4}''$

$1\frac{1}{8}''$

$\frac{7}{8}''$

$\frac{5}{8}''$

Styling Brush

Removing Tangles

Removing tangles from the hair is very important for successful hairstyling. To prevent damage, it is best to remove such tangles in a systematic manner.

Always begin in the nape area. With the coarse teeth of a comb, section off a small part of hair and comb across and down each strand. Fig. 1. Work across the back sections in steps, and gradually move up to the crown. Size of the sections depends on hair elasticity; for fine or lightened hair, pick up smaller sections.

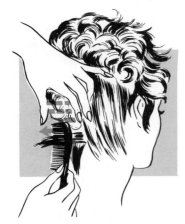

Fig. 1. Removing tangles
in nape area

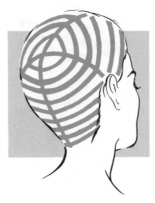

Fig. 2. Combing pattern
for removing tangles

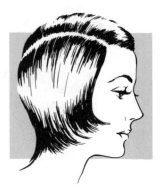

Fig. 3. Tangles removed

Making A Part

Combing pattern for removing tangles from hair is shown in Fig. 2. After tangles are removed, the hair is ready for setting or other service. Fig. 3.

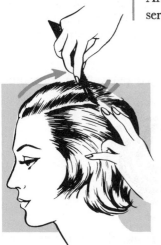

Fig. 1. Draw comb back
full length

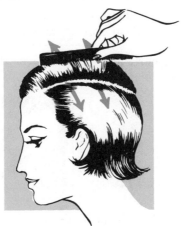

Fig. 2. Comb hair above and
below part

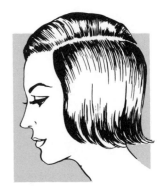

Fig. 3. Hair combed with
straight part

Making clean partings is essential for good hairstyling. Comb hair straight back. Hold the comb slightly angled and place it in front of the hairline. Draw the comb in an even line toward the back of the head until the length of the part is reached. Fig. 1.

Hold the lower side of the part with the left hand while combing the hair towards the right; then comb the hair down below the part. Fig. 2. A clean, straight part is illustrated in Fig. 3.

Finding The Natural Part

If a natural hair part is desired in a hairstyle, it may be made in the following manner:

After you have shampooed and towel-dried the hair, comb it straight back. Place the palm of the left hand on the head and push the hair forward. The hair will separate at the natural part. Fig. 1.

Separate and comb the hair over to the right. Fig. 2. Then comb the hair below the part. Fig. 3 illustrates a clean, straight part.

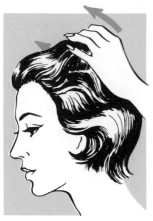

Fig. 1. Finding natural part

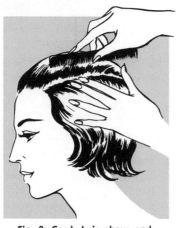

Fig. 2. Comb hair above and below part

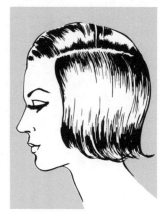

Fig. 3. Hair combed with straight part

PIN CURLS

Pin curls (also called sculpture curls), when carefully planned in exact patterns, will result in good lines, waves, ringlets, curls or rolls. Pin curls are suitable for naturally or permanently waved hair. The hair should be properly tapered and pin curls wound smoothly in order to make them springy and longer lasting.

Parts Of A Curl

Pin curls are constructed of three principal parts: **base**, **stem** and **circle**.

Parts of a Curl

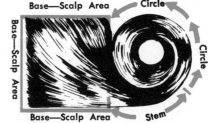

The **base** is the stationary or immovable foundation of the curl and is attached to the scalp.

The **stem** is that part of the pin curl, between the base and the first arc (turn) of the circle, which gives the circle its direction, action and mobility.

The **circle** is that part of the pin curl which forms a complete circle. The size of the curl governs the width of the wave and its strength.

Mobility Of A Curl

The **mobility of a curl** is determined by the **stem,** and depends on the amount of movement that takes place in the stem and circle. Curl mobility is classified as no-stem, half-stem and full-stem.

No-Stem Curl

1. The **no-stem curl** gives the base of the curl a firm, immovable position, permitting only the curl to move. It produces a strong, long-lasting curl. The curl is placed in the center of the base.

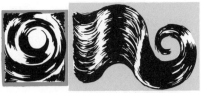

Curl opened out

Half-Stem Curl

2. The **half-stem curl** permits freedom of movement, since the half-stem allows the circle to move away from its base. It gives good control of the hair and produces softness in the finished wave pattern. The curl is placed one-half off its base.

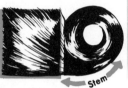
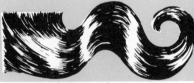

Curl opened out

Full-Stem Curl

3. The **full-stem curl** permits the greatest mobility to the curl. It gives the lines and directions as much freedom as the length of the stem will permit. It is used when a strong direction of the hair and a weaker wave pattern are desired. The base may be parted in a square, triangular, half-moon or rectangular section, depending on the area of the head in which the full-stem curls are used. The circle is placed completely off its base.

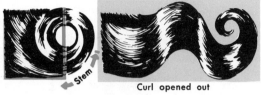

Curl opened out

The type of curl used will determine whether the design is to be close to the head or away from the head.

Pin Curl Comb-Outs

The size of the curl determines the size of the wave.

Note the difference between the combed out wave of a pin curl set with a closed center and one with an open center.

To obtain an even, smooth wave and a uniform end curl, use the **open center curl.**

A **closed center** is recommended for **fine** hair when a **fluffy** comb-out is desired.

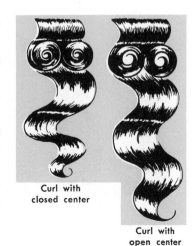

Curl with closed center

Curl with open center

**Curl And
Stem Direction**

The stem direction may be toward the face, away from the face, upward, downward or diagonal. However, the stem direction is determined by the finished hairstyle desired.

Curl and stem direction in relation to the face is spoken of in two ways:

1. **Forward movement** — toward the face
2. **Reverse (backward) movement** — away from the face

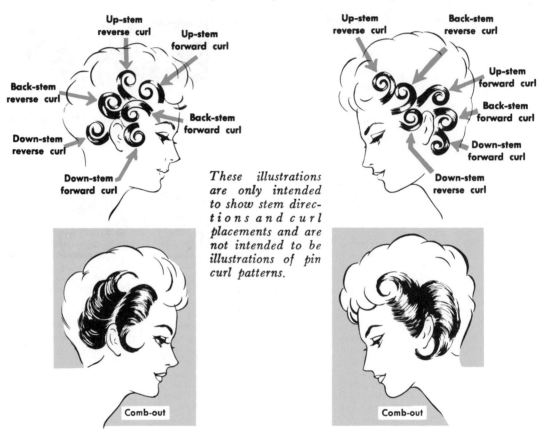

These illustrations are only intended to show stem directions and curl placements and are not intended to be illustrations of pin curl patterns.

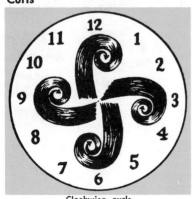

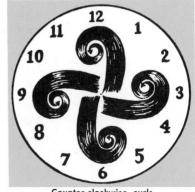

**Clockwise And
Counter-Clockwise
Curls**

Some hairstylists prefer to use the terms, clockwise curls and counter-clockwise curls.

Curls formed in the same direction as the movement of the hands of a clock are known as clockwise (C) curls.

Curls formed in the opposite direction to the movement of the hands of a clock are known as counter-clockwise (CC) curls.

Clockwise curls

Counter-clockwise curls

SHAPING

A **shaping** is the way in which hair is directed to create a guideline for the formation of a curl or wave pattern.

Shapings may be classified as **forward** and **reverse.**

Forward Vertical Shapings

A forward shaping is one in which the hair is directed toward the face. This type of shaping is oval in form and is larger in size at its **closed end** than at its **open end.**

Side Shaping

Side forward shaping. The hair is directed in a circular motion, following the side hair part, downward and towards the face, as shown on the illustration. The size of the shaping depends on the setting for the hairstyle that is being created.

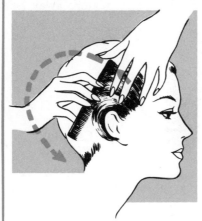
Oval shaping for right side

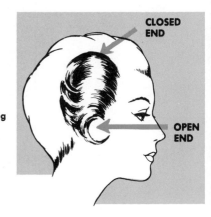
CLOSED END
OPEN END

Top Shaping

Top forward shaping. The hair is comb-directed in a circular motion away from the forehead and towards the face.

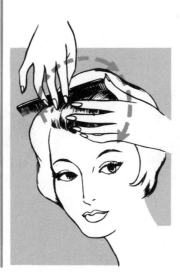
Oval shaping for top forward movement

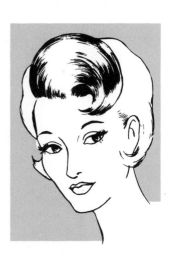

Diagonal Shaping

Diagonal shaping is similar to side forward shaping, with the exception that the shaping is formed in a diagonal manner to the side of the head.

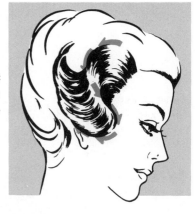

Reverse Vertical Shaping

Vertical side shaping is one in which the hair is comb-directed in a downward-upward circular motion, away from the face.

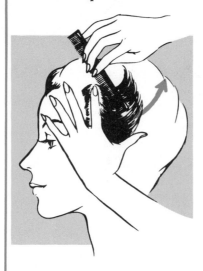

Left side vertical shaping

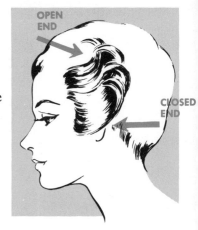

Horizontal Shaping

Horizontal oblong shaping is one in which the hair is comb-directed parallel with the parting. It is recommended for pin curl parallel construction and may be used for the first movement in finger-waving design.

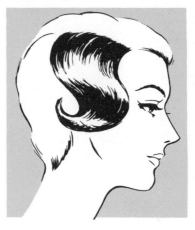
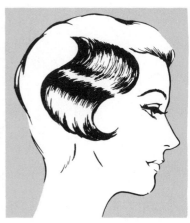

PIN CURL FOUNDATIONS OR BASES

The hair is first divided into sections or panels and then sub-divided into the foundations or bases required for the various curls. The most commonly shaped bases in use are triangular, rectangular, arc (half-moon or "C" shape) and square.

In order to avoid splits in the hair, the hairstylist must use care in selecting and forming the curl base. Furthermore, uniformity of curl development can be achieved only if the sections of hair are as equal as possible.

It is important to make certain that each curl lies flat and smooth on its base. If extended too far off the base, a curl that is loose near the scalp will result.

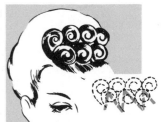

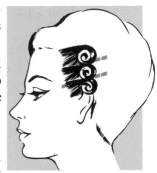

Triangular base

Triangular Base

Triangular base pin curls are recommended along the front or facial hairline to prevent **breaks or splits** in the finished hairstyle. The triangular base allows a portion of hair from each curl to overlap the next and comb into a uniform wave without splits.

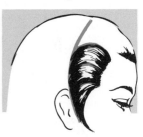

Rectangular base

Rectangular Base

Rectangular base pin curls are usually recommended for the side front hairline when a smooth upsweep effect is desired.

To avoid splits in the comb-out, the pin curls must overlap.

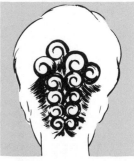

Arc base — side

Arc Base

Sides. Arc base, also known as **half-moon** or **"C" shape base,** pin curls may be carved out of a shaping at the sides of the head.

Back of head. Arc base pin curls may also be used for an upsweep effect or French twist at the lower back of the head.

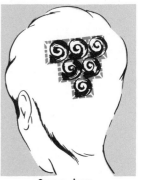

Arc base — back of head

Square Base

Square base pin curls are used for even construction suitable for combing and brushing into curls or waves. They can be used on any part of the head and will comb out with lasting results.

To avoid splits, stagger the sectioning as shown in the illustration.

Square base

PIN CURL TECHNIQUES

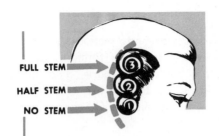

FULL STEM →
HALF STEM →
NO STEM →

Pin curls can be made in several ways. The following drawings illustrate several methods of forming them. Your instructor may demonstrate other methods which are equally correct.

Pin Curls For Right Side

Pin curls, carved out of a shaping without disturbing the shaping, are usually referred to as carved curls. To form these curls on the right side of the head, the following procedure is followed.

Procedure

Wet the hair with water or setting lotion; comb smooth and form shaping. Start making curls at the open end of the shaping.

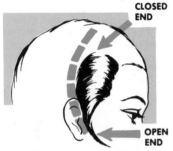

CLOSED END

OPEN END

1. Right side — symmetrical curve of shaping.

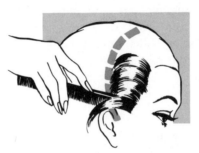

2. Slice strand for first curl.

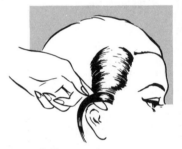

3. First strand ready for curling.

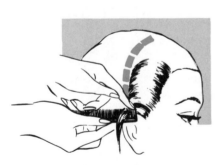

4. Ribbon strand for smoothness.

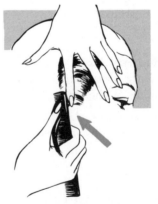

5. Strand stretched by pulling through comb.

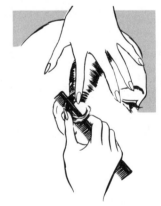

6. Form the curl forward.

Very Important!

Whenever a longer-lasting curl movement is desired, the strand should be stretched or tensioned.

This is accomplished by ribboning and stretching the strand. Firmly comb it between the spine of the comb and the thumb in the direction of the curl movement, as in Figs. 4, 5 and 6.

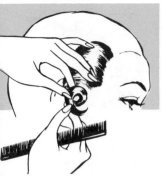

7. Wind curl.

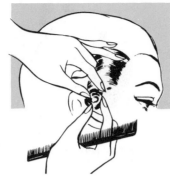

8. Mold and close the curl.

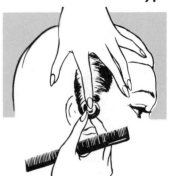

9. Place the curl in the shaping.

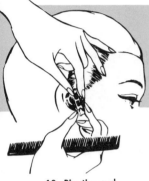

10. Pin the curl.

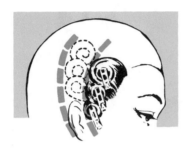

11. Sculpture curl arrangement backed up with a second row of curls.

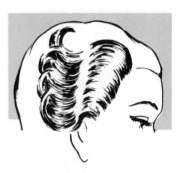

12. Unfurl into waves with a strong ridge.

Pin Curls For Left Side

Making pin curls on the left side of the head requires a different technique than making them on the right side.

Procedure

Wet the hair with water or setting lotion, comb smooth, and form the shaping. Start at the open end of the shaping.

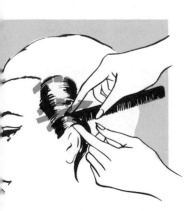

1. Slice strand out of shaping.

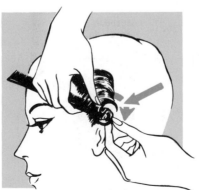

2. Smooth ends of strand before rolling them inside the circle of the curl.

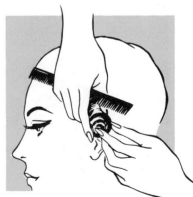

3 Roll and pin curl into place.

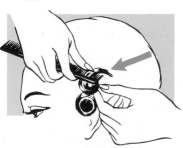

4. Smooth ends for second curl, without disturbing first curl.

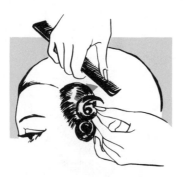

5. Complete curl and pin, overlapping first curl.

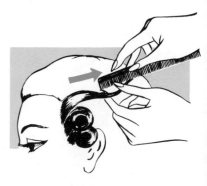

6. Pick up third strand. Comb through without disturbing shaping.

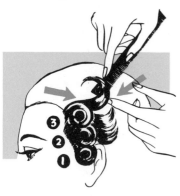

7. Note: Curls overlap and fit within curvature of shaping. Size of curls are graduated.

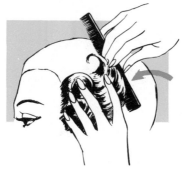

8. Reverse shaping for back-up curls.

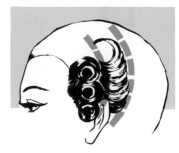

9. Reverse shaping ready for curls.

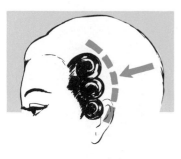

10. To slice strand, touch tip of comb with tip of finger.

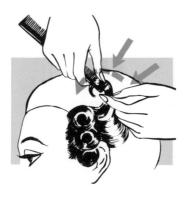

11. Ribbon curl, use coarse or fine teeth of comb, depending on the texture of the hair.

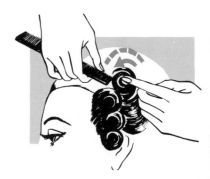

12. Ribbon tip of strand for neat closing of curl with fine teeth of comb.

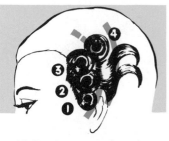

13. Top reverse curl completed and the shaping divided into strands for next two curls.

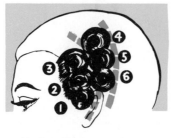

14. Completed second row of curls within curve of shaping.

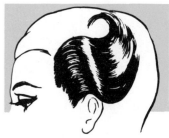

15. Comb out forward and reverse pin curl setting into a full, wide wave.

ANCHORING PIN CURLS

A hairstylist must know how to anchor pin curls in order to achieve success in hairstyling. It is essential that the curls hold firmly as placed, so that the planned pattern can be followed and developed into the desired coiffure.

Every hairstylist or instructor has his or her own favorite method for inserting clips or clippies. Each one of these professional methods can be considered equally correct. However, it is essential that **good common sense** be used at all times in the insertion of clips or clippies so that pin curls are anchored properly.

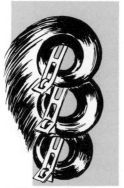

Hairline forward pin curls
(Clockwise curls)

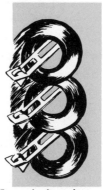

Forward pin curls
Equal in size. Any place
on the head

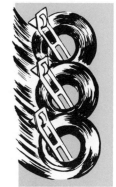

Reverse pin curls
(Counter-clockwise curls)
Equal in size. Any place
on the head

Procedure

To anchor the pin curl correctly, gently slide the clip or clippie through part of the base and/or stem, at an angle and across the ends of the curl. This will hold the curl securely without it unfurling, sagging or flipping over.

Caution

1. Clips should be anchored so that they will not interfere with the formation or placement of other curls, or with any other step in setting the hair.
2. To avoid indentations or impressions, it is advisable **not** to pin across the center of the entire curl.
3. The size of clips used should be governed by the size of the curl.
4. To avoid discomfort to the patron during the drying process, do not permit the clips to touch the ears, skin or scalp. In the event the clips do touch the skin, place cotton under the part of the clips touching these areas.

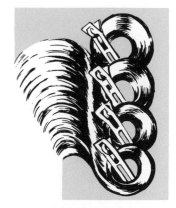

Ridge reverse pin curls
(Counter-clockwise curls)

EFFECTS OF PIN CURLS

There are a number of pin curl patterns designed to achieve specific effects, several of which are illustrated here.

However, care must be taken that the curls lie evenly and are placed in the direction in which they are intended to be combed; otherwise, a haphazard setting will result, with uneven wave or curl design.

Vertical Waves

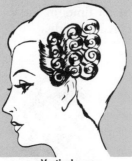

Vertical wave
pin curl pattern

To achieve vertical wave effects on the left side of the head, first give a reverse shaping; then follow pin curl pattern as illustrated.

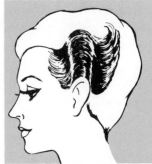

Vertical wave comb-out

Horizontal Waves

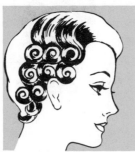

Horizontal wave
pin curl pattern

To achieve horizontal waves, first shape the hair to achieve a forward semi-circular effect from the hair part downward. Then, set the pin curls as illustrated. A long-lasting wave close to the head is created.

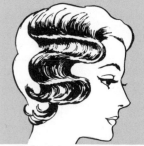

Horizontal wave comb-out

Interlocking Movement

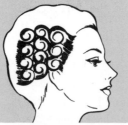

Setting pattern

1st Row — Back-stem with forward curls.

2nd and 3rd Rows—Forward stem with reverse curls.

Comb-out — The back curls are combed and interlocked with the front row of curls.

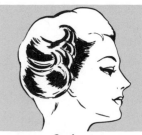

Comb-out

Waved Top

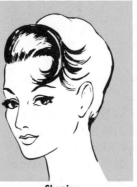

Shaping

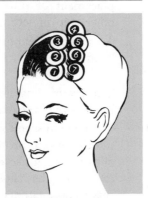

Setting pattern

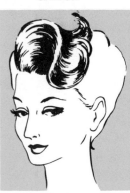

Comb-out

Diagonal Waves

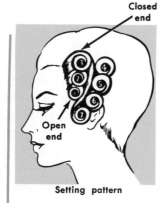

Closed end

Open end

Setting pattern

Shape hair—Oval forward shaping.
Set—Start at open end.
Comb-out—Diagonal waves.

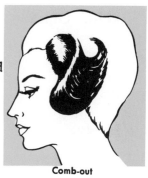

Comb-out

Waved Bangs

Fine Hair

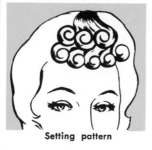

Setting pattern

Setting for fine hair
Shape hair.
Set—1st row.
Set—2nd row.
Comb-out.

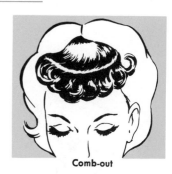

Comb-out

Normal Hair

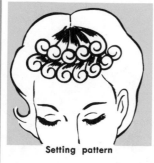

Setting pattern

Setting for normal hair
Shape hair.
Set—1st row.
Set—2nd row.
Comb-out.

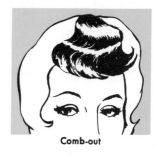

Comb-out

French Twist

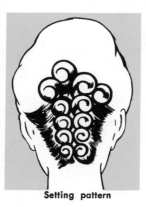

Setting pattern

Setting for normal hair
Part off back area and make vertical center part. Comb both sections toward center.

Start at top or bottom of nape section and make large, **smooth** pin curls as shown in illustration.

Comb - out. Back-comb each side. Brush or comb one side, fold in ends and pin.

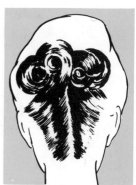

Comb-out and pinning

Brush or comb the other side and fold ends over first section. Pin hair in herringbone fashion, so ends do not show.

RIDGE CURLS

Procedure

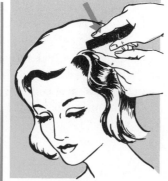

1. Slice strand

Ridge curls are pin curls placed behind the ridge of a shaping or finger wave. Care must be taken **not to disturb the ridge** when slicing out the strands for the curls.

Prepare hair. Shape hair and make ridge as for vertical finger wave. Slice strand without disturbing the ridge, as in Fig. 1.

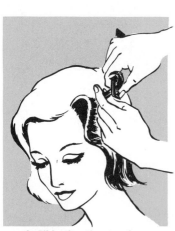

2. Ribboning the strand

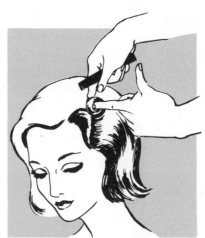

3. Winding the strand

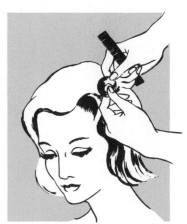

4. Sliding curl off tip of finger

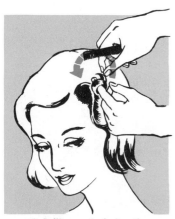

5. Rolling and placing the curl in back of ridge

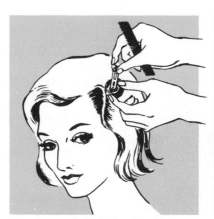

6. Anchoring the curl

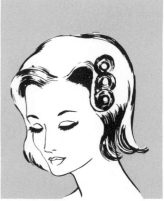

7. Completed ridge curls properly placed and pinned

Ridge curls are used in conjunction with finger waves, when a loose wave is desired.

SKIP WAVE

The skip wave is a combination finger wave and pin curl pattern, the pin curls being placed in alternate finger wave formations. This technique is recommended when wide, smooth-flowing vertical waves are desired.

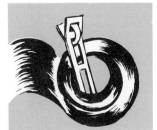

Pin curl properly pinned

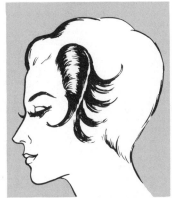

Shaping and ridge as for
vertical finger wave

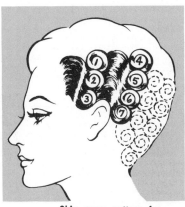

Skip wave pattern for
fluff ends

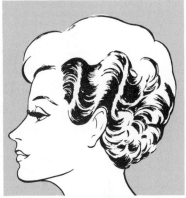

Comb-out with fluff ends

In order to obtain best results in skip waving, the hair should be three to five inches in length. It is not recommended for hair that has a tight permanent wave or for hair that is fine.

ELONGATED STEM PIN CURLS

When extremely wide, soft waves are desired, use elongated stem pin curls.

An elongated stem is usually $1\frac{1}{2}$ times the width of the curl.

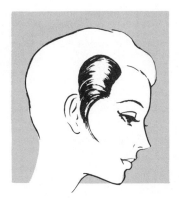

Shaping

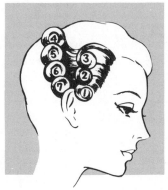

Setting pattern

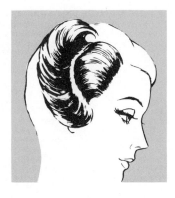

Comb-out

STAND-UP OR CASCADE CURL

The stand-up curl, sometimes referred to as a cascade curl, is wound from the hair ends to the scalp. The center opening is made large, and the curl is pinned in a standing position.

The stand-up curl provides a great deal of lift to the hair. It can either be used in conjunction with rollers, or by itself, when maximum volume is desired.

Note: In order to become proficient in hairstyling, the student must learn to make stand-up curls with ease and proficiency.

Procedure

Wet the top front section with water or setting lotion.

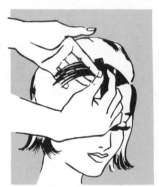

Combing, dividing and smoothing strand

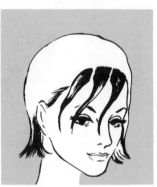

Dividing section into strands for easy pickup

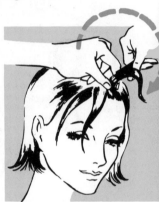

Ribboning strand

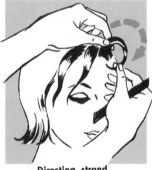

Directing strand

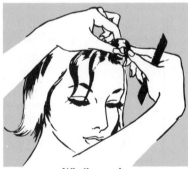

Winding curl

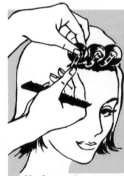

Pinning curl

Effects Of Stand-Up Curls

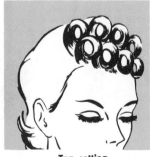

Top setting

Setting—Stand-up curls in a forward (clockwise) movement.

Comb-out—The hair is brushed from the hairline, then sliced off in small sections and flipped over the forehead as shown in the illustration.

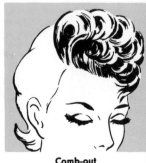

Comb-out

Semi Stand-Up Curls

Semi stand-up curls are pin curls carved out of a shaping and pinned into a semi-standing position.

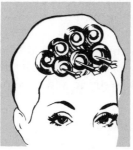 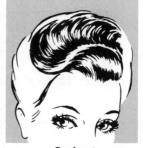 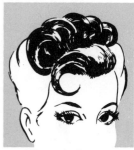

Semi stand-up curl   Comb-out   (Alternate) Comb-out

Setting—Top wave effect may be achieved with semi stand-up curls by the following procedure:

1. Shape top hair.
2. Make three counter-clockwise curls.
3. Back up with four clockwise curls.

Comb-out—The hair may be combed out as shown in the two illustrations.

ROLLER CURLS

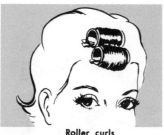

Roller curls

Roller curls are designed to create the same effects as stand-up curls. They are formed over special rollers that come in various sizes to fulfill special needs in a hair design.

The rollers are in effect molds around which curls are formed to create added lift or volume. They are especially effective in creating a straight line design with more height and stability than is usually achieved with stand-up curls.

An important difference between roller and stand-up curls is that stand-up curls are formed one at a time, while rollers can accommodate at one time the equivalent of from two to four stand-up curls. In addition, the rollers give far more security to the rolled hair while it is in a wet state.

Sectioning The Hair

First, the hair is sectioned into panels; then, subdivided into roller bases. The size of the bases should be as near as possible to the length and diameter of the roller.

A good example to follow: if a roller is 3″ long and 1″ in diameter, the base should be 1″ wide by 2¾″ long, about one-quarter of an inch shorter. If this proportion is followed with the various sizes of rollers, the hair will not be over-crowded, nor will the hair slip off the sides of the rollers.

Preparation

The hair is moistened with water or setting lotion in the same manner as it is for conventional curls. The hair is then sectioned according to the number of rollers that must be used to achieve the hairstyle desired. End papers may be used for easier winding as in cold waving.

Roller Setting Technique

Hold strand at 45° angle and roll in the same manner shown in illustrations 1-3. The roller will sit directly over the base of the rectangle. The curl will be strong and have maximum volume or body.

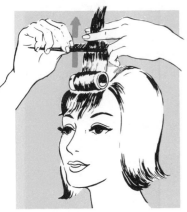

1. Preparing strand

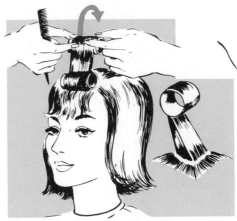

2. Hand position while winding roller

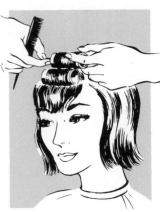

3. Holding roller in position while pinning

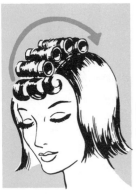

Set roller curls from hairline to crown with pin curls for bang effect

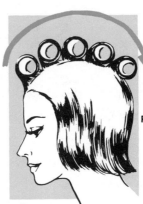

Roller setting for off-the-face effect

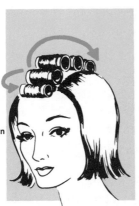

Roller curl pattern for bang effect

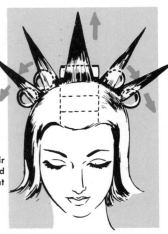

Angle at which hair is held from head for roller placement

**Effects Of Hair
Length On Rollers**

The length of the hair and the size of the rollers affect the finished hairstyle in the top front area in the following manner.

1.

A 4½″ strand will wrap around a roller one inch in diameter one full turn. Result: three roller curls will produce a soft puff with minimum curl turned in ends.

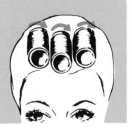
Pattern

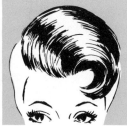
Comb-out

2.

A 4½″ strand will wrap around a roller ¾″ in diameter about one and one-half times. Result: four rollers will produce a curl fluff with turned in ends.

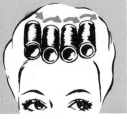
Pattern

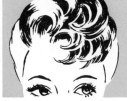
Comb-out

3.

Should the size of each roller be small enough to permit the hair strand to be wrapped around twice, five rollers will be needed to adequately curl the area. The use of these rollers will result in a deep, soft wave, because the hair ends are in the opposite direction from the original movement of the hair.

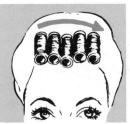
Pattern

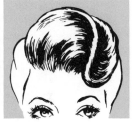
Comb-out

BARREL CURLS

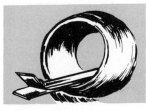
Barrel curl

A **barrel curl** serves as a substitute for a curl formed around a roller. It may be used where there is insufficient room to place a roller. However, it does not provide the tension that is present in roller wrapping.

The barrel curl is made in a similar manner as the stand-up curl, having a flat base and containing much more hair.

VOLUME AND INDENTATION
(With Cylinder Rollers)

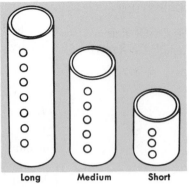

Modern hairstyling incorporates the use of various devices and methods in order to achieve special designs and effects. One of the most effective devices employed in this area is the roller, which is available in various sizes and lengths. Rollers are especially important in the creation of volume (lift) and indentation (valleys and hollowness) in the hairstyle.

Long   Medium   Short

NOTE: In order that the rollers are used to their maximum efficiency, be sure the hair length is over three times the diameter of the rollers.

Volume and Indentation

Full volume is created by directing the hair up from the head, rolling the ends under the rollers, and then rolling the hair down to the scalp onto its base. Fig. 1. For other degrees of volume, see Figs. 3-5.

Indentation is created by keeping hair at scalp level and rolling hair over to one-half off its base as in Fig. 2.

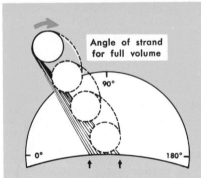
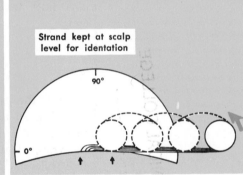

Fig. 1. To create full volume—rest the roller on its base.

Fig. 2. To create indentation or hollowness, keep hair low on head and roll to one-half off its base.

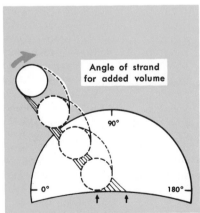
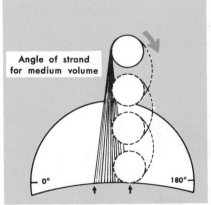
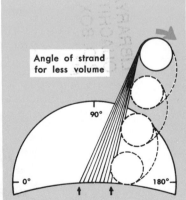

Fig. 3. To create maximum volume—rest roller one-half off left side of base.

Fig. 4. To create a medium amount of volume—rest roller one-half off the right side of base.

Fig. 5. To create a small amount of volume—rest roller off right side of base.

Setting For Volume And Indentation

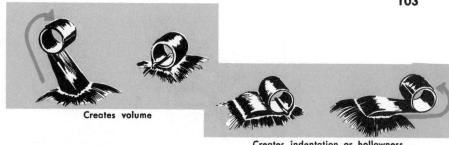

Creates volume

Creates indentation or hollowness

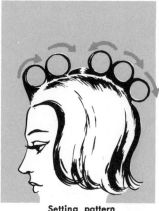

Setting pattern

Illustrates

1st two rollers— volume

3rd roller— indentation

4th and 5th rollers— volume

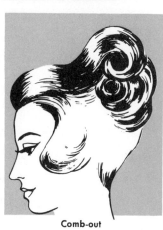

Comb-out

CYLINDER CIRCULAR ROLLER ACTION

The hair that is directed in a circular manner is referred to by many hairstylists in various ways, such as: radial motion, circular movement; curvature roller action; rotary motion or movement; spotmatic movement; contour movement, and others.

The spot or area from which the hair is directed to form a circular movement is also referred to by any of the following terms: balance point, swing point, terminal point, pivot point, pendulum point, radial point, fulcrum point, radiation point, rotary point and spotmatic.

Side Effects Of Hair Lengths On Cylinder Rollers

Short Hair

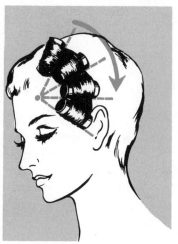

Pattern

Short hair — slender rollers

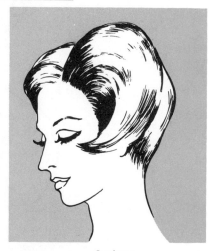

Comb-out

Medium Length Hair

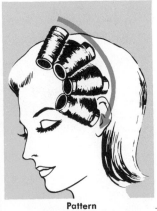

Pattern

Medium length hair—medium size rollers

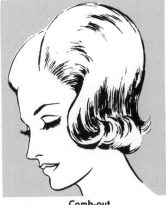

Comb-out

Long Hair

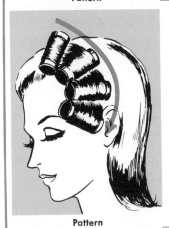

Pattern

Long hair — large rollers

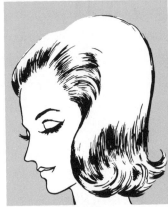

Comb-out

Effects Of Circular Roller Action

Top

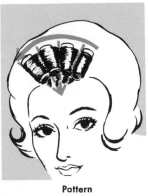

Pattern

Cylinder rollers set in wedge-shape partings in a circular manner. Comb-out in a forward shell effect with bangs.

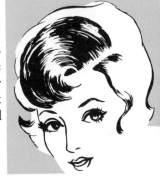

Comb-out

Side

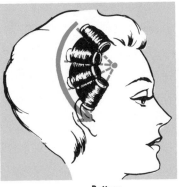

Pattern

Cylinder rollers set in wedge-shape partings. The comb-out gives a circular movement towards the face.

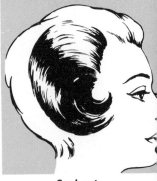

Comb-out

Special
Side Effects

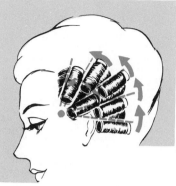

Special Side effects

Side volume roller setting with sculpture curl in front of ear.

The comb-out produces an "S" wave formation effect.

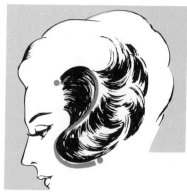

Pattern   Comb-out

Creating
A Ridge

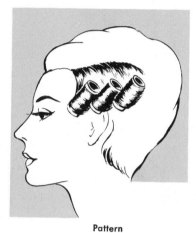

To create a ridge line and indentation (hollowness), set the hair on rollers at an angle, as shown in illustration.

This setting will produce the waved effect in the comb-out.

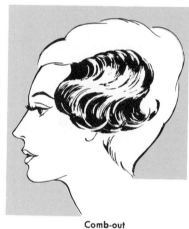

Pattern   Comb-out

TAPERED ROLLERS

Tapered circular roller setting. Practically the same styling results may be achieved by using either cylinder or tapered rollers. However, since the tapered rollers may be placed closer to the point of distribution in a pie-shaped parting, it is possible to develop a tighter curvature movement Whereas the cylinder rollers must be placed slightly further back from the point of distribution, this makes the movement a little weaker. The cylinder roller, on the other hand, is superior for the creation of straight lines, and may be used with good results in a curvature movement where a looser pattern is desired.

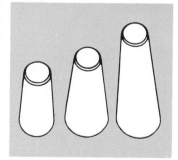

REMINDER

All rollers are implements or aids designed to assist the hairstylist in achieving a predetermined hairstyle. The choice of rollers to be used must be governed strictly by the preference of the hairstylist.

**Size Of
Tapered Rollers**

Size of rollers for curved lines is governed by the texture of the hair. Example: fine hair takes smaller rollers; coarse hair, larger rollers. Let your instructor be your guide.

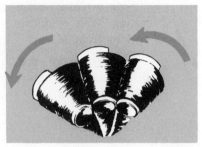

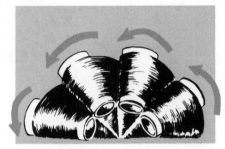

One-quarter circle setting, using thinner rollers, produces tighter comb-outs.

One-half circle setting, using larger (thicker) rollers, produces looser comb-outs.

Top Effects

Top hairline tapered roller setting combs out like a shell shaped front with bangs or curled up ends.

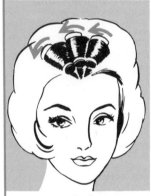

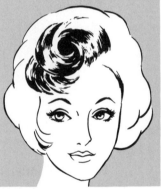

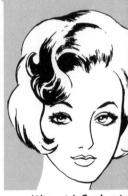

Setting

Comb-out

(Alternate) Comb-out

Side Effects

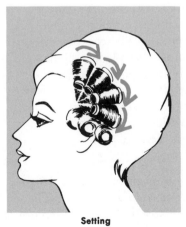

Side tapered roller setting and sculpture ear curls comb out in a forward movement with side fluff.

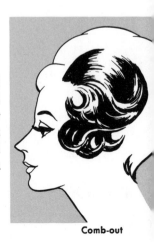

Setting

Comb-out

HAIR PARTINGS

The manner of parting the patron's hair should be adjusted to her facial type and the desired hairstyle. The hairstylist should be guided by the natural parting of the patron's hair.

The following illustrations reveal the best hair partings for various facial types and hairstyles.

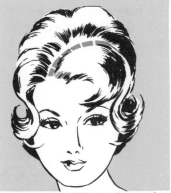

Diagonal part, used to give height to a round or square face.

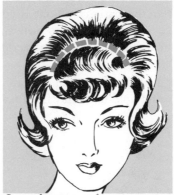

Curved rectangular part, used for receding hairline or high forehead.

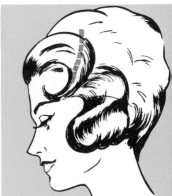

Concealed part, used for height and a one-sided style effect.

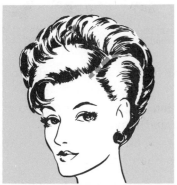

Side part, used for styles to be directed to one side. Helps to create the illusion of decreasing the width of forehead.

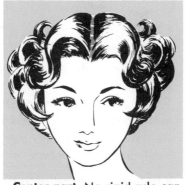

Center part. No rigid rule can be made for a center part hairstyle. Always try to create a hairstyle that will give an optical illusion of ovalness to the face.

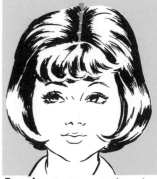

Popular center parting for children's hairstyles with bangs.

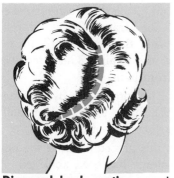

Diagonal back parting, used to create the illusion of width to crown and back of head.

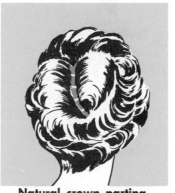

Natural crown parting.

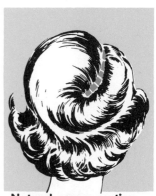

Natural crown parting.

BACK-COMBING AND BACK-BRUSHING TECHNIQUES

Back-Combing

Back-combing and **back-brushing** are processes of tangling or matting the hair by combing or brushing it toward the scalp, so that the shorter hair tangles to form a cushion or base for the top or covering hair.

Back-combing is also called **teasing, ratting, matting** or **French lacing.**

After the basic comb-out is completed, you may have to back-comb or back-brush the hair to achieve the planned hairstyle. After brushing and relaxing the hair, analyze the areas that must be raised.

Procedure

1. Pick up a section of hair about three-quarters of an inch wide and hold up firmly from scalp.

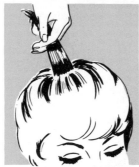 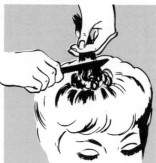 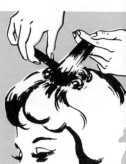

| The hair properly held between the index and middle fingers | Back-combing on top of strand | Back-combing in back of strand |

2. Insert the comb into the strand near its base, press to scalp and remove.
3. Repeat Step 2 by inserting the comb into the strand a little further away from the scalp, press to scalp and remove.
4. Repeat Step 3 as many times as necessary, using very small strokes, until the desired volume of cushioned hair has been achieved.

Back-Brushing

Back-brushing, also called **ruffing,** is a technique used to build a cushion at the scalp to a desired volume for the top or covering hair.

Procedure

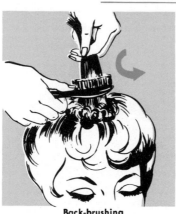

Back-brushing

1. Pick up and hold strand straight out from scalp.
2. With a slight amount of slack in the strand, place the brush near the base of the strand. Push and roll brush with the wrist until brush touches the scalp. Then remove brush from hair.
3. Repeat this procedure by moving the brush back to about one-half inch further away from the scalp.
4. Repeat this procedure until the desired volume has been achieved.

NOTE: Only the inner edge of the brush is used. The shorter ends of tapered hair have been interlocked to form a cushion at the scalp. In order for interlocking to occur, the brush must be rolled.

COMB-OUT

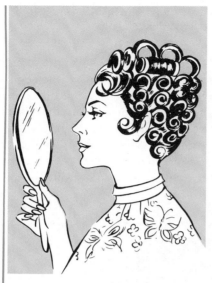

To achieve success as a hair-stylist, the cosmetologist must first master the art and technique of combing and brushing the hair. The creative skills of the hairstylist are realized when the hair has been properly shaped and molded and an attractive and fashionable coiffure is produced.

The imaginative cosmetologist, applying the skills of combing and brushing, can artistically create almost any hairstyle desired. It is this skill, this technical ability to handle the comb and brush, which forms the foundation for success as a professional hairstylist.

Suggested Procedure

Effectiveness in combing-out is based on a system or plan, indicating where to start and the procedure to follow, which will develop the desired coiffure. A suggested procedure is outlined here:

1. Brush out curls. (Relaxing the set)
2. Wave placement.
3. Accentuate and develop lines and style.
4. Finishing steps (Structural balance)

Brush Out Curls

Remove the rollers and clips and brush out the curls, thus relaxing the set. The objective of this technique is to smooth and brush the hair into a semi-flat condition and to remove excess curl, Figs. 1 and 2. This permits the stylist to properly position the lines for the planned hairstyle. It is essential that this procedure be properly executed in order to achieve a smooth, flowing, finished coiffure.

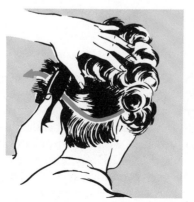

1. Brush back area.

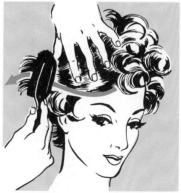

2. Brush sides.

Wave Placement

When the brushing is completed, the hair should be combed into the general pattern desired. Blend the basic lines and form the general style pattern.

Lines and direction should be slightly over-emphasized, to allow for some expected relaxation during the comb-out process. This may be accomplished by placing the hand on the head and gently pushing the hair forward, in order that the waves fall into the planned design. Any necessary teasing is performed, volume indentation and ridges are created, as part of the overall arrangement, Fig. 3. The entire coiffure is created in exaggerated and over-emphasized lines to provide for the final combing and styling.

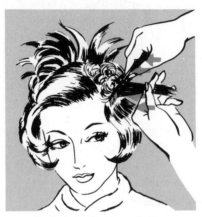
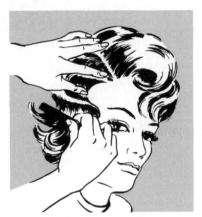

3. If desirable, tease from scalp out to two inches from hair ends.

4. Mold and comb hair to the desired hairstyle.

Developing Lines And Styles

Accenting and developing lines and style. Accentuate the lines to develop and arrange the desired style, taking one section at a time, the proper lines, ridges, volume and indentations are combed and brushed into the finished coiffure. Softness and evenness of flow are created by blending, smoothing and combing. Exaggerations and over-emphasis are carefully removed. Finished patterns are created and final evenness and smoothness of line are combed into the final silhouette.

Finishing Steps

After the creation of the style has been completed, it is time for the finishing touches. Lightly spray the hair to hold it in place for the final placement. Using the tips of the teeth of the comb, lightly fit any small hairs or loose ends into place. If necessary, lift and blend disarrayed hair with the tips of the fingers or by carefully lifting with the comb, Fig. 4. Every movement and touch during the final stage must be very carefully executed. The objective, at this point, is to smooth out any visible imperfections. When the finishing touches have been completed, check the entire set for structural balance and lightly spray the hair for the desired holding effect.

ARTISTRY IN HAIRSTYLING

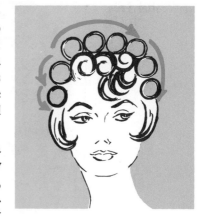

The principles of modern hairstyling and makeup are guides to the cosmetologist in selecting what is most appropriate in achieving a beautiful appearance. Best results are obtained when each facial type is analyzed for its own merits and defects.

Each type of face demands a distinctive coiffure that is rightly proportioned, has a balanced line, and correctly frames the face. Every accomplished cosmetologist possesses a sense of balance and harmony in visualizing and creating coiffures. The essentials of an artistic and suitable hairstyle must, therefore, be based upon the following general characteristics:

1. Shape of the entire head:
   a) Front view
   b) Profile (side view)
   c) Back view

2. Characteristics in features:
   a) Perfect as well as imperfect features
   b) Defects or blemishes

3. Body structure, posture, and poise

FACIAL TYPES

The facial type of each patron is determined by the position and prominence of the facial bones. There are seven facial types: oval, round, square, oblong, pear-shape, heart-shape and diamond.

To recognize each facial type and be able to give correct advice, the cosmetologist should be acquainted with the outstanding characteristics of each.

Oval Facial Type

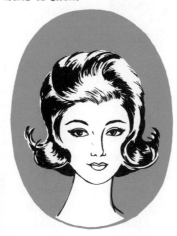

The **oval type** is generally accepted as the perfect face. The contours and proportions of the oval face form the basis for modifying all other facial types.

Facial Contour: The oval face is about one and a half times longer than its width across the brow; the forehead is slightly wider than the chin.

Aim: To maintain the oval contour.

Any style can be worn as there are no features to minimize.

Round Facial Type

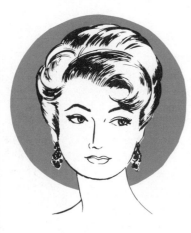

Facial Contour: Round hairline and round chin line.

Aim: To create the illusion of length to the face.

Arranging the hair high on top of the head, and leaving the ears exposed or dressed flat over the ears, will help to minimize the roundness of the face.

Square Facial Type

Facial Contour: Straight hairline and square jawline.

Aim: To create the illusion of length and offset the squareness of the features.

The problems of the square facial type are similar to those of the round. The style should lift off the forehead and come forward at the sides and jaw, to create the illusion of narrowness and softness in the face.

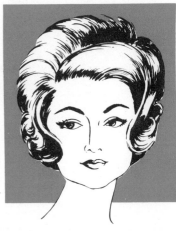

Pear-Shape Facial Type

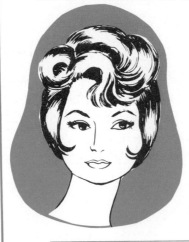

Facial Contour: Narrow forehead, wide jawline and chin line.

Aim: To create the illusion of width in the forehead.

Keep the hair dressed fairly full and high. Partially cover the forehead with a fringe of waved hair. The hair should be worn with a semi-curl or soft-wave effect over the lower jawline. This arrangement will add apparent width to the forehead.

Oblong Facial Type

Facial Contour: Long, narrow face with hollow cheeks.

Aim: To make the face appear shorter and wider.

The hair should be styled fairly close to the top of the head with a fringe of curls or bangs, combined with fullness at the sides. The length of the face will appear to be reduced.

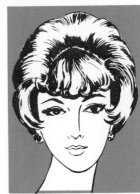

Diamond Facial Type

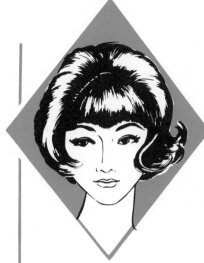

Facial Contour: Narrow forehead, extreme width through the cheekbones, and narrow chin.

Aim: To reduce the width across the cheekbone line.

Increasing the fullness across the forehead and at the jawline, while keeping the hair close to the head at the cheekbone line, will help to create the illusion of ovalness to the face.

Heart-Shape Facial Type

Facial Contour: Wide forehead and narrow chin line.

Aim: To decrease the width of the forehead and increase the width of the lower part of the face.

To reduce width of forehead, a hairstyle slanted to one side is recommended. Add width and softness at the jawline by brushing the sides forward onto the cheeks.

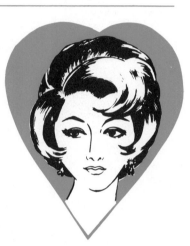

SPECIAL CONSIDERATIONS

Plump With Short Neck

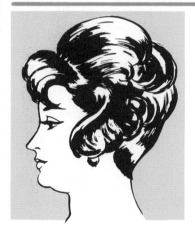

Aim: To creat illusion of length.

Corrective Hairstyle: For the forehead, use forward bangs. Style the crown high to lend the illusion of length. Waved-in sides create a slender effect. A smooth head-hugging napeline emphasizes slenderness from the back and side view.

Avoid hairstyles that give fullness to the nape area.

Long, Thin Neck

Aim: To minimize the long appearance of the neck.

Corrective Hairstyle: Cover the neck with soft waves or curls. Avoid styling the hair up from back of neck. Keep the nape hair long.

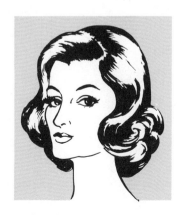

Thin Features

Aim: To minimize thinness of facial features and neck length.

Corrective Hairstyle: A high, soft crown line, with the sides lifted up and out from the hairline, and brushed loosely forward onto the cheeks, will create a softening effect for the face and develop a soft, fluffy effect at the forehead. Keep the nape hair long and full, to offset the long, thin neck.

Negroid Features

Follow styling rules that relate to each particular facial type.

Styling the hair. It may be accompanied by one of two different methods of hair straightening or relaxing.

Chemically relaxed. The hair should be wet set with rollers and pin curls. It is then dried and combed out in the usual manner.

Thermal straightened (pressed). Use large barrel curls or curl with thermal (marcel) irons. Then comb the hair into a suitable hairstyle.

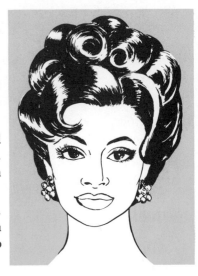

Uneven Features

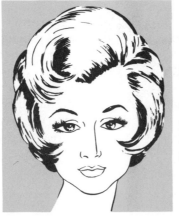

Aim: To minimize the imperfect features.

Corrective Hairstyle: Uneven features can be minimized by selection of the proper hairstyle. The suggested hairstyle recommended for this model is a soft effect over protruding features, thereby creating evenness on both sides of the face.

Oriental Features

Follow hairstyling rules that relate to the particular facial shape. The oriental hairstyle is very versatile in that it may be combed into a side-upward movement, or into a loose, fluffy page-boy style. This is achieved by rolling the hair outward or inward.

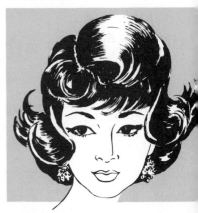

Straight

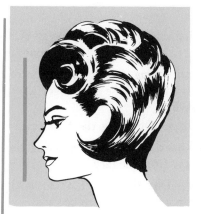

Usually, all hairstyles are becoming to the straight or normal profile.

A normal profile is neither concave nor convex. It contains neither a prominent protrusion nor a receding feature.

**Concave
Prominent Chin**

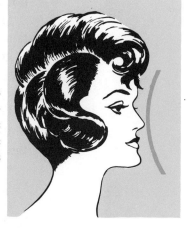

A close hair arrangement or bangs over the forehead minimizes the bulginess of the forehead. The hair at the sides and nape of the neck should be dressed in small, soft curls or waves to soften the features.

Convex

**Receding Forehead,
Prominent Nose
And Receding Chin**

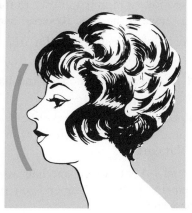

Curls or bangs should be placed forward on the forehead to conceal the receding forehead and irregular hairline. The hair at the sides and nape of the neck should be dressed close to the head to give it perfect balance.

**Low Forehead,
Protruding Chin**

To create the illusion of height to a low forehead and length to the face, the hair should be dressed high on the top of the head with curls or bangs on the forehead. An upsweep movement in the temple area with a soft hair arrangement over the jawline will soften the sharpness of the chin.

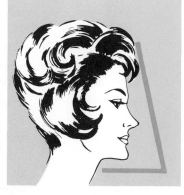

Shaping (in haircutting)—The process of shortening and thinning the hair to a particular style or to the contour of the head.

Shaping (in hairstyling)—The formation of uniform arcs or curves in wet hair, providing a base for finger waves, pin curls or various patterns in hairstyling.

Forward shaping—Directing the hair towards the face.

Reverse (backward) shaping—Directing the hair towards the back of the head or away from the face.

Down-shaping—Directing the hair in a **downward** movement in preparation for a particular pattern or style.

Up-shaping—Directing the hair in an **upward** movement in preparation for a particular pattern or style.

Slicing—Carefully removing a section of hair from a shaping, in preparation for making a curl. (The remainder of the shaping is not disturbed.)

Forward curl—A curl which is directed **toward** the face.

Reverse (backward) curl—A curl which is directed **away** from the face.

Clockwise—The movement of hair, in shapings or curls, in the **same** direction as the movement of the hands of a clock.

Counter-clockwise—The movement of hair, in shapings or curls, in the **opposite** direction to the movement of the hands of a clock.

Direction—The moving of hair in order to form a particular pattern or style. **Forward:** toward the face. **Reverse:** away from the face.

Under-directed—Insufficiently directing the hair in the formation of finger waves, curls or shapings.

Over-directed—Excessive direction of the hair in the formation of finger waves, curls or shapings.

Pin curl (sculpture curl)—A strand of hair which is combed smooth and ribbon-like, and wound into a circle, with the ends on the inside. Usually called a **flat** curl.

Overlapping curl—A strand of wet hair wound around the finger in a spiral movement, with the hair ends on the outside. Also known as **Maypole** or **post** curl.

Stand-up curl (cascade curl)—A curl with the stem directed straight up or out from the head and pinned in a standing position.

Ridge curl—A curl placed behind and close to the ridge of a finger wave.

Pin curl wave—Alternating the direction of rows of pin curls in order to form a wave pattern.

Finger wave—A wave formed in wet hair with the use of fingers and comb.

Skip wave—A pattern formed by a combination of finger wave and pin curl patterns, the pin curls being placed in alternate finger wave formation.

Roller curl—A section of wet hair wrapped around a roller.

Strand—A lock or section of hair.

Base—The stationary or immovable foundation of the curl, which is attached to the scalp.

Stem—That part of the pin curl between the base and the first arc of the circle.

Circle—That part of the pin curl forming a complete circle.

Curl—A circle, or circles, within a circle. The size of the curl governs the width of the wave.

Stem direction—The direction in which the stem moves from the base to the first arc. (Stem direction may be forward, backward, upward or downward.)

Back-combing—Combing small sections of hair from the ends toward the scalp, causing the shorter hair to form a cushion at the scalp. Also known as teasing, ratting, matting or French lacing.

Back-brushing, also called **ruffing**—The brushing of the hair toward the scalp so that the shorter hair tangles to form a cushion at the scalp for top covering hair.

Molding (**moulding**)—The forming or directing of the hair in order to create a desired shape or style.

Bouffant—The degree of height and fullness in a finished hairstyle.

Hair shaping pivot—The exact point from which the hair is directed in forming a curvature or shaping.

Extended or elongated stem—A space area between two rows of pin curls, which permits the first row of curls to unfold without buckling.

Panel—The area between two partings; also called **sections.**

Carved curls—Pin curls, carved out of a shaping without disturbing the shaping, are usually referred to as carved curls.

French lacing—Term used for back-combing or back-brushing the top part of the strand.

Molded (**moulded**) **curl**—Same as carved curl.

Semi-standup curl (**flair curl**)—A pin curl carved out of a shaping and pinned into a semi-standing position.

Barrel curl—A curl which is wound like a roller curl without the use of a roller.

Flat curl (**pin curl**)—Gives close to the head movement and no lift.

Movement—Directing and changing the direction of hair.

Volume—Indicates lift or height created in the formation of hairstyle design.

Indentation—Indicates a curved hollow or valley created in the formation of hairstyle design.

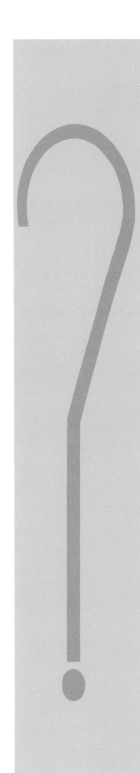

1. Why is it important that a cosmetologist know basic hairstyling?
2. Why is it important that the cosmetologist consider the patron's features and personality?
3. What is the foundation upon which a well-groomed hairstyle is designed?
4. What are the three primary factors which a cosmetologist must understand in order to become a proficient hairstylist?
5. What should be the condition of hair in order to obtain successful results in hairstyling?
6. Why is the correct removal of tangles important for successful hairstyling?
7. How should the hair be combed before a part is made?
8. By what other name are pin curls known?
9. What prior treatments should the hair receive in order to insure long-lasting and springy curls?
10. What type of hair is best suited for pin curling?
11. List the three principal parts of a pin curl.
12. Define the base of a curl.
13. Where is the stem of a curl located?
14. What is the function of the curl stem?
15. What is the function of the pin curl circle?
16. Which part of the pin curl determines its mobility?
17. Name three lengths of stems that affect the mobility of curls.
18. When is a no-stem curl used?
19. How does a no-stem curl affect its base?
20. When is a half-stem curl formation used?
21. How does a half-stem curl permit movement?
22. When is a full-stem curl used?
23. List the four most commonly shaped bases used in hairstyling.
24. What effect, if any, does the shape of the base have upon the resulting curl?
25. How can the greatest curl mobility be achieved?
26. What determines the size of the wave?
27. When is an open center curl used?
28. When is a closed center curl recommended?
29. Explain the directions of a forward curl and of a reverse curl in relation to the face.
30. What is a shaping?
31. How may shapings be classified?
32. How is the hair directed in a side forward shaping?
33. Why are triangular base pin curls used along the front, or facial, hairline?
34. When are square-base pin curls recommended?
35. Which type of pin curl base is used when an upsweep effect at the back of the head is desired?
36. How is a longer-lasting curl movement achieved?
37. Why must a cosmetologist know how to anchor a pin curl properly?
38. Describe the correct method for anchoring a pin curl?
39. In what direction are pin curls placed?
40. How is a vertical wave effect achieved for left side?
41. What are ridge curls?
42. Describe the formation of a skip wave.

43. When and where is the use of skip waves recommended?
44. What hair length is most likely to obtain the best results in skip waving?
45. By what other name is the cascade curl known?
46. Which hairstyle effects may be created with the use of cascade curls?
47. For what purpose are roller curls used?
48. Name one important difference between a roller curl and a stand-up curl.
49. How can a cosmetologist keep hair from slipping off the rollers?
50. How is the hair sectioned for roller curling?
51. What is the function of end papers when used with rollers?
52. When is a barrel curl used?
53. How is a barrel curl made?
54. What is meant by "volume" in a hairstyle?
55. What is meant by "indentation" in a hairstyle?
56. How is full volume created?
57. How is indentation achieved?
58. Name six ways in which cosmetologists refer to hair that is directed in a circular manner.
59. What type of roller is recommended for creating straight lines?
60. What governs the size of the roller used?
61. What three factors determine the patron's type of hair parting?
62. For which types of facial shapes is a diagonal hair parting usually given? Give reason.
63. When is a side hair parting recommended?
64. What is achieved by the use of back-combing and back-brushing techniques?
65. Give 4 alternate names for back-combing.
66. What other name is used for back-brushing?
67. Name the four basic steps to follow when combing out the hair.
68. Why is hair spray applied to the hair after a comb-out?
69. List the three general characteristics upon which an artistic and suitable hairstyle may be based.
70. Which is the ideal type of face for any hairstyle to be created?
71. How should the hair be styled for the square and round facial types?
72. In styling a pear-shaped facial type, what illusion should be created in the forehead and jawline areas?
73. In styling a heart-shaped facial type, what illusion should be created in the jawline and forehead areas?
74. For a short, thick neck, how should the hair at the back of the head be styled?
75. To minimize the long appearance of the neck, how should the hair be styled?
76. Define the following terms: a) curl; b) strand; c) slicing.

STYLING LONG HAIR

INTRODUCTION

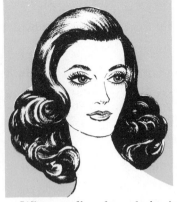

The special features of long hair give a hairstylist the opportunity to use fully his or her artistic ability and imagination to create attractive, modern hairstyles. The great versatility of long hair permits the designing of special versions of every long hairstyle to suit the individuality of the patron.

When styling long hair, it is important for the cosmetologist to set curls and rollers only in those areas where a fluff and curl design is desired. Where many curls are planned, she should set the entire head in smaller size rollers. Areas that are intended to be smooth should be shaped and combed close to the head. Exaggerated height should be carefully avoided.

Reminder: In order to achieve long lasting "holding action" when styling long hair, a body permanent should be given to straight hair where needed.

THE SWING FLIP

OBJECTIVE
To create a style which will permit the hair to fall and swing about the head in a free manner.

SETTING
Top: Part hair in the middle, from forehead to crown. Set one large stand-up curl with a large center on each side of the part. Set a smaller curl next to each large curl for a smooth, high front.

Side Hairline: Set large sculpture curls on each side hairline for width. Fig. 1.

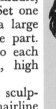

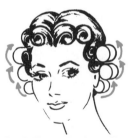

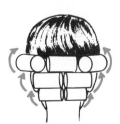

Fig. 1. Top and side hairlines

Fig. 2. Sides and back

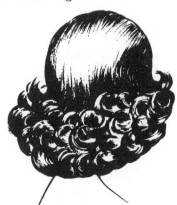

Fig. 3. ¾ back view

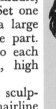

Fig. 4. Front view

Sides and Back: Use extra large rollers for sides and back, as shown in setting pattern. Fig. 2.

COMB-OUT
Comb and brush out hair with a limited amount of teasing. In the comb-out, flip up the curl ends to achieve added fullness. Fig. 3.

The finished, wide look is that of thick, un-razored hair, flowing and swinging about the head in a free manner. Fig. 4.

CASUAL ELEGANCE

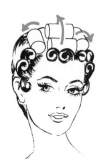

Fig. 1. Top and sides

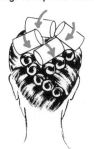

Fig. 2. Back

OBJECTIVE

To create a long "done up" hairstyle, from the turn of the century, in a modern manner.

SETTING

Top: Set 3 sculpture curls at the hairline. Fig. 1.

Sides: Set sculpture curls on each side along hairline. Fig. 1.

Rollers: Use 4 medium size rollers on top of head and 4 larger rollers in the crown area, as shown in the setting pattern.

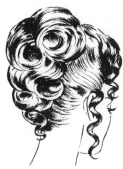

Fig. 3. ¾ back view

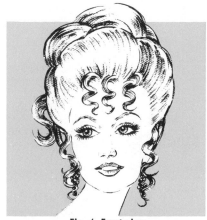

Fig. 4. Front view

Back: Set angled rows of curls in an upward direction, as shown in the setting pattern. Fig. 2.

COMB-OUT

Gather the hair at the crown in a double bun. Comb and brush the sides and back hair in an upward direction and roll curled ends into the buns. Fig. 3. Comb side hairline sculpture curls into long ringlets or tendrils that frame the face in a graceful manner. Fig. 4.

CLASSIC PAGE BOY

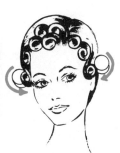

Fig. 1. Top and sides

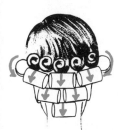

Fig. 2. Sides and back

OBJECTIVE

To create an overall "smooth-to-shoulders" hairstyle.

SETTING

Top: Set stand-up curls on forehead—on heavy side of part —backed up by another row of stand-up curls for volume. Fig. 1.

Sides: Set flat forward curls on each side of hairline.

Shaping: Form shaping in back of head area. Create a row of sculpture curls out of shaping, which will flow into a richly formed page boy formation in the finished comb-out.

Rollers: Set large rollers in a

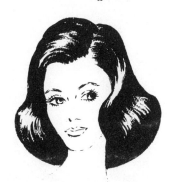

Fig. 3. Front view

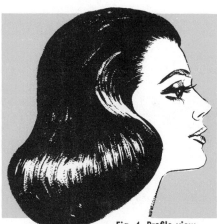

Fig. 4. Profile view

downward direction on the sides and back. Fig. 2.

COMB-OUT

Comb and brush the hair close to the face, to form a deep wave around the head. Fig. 3. Turn the curls under to frame the face and to lie gracefully on the shoulders. Fig. 4.

The Classic "Page Boy" is suitable for girls who like comfortable fashion in clothes. It goes with everything, and is perfect for the office or a party.

THE CORONET

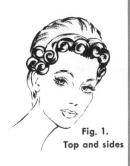

Fig. 1.
Top and sides

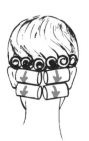

Fig. 2. Back

OBJECTIVE

To create a hairstyle using a braid to achieve a coronet effect.

SETTING

Top: Make a short center part. Comb section on each side of part. Set two large sculpture curls on each side of part.

Sides: Set large reverse curls on the sides, to create a wide wave on each side. Fig. 1.

Back: Comb and shape crown area and back of head. Set a row

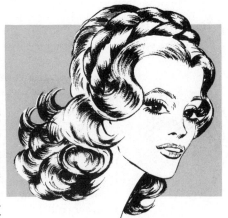

Fig. 4. ¾ front view

of flat curls in the shaping at the back of the head. Set four large rollers under, at back and nape. Fig. 2.

COMB-OUT

Comb and brush the hair in a cluster of loose curls reaching to the shoulders. Fig. 3. Attach the braid high on the head and pin closely on sides. Let curls flow out of the braid behind the ears. Fluff up hair on top by teasing. Fig. 4.

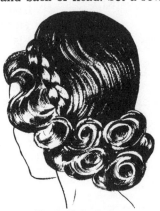

Fig. 3. ¾ back view

THE MODERN GODDESS

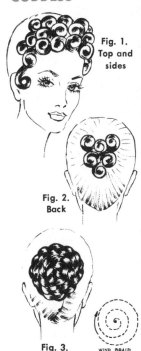

Fig. 1.
Top and sides

Fig. 2.
Back

Fig. 3.
Back view

WIND BRAID

OBJECTIVE

To create a modern version of a Grecian goddess hairstyle.

SETTING

Hair should be very long; if not, a separate, full, thick braid may be used.

Top: Part hair across top of head, from ear to ear.

Top and Sides: Set numerous flat sculpture curls on top and sides. Set one long stem curl at each ear for long ringlets, as shown in the setting pattern. Fig. 1.

Back: Draw and shape sides and back hair onto crown area. Tie off securely with a clasp. Make 6 or more large sculpture curls on crown. See setting pattern. These curls may be braided into the comb-out with the extra braid. Fig. 2.

COMB-OUT

Comb, tease lightly and braid own hair at crown and let fall

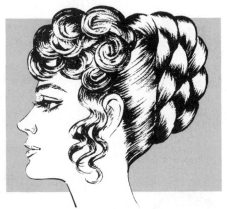

Fig. 4. Profile view

out of the way. Brush top and side sculpture curls out and arrange into a cluster of curls. Fig. 3. Arrange 3 long tendrils to fall on each side of face.

If necessary, set on a pillow of hair wool to build the braid out and away from crown into a full effect. For extra glamour, insert separate small jeweled ornaments into braid. Fig. 4.

THE MONA LISA LOOK

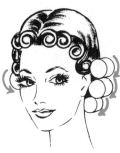

Fig. 1. ¾ front and sides

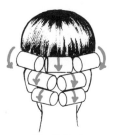

Fig. 2. Back

OBJECTIVE

To create the modern version of a Mona Lisa look.

SETTING

This romantic style has 3 sections in which the hair is first cut only in the outer layers, beginning at the nape area. Hair remains long.

Top: Make center part from front to crown. Set large sculpture curls around entire front hairline. Fig. 1.

Sides and Back: Set with extra large rollers. Fig. 2.

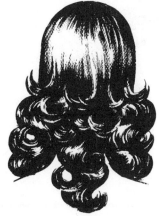

Fig. 3. Back view

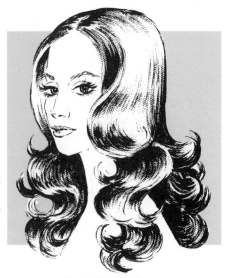

Fig. 4. ¾ front view

COMB-OUT

Comb into three sections, to fall forward on each shoulder and down in back. Fig. 3. Top is teased softly and brushed down, to fall smoothly into a curl and wave combination.

Wispy flips turn up gracefully about the shoulders and down the back. Fig. 4.

HIGH FASHION

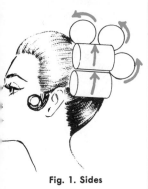

Fig. 1. Sides

Fig. 2. Top, sides and back

OBJECTIVE

To create a high fashion hairstyle with long hair.

SETTING

Top: Comb hair straight back.
Sides: Place a single curl in front of each ear. Fig. 1.
Back: Set extra large rollers on and around crown, as indicated in setting pattern. Fig. 2.

COMB-OUT

Comb and tease front into a smooth pompadour with a lift on hairline. Comb a long curl forward on each cheekbone. Bring hair together in the crown area and arrange into huge poufs of curls that are pinned on base. Tie and pin under a wide scarf. Fig. 3.

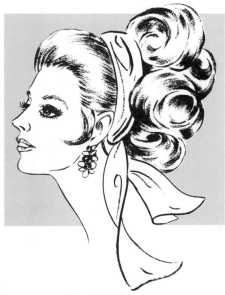

Fig. 3. Profile view

PAGE BOY FLIP

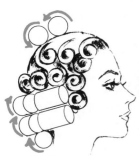

Fig. 1. Sides and back

OBJECTIVE

To create a modern and free flowing version of a page boy hairstyle.

SETTING

Top: Part off about 2 inches in front for center part.

Sides: Set both sides in large sculpture flat curls.

Back: Follow across back with one row of curls.

Rollers: *Top of head*: Set two or more extra large rollers for height or pouf. Set back and

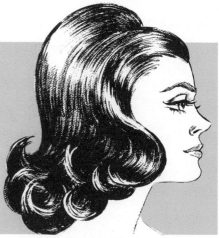

Fig. 3. Profile view

nape areas in extra large rollers, turned up. Fig. 1.

COMB-OUT

Brush the hair and side waves will appear. Follow through, and blend the hair into the back area. All hair should turn up gracefully. Fig. 2.

(Note front view illustration.) The wide effect is achieved by bringing the hair forward onto the cheeks and arranging it into immense waves, flipping out to the sides. Fig. 3.

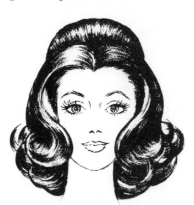

Fig. 2. Front view

THE SOPHISTICATE

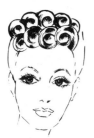

Fig. 1. Top

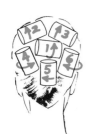

Fig. 2. Crown and back

OBJECTIVE

To create a sophisticated hairstyle for a young lady.

SETTING

Top: Set two rows of extra large stand-up curls on front hairline, to comb out into a high, wide wave. Fig. 1.

Back: Set crown and back area with extra large rollers, as shown in setting pattern. Fig. 2.

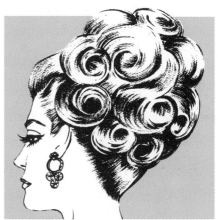

Fig. 4. Profile view

COMB-OUT

Brush, comb and arrange high front wave. Fig. 3. Brush out roller set. At nape, make a smooth French twist. Brush and form crown into an elaborate arrangement of extra large, fluffy, airy curls. Fig. 4. In back of high ridge of the wave, place long curls into a halo effect, from side to side of the head. See Fig. 3.

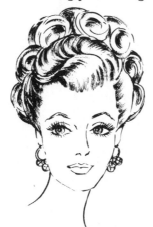

Fig. 3. Front view

THE POMPADOUR

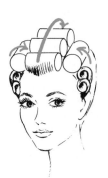

Fig. 1. Top and sides

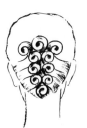

Fig. 2. Back

OBJECTIVE

To create an "up-do" hairstyle with a French twist.

SETTING

Top: Set 5 or more rollers on top and crown. Fig. 1.

Side Hairline: Set reverse curls on each side hairline. Fig. 1.

Back: Shape back and nape and set sculpture curls, as shown in setting pattern. Fig. 2.

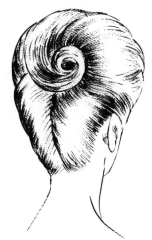

Fig. 3. ¾ back view

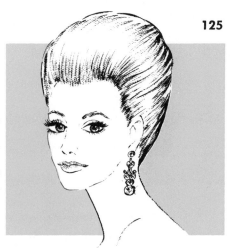

Fig. 4. Front view

COMB-OUT

The entire effect should be one of smoothness. Tease top hair into a high, smooth pompadour. In the back and nape area, arrange the hair in a French twist. Elegant simplicity is the keynote of this style. Fig. 3.

For evening wear, the pompadour should be worn with elaborate jewelry. Fig. 4.

PONYTAIL CHIGNON

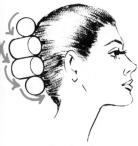

Fig. 1. Sides

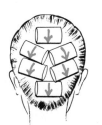

Fig. 2. Back

OBJECTIVE

To create a smooth hairstyle with an extra large pouf.

SETTING

Comb all hair back and up toward crown, and hold in place with a string or rubber band.

Use extra large rollers, and follow formation as shown in setting pattern. Figs. 1 and 2.

If hair is long and thick, use more rollers.

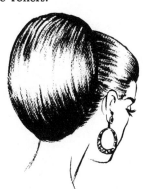

Fig. 3. Back view

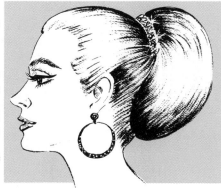

Fig. 4. Profile view

COMB-OUT

Comb and brush hair towards crown. Tease each section and brush into an extra large pouf. Pin outer part of pouf down to back of head. Fig. 3.

A jeweled ornament may be used to hold the base in place. Fig. 4.

PONYTAIL FLIP

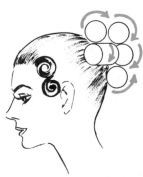

Fig. 1. Top, sides and back

OBJECTIVE

To create a ponytail hairstyle with turned up hair ends.

SETTING

Top: Shape hair smoothly toward crown and up from nape area. Tie securely the gathered hair at the crown.

Sides: Set 2 sculpture curls on each side hairline for ringlets. Set ponytail section in 5 or 6 extra large rollers. Fig. 1.

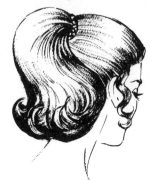

Fig. 2. Back view

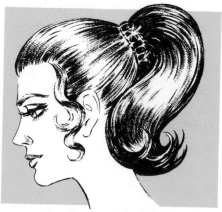

Fig. 3. Profile view

COMB-OUT

Comb through all the hair, keeping ponytail sections separated. Tease each section of the ponytail for fullness; then, brush smoothly through the ponytail. Turn up ends. Fig. 2. Place barrette or jeweled band at base of ponytail. Comb out side ringlets to fall in front of ears. Fig. 3.

PONYTAIL FORMAL

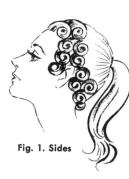

Fig. 1. Sides

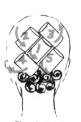

Fig. 2. Back

OBJECTIVE

To create a ponytail in a formal manner.

SETTING

Comb hair smoothly back; tie off all long hair at crown.

Separate nape hair for sculpture curls.

Set front and sides in large, flat sculpture curls, and cheek curl at ear. Refer to setting pattern. Fig. 1.

Set crown hair on 6 extra large rollers, in even formation, as shown in setting pattern. Set nape in curls. Fig. 2.

COMB-OUT

Brush out hair. Create a little height on top and fluffiness

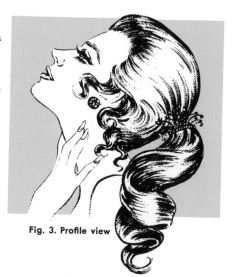

Fig. 3. Profile view

around sides and nape by limited amount of teasing. Tie off mass of long hair below crown. At nape, comb a fringe of tendrils to hang down neck.

Tease the tied-off back hair; brush through. Tease and blend hair together into a solid twisted coil to be worn over shoulder, or to fall free. A sparkling ornament may be worn for evening highlights. Fig. 3.

THE GRAND CASCADE

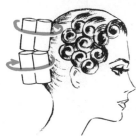

Fig. 1. Sides

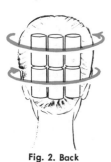

Fig. 2. Back

OBJECTIVE

To create a long, wavy hairstyle to fall over the shoulder.

SETTING

Top: Part hair in the middle, from hairline to crown.

Sides: Set each side in long stem large curls, as shown in setting pattern. Comb back rest of hair. Fig. 1.

Back: Set back area in two rows: top row, 3 extra large rollers directed to the right; bottom row, 3 extra large rollers directed to the left, creating a wide wave. Fig. 2.

COMB-OUT

Top and Sides: Brush through hair. Comb each side into deep waves at temples. Brush through longer hair and attach an ornament to hold the base on the crown. Slightly tease the rest of

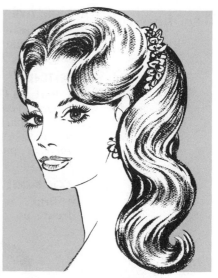

Fig. 3. Profile view

the long hair and brush it into a large coil, twisting as you comb. Spray lightly to keep its form. The strong roller action will give the twisting an undulating effect. It is worn down the back or resting over the shoulder. Fig. 3.

SPLIT PONYTAIL

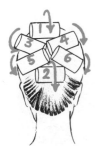

Fig. 1. Crown

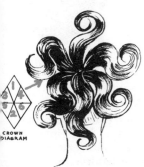

Fig. 2. Crown diagram

OBJECTIVE

To create a style with an unusual high crown effect and a number of ponytail tendrils.

SETTING

Comb hair straight back and up, from nape to crown, and tie or pin down securely.

Crown: Make a crown setting of extra large rollers, as shown in setting pattern. Fig. 1. Separate tied hair into 6 to 8 sections, depending on the texture (coarse, medium or fine) of the hair. Fig. 2. Set hair, using extra large rollers, as shown in the setting pattern.

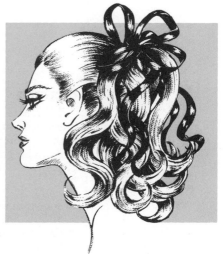

Fig. 3. Profile view

COMB-OUT

Brush hair thoroughly. Comb each section of the ponytail individually, until hair falls naturally into slim hanging tendrils. Decorate with double bows of slim ribbon. Let long ends of the ribbon fall gracefully among the curly tendrils. Fig. 3.

CLASSIC CHIGNON

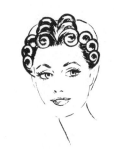

Fig. 1. Top

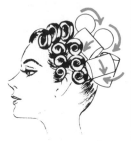

Fig. 2. Sides

OBJECTIVE

To create massive curls gathered at the crown into a classic chignon.

SETTING

Part the hair in the middle. Set 3 large stand-up curls on each side of part. Fig. 1. Shape and set sides in alternate reverse and forward pin curls. Fig. 2. Use large rollers for the crown.

COMB-OUT

Brush back hair first; then front and sides. Pick up and re-

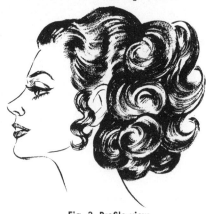

Fig. 3. Profile view

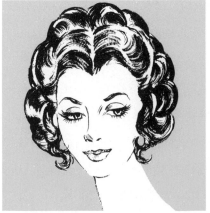

Fig. 4. Front view

trace a free wave pattern with comb. For side hanging tendrils, borrow hair from middle and last curl. Tease and lock ends to fall loosely. Fig. 3.

Notes: For a slender or oval face, dress crown hair curls to fall forward over ears for a fuller effect. Fig. 4.

For a wide or round face, hold crown chignon smoothly back of ears.

Increase height by teasing crown chignon higher on the head.

THE OUTDOOR GIRL

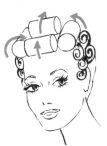

Fig. 1. Top and sides

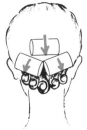

Fig. 2. Back

OBJECTIVE

To create a hairstyle for girls interested in outdoor activities, such as horseback riding, tennis, and walking.

SETTING

Top: Use extra large rollers, as shown in setting pattern. Fig. 1.

Sides: Set a row of forward curls on each side hairline. Back them up with two reverse curls on each side. Fig. 1.

Back: Use extra large rollers, as shown in setting pattern. At the nape, set curls with change of direction from the center curl. Fig. 2.

COMB-OUT

Comb and brush hair into a high, smooth pouf pompadour. Gather hair at the back of

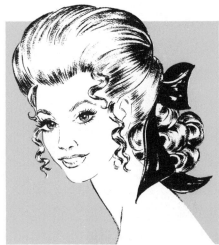

Fig. 3. ¾ front view

head with a large bow or ornament. Style nape hair into a cluster of fluffy curls. At sides, comb ringlets or tendrils to frame the face gracefully. Fig. 3.

SWEET SEVENTEEN

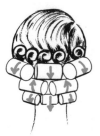

Fig. 1. Top and sides

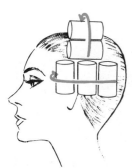

Fig. 2. Back

OBJECTIVE

To create a youthful hairstyle that moves easily about the face.

SETTING

Top: Make a side part. Set stand-up curls on front hairline. Fig. 1.

Sides: Set long stem curls on each side hairline, as shown in the setting pattern. Fig. 1.

Back: Just below the crown, set a row of 4 large flat curls directed to the right; reverse the direction of the fifth curl. Complete the back and nape areas with roller curls. Use large rollers

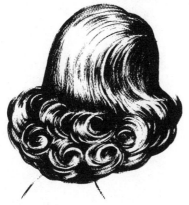

Fig. 3. ¾ back view

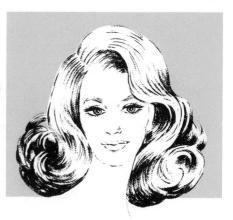

Fig. 4. Front view

in the back and medium size rollers at the nape, as shown in setting pattern. If hair is thick and full, use all large rollers. Fig. 2.

COMB-OUT

Starting at right part, brush top smooth, ending in very wide waves that move away from the face. In the back, brush the hair full and deep, to fall over the shoulders, Fig. 3, turning into a mass of curls and flips. Fig. 4.

TWIN PONYTAILS

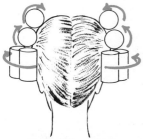

Fig. 1. Sides

Fig. 2. Sides and back

OBJECTIVE

To create a ponytail on each side of the head.

SETTING

Top: Make a middle part from forehead to nape.

Sides: Comb all hair on each side toward respective side of the head and pin down. Separate ponytail into sections and set extra large rollers on both sides, as shown in setting pattern. Figs. 1 and 2.

COMB-OUT

Brush hair smoothly and gather curls; pin or attach securely to each side. Tease and comb through falling curls; arrange them to fall neatly down the sides. Tie wired ribbon around at base of ponytail; make round bows to look attractive in the falling curls. Fig. 3.

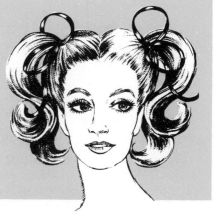

Fig. 3. Front view

JUNIOR MISS

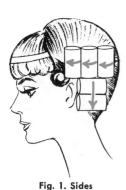

Fig. 1. Sides

OBJECTIVE

To create a hairstyle for girls who desire to look younger.

SETTING

Parting: Part off a full front section for bangs. Hold down with tape while drying. Make a middle part from top of head to nape.

Sides: Set side sections in 5 extra large rollers, as shown in setting pattern. Set a long stem ringlet curl in front of each ear. Fig. 1.

COMB-OUT

Brush out curls on each side. Recomb bangs. Comb side sections and pin or tie braid section. Divide side sections into 3 uni-

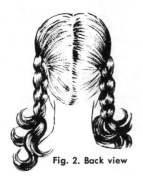

Fig. 2. Back view

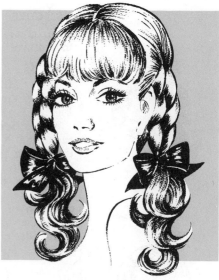

Fig. 3. ¾ front view

form strands. For a full braid, slightly tease each strand and brush it down softly.

Pleat braid and tie off, leaving ends to curl. Repeat same procedure on the other side of the head. Fig. 2. Dress up with ribbon bows, or other ornament, like a barrette. Fig. 3. For curl at ear, comb down loosely, or brush into the side section, as desired.

DEBUTANTE

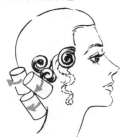

Fig. 1. Sides

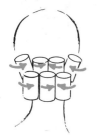

Fig. 2. Back and nape

OBJECTIVE

To create a hairstyle for a special occasion.

SETTING

Comb and shape hair back from hairline to crown area. Set a large size side curl over each ear. In back of each ear, make two reverse curls. Fig. 1.

On back and nape area, set two rows of rollers. Fig. 2.

COMB-OUT

Comb roller curls down in a cluster of long curls, held together with a clamp, comb, or for the evening, an ornament or large bow. It is a matter of choice.

Ear curls can be combed into a full, undulating motion, or can be split into several slender tendrils. Fig. 3.

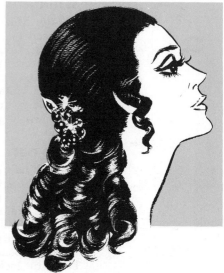

Fig. Profile view

THE FRENCH TWIST

Introduction

You can discover many interesting ways in which to create this versatile and popular hairstyle. Working on medium-length hair is ideal, since the hairstyle can be completed faster and is easily maintained by the patron. However, very long hair can look glamorous and can be styled into many unusual and exotic effects.

Avoid excessive and distorted height. Plan the style to harmonize with the patron's features, taking into consideration her nape hairline, length of neck, hair texture, etc.

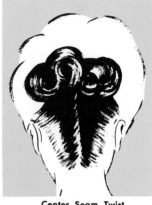

Center Seam Twist

Use ingenuity and control in pinning. Secure pinning may be achieved with bobby pins, hairpins, or both. Some hairstylists prefer the exclusive use of bobby pins. But, whichever you use, all pins must be concealed. Invisible pinning is the art you must learn.

For extra hold, use small, ornamented combs—many patrons prefer them. For formal evenings, an up-style can be decorated glamorously.

The following illustrations show a series of beautiful results that can be accomplished in styling French Twists.

FRENCH TWIST FOR SHORT HAIR

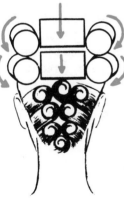

Fig. 1. Crown and nape

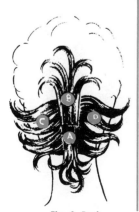

Fig. 2. Back

OBJECTIVE

To achieve a French Twist with short hair.

SETTING

Set the top on large rollers. Set the back and nape areas in long stem pin curls, in a diagonal pattern toward center. Fig. 1.

COMB-OUT

After drying and brushing the hair, part at nape into four sections. Fig. 2.

Tease and fold Section C diagonally and smoothly over

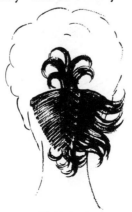

Fig. 3. Back

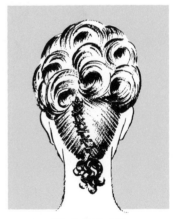

Fig. 4. Back view

Sections A and B in a rolling action. Pin securely with bobby pins. Teasing (back-combing) prevents hair from slipping. Top ends will blend into finished style. Fig. 3.

Tease and brush Section D diagonally and smoothly over Section C in a rolling action. Pin securely in invisible herringbone manner with hair pins. Fig. 4.

Note: Style top and sides last.

FRENCH ROLL TWIST

OBJECTIVE

To create a simple French Roll Twist with shoulder-length hair.

SETTING

Set the crown on large rollers. Wind side rollers up and down, providing a greater directional movement of hair in comb-out. Set pin curls in a diagonal arrangement, starting at top of back section as shown. Fig. 1.

COMB-OUT

After drying and brushing the hair, part off crown section and

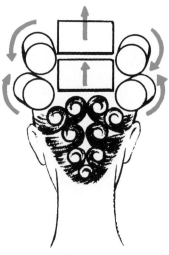

Fig. 1. Crown and nape

hold out of way with clamps. Part back hair in center from crown to nape. Fig. 2.

Tease Section A. Brush and fold smoothly in a rolling action on center back. Pin securely with bobby pins. Leave hair ends out. Conceal bobby pins as shown with dotted line. Fig. 3.

Tease and fold Section B over Section A in a rolling action, Fig. 3, and place directly on center of back in cone shape. Fig. 4.

Top hair: Style hair as desired.

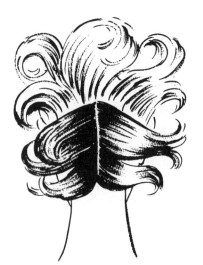

Fig. 2. Back

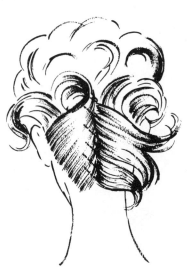

Fig. 3. Back

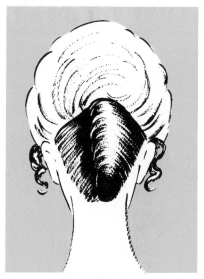

Fig. 4. Back view

SIDE SEAM TWIST

OBJECTIVE

To create a beautiful high hairstyle with a Side Seam Twist.

SETTING

Arrange the entire crown in angled rollers for a variety of comb-out effects. Set back and nape in diagonal, long stem pin curls, starting at the top. Fig. 1.

COMB-OUT

After the hair has been dried and brushed, part crown hair off and hold out of the way with clamps.

Back area. The entire back area is teased in the direction of the pinning. Teasing (back-combing) keeps the hair from sliding.

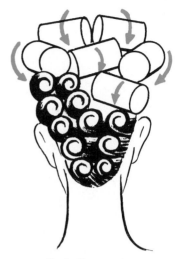

Fig. 1. Crown and nape

Shape and pin the back area to the left. The extra hair ends may be done into large pin curls, set in a cluster to the side, which will be combined with the crown hair in the comb-out. Phantom dotted lines show herringbone invisible pinning. Fig. 2. Diagram of herringbone pinning shows how the hair pins are interlocked. Fig. 3.

Top hair is done last. Figs. 4 and 5 show the profile and back views of a beautiful high hairstyle with a back Side Seam Twist.

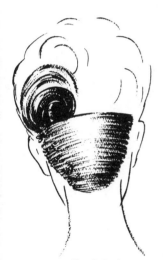

Fig. 2. Back

Fig. 3.

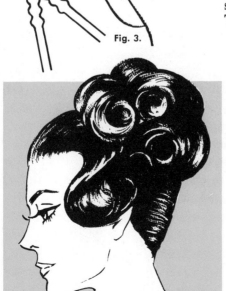

Fig. 4. Profile view

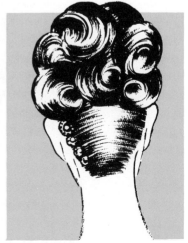

Fig. 5. Back view

HIDDEN SEAM TWIST

OBJECTIVE

To create a twist with a hidden seam.

SETTING

Set crown hair on rollers. Style back section without a complete setting. Set only the ends of the hair in large pin curls.

COMB-OUT

After the hair has been dried and brushed, it is ready for styling.

Section A: Part hair diagonally. Tease Section A and fold

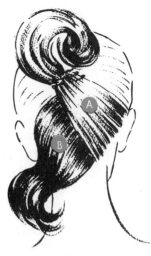

Fig. 1.

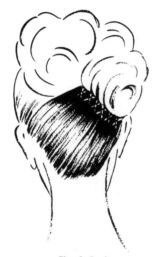

Fig. 2. Back

diagonally over to the left. Pin securely with bobby pins; hold ends of hair out of the way with clamps. Fig. 1.

Section B: Tease and arrange Section B diagonally over to the right. Pin with hairpins, as shown in dotted lines, in an invisible herringbone pattern. Fig. 2.

Combine hair ends of Sections A and B with crown hair, to create an elegant asymmetrical hairstyle as shown in Figs. 3 and 4.

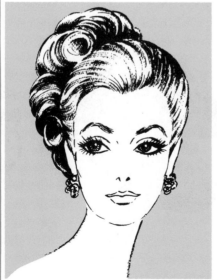

Fig. 3. Front view

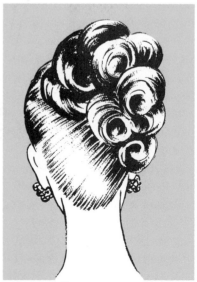

Fig. 4. Back view

UPDO HAIRSTYLE

OBJECTIVE

To create a smooth swirl updo hairstyle with shoulder-length hair.

SETTING

Top: Set on large rollers.

Back: Set in long stem curls, below crown to nape, in three rows of graduated size curls. Fig. 1.

COMB-OUT

After the hair has been dried and brushed, it is ready for styling. Part back hair diagonally

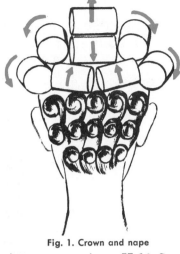

Fig. 1. Crown and nape

into two sections. Hold Section A out of the way with hair clamp. Fig. 2. Tease Section B at base in narrow sections through the entire section. Figs. 3 and 4.

Begin teasing Section A in a fanned out manner, bringing hair upward with each motion. Pick up sub-sections as shown by dotted line. Fig. 3. Lock hair at base on scalp. Brush the hair up into a swirled back design.

Top, sides and front hair may be styled in many ways. Fig. 5.

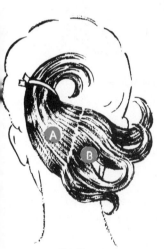

Fig. 2.

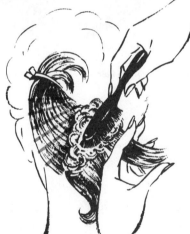

Fig. 3.

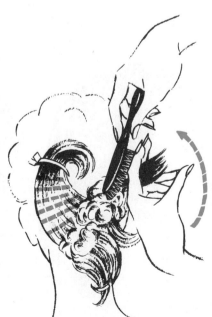

Fig. 4.

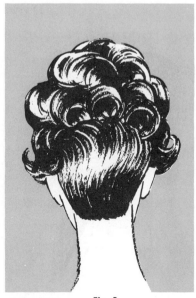

Fig. 5.

PERMANENT WAVING MEDIUM LONG AND LONG HAIR

Introduction

The permanent waving of medium long and long hair is a very important phase of beauty culture training. You will note from the two illustrations shown here that the one with a permanent wave is much more attractive than the one with straight hair.

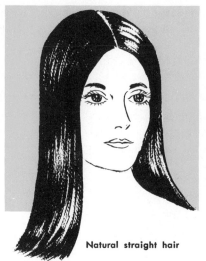

Natural straight hair

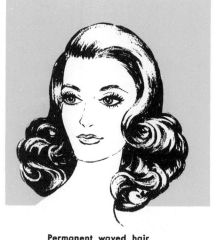

Permanent waved hair

BODY PERMANENT FOR MEDIUM LONG HAIR

OBJECTIVE

To section medium long hair for wrapping on curling rods in order to achieve a tighter curl.

SECTIONING

Divide hair into 6 sections.

Gather each section to form ponytails. Secure each one with rubber bands. Figs. 1, 2 and 3. Leave the rubber bands on throughout the entire permanent waving process.

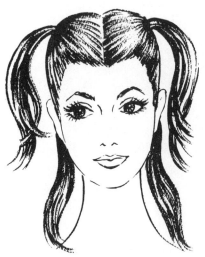

Fig. 1.

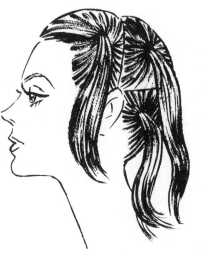

Fig. 2.

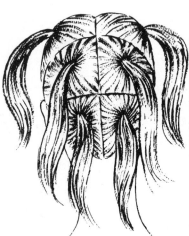

Fig. 3.

SUB-SECTIONING AND WRAPPING

Sub-divide into as many block-ings as are required for the number of curling rods em-ployed. Figs. 1, 2 and 3. Wrap the hair close to the scalp. In the nape area, use smaller and addi-tional rods, if a tighter curl is desired.

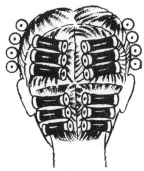

Fig. 1.

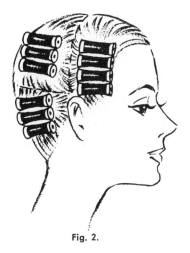

Fig. 2.

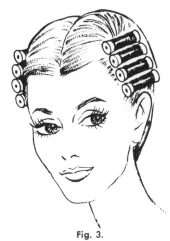

Fig. 3.

SETTING

After the permanent wave, set both sides in the same manner on large rollers. Fig. 4. Set front in large, forward stand-up curls. These curls will comb out into full, strong bangs, or they may be arranged into various pat-terns to create the desired hair-style.

COMB-OUT

Fig. 5 illustrates the final comb-out.

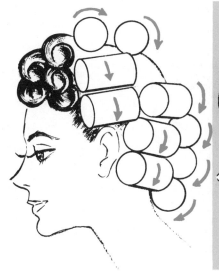

Fig. 4. Setting

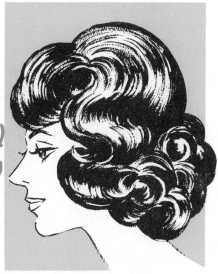

Fig. 5. Comb-out

BODY PERMANENT FOR LONG HAIR

OBJECTIVE

Wrapping long hair on curling rods to achieve a looser curl.

SECTIONING AND WRAPPING

Part the entire head into six large sections. Use the largest curling rods. Wrap sub-sections in hanging clusters of 3 or more curling rods, depending on the amount of hair. The heavier the hair, the more curling rods will be required. Figs. 1, 2 and 3.

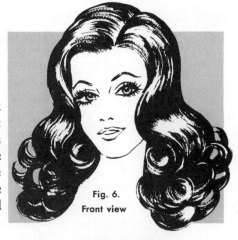

Fig. 6.
Front view

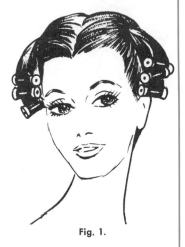

Fig. 1.

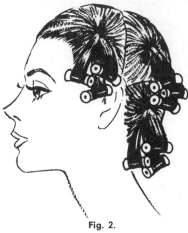

Fig. 2.

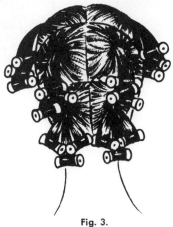

Fig. 3.

SETTING

Form a left side part. Set large stand-up curls. On temples, set two large reverse curls which will create a wave effect. Fig. 4.

Give a crown-back shaping; set the rest of the head with jumbo rollers, patterned as shown in Figs. 4 and 5.

COMB-OUT

The final comb-out is illustrated in Fig. 6.

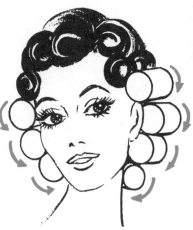

Fig. 4.

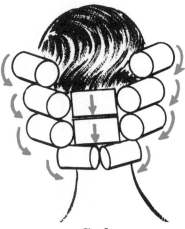

Fig. 5.

BRAIDING

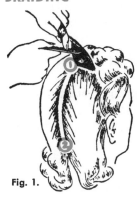

Fig. 1.

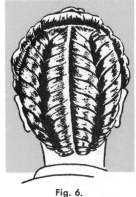

Fig. 2.

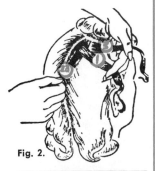

Fig. 6.

OBJECTIVE

Braiding is popular with both adults and children. The hairstylist should be able to form a Regular French Braid by overlapping the strands on top.

PROCEDURE

1. Part crown section off. Hold out of way with clips or clamps. **Back hair:** Part hair from center of crown, 1, to nape, 2, Fig. 1.

2. Divide section evenly into three strands. Start to braid by bringing strand 1 (on the left) over strand 2a (in the center). Fig. 2. Draw strands tightly.

3. Pick up another strand from the left, about ½ inch wide, as indicated by 2b. Fig. 3. Join strands 2a and 2b. Tighten strands.

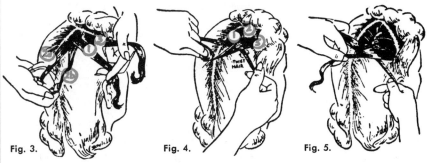

Fig. 3.   Fig. 4.   Fig. 5.

4. Bring strand 3 over strand 1 and tighten. Fig. 4. Pick up another strand on the right, about ½ inch wide, and place with strand 1.

Note: To insure a neat braid with all short hair ends in place, twist each strand toward the right or left with the thumb and index finger.

5. Continue to pick up strands and braid, Fig. 5, finishing with braiding of hair ends at nape. Fasten with a rubber band or string.

Braid the left side of the head, following the same procedure. The final Regular French Braid is illustrated in Fig. 6.

ALTERNATE METHOD

The Regular French Braid may also be started at the nape and braided toward the top of the head. The ends may be finished into rolls or curls.

FASHION

The braids may be crossed and tucked neatly underneath and held in place with hairpins or bobby pins.

When hair is long enough, braids can be crossed and extended up the back of the head.

Another attractive effect may be obtained by tying the braids with ribbons at the hairline and allowing the ends to fall into clusters of curls.

INVERTED FRENCH BRAID

OBJECTIVE

To form an inverted French Braid by pleating the strands under, thus making the braid visible.

PROCEDURE

Part and section hair in the same manner as for Regular French Braid.

1. Divide top right section evenly into three strands. Start to braid the hair strands by placing the right side strand **under** the center strand, and the left side strand **under** this one. Draw strands tightly. Fig. 1.

2. Pick up ½ inch strand on right side and combine with right side strand. Place this combined strand under the center strand. Pick up ½ inch strand on left side and combine with left side strand. Place this combined strand under center strand. Fig. 2.

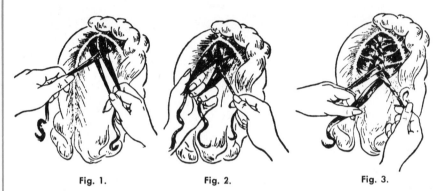

Fig. 1.   Fig. 2.   Fig. 3.

3. Continue to pick up hair and braid as above. Fig. 3. Finish braiding at nape, and hold in position with rubber bands.

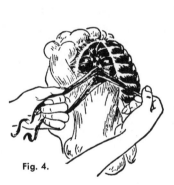 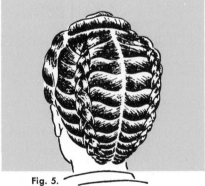

Fig. 4.   Fig. 5.

4. Braid left side of head in the same manner as right side. Fig. 4.

Appearance of finished Inverted French Braid with braids tucked under and held in place with hairpins or bobby pins.

FASHION

The same suggestions recommended for the Regular French Braiding can be utilized for the Inverted French Braiding.

CHAPTER 12

CARE AND STYLING OF WIGS

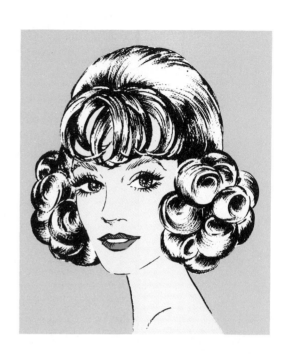

INTRODUCTION

Throughout history, wigs have served to enhance milady's charm and beauty. The ancient Egyptians first wore wigs in 4,000 B.C., primarily to protect their own hair from the sun. From Europe, wigs spread to America, where they have grown in popularity over the years.

The use of wigs, hairpieces, wiglets or falls, which started as a fad only a few years ago, has grown to such a great extent that hairpieces of all kinds are now a very important part of the beauty industry.

Wigs and hairpieces give patrons the opportunity to change the appearance of their hair to suit the fashion, styling and coloring needs of the moment. They present to alert cosmetologists an opportunity to expand their services and increase profits by selling, styling and servicing wigs and hairpieces.

In order for cosmetologists to offer the best possible wig services, they must be familiar with the following subjects:

1. How wigs can benefit patrons and improve their appearance.
2. How wigs are made and fitted.
3. How to select and style wigs to the patron's advantage.
4. How to clean and service wigs for patrons.

Why Wear Wigs

Wigs may be worn for three principal reasons:

1. **Necessity**—to cover up baldness, sparse or damaged hair.
2. **Fashion**—for changes in everyday hairstyles, for decorative purposes and for special occasions.
3. **Practicality**—for quick changes in hair shades and styles to accommodate the busy woman.

Quality Of Wigs

The quality of a wig varies with the type of hair it contains, the way it is constructed and how it is fitted to the patron's measurements.

Modern wigs are so expertly made that they closely resemble a real head of hair. Wigs may be made from human hair, synthetic (man-made) hair, animal hair, or a blend of each.

Match Test

A simple **match test** will tell the difference between human and synthetic hair. Cut a small piece of hair from the back area of the wig. With a lighted match, burn this hair and observe the following:

1. **Human hair** burns **slowly** and gives off a strong odor resembling burnt chicken feathers.
2. **Synthetic hair** burns **quickly** and gives off little or no odor. Besides, tiny hard beads can be felt in the burnt ash.

TYPES OF WIGS

In addition to the type of hair being used, the quality of the wig also depends on whether it is constructed by hand or machine. Expensive, custom-made wigs are hand knotted and have a fine mesh foundation. In the cheaper "weft wigs," the hair is sewn by machine onto the net cap in circular rows.

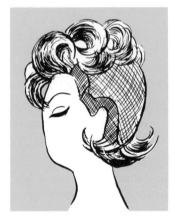

HANDMADE WIGS
(Ventilated Wigs)

DETAIL CUTAWAY shows hair crocheted and hand knotted onto the mesh foundation.

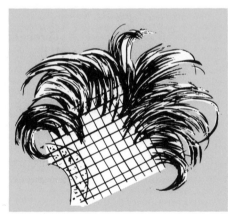

MACHINE-MADE WIGS
(Wefted Wigs)

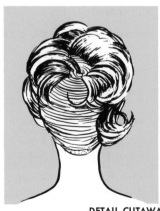
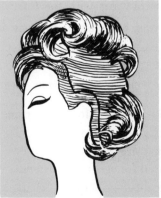
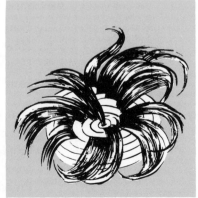

DETAIL CUTAWAY. Hair is sewn by machine onto net cap or weft in circular rows.

HAIR FOR WIGS

HUMAN AND ANIMAL HAIR

Type	Where Obtained	Qualities	Color	Advantages	Disadvantages	Future Outlook
HUMAN HAIR **1—European** A. First Quality	Italy Germany	(Cut in lengths directly from head) Good lustre Finest quality Good elasticity Soft, well-bodied texture	Whole range of colors in all shades	Very good quality for wigs Beautiful to handle	Very scarce Expensive	More difficult to obtain Very costly
B. Second Quality	Spain Portugal France Middle Europe	(Obtained from combings, not directly from head) Too soft—difficult to hold curl Requires hackling to untangle and align shafts	Range of colors fair	More plentiful than first quality Less costly	May be chemically damaged Dry and dull looking	This type of hair is becoming difficult to obtain
2—Oriental	Japan China Far East Countries	Coarse texture Straight Dry and brittle	Dark colors only	More plentiful Easily accessible Less expensive When properly refined, can have good setting characteristics	Dry and brittle	Modern processing may produce a wide range of colors
3—Indonesian	Indonesia	Not as coarse as Oriental hair Better body than second quality European hair	Dark colors only	More plentiful Fair quality	Inferior processing results in dry, dull hair Some qualities are too fine to hold set Unsatisfactory for wigs	Modern techniques may develop full range of colors
4—Indian	India	Very poor texture Very limp	Dark colors only			
NOTE:	American hair is usually unsuitable for wig work, due to cutting, coloring and permanent waving.					
ANIMAL HAIR **1—Angora**	Angora goat	Very soft and fine	Pure silvery white	Very fine quality	Fairly difficult to work with	Wider use, mixed with human hair
2—Syrian	Mixture of yak and angora	Good body and substance Straight	White	Good body and texture Good to handle	Straight hair	New uses being developed by new techniques and blending
3—Yak	Tibet—(Type of ox)	Straight Good body	White	After special processing—straight, white, good body	Limited supply	New processing and techniques develop new colors and uses
4—All Long Haired Animals	Horses, Sheep, etc.	Straight Coarse	Color limitations	Plentiful Cheap	Very coarse and straight	New techniques and combination will develop new uses and colors

WIG MEASUREMENTS

Take correct measurements of the patron's head to assure a comfortable and secure fit. First, brush the hair down smoothly and pin it as flat and tight as possible. Keeping close to the head without applying pressure, take flat measurements with a tape, as follows:

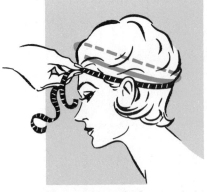

Place tape completely around the head: start at hairline, at middle of forehead; place tape above the ears, around back of head, and return to starting point.

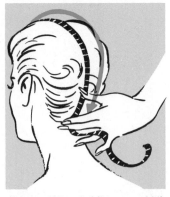

Measure from hairline at middle of forehead, over top, to nape of neck. Bend head back and measure to point where wig will ride on base of skull at the nape.

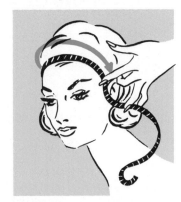

Measure from ear to ear, across forehead.

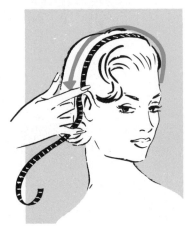

Measure from ear to ear, over top of head.

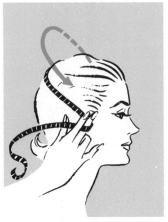

Place tape across the crown, temple to temple.

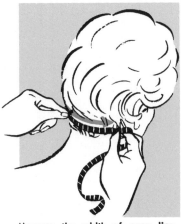

Measure the width of nape line, across nape of neck.

CHECK TO MAKE CERTAIN THAT THESE MEASUREMENTS ARE ACCURATE.

WIG ORDERING

When ordering the wig, keep a written record of the patron's head measurements, and forward a copy to the wig dealer or manufacturer. Also specify what is desired, as to:

1. The hair shade (natural or artificial). If necessary, submit samples of patron's hair to the manufacturer. Hair samples should be of hair that has been freshly shampooed, tinted or color rinsed.

2. The quality of hair.

3. The length of hair.

4. The type of hair part and hair pattern.

BLOCKING A WIG

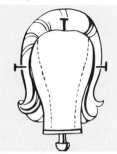

One pin is placed at center of forehead and one at each side.

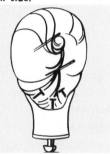

One pin is placed at center of nape and one pin at each corner.

WIG CLEANING

Procedure

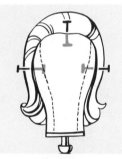

FRONT VIEW

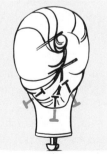

BACK VIEW

To retain same size after wig is cleaned a pin is placed at edge of cap next to the six pins securing wig.

Good blocking helps obtain professional results when shaping, setting and combing out the wig. It also reduces the possibility of disrupting the comb-out when T-pins are removed.

Use **canvas blocks** for all wig services, because they stand up under continuous pinning and rough handling. You can use **styrofoam blocks** for storing the wig, and a **swivel clamp,** for better block control.

There are six sizes of canvas blocks available in wig styling: from smallest to largest — 20, 20½, 21, 21½, 22, 22½.

The wig should be placed on a block comparable to it in size, since they come in many sizes. The wig should not be either stretched or hung loosely on a block, but it should fit comfortably. A wig that is stretched and pinned may become larger when the cap is wetted. If it is hung loosely, the cap may shrink when wetted.

Mount the wig on a block of the correct head size.

Pin the wig at six points in the following order:

    a) Center of the forehead

    b) At each side (temple side)

    c) At the center of the nape

    d) At each corner of the nape

A human hair wig should be dry-cleaned every two to four weeks, depending on how often it is worn. Also, when a wig is ready for restyling, it should be dry-cleaned.

Block wig. Remove back combing. Direct hair off the hairline. Brush the hair to loosen dirt and hair spray.

Before taking the wig off the block to be cleaned, mark the size of the wig on the block in order to retain the same size after it has been cleaned. This is done by placing a T-pin into the block on an angle next to the edge of the cap and directly in front of the six T-pins securing the wig. Remove the wig and proceed with the cleaning.

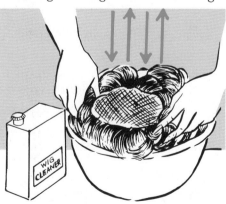

Saturate the wig in a large plastic or glass bowl containing about three ounces of non-inflammable liquid cleanser. With the hair side down, dip the wig up and down until it is clean. AN ALTERNATE METHOD. Swirl the wig around in the liquid cleanser. If necessary, clean edges and inside foundation with a cotton ball or toothbrush.

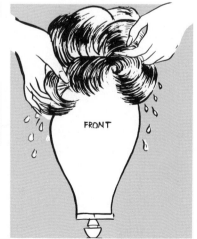

Squeeze the clean wig gently to remove excess fluid. Place wet wig immediately on a canvas block. Stretch wig lightly and pin securely to block. When dry, set and style the wig.

WIG CONDITIONING

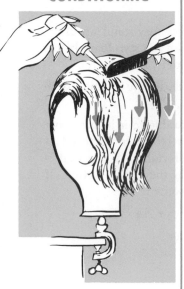

Apply a conditioner to the wig whenever the hair is dry and brittle or when the foundation is dry.

In order to keep the wig in good condition, apply a conditioner to the wig hair every time you clean and restyle it.

There are two methods of reconditioning:

1. The wig hair only
2. The entire wig (wig and foundation)

Conditioning wig hair only. Protect block with plastic covering and block the wig properly.

Apply conditioner to damp, clean hair.

Distribute conditioner evenly with a wide tooth comb. Keep conditioner in hair according to instructions accompanying the conditioner you are using. Set and style the hair.

Conditioning entire wig. Clean the wig before conditioning.

The procedure is the same as for cleaning the wig. The only difference is that conditioner is used instead of wig cleaner. Mix conditioner in luke-warm water and immerse the entire wig in the mixture for about ten minutes. Then rinse thoroughly in clean water.

ADJUSTING THE WIG

After the wig has been prepared according to specifications, it may require shrinking, stretching or other adjustments, in order to obtain a secure fit on the patron's head.

Shrinking The Wig

Wig shrinkage is accomplished by wetting the net foundation of the wig with hot water, pinning it on a smaller size block, and allowing it to dry naturally.

In fitting the shrunken wig to the patron's head, the staves must be bent slightly inward to conform to the shape of the patron's forehead. The elastic mesh must be adjusted with needle and thread, and excess parts tucked in.

Stretching The Wig

If the wig feels too tight, it may require some stretching. The net foundation of the wig is wetted with hot water, the wig is pinned on to a larger size block, and then allowed to dry naturally.

Tucking

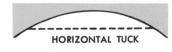

HORIZONTAL TUCK

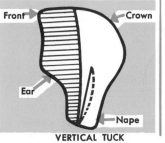

VERTICAL TUCK

If it is necessary to improve the fit of the wig in specific areas, tucking is employed.

Horizontal tucks shorten the wig from front to nape. They are taken across the back of the wig in order to remove excess bulk.

Vertical tucks remove width from the wig, from ear to ear.

It is essential to check both earpieces to be certain they are directly across from each other and do not touch the ears. If the wig is touching the ear, it is necessary to make a small horizontal tuck over the ear, in order to raise the wig off the ear. If the wig is rubbing or touching the side of the ear, a small vertical tuck behind the ear will pull the wig back and eliminate the problem.

Great care must be exercised during the tucking process by checking the cap fit after each tuck. Excessive tucking will cause the wig to "ride up" and create new fitting problems.

SHAPING THE WIG

Introduction

Basically, a wig may be shaped (cut) in the same manner as natural hair on the head is cut. However, consideration must be given to the fact that a wig has a great deal, about twice as much hair as the normal human head. As a result of this large quantity of hair, the failure to thin and taper the wig properly will cause it to look bulky and artificial.

Hair shaping (cutting) is one of the most important operations in the styling process; therefore, it must be considered and planned carefully and in great detail.

In cutting the wig, special care and caution must be exercised, because once a wig has been cut it will never grow back to cover any error in judgment or a technical failure.

The wig may be cut either on the head, to fit in with the natural hair, or on a canvas block, to facilitate ease and freedom of the hairstylist's movements. Cutting on the block also has the advantage of permitting the wig to be pinned securely, thus avoiding possible slippage during the cutting process.

In placing the wig on the canvas block to be cut, it is important that it be carefully set on the block evenly and at proper hairline distances.

Procedure

Section hair as shown on diagrams.

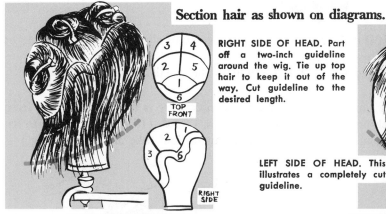

RIGHT SIDE OF HEAD. Part off a two-inch guideline around the wig. Tie up top hair to keep it out of the way. Cut guideline to the desired length.

LEFT SIDE OF HEAD. This illustrates a completely cut guideline.

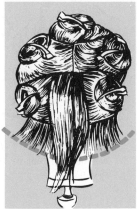

BACK OF HEAD. Let down center back hair. Cut to same length as guideline.

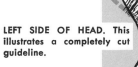

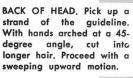

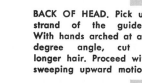

BACK OF HEAD. Pick up a strand of the guideline. With hands arched at a 45-degree angle, cut into longer hair. Proceed with a sweeping upward motion.

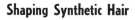

Shaping Synthetic Hair

Use only scissors and thinning shears on either synthetic fiber, or on a mixture of synthetic and human hair. The durable fiber is extremely dulling to the razor.

WIG SETTINGS AND COMB-OUTS

Setting wig hair is similar to setting hair on the human head, except for hairline coverage, and the need for a tight curl at the nape area.

The added fullness of the patron's hair, plus the hair and foundation of the wig are factors to be considered when setting and styling the wig. **Reminder:** Keep in mind that pin curls replace rollers in certain parts of the head, in order to keep the style close to the head.

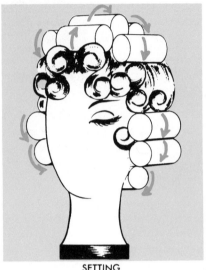

SETTING

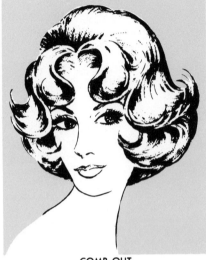

COMB-OUT

It is desirable to use T-pins instead of clippies or bobby pins to hold both rollers and curls.

Set, dry and style the hair in the usual manner.

PUTTING ON WIG AND TAKING IT OFF

A simple but very important procedure is removing the wig from a block and placing it on the patron's head. (It is a good policy to show the patron the proper way to put on and take off her own wig.)

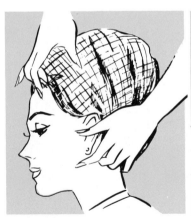

First, comb patron's hair away from her face. Pile hair on top. For long hair, put on a fine net.

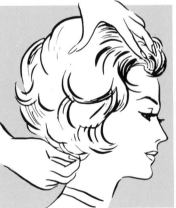

Place wig on front of patron's head. While holding wig securely on top, glide it back to nape. Pull wig securely over sides, front and back.

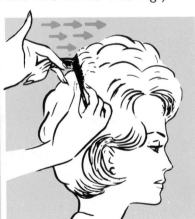

Recomb and adjust style to suit patron.

To remove the wig from the head, place only the thumb of your right hand under the cap at the nape. **Do not put fingers into hair.** Have patron bend her head down and slide wig off, catching it in the palm of the left hand.

COMBING PATRON'S HAIR INTO WIG

First comb patron's hair away from her face. Set a flat row of pin curls at the nape. Anchor pin curls with criss-cross bobby pins. Secure wig at nape. Bring it forward and adjust it to the front hairline.

When wig feels comfortably adjusted, draw out approximately 1 inch of the patron's hair from around the front hairline; then comb and blend the hair into the style of the wig.

WIG COLORING

Color Rinses

Color rinses are used as a temporary coloring and must be reapplied everytime the hair is cleaned. Color rinses only darken the hair, so a lighter wig must be used to obtain desired color.

Prepare block for wig by covering it with either Saran Wrap or a plastic cap.

Place wig on block. Holding it firmly, pin it securely at front, sides and back.

The following method is one way to apply a color rinse. Your instructor's method is equally correct.

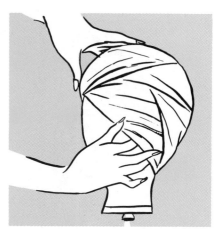

Protect block by covering it with either Saran Wrap or a plastic cap.

Procedure

Dampen clean hair using a spray applicator bottle.

Whenever in doubt of which color to use, strand test the color rinse on the back of the wig.

If color rinse is applied on dry hair, additional rinse is required for complete coverage.

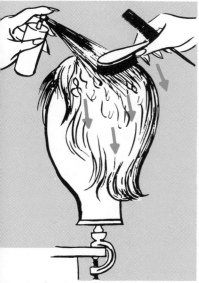

Spray hair with a color rinse. Distribute it evenly with a *downward motion* using a small brush and a wide tooth comb.

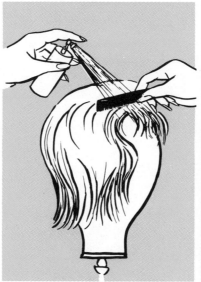

Apply setting lotion in usual manner.

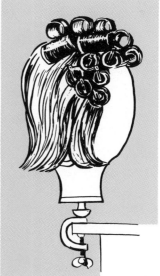

Set, dry and comb out hair to desired style.

HAIRPIECES

A variety of hairstyles may be created with hairpieces which can be dressed for either daytime or evening wear.

These hairpieces come in various forms, such as:

1. **Switches**—long wefts of hair mounted with a loop at the end. They are constructed with one to three stems of hair. The better switches are constructed with three stems to provide greater flexibility in styling and braiding. They may be worked into the hair or braided to create special styling effects.

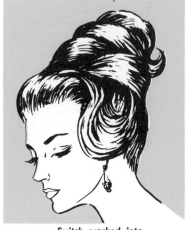

Switch worked into
patron's hair

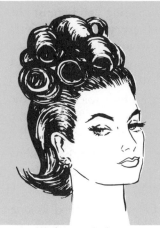

Wiglet attached to
patron's hair

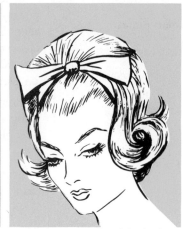

Bandeau type placed back of
patron's hairline

2. **Wiglets**—hairpieces with a flat base which are used in special areas of the head. They are used primarily to blend with patron's own hair in order to extend the range of the hair. Wiglets can be worked into the top of the hair in curls or under the hair to give it height and body. They are also employed to create special effects.

3. **Bandeau type**—a hairpiece which is sewn to a headband. The headband, which may be replaceable and comes in different colors, serves as an excellent disguise for the hairline. The bandeau type hairpiece is usually worn over the hair and is dressed in a casual, relaxed manner.

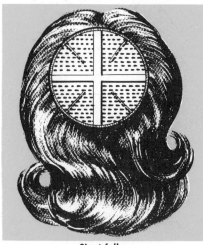

Short-fall

4. **Fall** — a section of hair, machine wefted on a round base, running across the back of the head and available in various lengths. Falls have a thick, full and plushy look.

Short-falls range from 12 to 14 inches in length.
Demi-falls, 15 to 20 inches.
Long-falls, 18 to 24 inches.

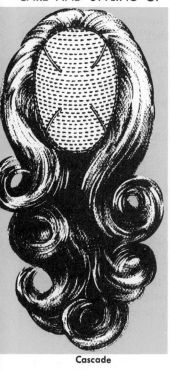

Cascade

5. **Demi-fall or Demi-wig**—a large base hairpiece which is designed to fit to the shape of the head, and generally ranges in length from 15 to 20 inches.

6. **Cascade**—a hairpiece on an oblong base which offers an endless variety of styling possibilities.

7. **Braid**—a switch whose strands are woven, interlaced or entwined together. Some are prepared with a thin wire inside in order that they be formed into various shapes. Others, without wire, are permitted to hang loose on the head.

8. **Chignon**—a knot or coil of hair that is created from synthetic hair and worn at the crown or nape of the head. A chignon is most effective when worn in combination with another hairpiece.

9. **Crown curls**—a bunch of light curls worn on top of the head.

10. **Frosting curls**—segments of frosted or blended hair are pinned into any head of hair to simulate a frosted or streaked head of hair.

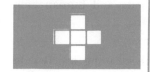

SAFETY PRECAUTIONS

1. Great care must be taken when combing or brushing wigs, to avoid matting and loss of hair.

2. Never rub or wring the cleaning fluid from a wig or hairpiece when dry-cleaning it.

3. Use great care when shaping (cutting) a wig or a hairpiece; once the hair has been cut, it cannot grow back.

4. Use a wide-tooth comb when combing a freshly set wig, to avoid abuse to the foundation and to gain greater control in combing.

5. When cleaning or working with a wet wig, it must always be mounted on a block the same head size as the wig, to avoid stretching or shrinking.

6. Correct measurements must be taken of the patron's head to assure a comfortable and secure fit.

7. Recondition wigs as often as necessary, to prevent dryness or brittleness of the hair.

8. Dry-clean wigs before setting and styling, if required.

9. Brush and comb wigs and hairpieces with a downward movement.

10. **Never lighten** (bleach) a wig or hairpiece.

11. Never give a permanent to a wig or hairpiece.

12. If hair coloring is necessary, it must be done with great care.

SYNTHETIC WIGS AND HAIRPIECES

Great improvements have been made in the manufacture of synthetic fibers. Modacrylic fibers, such as dynel, kanekalon, venicelon, and others, have eliminated most of the disadvantages of synthetic hairs. Hair fiber research has developed synthetic hair which closely resembles human hair in texture, resiliency, color acceptance, pliability, durability, sheen and feel. The fibers have good curl retention and are nonflammable; and they do not oxidize and change color in sunlight. In fact, some synthetic fibers so closely resemble human hair that it is difficult to distinguish between them.

Synthetic hair has a number of additional advantages which have contributed to their acceptance for the manufacture of wigs and hairpieces. Since the hair is synthetically produced, it is very economical. The supply is unlimited. The wigs and hairpieces are made from long threads that have been rolled on spools, permitting great efficiency in use. They are made with color fasteners in any color or shade desired.

Synthetic wigs are available as handmade stretch wigs, as machine made stretch wigs, and as handmade fitted wigs. Whatever the type of wig, careful selection of quality, fit and workmanship will give satisfaction in wear, comfort and style.

Synthetic Hairpieces

The development of fine quality, easy to handle hairpieces has opened a new fashion trend in hairstyling.

Synthetic hairpieces are available in such varieties as wiglets, demi-wigs, braids, chignon, cascades and falls.

Shaping Synthetic Wigs

In shaping synthetic wigs, use only scissors and thinning shears on either synthetic fiber or on a mixture of synthetic and human hair. The durable fiber is extremely dulling to a razor.

Cleaning Synthetic Wigs

Synthetic wigs and hairpieces do not require cleaning as often as human hair wigs. Synthetic fibers are nonabsorbent (lack porosity) and do not attract dust and dirt. Synthetic wigs and hairpieces require cleaning about every three months, depending on the amount of wear and styling. Use tepid or cool water to clean wig, as hot water will take the curl out of the synthetic wig.

Procedure

1. Mount wig on appropriate canvas block.
2. Brush wig free of tangles and wig spray before cleaning.
3. Fill container with mild shampoo, or specially formulated cleaner (read directions). Use tepid or cool water.
4. Swish wig thrugh cleaning solution for a few minutes. Rinse thoroughly in cool water.
5. Use a towel, toothbrush or cotton to clean the foundation.
6. Squeeze out excess water.
7. Towel blot.
8. T-pin wig on proper size block and let dry naturally.
9. Do not brush a synthetic wig when it is wet.
10. Do not expose a synthetic wig to heat.

GLOSSARY

This glossary is a list of technical words commonly used in connection with wig work.

angora: long, silky hair of the Angora goat. It is used primarily in fantasy work.

band wig: a hairpiece which is sewn to a head band that covers the hairline. The foundation of the hairpiece covers about $2/3$ of the head, and the overhanging hair covers all of the patron's hair. This can be used instead of a full wig.

base: the foundation of a hairpiece.

binding: a ribbon used to protect and reinforce the edges of netting.

block (foundation block): a head-shaped block made to hold a wig upon which work is to be done.

cap (wig cap): the combined netting and binding of a wig.

capless wig: wefts of synthetic hair sewn on a cap made of wide straps. Also referred to as "synthetic wig cap."

carbon tetrachloride (or carbon tet): a chemical used for dry cleaning wigs.

caul: an open weave netting used in the crown of a wig.

chignon: a knot or coil of hair worn at the crown or nape.

clamp: a device which can be attached to a table and upon which a wig block can be mounted. A **swivel clamp** can be adjusted to hold the block at different angles.

custom-made wig: a wig that is fitted to the exact measurements of a patron's head, and styled to her specifications.

dart: a tapered seam formed by cutting into a piece of wig net foundation and sewing the cut ends together. A dart is used to reduce the size of a wig cap.

drawing brushes: the brushes used to hold hair for mixing, matching, ventilating or weaving.

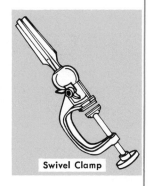

Swivel Clamp

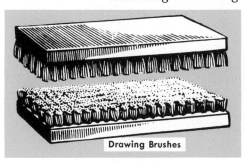

Drawing Brushes

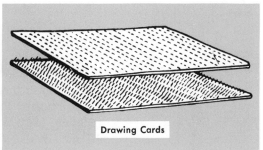

Drawing Cards

drawing cards: two identical rectangles of leather with bent wire protruding throughout the surface area. They are held with the teeth pointed away from the operator so as to create a resistance while the hair is being pulled through. They are used to hold hair and keep it from tangling while a small quantity is being drawn off.

fantasy: a hairpiece used for its artiness rather than for its practicality. The stylist uses any design and color combination to achieve an effect.

foundation (base): any supporting material used as a base to attach hair to.

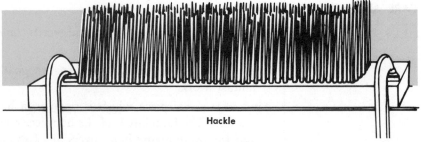

Hackle

hackle: a board with long metal teeth used for combing and mixing hair.

hackling: using a hackle to mix or blend hair.

hairpiece: a small wig used to cover the top or crown of the head.

hair roll: a sausage-like shape, in various lengths, used to fill in under the natural hair in order to create special effects.

halo: lengths of layered hair, on a ventilated or wefted foundation band, used either over the top of the head or to encircle the head.

hem: the bent over edge of a piece of material which has been turned under to avoid fraying; in wig work, the netting is so hemmed in order to place the raw edge between the outside netting and the binding.

hand-made wig (or **hand ventilated**): a wig that is made by hand-knotting hair onto a fine mesh net.

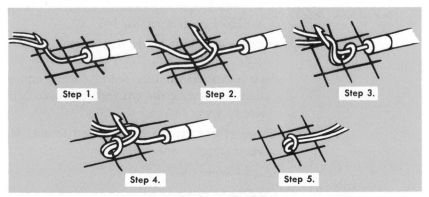

Step 1.   Step 2.   Step 3.   Step 4.   Step 5.

Single Knotting or Ventilating

knotting (or **ventilating**): the process by which hair is attached to the foundation in the creation of a wig or hairpiece; the actual knotting is also referred to as "ventilating." There are two types of knotting generally used, single and double. **Single knotting** fastens the hair to the net by a single knot. **Double knotting** uses a double knot.

knotted hair: hair that has been knotted to a wig or hairpiece foundation.

machine-made wig (or **wefted wig**): hair is sewn on to strips of material by machine, and then the strips of material are sewn onto a net by machine. The strips of material are also called "wefts."

mesh: an open weave foundation used in wig and hairpiece construction.

mixing: the intermingling of hair of different shades or lengths.

net (or **netting**): See mesh.

refined hair: oriental hair, being coarse in texture, is often chemically treated to make it more workable and usable.

semi-handmade wig: the front of this wig is handmade and the top and back are machine made.

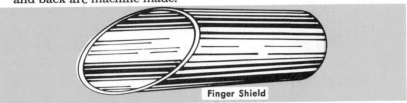

Finger Shield

shield (finger shield): a long, pointed metal cap, worn to protect the finger from the needle—used in a similar manner to a thimble. It is used to work in difficult wig areas.

smocking: a length of weft sewn in triangles, diamonds or loops in order to create the flat, airy base of a hairpiece.

spring (wig spring): spring inserted into a wig or hairpiece foundation to hold the foundation close to the head.

stretch base wig: a wig cap (foundation) made of elastic material that stretches to fit various size heads.

styrofoam: a lightweight plastic foam used for a wig block; recommended for storing wigs.

switch: a long length of wefted hair mounted with a loop on the end; usually constructed with three stem strands to provide flexibility in styling.

synthetic hair: artificially produced hair fibers used in the manufacture of wigs and hairpieces.

Syrian hair: a mixture of angora and yak hair.

T-pin: a pin resembling the letter "T." It is used to secure the hairpiece to the block. It is also called a "block point" or "wig point."

topper: a hairpiece, generally made on a round or oval base, designed for use on the top of the head.

tuck: reducing the size of the wig cap by folding the netting into a tuck formation and sewing the fold together.

turning (root): the process by which hair cuttings or combings are arranged in order so that all root ends are together and the imbrications face in the same direction.

ventilate: See knotting.

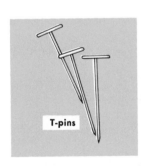

T-pins

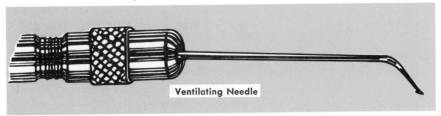

Ventilating Needle

ventilating needle: a miniature crocheting needle made of spring steel and used in attaching hair to a foundation.

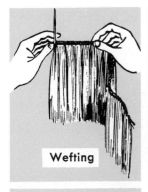

Wefting

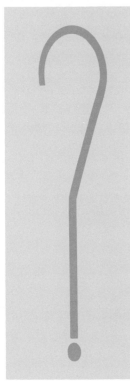

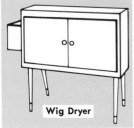

Wig Dryer

weft: an artificial section of woven (or sewn) hair used for practice work or as a substitute for natural hair.

wefted wig (machine made): a wig made of wefts of hair sewn into a wig base.

wefting: the art of weaving, or sewing, hair strands side by side to form a length of hair,

wig dryers: wig cabinet dryers used for drying wigs and hairpieces. They provide regulated heat and can dry many wigs and hairpieces at one time.

wiglet: a hairpiece with a flat base which is used to extend the area of hair.

yak: a long-haired ox of Tibet and Central Asia. It has long, coarse, silvery hair which is used in the manufacture of wigs.

REVIEW QUESTIONS

1. Give at least three reasons which might induce a person to wear a wig or hairpiece.
2. What four areas of knowledge are required by the cosmetologist in order to give the best possible wig service?
3. In what three ways do the quality of wigs vary?
4. Of what four types of materials are wigs usually made?
5. How can one distinguish between synthetic and human hair?
6. Why is it important to always work with the proper sized block?
7. In what two ways are wigs made?
8. How is the patron's hair prepared before her wig measurements are taken?
9. If it becomes necessary to shrink a wig, how is this best accomplished?
10. What treatment should be given before human hair wigs can be tinted?
11. How often should a wig be dry-cleaned?
12. What are switches?
13. What are wiglets?
14. What are bandeau type hairpieces?
15. How long will a style set last on a synthetic wig?
16. Will wearing a synthetic wig cause damage to the wearer's natural hair?
17. Which type of synthetic fiber is best suited for wigs and hairpieces?
18. How will the color of a modacrylic fiber wig react to sunlight?
19. How does the weight of a modacrylic wig compare to a human hair wig of the same quality?
20. Define the following: a) turning; b) hackling.

CHAPTER 13

BLOW CURLING AND WAVING

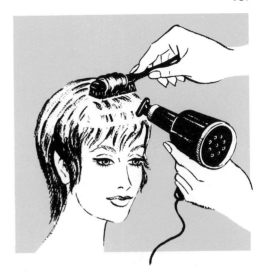

INTRODUCTION

The popularity of blow waving and curling has grown tremendously in recent years. Because it helps to create free and natural effects, and is timesaving, blow waving and curling has special appeal to both cosmetologists and patrons. However, like all hairstyling, pre-planning and a step-by-step development of the design are required.

To be successful, you must master the proper techniques in the use of combs, brushes and blowers, in order to produce good wave and curl formations.

Better natural waves and curls are produced with hair that has a natural wave, rather than with straight hair.

Caution. Blow waving and curling should be done with caution on permanently waved hair, to avoid damage to the permanent.

IMPLEMENTS

Use metal combs and cushioned metal, bristle brushes during the blow waving and curling procedure. Metal instruments concentrate the heat on the hair where it is most needed.

Caution. Rubber combs and some bristle brushes **should not be used** because they cannot withstand the intense heat coming out of the blower.

REMINDER. The procedures given here are different ways to perform comb, brush and blower techniques. However, your instructor's method is equally correct.

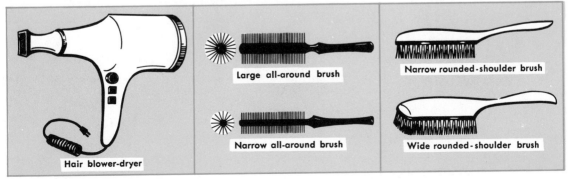

Hair blower-dryer

Large all-around brush

Narrow all-around brush

Narrow rounded-shoulder brush

Wide rounded-shoulder brush

BRUSH BLOW CURLING A SHORT HAIRSTYLE

OBJECTIVE

To create a natural looking, easy-to-wear, informal style on short hair with brush and blower.

PROCEDURE

Shampoo and towel dry the hair. When necessary, redampen it with spray-on setting lotion. During styling, comb the hair free of all tangles.

1. Pre-plan the style. Start at the crown or top of the head, as desired. Section the hair, pick up a wide strand, and comb through. (Fig. 1)

2. Bring the comb out to the hair ends and insert the brush. Brush through the strand, bringing the brush out to the ends. (Fig. 2)

3. Roll the hair with the brush, making a complete downward turn away from the face, until the brush rests on the scalp. (Fig. 3)

   Maintain the hair over the brush and start the blower. Direct the blower off the scalp and through the curl in a back-and-forth movement. (Fig. 3)

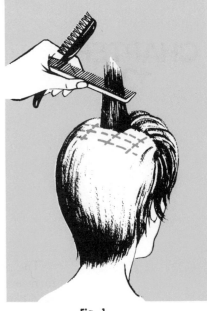

Fig. 1

When the hair section is completely dry, release the brush.

4. Continue making curls in the same manner, across the crown and back of the head. (Fig. 4) Shape the neckline curls with a comb, or make pin curls on the nape for a finished, close-to-the-head look.

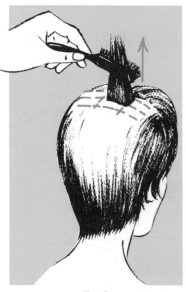

Fig. 2

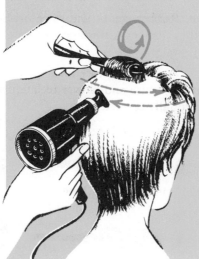

Fig. 3

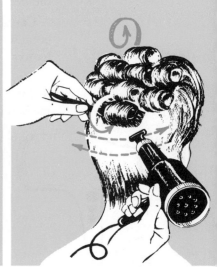

Fig. 4

5. For the front-top and bangs, make about 5 or 6 forward-directed curls, depending on the length of the hair. Part, pick up section, and comb. Place the brush in front of the section and make a complete turn forward, until the brush is resting on the scalp. Start blower and direct air stream off the scalp and through the curl in a back-and-forth movement, until it is dry. (Fig. 5)

6. Complete the front sections with five curls. (Fig. 6)

7. **Comb-out:** After curling the entire head, recomb the hair. Lift the hair and apply a small amount of teasing.

   The finished style: If desired, arrange the hair into a short, casual style. (Fig. 7). For a longer-lasting style, apply hair spray lightly.

8. **Alternate style:** Rearrange the hair into a new pattern. A short, casual style can feature a center part and "brow" bangs. (Fig. 8)

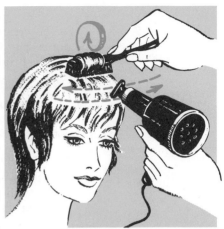

Fig. 5

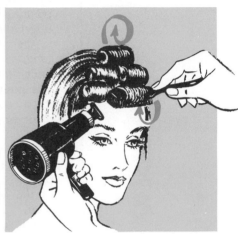

Fig. 6

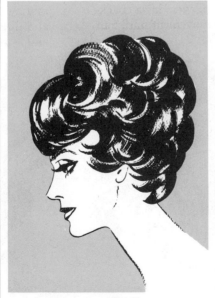

Fig. 7

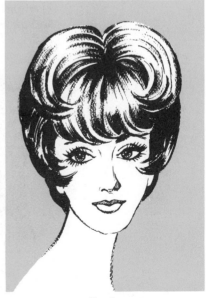

Fig. 8

THE WAVED BACK "FLIP"

OBJECTIVE

To create a loose wave effect for a long hairstyle by using the comb, brush and blower.

PROCEDURE

Shampoo, towel dry, re-dampen the hair with setting lotion and comb free of tangles.

1. When forming the first ridge and wave, carefully comb through the hair, shaping it as in fingerwaving. Starting at the right side, insert the metal comb into the hair, turn the comb with teeth pointing slightly upward, and direct the hair with the comb to the right, forming a ridge. (Fig. 1.) Push the comb under the ridge and hold in this position. Use the blower in a back-and-forth movement until hair is dry.

2. After the first ridge and wave formation has been completed, start the second ridge at the left side, working toward the right. Use the metal comb in the same manner, except that the ridge is directed toward the left. Use the blower in a back-and-forth movement until hair is dry. (Fig. 2)

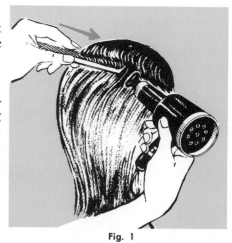

Fig. 1

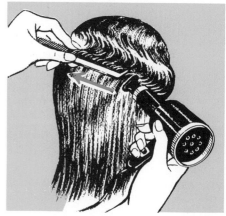

Fig. 2

3. Develop the third wave formation in the same manner and direction as the first ridge and wave. (Fig. 3)

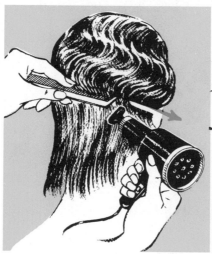

Fig. 3

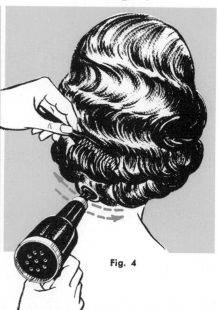

Fig. 4

4. Upon completion of the three ridges and wave formations, curl the nape hair with a brush into 2 or 3 rows to form a flip. (Fig. 4)

   Retrace and blow wave or curl through the entire style to assure complete dryness of the hair.

5. **Comb - out:** Complete the hairstyle with a high pompadour, waved at the back and curled at the nape area, to achieve a loose, flip-ends effect. (Fig. 5)

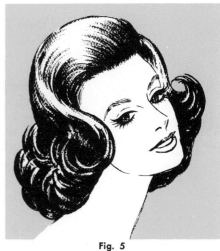

Fig. 5

THE PAGE BOY STYLE

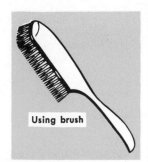

Using brush

OBJECTIVE

To create a smooth crown and page boy style with brush and blower.

PROCEDURE

1. Comb and shape the entire crown area, ending in a wave formation at the back of the ears. Form a row of upward directed curls at the end of the wave. Roll the curls over the brush and blow dry. (Fig. 1)

2. When creating the **Page Boy**, form two rows of downward curls below these curls. (Step 1). Pick up wide strands for each curl with the comb and hold between index and middle fingers. Place brush under the curl, near the scalp, and slide through hair to the ends. Roll under in a complete circle toward the scalp. (Fig. 2)

3. Use blower in an over-and-under, back-and-forth movement to dry each curl.

   The entire lower section of the hair should be curled and blower dried in the same manner. (Fig. 3)

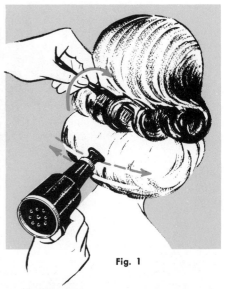

Fig. 1

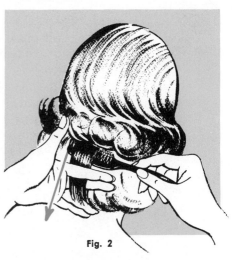

Fig. 2

4. To finish the style with a **Page Boy** effect, smooth and brush the lower section of hair under with a styling brush. The hair should be brushed over the palm of the hand, using a half-circular movement. Incorporate the fullness of the two rows of curls into a single, full formation. (Fig. 4)

5. **Comb-out:** The page boy with a high side waved pompadour and shoulder length hair is suitable for all occasions. (Fig. 5)

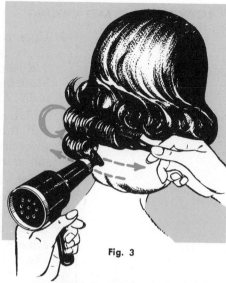

Fig. 3

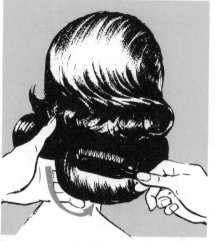

Fig. 4

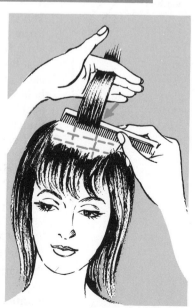

Fig. 5

HIGH CROWN POMPADOUR

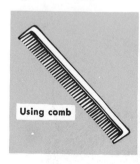

Using comb

OBJECTIVE

To create a high top with a comb and blower.

PROCEDURE

Shampoo, towel dry the hair, and redampen it with setting lotion.

1. Beginning at the crown, pick up a wide section of hair with a metal comb, ribbon and smooth strand to the ends. (Fig. 1)

2. Roll the hair firmly over with the comb, making a complete turn. The comb should be parallel to the scalp, but not resting heavily on it. (Fig. 2)

Fig. 1

Direct the blower away from the scalp in a back-and-forth motion, until the curl is completely dry. (Fig. 3)

3. Follow the same procedure in the formation of all the curls on the top of the head. (Fig. 4)

4. Respray each strand lightly before rolling into a curl. Continue the rolling process to form complete, firm curls. Blow each curl until it is thoroughly dried. (Fig. 5)

5. The completed curling formation contains 6 or 7 large curls, depending on the length and bulk of the hair.
   The rest of the hair is curled in the same manner as for the **Page Boy** style.

6. **Comb-out.** The high pompa-

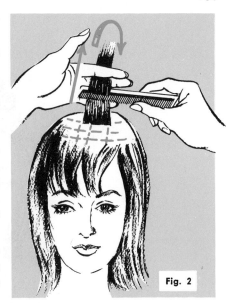

Fig. 2

dour is swept to the left side, creating a wave effect, and blended into a **Page Boy** style. (Fig. 6)

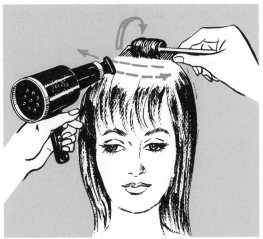

Fig. 3

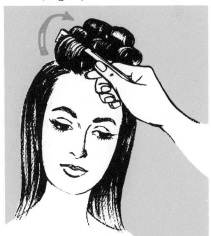

Fig. 4

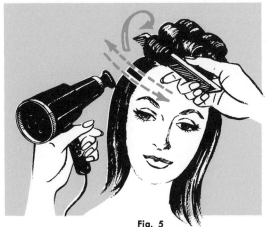

Fig. 5

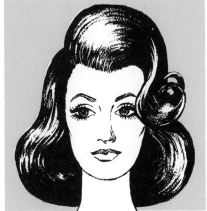

Fig. 6

ALTERNATE HAIR STYLE

POMPADOUR WITH FLIPPED HAIR ENDS

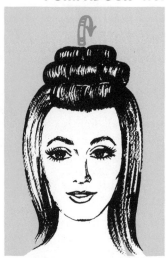

Top Pattern: Hair ends are flipped up with brush and blower.

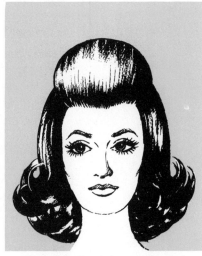

Comb-out: Top hair may be tied below the crown with a clamp or held with velvet or silk ribbon.

REVIEW QUESTIONS

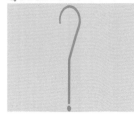

1. Why does blow waving and curling appeal to cosmetologists and patrons?

2. What techniques must be mastered in order to produce good wave and curl formations?

3. In what type of hair are better natural waves produced?

4. Why is the use of metal instruments preferred for the blow waving procedure?

5. Why should the use of rubber combs be avoided during blow waving?

CHAPTER 14

PERMANENT WAVING

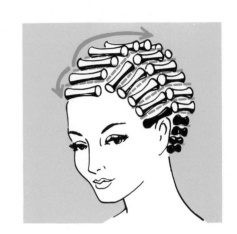

SHORT HISTORY

A crude system of permanent waving was practiced by the early Egyptians and Romans. The first real progress in permanent waving was made in 1905, when Charles Nessler invented the heat permanent waving machine.

Spiral Permanent Wave

The **spiral permanent wave** was the first method used. It involved winding the hair from the scalp to the ends and was suitable only for long hair.

Croquignole Permanent Wave

The **croquignole permanent wave** was introduced in 1926 to meet the needs of short hair. It required that the hair be wound from the hair ends towards the scalp. The hair could be formed into waves with end curls.

Combination Permanent Wave

A **combination** (spiral and croquignole) **permanent wave** soon came into vogue. The crown of the head was given a **spiral wave** to take care of the longer hair, while the rest of the head received a **croquignole wave**.

Pre-Heated Method

In 1931, the **pre-heat method** of permanent waving was introduced. The procedure was the same as the croquignole method with the difference being the source of heat. Unlike the machine method, the heaters were heated by means of electricity, disconnected from the machine, and then clamped over the prepared curls.

Machineless Method

Another advance in permanent waving was the **machineless method**, which was publicly introduced in 1932. This method required no electrical wires or machines. The heat was obtained through the use of chemical pads.

COLD WAVING
(Permanent Waving)

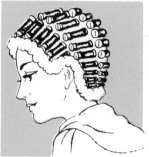

Cold waving was first introduced in California in 1938 and 1939. However, by 1940, the nationwide promotion of cold waving got underway.

Why Cold Waving Is So Called

Since cold waving employs no heat and is given at room temperature, the manufacturers had to find a suitable name to distinguish this chemical method of permanent waving from the heat method, and so the name of cold waving was adopted. Compared to heat permanent waving, cold waving has the following advantages:

1. It is relatively inexpensive, as no high priced equipment is necessary.

2. It is more comfortable to the patron, because no heavy heating clamps attached to curlers are necessary.

Term "Perm" Is Now Popular

Modern permanent waving is performed solely by the cold waving method and the words "Perm" and "Permanent" are now popularly used to indicate this service.

Progress In Cold Waving

From its beginning, cold waving has made considerable progress in materials and techniques used. Both cosmetologists and chemists have contributed many improvements to the cold waving methods in use today. For best results, it is always important that cosmetologists follow carefully manufacturers' directions.

Today, cold waving is the accepted method of permanently waving nearly all types of hair. Exceptions are persons who may be allergic to the waving lotion and those whose hair does not take a cold wave satisfactorily.

PRINCIPAL ACTIONS IN COLD WAVING

Cold waving is a system of permanent waving involving two major actions on the hair, namely:

1. Physical action
   a) The wrapping of hair around rods
2. Chemical action
   a) Processing—softening of the hair
   b) Neutralization—rehardening the hair into its new shape

Knowing just what takes place as the hair is wrapped around the rods, the chemical action of the cold waving lotion when applied to the hair, and how the neutralizer rehardens the hair in its newly formed position, is vital to successful cold waving.

Physical Actions
Wrapping

This physical action consists of wrapping the hair around the rods without stretching and with an absolute minimum of tension. By being so wrapped, the hair can expand when completely saturated by the permanent wave solution during processing.

Chemical Actions

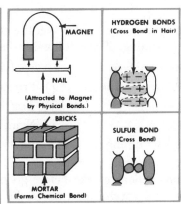

Hair develops and maintains its natural form by means of physical and chemical cross-bonds in the cortical layer, which hold the hair fibers in position and give the hair its strength and firmness. These physical (hydrogen) and chemical (sulfur) bonds must be broken before the shape or contour of the hair can be changed. For additional information on the chemistry of cold waving, see **Chemistry Chapter.**

Processing

The physical bonds are much the weaker of the two types of bonds and are easily broken by the shampooing and rinsing processes. However, the chemical action of the permanent waving lotion is required to break the chemical bonds and thus soften the hair. This chemical action permits rearrangement of the hair's inner structure so that it can assume the form of the curlers around which it is wound.

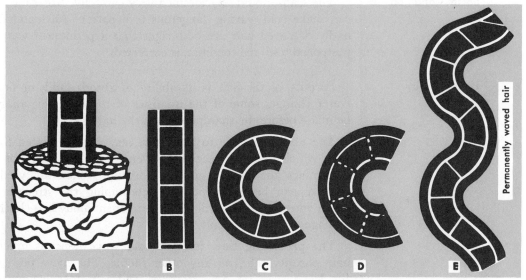

A. Each hair strand is composed of many polypeptide chains. This series of illustrations shows the behavior of one such chain, relative to an adjacent chain.

B. Hair before processing: A single polypeptide chain being held together with chemical cross bonds (links) which give hair its strength and firmness.

C. Hair wound on rod. The hair bends to the curvature and size of the rod.

D. During processing, waving lotion breaks the chemical bonds (links), permitting the hair to adjust to the curvature of the rod while in this softened condition.

E. The neutralizer re-forms the chemical bonds (links) and rehardens the hair, thus creating the permanent wave.

Neutralizing

After the hair has assumed the desired shape, it must be chemically neutralized so that the hydrogen and sulfur cross-bonds in the cortical layer are re-formed. This action also rehardens the hair into its newly curved form. When this action is completed, the hair is unwrapped from the rods and assumes its newly curled formation.

BASIC REQUIREMENTS

Before attempting to give a cold wave, the cosmetologist must have a thorough understanding of the following basic requirements:

a) Scalp and hair analysis f) Applying waving lotion
b) Hair sectioning patterns g) Processing
c) Chemical solutions h) Test curls
d) Curling rods i) Neutralizing
e) Blocking and wrapping j) Safety measures

Scalp And Hair Analysis

A very important action to take before giving a permanent wave is to make a **correct** and **careful analysis** of the patron's scalp and hair condition. The intelligent and professional approach is to learn all the pertinent facts about the patron, such as:

1. Scalp condition 4. Hair elasticity
2. Hair porosity 5. Hair density
3. Hair texture 6. Hair length

Scalp Condition

The scalp should be examined very carefully. Abrasions on the scalp can make cold waving dangerous to a patron. An irritated scalp and badly damaged hair are both signs that a permanent wave should be postponed until the condition is corrected.

Hair Porosity

Porosity of the hair is its ability to absorb fluids or liquids. Since water changes some of the qualities of the hair, this analysis should be made before the shampoo, when the hair is dry.

The ability of hair to absorb is very closely related to the speed with which hair can receive a given fluid. This speed of absorption determines the degree of hair porosity. When analyzed properly, porosity can be a measure of determining the strength of waving lotion you should use. Unless pre-permanent analysis is closely observed, damaged hair may result.

The **processing** time for any cold wave depends much more on **hair porosity** than on any other factor. The more porous the hair, the less processing time it takes, and a milder waving solution is required. **The degree at which hair absorbs the cold waving lotion is related to its porosity, regardless of texture.**

Hair porosity is **affected** by such factors as the patron's health, climate, altitude, humidity, excessive exposure to sun and wind, and the continued use of harsh shampoos, tints and lighteners.

Porosity Classified

Before giving a cold wave, determine the degree of porosity. Porosity may be classified as:

Good porosity—hair with the cuticle layer raised from the hair shaft. Hair of this type can absorb moisture or chemicals in average time.

Moderate porosity (normal hair)—hair that is less porous than hair with good porosity.

Poor porosity (resistant hair)—hair with the cuticle layer lying close to the hair shaft. This type of hair absorbs waving lotion more slowly and usually requires a **longer processing time.**

Extreme porosity (tinted, lightened or damaged hair)—hair that has been made **extremely porous** by various hair treatments and abuse. It absorbs the lotion very quickly and requires the shortest processing time. Use only mild or a very mild lotion for such hair.

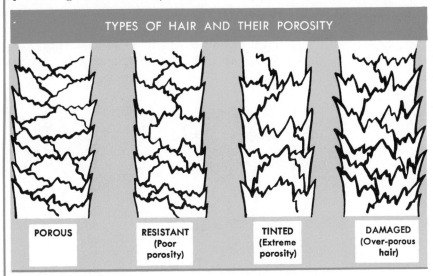

TYPES OF HAIR AND THEIR POROSITY

POROUS

RESISTANT
(Poor
porosity)

TINTED
(Extreme
porosity)

DAMAGED
(Over-porous
hair)

Over-porous hair—a result of over-processing. Such hair is extremely damaged, dry, fragile and brittle. Until the hair has been reconditioned, or removed by cutting, **it should not receive a permanent wave.**

Porosity Test

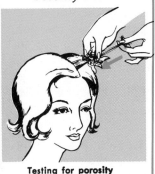

Testing for porosity

In order to test accurately for porosity, use three different areas: front hairline, in front of ears, and near the crown.

Grasp a small strand of dry hair and comb smoothly. Hold the ends firmly with the thumb and index finger of one hand and slide the fingers of the other hand from the ends toward the scalp. If the fingers do not slide easily, or if the hair ruffles up as your fingers slide down the strand, **the hair is porous.**

The more ruffles formed, the more porous is the hair. The less ruffles formed, the less porous is the hair.

If the fingers slide easily and no ruffles are formed, the cuticle layer lays close to the hair shaft. This type of hair is least porous, is most **resistant** and will require a **longer processing time.**

---

*Other Ways To
Test For Porosity*

1. **Cutting dry hair with scissors.** If the scissors cut through dry hair very easily, meeting little resistance, **that hair is porous.**

2. **Cupping the hair.** If the hair is squeezed and released in the hand and feels completely soft, showing little or no spring, **that hair is porous.**

3. **Wetting the hair** at the shampoo bowl. If the hair wets easily and thoroughly with the initial spray of water, **that hair is porous.**

4. **Drying the hair under dryer.** If hair takes longer than usual to dry, **it is porous.** The faster the hair dries, the less porosity it has.

Hair Texture

Hair texture refers to the individual size of the hair strand and its degree of coarseness or fineness. **The texture and porosity are judged together in determining the processing time.** Although porosity is the most important of the two, texture does have a part in judging processing time. Coarse hair that is very porous will process faster than fine hair that is **not** porous.

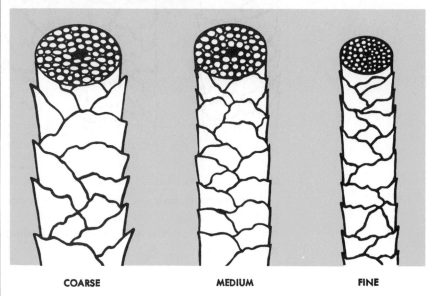

COARSE   MEDIUM   FINE

Hair texture should also be a factor when deciding the size of the **wave pattern.** The texture and density of the patron's hair must be taken into consideration when planning a hairstyle.

Variations in hair texture are due to the following:

1. **Diameter of the hair shaft:** coarse, medium, fine or very fine
2. **Feel of the hair:** harsh, soft or wiry

Hair Elasticity

Hair elasticity is a very important factor to consider when giving a permanent wave. Elasticity is the ability of the hair to stretch and contract. All hair is elastic, but its elasticity ranges from very good to poor. Without elasticity, there will be **no curl in the hair.** The greater the degree of elasticity, the longer the wave will remain in the hair, because less relaxation of the hair occurs.

The elastic qualities of hair will determine the success of a cold wave.

1. **Hair with very good elasticity** will produce a resilient curl.
2. **Hair with good elasticity** will produce a curl with average resilience.

3. **Hair with fairly good elasticity** will produce a slightly less resilient curl.

4. **Hair with poor elasticity**, also known as **limp** hair, will result in a very small amount of resiliency in the curl.

Testing For Elasticity

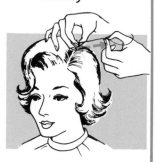

A simple test for elastic qualities of the hair. Take a single dry hair and hold it between the thumb and forefinger of each hand. **Slowly** stretch it between them. The further it can be stretched without breaking, the more elastic is the hair. If the elasticity is good, **the** hair slowly contracts after stretching. Hair with **poor** elasticity will **break** quickly and easily when stretched.

Normal dry hair is capable of being stretched about one-fifth its length, and will spring back when released. However, wet hair can be stretched 40 to 50% of its length. Porous hair will stretch more than hair with poor porosity.

Poor Elasticity

Signs of poor elasticity are limpness, sponginess and hair that tangles easily.

Limp hair will **not** develop a firm, strong cold wave. This hair requires a **smaller** diameter rod than hair having good elasticity and special waving lotions must be used.

Hair will change its elasticity from time to time. Usually, the over-porous hair loses its elasticity faster than non-porous hair. This change may be temporary, due to humidity and temperature, the type of shampoo used, the amount of hair lacquer or spray-net used, and drying action of wind and sun.

Hair Density

The density of the hair is the amount of hair strands per square inch on the scalp. Density has nothing to do with the hair's texture. **Smaller blockings** (sub-sections) and **larger rods** are often required for thickly growing hair. However, if the **hair is thin** per square inch, **smaller blockings** and **smaller** (**thinner**) **rods** are required in order to form a good wave pattern close to the head.

Avoid large blockings on thin hair growth, as the strain may cause breakage.

Hair Length

Hair length is another important factor that must be considered. Waving hair of average length presents no real problem. However, if the patron wears her hair six inches or longer, a number of waving and wrapping problems may be created. Because of its excessive length, the hair cannot be wrapped close enough to develop a good, strong wave pattern near the scalp. In addition, the extra pull of the excessive hair weight may pull the curl out of the hair very **quickly**. Therefore, in selecting a hairstyle, it is very important to consider carefully hair length, texture, elasticity and density.

CURLING RODS

Rod Sizes

Proper selection of curling rods is essential for successful permanent waving.

The size of the rods control the shape of the hair during the waving process. Rods are made of a canvas and plastic composition, and they vary in diameter, length, and design.

1. Diameter is the distance through the center of the rod.

2. Circumference is the distance around the rod, which is 3.1416 times the diameter of a rod. The circumference is the important factor in determining the size of the wave or curl formation.

Curling rods are available in various **lengths**: long, medium and short ($3\frac{1}{2}''$ to $1\frac{3}{4}''$ in length).

They also come in varying **thicknesses**. These range in diameter from large to very thin (size $\frac{3}{4}''$ to $\frac{1}{8}''$).

Securing The Rods

All rods must have some means of securing the hair and the rod into the desired position to prevent the curl from unwinding.

Type Of Rods

Concave Rods

The two types of rods in general use are the concave and straight.

Concave rods are usually thinner in diameter than the straight rods. They are formed with a smaller circumference in the center area, which gradually increases to their largest circumference at both ends.

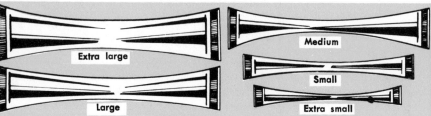

Extra large

Medium

Large

Small

Extra small

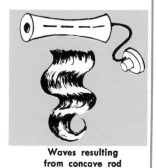

Waves resulting from concave rod

Concave rods are used when a definite wave pattern, close to the head, is desired.

When hair is wound on a rod, the outside hair of the winding forms a larger curl or wave than the hair next to the rod. This creates a tighter curl, or ringlet, at the hair ends, which gradually becomes slightly wider as it nears the scalp.

Straight Rods

Straight rods are made so that their circumference and diameter are almost the same throughout their entire length. They may, however, taper very slightly toward the center.

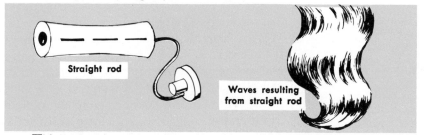

Straight rod

Waves resulting from straight rod

This type of rod usually creates the same size curl throughout the entire hair strand.

Large, straight rods are usually employed to give a "body wave" or "style wave." They permit the formation of a strong permanent with a large enough wave to be dressed into any hairstyle desired.

CHEMICAL SOLUTIONS

For success in permanent waving, it is absolutely essential that the curling rods and lotion be properly selected. The chemical compounds contained within the waving lotion will have an important influence on the procedure to be followed in the waving process.

Waving Lotions

Cold waving lotions in general use today have as their basic ingredient ammonium thioglycolate, commonly referred to as "thio," that permanently changes the structure of the hair. This compound is prepared by combining ammonia and thioglycolic acid. Other ingredients included in the waving lotion may be lanolin and its derivatives, wetting agents, proteins, and conditioners. Excess ammonia is added to make the solution alkaline.

Preconditioning

Over-porous or damaged hair may require a preconditioning treatment before the application of waving lotion. Special fillers that contain protein are now available which condition the hair and equalize its porosity. Some fillers also contain lanolin and cholesterol, which may help to protect the hair against the harshness of the cold waving lotion.

Conditioners

The alkaline permanent waving solution has a tendency to remove natural oils from the hair, causing it to dry out rapidly through loss of moisture. Mineral oils, lanolin, or lanolin derivatives are added to the waving lotion, or may be used in a separate application to replace natural oils. By the conditioner remaining in the hair after the lotion has been rinsed out, the moisture content is somewhat preserved, and the feel and appearance of the hair are improved.

Strengths Of Waving Lotions

The strength of the waving lotion can be adjusted by either increasing its pH (alkalinity) or by increasing the amount of active ingredient (ammonium thioglycolate). To adjust the pH of the lotion, the ammonia content is either increased or decreased, not to exceed pH 9.6, which is a strong solution.

Most manufacturers of cold waving products market three or more strengths to be used as follows:

1. **Damaged** or **porous hair**—weak or mild strength
2. **Normal hair** (having good porosity)—average strength
3. **Resistant hair** (less porosity)—a stronger strength
4. **Over-lightened** or **tinted hair** (over-porous)—extra mild strength

Important reminder. Manufacturers of cold waving products are constantly improving their formulas. It is advisable to follow their directions explicitly.

Neutralizers

Neutralizers contain peroxide, lanolin and other special ingredients. They come in various forms, such as liquids, powders and crystals. Depending on the method of application, they may have a thick consistency and may have to be diluted. **Conditioners** are often incorporated in the prepared liquid neutralizer to give some protection to the hair.

SECTIONING AND BLOCKING

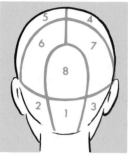

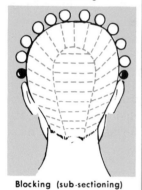

Sectioning

Blocking (sub-sectioning)

Wave Formation

SUGGESTED HAIR BLOCKINGS AND ROD SIZES

Sectioning is dividing the head into uniform working panels.

Blocking, also known as **sub-sectioning,** is the subdividing of the panels into uniform individual rectangular rod sections. Uniform wave patterns depend on the following:

1. Uniformly arranged sections
2. Equally subdivided sections (blockings)
3. Clean and uniform partings (length and width)

The size of the blockings is determined by the diameter of the rods, the density and texture of the hair.

Depending on the pattern used in hair sectioning, the number of hair blockings may vary with each patron.

The **average blocking** for a standard wave should match the diameter (size) of the rod being used. However, the length of the blocking can be a little shorter (about one-half inch) but no longer than the length of the rod. If the rod is shorter than the length of the blocking, the hair will not wave evenly.

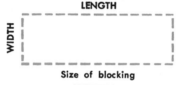

LENGTH denotes span of blocking.

WIDTH refers to the depth of the blocking. Small or large blockings usually refer to its width.

The **size of the rods and blockings** determines the size of the wave formation. **Processing time** has no bearing on the size of the wave pattern. Thicker hair with good elasticity gives a deeper wave formation. Thinner hair, usually fine in texture, gives a more shallow wave. The loss or increase of elasticity also affects the depth of the wave pattern.

Although the hair elasticity and texture must both be considered in the choice of rods, the texture should be the determining factor.

Coarse hair—good elasticity. Thickly growing hair requires smaller (narrower) blockings and larger rods to permit better arrangements for a definite wave pattern.

Medium hair—average elasticity. Medium or average textured hair requires smaller blockings and medium size rods.

Fine hair—poor elasticity. Thin hair requires smaller blockings and smaller (thinner) rods to prevent strain or breakage and to form a good wave pattern close to the head.

Lightened or tinted hair—very poor elasticity. Use smaller hair sub-sections and larger rods. If the lightened or tinted hair is fine in texture, use smaller hair sub-sections and medium rods.

Hair in nape area. Use smaller sub-sections and smaller rods.

Long hair. To permanently wave hair longer than six inches, wrap it smoothly and close to the scalp in smaller blockings. The use of smaller blockings permits the waving lotion and neutralizer to penetrate more easily and thoroughly.

PATTERNS FOR SECTIONING AND BLOCKING

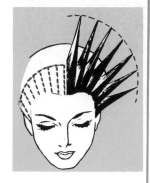

By knowing the texture, elasticity, porosity and condition of the patron's hair, the cosmetologist is better able to judge how the hair is to be sectioned, blocked, which rods to use, and where the application of waving lotion should begin. (**Be guided by your instructor.**)

> **REMINDER**
>
> The size of the rods and blockings determines the size of the curl or wave pattern. Processing time has no bearing on the size of the wave pattern.

Four popular blocking (sub-sectioning) patterns:

1. Single Halo
2. Double Halo (Double Horseshoe)
3. Straight Back
4. Dropped Crown

These are known by other names in various areas of the country.

The following patterns are suggested blockings. However, your instructor may suggest different patterns, which are equally correct.

Single Halo

The **Single Halo** wrap is one commonly used for average size heads.

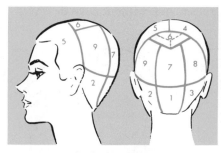

Sectioning diagram   Blocking (sub-sectioning) pattern

Double Halo (Double Horseshoe)

The **Double Halo** wrap is usually used for larger size heads.

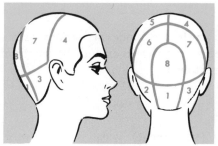

Sectioning diagram   Blocking (sub-sectioning) pattern

Straight Back

The **Straight Back** wrap is used when it is desired to create a soft, full and high style effect, directed off the face.

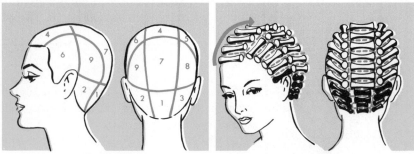

Sectioning diagram   Blocking (sub-sectioning) pattern

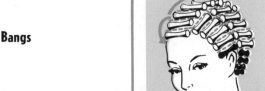

Bangs

To create **bangs** on the forehead, wrap the first two top curls in a forward direction.

Dropped Crown

The **Dropped Crown** wrap is usually used for longer hair and for a smooth crown effect. As indicated in the illustration, no curls are wrapped in the crown area. This permits the long hair in this area to be combed smooth, without curls or waves.

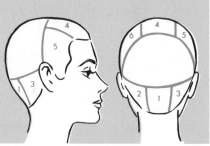

Sectioning diagram   Blocking (sub-sectioning) pattern

If necessary, the ends of the dropped crown area may be wrapped to blend with nape area. (Be guided by your instructor.)

Pick-Up Curls

Pick-up curls are made at various areas, such as the nape and over the ears, in order to extend the length of time between complete waving treatments.

Body Waves

A **body** (permanent) **wave** is given with extra large rods solely for the purpose of adding slight "body" or wave pattern to the hair.

WINDING OR WRAPPING THE HAIR

To form a uniform wave with a firm ridge, you must wrap the hair smoothly and neatly on each rod, without stretching the hair. It is not stretched because the penetration of waving lotion causes the hair to expand. Tight wrapping or stretching interferes with this expansion and prevents penetration of the waving lotion and neutralizer, resulting in hair breakage.

End Papers

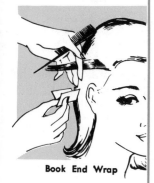

Book End Wrap

Porous end papers are very important aids in the proper wrapping or winding of the hair around curling rods. Properly used, end papers may help in the formation of smooth, even curls and waves. They help to eliminate "fishhooks" and minimize the danger of hair end breakage. They are especially important in helping to facilitate the wrapping of uneven hair length.

There are three methods of end paper application in general use in the practice of permanent waving. Each method may be equally effective, if properly used.

1. The book end paper wrap
2. The single end paper wrap
3. The double end paper wrap

Book End Paper Wrap

Hair should be moistened (not saturated) with a weak solution of the waving lotion in the area starting one-half inch from the scalp and up to one inch from the hair ends. However, water should be used instead of waving lotion while practicing and until the student has become proficient in the technique of winding or wrapping the hair.

Procedure

Step-by-step procedure for the book end paper wrap method.

Note: The blocking (sub-section) should not be wider than the rod is long. If it is, the hair will not wave evenly.

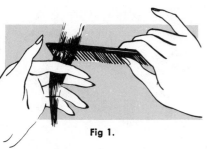

Fig 1.

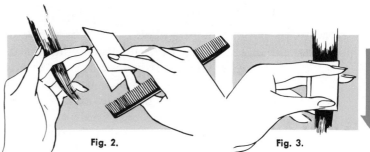

Fig. 2.

Fig. 3.

1. Part and comb sub-section up and out until all hair is evenly directed and distributed.

2. Hold strand between the index and middle fingers; fold and place the end paper over the strand, forming an envelope.

3. Hold the strand smoothly and evenly; slide the paper envelope a small fraction beyond the hair ends.

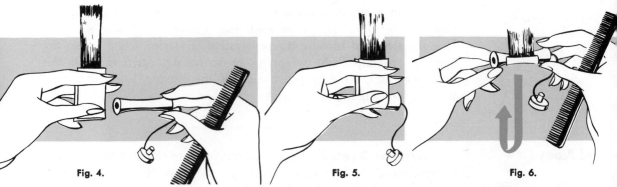

Fig. 4.   Fig. 5.   Fig. 6.

4. Pick up rod with the right hand. 5. Place the rod under the folded end paper, parallel to the parting. Draw end paper and rod toward hair ends until hair ends are visible above the rod. Start winding end paper and hair under and toward the scalp. 6. Wind the hair smoothly (without tension) to the scalp.

CAUTION. When wrapping hair, always avoid bulkiness on the rod. Bulkiness prevents the formation of a good curl because the hair cannot conform to the shape of the rod.

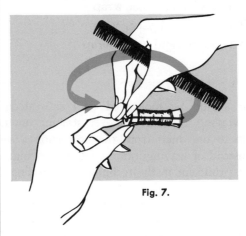

7. Fasten the rod band evenly across the wound hair at the top of the rod.

Fig. 7.

CAUTION. To prevent breakage the band should not cut into the hair or be twisted against the curl.

Placement Of Curl In Blocking

Regardless of the type or size of rod used, it should be placed slightly off its base in order to give a close-to-the-head permanent and to leave the hair easy to wave. Placing the rod slightly off its base helps to prevent the creation of excessive tension and hair breakage.

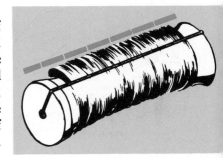

**Single End
Paper Wrap**

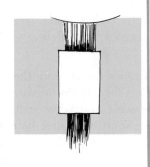

Hair preparation is the same as for Book End Paper Wrap.

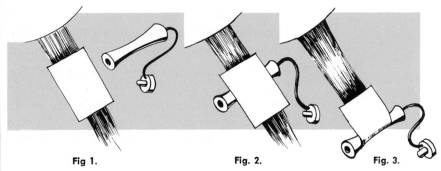

Fig 1.   Fig. 2.   Fig. 3.

Place the end paper on top of strand and hold it flat to prevent bunching. Fig. 1.

Place rod under the strand, holding it parallel with the parting; then draw the end paper and rod downward until hair ends are covered. Fig. 2.

Roll the end paper and strand under, using the thumb of each hand to keep the strand smooth. Fig. 3. Wind strand on the rod to the scalp without tension.

Fasten band at top of rod in the same manner as for Book End Paper Wrap.

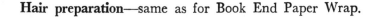

**Double End
Paper Wrap**

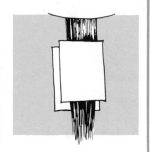

Hair preparation—same as for Book End Paper Wrap.

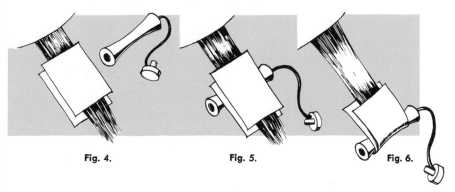

Fig. 4.   Fig. 5.   Fig. 6.

Place one end paper beneath the hair strand and the other on top. Fig. 4.

Place rod under double end papers, parallel with hair part. Draw both towards hair ends. Fig. 5.

Roll hair and end papers on roller to the scalp without tension. Fig. 6.

Wind the strand smoothly on the rod to the scalp without tension and fasten band at top of rod as for Book End Paper Wrap.

PRE-PERMANENT WAVE SHAMPOO

In order to help assure success, it is necessary that the hair be shampooed prior to permanent waving.

Dust, hair spray, hair lacquer, sebum and various cosmetics tend to accumulate on the hair between shampoos. Unless these are removed and the hair and scalp thoroughly cleansed, it will be extremely difficult to give a successful permanent.

The proper and even penetration of the waving lotion and the neutralizer are essential to successful permanent waving. If the waving lotion penetrates the hair evenly, the resulting curls and waves will be more uniform and manageable. Uneven or spottily curled hair is quite difficult to control and style. Even, longer-lasting waves can only be attained in clean hair.

Procedure

The procedure for the pre-permanent shampoo is somewhat different from that followed for the regular shampoo.

1. Use an **acid-balanced** or **mild shampoo,** one that will cleanse the hair without leaving a coating or film.

2. **Do not brush** the hair, as the patron's scalp may become sensitive or irritated.

3. **Do not massage** the scalp **vigorously,** to avoid irritating the scalp.

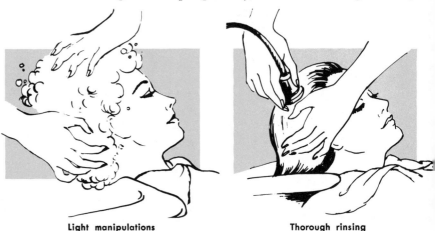

Light manipulations   Thorough rinsing

4. Use **extreme care in rinsing**, to make certain that all the shampoo is removed. A residue of shampoo could destroy the effectiveness of the waving lotion. Proper rinsing equalizes the porosity of the hair.

5. While the hair is still wet, comb it smoothly and carefully, to avoid irritating the scalp. Thoroughly examine the scalp and hair for any signs of scalp irritation or hair damage.

6. While the hair is still wet, carefully examine for signs of previous permanent. Any hair which indicates that it has recently received a wave could be in a weakened condition and should be treated with extreme caution to avoid hair damage.

TEST CURLS

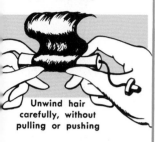

Unwind hair
carefully, without
pulling or pushing

Test curls help to determine in advance how the patron's hair will react to the cold waving process. A **test curl** gives the cosmetologist information on how to protect the patron's hair and how to obtain the best possible results.

Regular testing enables the cosmetologist to observe the following aspects of the hair:

a) Speed of wave formation
b) Overall picture of wave formation
c) Exact time when peak of wave formation has been reached
d) Resistant areas

Test curls may be given **before** or **while waving** the entire head.

Pre-Permanent Test Curl Method

Pre-permanent test curls should be given if the hair presents any problem, such as damage, poor texture or elasticity. If the patron has an illness, or if there is **any doubt in the mind of the cosmetologist** concerning the final results, pre-test curls are important.

Procedure

After the hair has been shampooed and towel dried, wrap two or three curls on the upper back of the head. Give each curl a complete treatment of varying strengths of the waving lotion. Time the action of the lotion and examine the curl according to manufacturer's directions. After neutralizing and rinsing the curls, analyze and record the results.

Test Curl-Wave Development Method

This procedure is part of the processing phase of a cold wave. Each head of hair is different. In fact, conditions may vary even on the same head of hair. A patron's hair will not always process in the same length of time. Neither will one type of curl always process in the same time on every head. **Curl-wave development should be tested:**

1. **Immediately after the last rod is secured.**
2. **Following the rewet application of lotion.**
3. **Every 30 seconds** thereafter **until wave formation has occurred.** Frequent testing for wave formation will prevent over-processing. While manufacturer's directions supply a general guide, the cosmetologist should carefully judge **individual** curl development.

Procedure

1. Thoroughly blot the waving solution from the curl to be tested.
2. Loosen the rod fastener. (Do not let the hair become loose or unravel on the rod. Hold it firmly with thumbs touching on the rod.)
3. Unwind the rod 1½ turns, without pulling on the strand. (Since the hair is in a softened condition, pulling or pushing the strand will spoil the test.) Permit the hair to relax into a firm "S" wave pattern without pushing or pulling at it.
4. If the curl has not reached the firm "S" pattern, rewind the test curl.

Continue testing for wave development at regular intervals (every 30 seconds is preferable) until the desired wave pattern has been reached. Test on different areas of the head each time. **Do not use the same curl for retesting.**

182

APPLICATION OF WAVING LOTION

Safety Measures

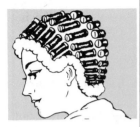

Protect Patron's Eyes

Applicator Bottle

Applying The Waving Lotion

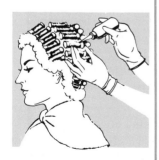

Safety measures protect the skin and scalp against chemical injury. The cosmetologist should wear **protective gloves,** or use a protective preparation to cover the hands.

For the **patron's safety,** apply protective cream around the hairline and neck, and cover area with a strip of cotton or neutralizing band. Use dry cotton pledgets or neutralizing band between curls to absorb any excess waving lotion. If cotton strips or the neutralizing bands become wet with lotion, remove, blot and replace with dry material. Be sure that the lotion does not drip on the skin or scalp. If this happens, absorb drips with cotton pledgets saturated with cold water or a neutralizer.

If the waving lotion gets into the patron's eye, rinse immediately with cold water or preparation recommended by your instructor, and then take patron to a doctor.

A **plastic bottle** with a nozzle makes the most efficient applicator. It dispenses liquid freely, yet permits good control. There is a minimum loss of lotion and a better distribution is achieved throughout the hair.

CAUTION. Bottles should be absolutely clean before being filled with waving lotion. Be certain that there are no traces of leftover chemicals in the bottle, since such leftover chemicals may weaken or spoil the waving lotion.

Pre-wrap wetting or moistening. Following shampooing and towel drying, moisten the hair with a weak solution of the waving lotion, to facilitate the wrapping procedure. Apply the lotion with a bottle applicator to an entire section at a time. Start about one-half inch from the scalp and extend the lotion to within one inch from the hair ends. To assure a complete and even distribution, apply the lotion from the top, and comb through the section from underneath using an upward motion.

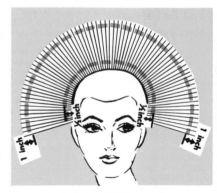

Apply lotion ½" from scalp to about 1" from hair ends.

Rewetting or saturation. After sub-sectioning and winding the curls over the entire head, the hair is ready for rewetting or complete saturation. This procedure is important and essential to assure complete penetration and processing of the entire hair shaft.

The lotion is thoroughly applied to each curl, following the same order as that employed in the pre-wetting step. It is most important to the success of the permanent that each curl be thoroughly and completely saturated.

CAUTION. Be careful not to disturb the wrapping or the placement of the curls by dragging the nozzle over the hair. Do not leave the patron alone while processing the hair. Do not interrupt the rewet or saturation step. Complete it as quickly as possible.

Processing Time

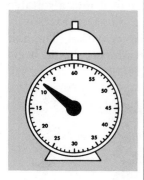

Processing time is the length of time required for the hair strands to absorb the waving lotion and complete the total rearrangement of the chemical bonds in the hair around the rod. The ability of the hair to absorb moisture may vary from time to time on the same individual, even while using the same lotions and procedures. A **record** of the previous processing time is desirable but should be used only as a guide. It is usually safe to anticipate the processing time to be **less** than that suggested by the manufacturer or a patron's previous record card.

The factors affecting processing time are the strength of the lotion; texture, porosity, length and condition of the hair; room temperature; patron's body heat and the working speed of the cosmetologist.

Resaturation Step

Resaturation step during the processing time. The lotion is applied in the same order as it is for the saturation step. Often, it is necessary to rewet all the rods a second time during the processing time. This may be due to the following:

1. Evaporation of the lotion or dryness of the hair
2. Hair poorly saturated by the cosmetologist
3. No wave development after the maximum time indicated by manufacturer
4. Improper selection of solution strength for the patron's hair
5. Failure to follow manufacturer's directions for a specific formula

A reapplication of the lotion will hasten the processing. Watch the wave development closely since **negligence may result in hair damage.**

Wave Pattern Formation

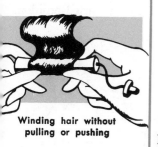

Winding hair without pulling or pushing

During the processing, the wave forms a deep-ridged pattern. The wave has reached its peak when it forms a firm letter "S". The size of the rod used determines the size of the "S" pattern. The time required to attain the proper firmness and depth of the "S" pattern governs the processing time.

The "S" pattern reaches a desirable peak only once. Shortly after the "S" is well formed, unless processing is stopped, the hair could become "frizzy." This indicates that the processing time has gone beyond its peak and the hair is **over-processed** and **damaged.**

Different conditions and textures of hair will form different wave patterns. Hair of **good** texture will show a firm, **strong** pattern, whereas hair that is **weak** or **fine** will **not** produce a firm pattern.

Over-Processing

Any lotion that can properly process the hair can also over-process it. Lotion left on the hair too long, beyond the best wave formation point, results in over-processing. Other causes of over-processing are the failure of the cosmetologist to make frequent test curls; or if they are made, the failure to judge them properly. **If neutralizer is used too sparingly,** the hair may continue to process, also causing over-processing.

Over-processed hair is easily detected. It is **very curly when wet, completely frizzy when dry** and **refuses to be combed into a suitable wave pattern.** The elasticity of the hair has been damaged excessively and the hair is unable to contract into the wave formation. The hair feels harsh after being dried. **Reconditioning treatments should begin immediately.**

Different Types Of Permanent Waved Hair

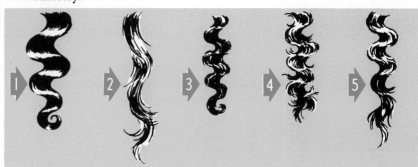

1. A good permanent wave looks like this. — 2. Under-processed curl. RESULT: Little or no wave. — 3. Over-processed curl. RESULT: Narrow waves when wet, no waves when dry. — 4. Porous ends over-processed. RESULT: Frizzy ends. — 5. Improper winding when hair ends are wound too tight. RESULT: No wave or curl at hair ends.

Under-Processing

Under-processing results in a limp or weak wave formation. The ridges are not well defined and the hair retains little or no wave formation. Under-processing may be corrected by giving one or two reconditioning treatments. After these treatments, rewrap the hair and apply a milder waving lotion, since the hair has already been softened somewhat. Watch the wave formation closely.

NEUTRALIZATION OF THE HAIR

The waving lotion produces the curl formation by rearranging the chemical bonds (links) in the cortex of the hair shaft into a new alignment. The rods hold the hair in this formation until it is "rehardened" or "fixed" by neutralization.

Preparation Before Neutralization

The neutralizer stops the action of the waving lotion, re-forms the chemical bonds and rehardens the hair in its newly curled position.

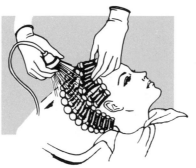
Rinsing waving lotion from the hair

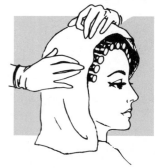
Towel blotting

Prior to the application of the neutralizer, most manufacturers require thorough rinsing with warm water to remove the waving lotion, followed by careful towel blotting of each curl to remove excess moisture. To obtain the best results from towel blotting, carefully press the towel with the fingers between each curl.

CAUTION. Do not rock or roll the rods while blotting. The hair is in a softened state and such movement may cause hair breakage.

Methods Of Neutralization

Neutralizers are packaged in the form of powders, liquids or crystals and must be prepared immediately before their use.

There are two methods of neutralizer application in general use: the **Direct** or **On-the-Rod Method** and the **Conventional** or **Splash-On Method.**

Direct Or On-The-Rod Method

Direct or **On-the-Rod Method** is also referred to as the **Applicator** or **Instant Method.** The neutralizer comes in two forms: ready-for-use and to-be-mixed.

1. **Ready-for-use neutralizer:** snip off tip of squeeze-applicator bottle and apply.
2. **Neutralizer to-be-prepared:** mix it according to manufacturer's directions, pour into the squeeze-applicator bottle and apply.

Procedure

Apply neutralizer directly to each curl in the same order as that followed in the application of the waving lotion. Start at the top center of the curl and apply in either direction; then apply to the bottom of the curl, making sure that each curl is thoroughly saturated. Repeat if necessary.

Note: A cotton pad saturated with neutralizer may be placed at the nape of the neck on the rim of the shampoo bowl, to assure that the neckline curls are in constant contact with the neutralizer.

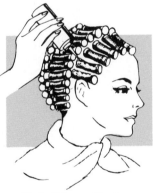
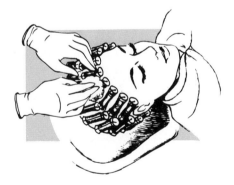

Neutralizing — Direct or
On-the-Rod Method

Neutralizing — Conventional
or Splash-On Method

Conventional Or Splash-On Method

Mix neutralizer with water in accordance with manufacturer's directions. Position patron at shampoo bowl in the same manner as for a shampoo.

Procedure

Using glass or plastic measuring cup, pour one-half of the neutralizer carefully over the curls, thoroughly saturating each curl. The neutralizer is caught in a plastic basin or pocket placed around the neck for this purpose.

Using large pads of cotton or sponge, reapply neutralizer, thoroughly saturating each curl. Repeat 2 or 3 times. (For removing neutralizer, see below.)

Methods For Removal Of Neutralizer

There are two general methods for removing neutralizers from the hair, whether it be the On-the-Rod or Splash-On Method that was used to apply the neutralizer. (Manufacturer's directions must be followed at all times.)

Method 1

After the neutralizer is thoroughly applied, allow it to remain in the hair for five to eight minutes. Rinse the hair with tepid water and follow it with a cool water rinse to reharden the hair. Lightly towel-blot the hair. Remove the rods carefully and proceed to set the hair.

Method 2

After the neutralizer is thoroughly applied, allow it to set for five to eight minutes. Carefully remove the rods without stretching the hair and apply the balance of the neutralizer. Permit an additional minute of neutralizing time and then rinse with cool water. Proceed with setting the hair.

UNLESS THE HAIR IS NEUTRALIZED THOROUGHLY AND CORRECTLY, THE COLD WAVE WILL NOT BE SUCCESSFUL AND ALL THE WORK DONE WILL BE WASTED. IN ADDITION, THE HAIR MAY BE DAMAGED.

**Examine Scalp And
Analyze Hair**

**Shampoo For
A Cold Wave**

**Shaping Suggestions
For A Cold Wave**

Shaping Precautions

Examine scalp. If patron's scalp has cuts, abrasions or scalp irritations, **do not give her a cold wave**, as waving lotion will aggravate the condition.

Analyze hair. Determine the condition of the hair by a thorough analysis, as previously described in this chapter.

Shampoo. Usually a shampoo is given before a cold wave. It is advisable to use an acid-balanced or mild shampoo as suggested by manufacturer. Avoid brushing or massaging, as the scalp may become sensitive to the cold waving lotion.

Shaping the hair may be done **before or after** a shampoo. A razor or scissors may be used for shaping the hair.

1. A **razor** may be used on damp hair after a shampoo.
2. **Scissors** may be used on **dry hair before** a shampoo, or may be used on **damp hair after** the shampoo. Fine, thin, damaged, or limp hair should be shaped with the scissors while in a dry condition.

The texture of the hair must be carefully considered in planning the shaping procedure.

Coarse or medium hair. Taper the hair ends sufficiently to form strong, resilient curls. Excessive tapering may make it difficult to wrap the hair, or may also cause the hair ends to frizz.

Fine or thin hair. Use a blunt cut or a short taper. Excessive thinning or tapering will result in frizzy hair ends.

Length of hair. The hair should be long enough to wind around the rods at least two full turns. Otherwise, there will be no wave pattern. If the desired hairstyle requires shorter hair, use smaller diameter rods. If necessary, trim the ends of the hair strands after the wave is completed.

Precaution. In order to avoid distorted wave formation, it may be advisable to thin the hair after the cold wave is given.

> ### IMPORTANT REMINDER
> The foundation for a professional permanent wave is the careful pre-shaping of the hair.

COLD WAVING PROCEDURE

A correct analysis for good cold waving results should include the following:

1. Strength of waving solution
2. Proper size rods
3. Blocking and winding the hair
4. Test curls
5. Processing time
6. Neutralization

Implements And Supplies

1. Applicator bottles
2. Porous end papers
3. Cold waving lotion
4. Neutralizer
5. Neutralizing bib
6. Shampoo cape
7. Curling rods
8. Protective cream
9. Cotton or neutralizing bands
10. Mild liquid shampoo
11. Neutral or cream rinse
12. Neck strips and towels
13. Combs
14. Hair clips and hair pins
15. Scissors or razor
16. Protective gloves
17. Record card

If the neutralizer is to be applied by the splash or pour-over method, a rinse pan, measuring cup and quart jar are also needed.

Preparation

1. Select and arrange required materials.
2. Wash and sanitize hands.
3. Seat patron comfortably; remove her earrings and neck jewelry; adjust towel and shampoo cape.
4. Remove all hairpins and combs from patron's hair.
5. Examine carefully condition of scalp and hair.
6. Seat patron comfortably at the shampoo bowl.

Draping Patron

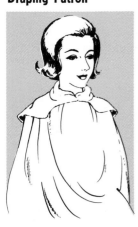

There are several ways in which a patron may be draped for a cold wave. The comfort of the patron, adequate protection of her person and her clothing are important considerations during the entire procedure. One way to drape a patron is to place a small folded towel around her neck, fasten the shampoo cape over it, then place another towel over the cape. Fasten the towels securely. (Your instructor may recommend another method, which is equally correct.)

REMINDER

It is important for the student to remember that there are many correct ways to give a cold wave. The method recommended in this section is merely one suggested way a cold wave can be given. Always be guided by your instructor.

Procedure

1. Shape hair before or after shampoo, as preferred.
2. Shampoo hair lightly (one soaping), rinse thoroughly. Towel dry.
3. If wrapping is to be done after the application of cold waving lotion, apply protective cream and cotton strips around patron's hairline. Wear protective gloves.

If wrapping is to be done after conditioner is applied, no protective cream is necessary, nor must you wear protective gloves. However, you must apply protective cream and wear protective gloves before you apply cold waving lotion to the wound curls.

4. Section the hair. Subdivide (block) section and wrap.

5. Apply cold waving lotion as recommended by manufacturer.

6. **Test curl immediately** after saturating hair with cold waving lotion. Take frequent test curls on different areas of the head.

7. Process hair for the required time. If rewetting the curls is necessary, apply the lotion in the same order followed originally. Protect patron with fresh protective cotton strips around hairline and neck.

8. Rinse out waving lotion thoroughly with warm water. Follow manufacturer's directions.

9. Blot excess moisture from hair wound on rods. **Do not** rock or roll the rods while blotting. Because the hair is in a softened state, any such movement may cause hair breakage.

10. Thoroughly apply neutralizer and retain for required time.

11. Rinse with tepid water; follow it with a cool water rinse to reharden the hair. Lightly towel blot.

12. Unwind rods and remove carefully.

13. Apply neutralizer again, if required.

14. Rinse hair again, if required.

15. Towel dry hair.

Important Reminders

A neutral or cream rinse, or a hair cream, may be applied to protect the permanent and to facilitate the styling of the hair. However, a cream rinse should not be applied to a shallow wave or body permanent wave, lest it relax the hair to the point where the wave is almost completely eliminated. If the manufacturer has included a special rinse with the product, it will prevent excessive stretching while combing and will counteract any alkaline residue. Setting lotion, if used, should be of a light consistency. **Avoid excess tension in styling the hair.**

Completion

1. Check for scalp abrasions.

2. Set, dry and style hair.

CAUTION. Do not use extreme heat when drying the hair. In handling soft, fine, limp or damaged hair, it is of utmost importance to use as little tension as possible.

Clean-Up

1. Discard used supplies.

2. Cleanse and sanitize equipment.

3. Wash and sanitize hands.

4. Complete cold wave record card.

BODY (PERMANENT) WAVE

A body (permanent) wave gives the hair softer, wider, longer-lasting waves. A body wave is given when a strong curl or wave effect is **not** desired.

A body wave gives a "holding action" to the hairstyle, thus permitting the setting to last longer, from one shampoo to another.

Reminder: Hair texture determines whether or not a body permanent wave should be given. If the hair is fine and soft, and the ultimate hairstyle requires curls, a body wave **must not be given**, as it will not give the hair the desired soft, wide wave effect.

Procedure

Since extra large, straight type rods are used, the procedure is somewhat different from that followed in using regular size rods. The wrapping should start in the front section. This should be followed by the crown section, leaving the nape section to be wrapped last. Smaller rods should be used in the nape area. (Hair on these rods does not require as much time to curl.)

In any event, the largest curls should be wrapped first, since they must be sufficiently strong to hold the large size wave.

Curling Rods

For a body (permanent) wave use straight rods to give uniform curl formation over the entire strand.

1. For crown and sides—use large (thick) rods.
2. For nape area—use small (thin) rods.
3. For intermediate areas—use medium size rods.

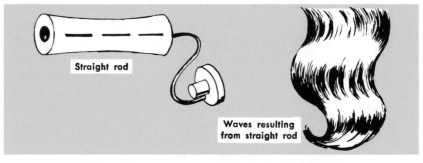

Straight rod

Waves resulting from straight rod

BODY WAVE EXTRA LONG HAIR

The permanent waving of long and extra long hair is a very important technique in beauty culture. Long and extra long hair can be made exceedingly attractive when properly permanent waved and styled. A wide variety of styles can be designed to suit the individuality and personality of the patron. For a discussion of the technique employed in performing this type of permanent wave, see page 136.

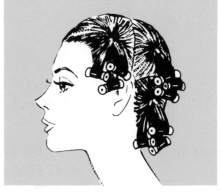

Long hair

NEUTRAL OR ACID-BALANCED PERMANENT WAVING SYSTEMS

For many years, manufacturers sought to develop a permanent wave solution that did not require the use of excess ammonia with thioglycolic acid (thio). They wanted to limit the damage caused to hair when permanent waved, and to permit hair that had been damaged by lightening or tinting to receive a permanent. To achieve these goals, they needed a waving solution that was not highly alkaline.

Neutral or acid-balanced permanent waving solutions have been introduced which use chemical compounds other than thio. These products have a pH of 5.5 to 7. Within this range lotions are slow to penetrate hair and processing speed is greatly reduced. To overcome this problem, heat must be applied.

Heated Clamp Method

There are two methods in use today to speed up the processing time:

1. The heated clamp method

With the heated clamp method, clamps are pre-heated and then placed over the rods, upon which hair has been wound and waving lotion applied.

Hair Dryer Method

2. The hair dryer method

When using the hair dryer method, hair is wound on the rods, lotion applied, and a thin plastic cap placed over the hair. The patron is then placed under a pre-heated hair dryer.

In both methods, processing does not effectively begin until heat is applied to the solution-dampened hair.

It is important to take notice of the fact that in both of these methods of permanent waving, the important new addition to the procedure is the application of heat into the process.

The chemical compounds employed are acid-balanced and therefore do not stimulate the relaxing or opening of the imbrications of the hair cuticle to permit penetration of the waving solution. This failure to stimulate penetration is the primary reason for the exceedingly slow action of the chemicals. In order to overcome this deficiency, heat must be employed as another method of opening the imbrications and permitting penetration into the cortex. Therefore, one method employs the heated clamps, while the other uses the hair dryer to bring heat directly to bear upon the patron's hair and thus create porosity.

Neutralizer

The techniques used for neutral and acid solution permanent waving are generally similar to those used for the alkaline method. However, manufacturers' directions vary somewhat with different products.

Follow Manufacturer's Directions

Because each manufacturer has his own formula and special features related to his product, it is essential that the manufacturer's instructions be followed carefully.

IMPORTANT REMINDER

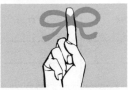

Cold waving is one of the most important services a cosmetologist is called upon to give. Proficiency in the techniques outlined in this chapter can only be achieved by constant practice and by taking painstaking care in all details. It is the meticulous worker who becomes the sought-after cosmetologist. So, remember, practice, practice and practice, following the instructions in this book and the guidance of your instructor.

RELEASE STATEMENT

A release statement is used for permanent waving, hair relaxing, or any other type of chemical treatment. It relieves the salon owner, to some extent, from responsibility for accidents or damages.

RELEASE FORM

Patron's Name .... Address ....

Condition of Hair ....

Permanent Wave: Kind .... Given by ....

   I fully understand that the permanent wave which I have requested and am about to receive is ordinarily harmless to normal hair, but may damage my hair because of its present condition.

   In view of this, I accept full responsibility for any possible damage that may result, directly or indirectly, to my hair.

Signature of Patron ....

Witnessed by .... Date ....

PERMANENT WAVE RECORD

A record of each permanent wave must be kept for each patron. It is referred to each time the patron takes a permanent. It contains all essential information. It eliminates guesswork. The following is a typical form of Permanent Wave Card.

PERMANENT WAVE RECORD

Name .... Tel. ....

Address .... City ....

DESCRIPTION OF HAIR

Form	Length	Texture		Elasticity	Porosity	
straight	short	coarse	soft	normal	very porous	less porous
wavy	medium	medium	silky	good	moderately porous	least porous
curly	long	fine	wiry	poor	normal	resistant

Condition:
☐ virgin   ☐ rewave   ☐ normal   ☐ dry   ☐ oily   lotion .... strength..............

If tinted or lightened, use: ☐ double end wrap   ☐ water   ☐ protein filler

previously waved with .... system

☐ original sample of hair enclosed   ☐ not enclosed

TYPE OF PERMANENT WAVE

☐ regular   ☐ body wave   ☐ other .... lotion .... strength ....

Curls — Roller sizes: Top .... sides .... crown .... nape ....

Results: ☐ good   ☐ poor   ☐ too tight   ☐ too loose
☐ sample of finished P.W. enclosed   ☐ sample not enclosed

Date	Operator	Price	Date	Operator	Price

SAFETY RULES AND REMINDERS

For the protection of both the patron and the cosmetologist, the following should be observed:

1. In giving a permanent wave, always follow manufacturer's directions.
2. Examine scalp for abrasions and lesions.
3. Analyze the hair before every permanent wave.
4. Obtain information concerning patron's cold wave history.
5. Protect clothing of patron by proper draping.
6. Have the patron remove her glasses, earrings and neck jewelry.
7. Select a mild shampoo and apply it without irritating the scalp.
8. Eliminate hair brushing or massaging before a permanent wave.
9. Always shape the hair before giving a cold wave.
10. Use protective cream around patron's hairline and neck.
11. Protect patron's face and neck with cotton strips or neutralizing band during processing.
12. Protect cosmetologist's hands with gloves or protective cream.
13. Use clean applicator bottles for **all** solutions. Use glass or plastic measuring cups and bowls. **Do not** use metallic cups or bowls.
14. Take pre-permanent test curls, when in doubt.
15. Sub-section hair evenly. Uneven blockings may produce uneven waves.
16. Select proper size rods and correct waving lotion for the hair.
17. **Do not** stretch the hair when wrapping, or stretch rubber bands over the curls, as hair breakage may result.
18. When applying waving lotion, be sure the curls are thoroughly saturated.
19. Avoid dripping of lotion on scalp and skin. For the removal of lotion drippings, blot with cotton saturated with cold water. Apply neutralizer, if necessary.
20. Immediately remove cotton strips or neutralizing band from hairline and neck if saturated with waving lotion.
21. If waving lotion gets into patron's eyes, wash immediately with cold water, or be guided by your instructor. (Take patron to doctor.)
22. **Do not** leave patron alone while the hair is processing.
23. Test wave formation every 30 seconds during processing.
24. Neutralize hair thoroughly, as directed by manufacturer.
25. Remove drippings from the floor as soon as possible.
26. **Do not** apply on the same day a color rinse, tint, lightener or any other cosmetic that may cause damage to a new permanent.
27. **Do not** give a permanent to a patron if she has experienced an allergic reaction from a previous cold wave permanent
28. **Do not** allow patron to sit in draft or near an air conditioner.
29. Complete permanent wave record card carefully and accurately.

SPECIAL PROBLEMS

Reconditioning Treatments

Dry, brittle, damaged or over-porous hair should be given reconditioning treatments. However, avoid any treatment requiring massage or heat just prior to a cold wave. Such treatment could create a sensitive scalp.

Cold Wave Conditioners

Over-porous or damaged hair must be preconditioned before the application of waving lotion. Special fillers that contain **protein** are now available which recondition the hair and equalize its porosity. Some fillers also contain lanolin and cholesterol, which may help to protect the hair against the harshness of the cold waving lotion.

After-Care

Reconditioning treatments for patrons also have a place in the **after-care** of a permanent wave and between permanents.

The aftercare of the patron's permanent wave helps to keep the hair in the best possible condition. It includes regular hair care as follows:

1. Shampoo hair weekly with mild shampoo and rinse.
2. Use appropriate hair conditioner as directed by manufacturer.
3. Comb and brush hair daily. Use type of brush best suited to the hair. Avoid excessive brushing or combing in the opposite direction.
4. Have hair trimmed and styled at regular intervals in order to make the hairstyle more serviceable.

To Tint Or Wave

If a patron requests both a permanent wave and a hair tint on the same day, **advise against it.** Give the following reasons to the patron:

1. If the tint is given first, the application of waving lotion will lighten hair and often cause an uneven color.
2. If the permanent is given first, the application of a tint will distort and weaken the wave pattern.
3. The combination of two chemical treatments on the same day may cause scalp irritation and/or hair breakage.

Recommended Sequence

First, give the permanent wave and postpone the tint treatment for a few days to avoid distorting the wave pattern. Suggest a reconditioning treatment before the tint application.

Do not give a color rinse immediately after a cold wave. It is likely to disturb the wave pattern. If required, use a color rinse having a weak strength.

If the hair is to be lightened after the permanent, it should be reconditioned first and lightened at a later date.

Waving Tinted Or Lightened Hair

The following special precautions are recommended when waving tinted or lightened hair:

1. Shampoo hair with a mild shampoo before waving.
2. Wrap the hair with a special conditioner, as required for damaged hair.
3. Use a special cold waving lotion according to directions.
4. Give test curls, using a milder waving solution and a shorter processing time than is employed for normal hair.

Hair Tinted With Metallic Dye

Hair tinted with a metallic dye must first be treated with a dye remover to avoid hair discoloration or breakage. **Do not** wave the hair if the test curls break or discolor. This type of discoloration is very difficult to remove.

Curl Reduction

Sometimes a patron is unhappy with her hair after a permanent because the hair appears to be too curly. If the hair is fine in texture, do not suggest curl reduction until after two or three shampoos. This type of hair relaxes to a greater extent than normal or coarse hair. Usually, after the second shampoo, the hair has relaxed enough to be satisfactory.

If the hair has a normal or coarse texture, curl reduction may be given either immediately following neutralization or after a few days.

Cold waving lotion may be used where required to relax the curl. Carefully comb it through the hair to widen and loosen the wave. When sufficiently relaxed, the hair is rinsed, towel blotted and neutralized.

If curl analysis and proper application is not pre-determined, hair could be damaged and breakage could occur. **Be guided by your instructor.**

CAUTION. Do not attempt curl reduction in hair which has been over-processed. Such a treatment will further damage the hair.

Cold Waving Hair With Partial Permanent

Hair previously permanent waved should be given a reconditioning treatment. Leave the conditioning agent over the old permanent and cover this hair with two or three end papers. Then proceed with the usual cold wave routine.

This is only one suggestion for permanent waving this type of hair. Your instructor's method is equally correct.

Items To Consider
Air Conditioning

Because of its cooling effect, air conditioning may slow down the action of the cold waving lotion. Additional time **may be** required.

Long Hair

Because of its excess length, long hair may require smaller blockings to assure thorough saturation of the waving lotion and neutralizer.

Permanent Waving

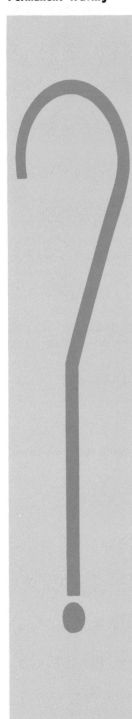

1. What is permanent waving?
2. The physical action involves the wrapping of the hair around ....
3. The application of which chemical follows the permanent waving lotion?
4. Name two types of chemical solutions used in permanent waving.
5. What is the main action of a permanent waving solution?
6. What is the main action of the neutralizer?
7. What is the most important step before giving a permanent wave?
8. List six factors which a scalp and hair analysis should include.
9. Which two hair factors determine the processing time during a permanent wave?
10. Why is hair elasticity so important in relation to permanent waving?
11. To achieve best results, what should guide the student?
12. What determines the size of the wave formation in permanent waving?
13. What determines the choice of rods in permanent waving?
14. Why should hair be wrapped smoothly and without tension on each rod?
15. Why do we avoid stretching the hair in wrapping for a permanent wave?
16. In permanent waving, what determines:
    a) The size of the blocking (sub-sectioning)?
    b) The length of rods used?
17. When may a permanent waving solution cause irritation to a healthy skin or scalp?
18. Why is it necessary to give test curls?
19. What determines the strength of waving lotion used?
20. Why are special hair conditioners recommended in permanent waving?
21. At what three points should wave development be tested?
22. Why should safety rules be observed in permanent waving?
23. What must be done if the waving lotion accidentally gets on the skin or scalp?
24. When does the complete wave formation reach its peak?
25. What kind of hair texture will not form a firm wave pattern?
26. How is over-processed hair detected?
27. How is the hair affected by the application of permanent waving lotion?
28. Why should a hair coloring treatment and a permanent wave not be given the same day?
29. Why should a color rinse not be given immediately following a permanent wave?
30. How may an over-curly permanent wave be relaxed?
31. What strength waving lotion is always recommended for tinted or lightened hair?
32. Why should a permanent wave record be kept for each patron?
33. Why is it a good practice to obtain a release statement from each patron before giving her a permanent wave?

CHAPTER 15

HAIR COLORING

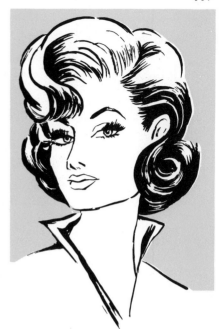

INTRODUCTION

Hair coloring (tinting) is both the science and art of changing the color of hair. **Hair coloring** involves the addition of an artificial color to the natural pigment in the hair, or the addition of color to lightened hair. **Hair lightening,** on the other hand, involves a partial or total removal of the natural pigment, or artificial color, from the hair. (The terms "tinting" and "coloring" are used interchangeably in this text.)

Hair tinting and lightening can be accomplished by continuous practice and long hours of study. They can become profitable sources of income in the beauty salon because they represent **repeat business.** The patron who has her hair tinted or lightened usually returns for retouching at regular intervals. Satisfactory service will encourage her to return to the same beauty salon.

Reasons For Coloring Hair

The following are the usual reasons given for coloring hair:

1. To change grey hair to its natural shade
2. To change the natural shade of hair to a more attractive color
3. To restore hair to its natural color
4. To create decorative effects, such as frosting, streaking or tipping

Advantages Of Hair Coloring

Hair coloring is advantageous for the following women:

1. Women with prematurely grey hair
2. Business women who may feel that the shade of their hair is a handicap to their business
3. Women who wish to maintain a youthful appearance

Knowledge Needed By Cosmetologist

The successful cosmetologist must know:

1. The general structure of the hair and scalp
2. The proper selection and application of hair tints and lighteners
3. The chemical reactions following their application

HAIR COLORING

Hair coloring is the application of artificial color to the hair.

Hair coloring falls into three main categories: **temporary, semi-permanent** and **permanent.** The professional cosmetologist must know how each group acts on the hair.

CLASSIFICATION OF HAIR COLORING

Temporary

1. **Color rinses** are prepared rinses used either to highlight the color or add color to the hair. These rinses contain certified colors and remain on the hair until the next shampoo.
2. **Highlighting color shampoos** combine the action of a color rinse with that of a shampoo. These shampoos generally contain certified colors, give highlights and impart color tones to the hair.
3. **Crayons** are sticks of coloring which are available in all shades and are compounded with soaps or synthetic waxes. They are used to retouch newly grown hair between tint treatments.
4. **Hair color creams** are used mostly for theatrical makeup. They rub off easily because of their greasy base.
5. **Hair color sprays** are generally used in gold and silver colors and are applied from aerosol containers for exotic effects.
6. **Mascara** is used to add color to the eyelashes and eyebrows.

Semi-Permanent

Tints that are formulated to last four to six weeks are semi-permanent hair coloring agents. They are self-penetrating and are applied without peroxide. They do not change the basic structure of the hair.

Semi-permanent tints are designed to do the following:

1. Cover or blend partially grey hair without affecting the natural color of the hair
2. Enhance the beauty of grey hair without changing its color
3. Highlight and bring out the natural color of the hair

Permanent
Aniline

1. **Aniline derivative tints** are also called **penetrating tints,** synthetic organic tints, peroxide tints, oxidation tints, para tints and amino tints. **Toners** are also classified as penetrating tints.

Vegetable

2. **Pure vegetable tints.** In the past, indigo, camomile, sage and Egyptian henna were used for hair coloring. They deposited a thin coating on the hair. These tints are no longer used professionally today.

Metallic

3. **Metallic** or **mineral dyes,** such as lead acetate or silver nitrate, are the **progressive type known as color restorers.** They form a metallic coating over the hair shaft and render the hair unsatisfactory for permanent waving, hair lightening or tinting. Successive applications are made until the proper shade has developed. These products are used in the home.

Compound

4. **Compound dyes,** such as compound henna, are combinations of vegetable dyes with certain metallic salts and other dyestuffs. The metallic salts fix the color. Compound dyes coat the hair shaft and render the hair unfit for permanent waving, lightening or tinting.

METALLIC DYES
Precaution

Metallic dyes and compound dyes are never used professionally. However, women do buy and apply such products to their hair. Therefore, the cosmetologist must be able to recognize and understand their effects. Such coloring agents must be removed and the hair reconditioned before the application of tints, lighteners or permanent wave solutions.

Hair treated with either a metallic dye or compound dye appears to be dull without highlights. It is generally harsh and brittle to the touch. These colorings usually fade into peculiar or unnatural shades. **Silver** dyes have a **greenish** cast; **lead** dyes have a **purple** color, and those containing **copper** dyes turn **red**.

Test For Metallic Salts

1. In a glass container, mix one ounce of 20 volume peroxide and 20 drops of 28% ammonia water.
2. Cut a strand of hair from the patron's head. Bind with scotch tape and immerse the hair in the above solution for 30 minutes.
3. Remove from container and observe.

Since most of these products contain lead, silver or copper, look for the following reactions:

Test For Lead

Lead. Hair will change color immediately. It often turns much **lighter** very rapidly.

Test For Silver

Silver. No reaction whatsoever at end of half an hour. A peroxide and ammonia solution cannot lighten because it cannot penetrate the silver coating, while the hair strand with no artificial coloring or penetrating tint will lighten to some degree.

Test For Copper

Copper. The solution will start to boil within a few minutes. The hair strand feels hot and gives off a very disagreeable odor. After a few minutes, the hair will pull apart easily.

If any of these conditions are present, the metallic coating must be removed before the hair can be successfully colored or given a permanent wave. After the coating has been removed, the strand should be checked again in 24 hours by stretching for breakage. If breakage occurs, recondition the hair before any aniline derivative tint, lightener or permanent waving solution is used.

Removing Metallic Dye

Preparations are available for the removal of metallic dyes and compound dyes. Follow manufacturer's directions.

ANILINE DERIVATIVE TINTS

The aniline derivative tints contribute the greatest success to hair tinting. Most permanent hair coloring is done with aniline derivative tints. These tints remain in the hair until they are removed by chemical means, or until the hair grows out. The coloring penetrates through the cuticle into the cortex of the hair and cannot be washed out.

An aniline derivative tint contains, as its essential ingredient, **paraphenylene-diamine,** or related chemical compound. With this type of preparation, it is possible to duplicate the various shades of human hair without impairing its luster. These tints may be applied successfully over permanently waved and chemically relaxed hair.

A small percentage of patrons are allergic to aniline derivative tints. To identify such individuals, a **skin or patch test** is required by law for all patrons 24 hours before each application.

Aniline derivative tints are sold in small bottles and in tubes. The stock of these tints should be kept fresh, as they deteriorate on standing.

When the developer (hydrogen peroxide) is mixed with the tint, a chemical reaction, known as **oxidation,** begins. For this reason, the tint mixture must be applied immediately to the hair. After the mixture is applied to the hair, the oxidation continues until the color has developed to the desired shade.

Timing the development of the applied tint requires a **thorough study** of the product being used.

Allergy

Allergy to aniline derivative tints is an unpredictable condition. Some patrons may be sensitive to aniline derivative tints. To identify such individuals, a **skin or patch** test is required for all patrons prior to the application of a tint or toner.

A person who has been free of an allergy may suddenly develop it. To be sure, give a patch test, to find out if the patron has become sensitive since her last tinting treatment.

The **U.S. Federal Food, Drug and Cosmetic Act** prescribes that a **patch test,** or **predisposition test,** must be given before each application of an aniline derivative tint, whether on a **virgin** head or **retouch.** This test is required to protect the patron, the cosmetologist, and the entire cosmetology profession.

CAUTION. Aniline derivative tints must **never** be used on the eyelashes or eyebrows. **To do so may cause blindness.**

PATCH TEST

The patch test must be given 24 hours before each tinting or toner treatment. The tint used for the skin test must be of the **same shade and mixture** as the tint intended to be used for the hair tinting treatment.

Procedure

1. Select test area, either behind ear, extending partly into hairline, or on inner fold of elbow.
2. Wash test area, about the size of a quarter, with mild soap and water.
3. Dry test area by patting with absorbent cotton or clean towel.
4. Prepare test solution by mixing one capful of tint and one capful of 20 volume peroxide, or as directed by the manufacturer.
5. Apply enough test solution with cotton-tipped applicator to cover the area previously cleansed.
6. Allow test area to dry. Leave uncovered and undisturbed for 24 hours.
7. Examine test area for either negative or positive reactions.

A **negative skin test** will show no sign of inflammation; hence, an aniline derivative tint may be applied.

A **positive skin test** is recognized by the presence of redness, swelling, burning, itching, blisters or eruptions. A patron showing such symp-

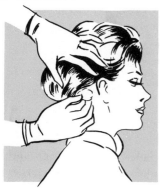

Wash patch test area behind ear.

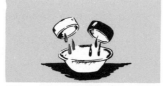

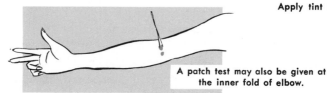

Mix one cap of tint and one cap of peroxide.

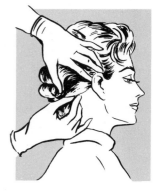

Apply tint mixture.

A patch test may also be given at the inner fold of elbow.

toms is allergic to an aniline derivative tint, and **under no circumstances should this particular kind of tint be used.**

Symptoms of hair tint poisoning are as follows:

1. Swelling
2. Itchy red spots spreading all over the body
3. Tiny blisters from which a liquid oozes
4. Patron suffering from headaches and vomiting

Immediate medical attention should be sought by a patron exhibiting the above symptoms.

PREPARATION FOR HAIR TINTING
Color Selection

What to consider in color selection. Always consult the patron and consider her color preference before starting to tint the hair. For this purpose, make use of a well-lighted room, providing either a strong natural light or incandescent lighting. Fluorescent lighting is not good for judging hair colors.

When talking to the patron, find out whether she knows what color suits her **age** and **skin tones.** You must consider that skin tones change with age. The natural color of her hair, which harmonized beautifully with her skin coloring at the age of twenty or thirty, may be harsh and unbecoming at the age of forty or fifty. For patrons in this age group, keep to the lighter shades of color.

Here are a few general guides to color selection.

1. Women, young in age or appearance, with **fair** or **creamy** complexions can afford to be as daring as they wish when it comes to color selection.
2. Women with complexions having a **florid** or **pinkish** hue should adhere to the ash tones, either in the pale or darker shades, depending on their skin texture and age.
3. Women with **clear olive** complexions have a cool-looking skin. The choice of colors ranges from blonde to the warm series of browns and sometimes to the very dark colors.

4. Women having a **yellowish** or **brownish** hue to their skin tones should **avoid** the ash colors. Careful study of skin texture is necessary for these skin tones to determine the amount of gold, copper or red color to be applied.

Basic Rules For Color Selection

The success or failure of a hair tint depends on a careful selection of the **right** color. Skill in color selection can best be developed by observing the following basic rules:

1. For color observation, the patron's hair should be clean and dry. If the hair is soiled or wet, the tendency is to select a color that is too dark.
2. Use a color chart to show the product's range of colors, their names and numbers.
3. Compare the patron's hair with the particular shade that is closest to it on the chart.
4. Determine if her particular shade, or one more becoming, is to be selected.
5. To match the hair color, examine the hair nearest the scalp at the back of the head. This is where the hair is darkest.
6. Always look through, rather than down on, the hair. To see depth as well as highlights, raise the hair by pushing the hair up with the hands against the scalp.
7. Know the properties and manufacturer's instructions concerning the particular product you are using.

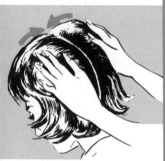

Checking hair color

Tint colors are usually divided into **four** groups, according to the basic tone values:

1. Shades with no red are classified as **drab.**
2. Shades with some red or gold tones are in the **warm** series.
3. Shades with a great deal of red are included in the **very warm** or **red** series.
4. Shades with silver or platinum are classified as **cool** series.

Testing For Color Selection

Before applying a hair tint, give a preliminary strand test, which will indicate the following:

1. Whether the proper color selection was made.
2. The correct length of time to leave the tint on the hair.
3. Whether the hair is subject to possible breakage or discoloration due to the excessive or faulty use of either a cold waving lotion, lightener, tint, metallic dye or compound dye. If the hair is in a damaged condition, have it reconditioned and retested before applying the tint.
4. Hair in a poor condition, having porous areas, or streaked or dark ends, needs reconditioning treatments. (For information on reconditioning treatments see section on **Fillers** in this chapter.)

Strand Test Procedure

1. Mix a small amount of equal parts of the tint selected and 20 volume peroxide.
2. Apply the mixture to a full hair strand. Retain it on the hair until the desired shade is developed.
3. Wash, dry and examine the hair strand. If the results are satisfactory, proceed with the tint treatment.

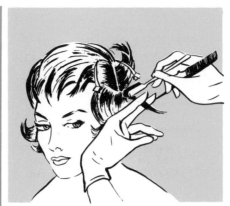

Give a color strand test.

Should the color produced on the test strand be different from the color desired, select another color and **strand test** again.

If the strand test shows discoloration, which might indicate the presence of a metallic dye, take corrective steps before tint application.

Examining Scalp And Hair

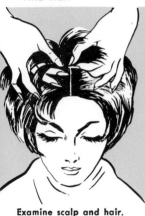

Examine scalp and hair.

Carefully examine the scalp and hair to determine if it is safe to use an aniline derivative tint and whether any special hair tinting problems exist.

The results of such an examination may indicate the need for any of the following:

1. Reconditioning treatments
2. Removal of color from the hair
3. Testing hair for discoloration
4. Testing hair for breakage

An aniline derivative tint **should not be used** if the following conditions are recognized:

1. Signs of a **positive skin test**
2. Scalp irritation or eruptions
3. Contagious scalp or hair disease
4. Presence of metallic or compound dyes

If the scalp and hair are in a **healthy condition,** observe carefully and record data on a permanent hair tint record card.

Use Soft Water

When water is used in connection with hair tinting or lightening, be certain that it is **soft** or **demineralized** water.

Follow Working Plan In Tinting

For successful hair tinting with aniline derivative tints, the cosmetologist must follow a definite procedure. Such a system makes for the greatest efficiency. A permanent record should be kept of each patron's hair tinting treatments. Without a plan, the work takes longer and mistakes may be made. Besides, the patron soon becomes dissatisfied and loses confidence in the cosmetologist's ability.

A working plan includes the materials and supplies needed for the tinting treatment, and a thorough knowledge of the product to be used.

KEEPING HAIR TINT RECORDS

It is of the utmost importance to keep an accurate record so that any difficulties encountered in one treatment may be avoided in subsequent treatments. A complete record should be made, containing information such as "dries out rapidly," "tint does not develop fast enough," or any other data connected with that particular head.

HAIR TINT RECORD

Name .... Tel. ....

Address .... City ....

Patch Test: Negative ☐ Positive ☐   Date ....

DESCRIPTION OF HAIR

Form	Length	Texture	Porosity	
straight	short	coarse	very porous	resistant
wavy	medium	medium	porous	very resistant
curly	long	fine	normal	perm. waved

Condition:

☐ Normal   ☐ dry   ☐ oily   ☐ faded   ☐ streaked   .... % grey

Previously lightened with .... for ....(time)

Previously tinted with .... for ....(time)

☐ original sample enclosed   ☐ not enclosed

CORRECTIVE TREATMENTS

Color filler used ....Corrective treatments with ....

HAIR TINTING PROCESS

whole head ....   retouch .... inches   shade desired ....

Formula: Color .... Lightener ....

Results: ☐ good   ☐ poor   ☐ too light   ☐ too dark   ☐ streaked

Date	Operator	Price	Date	Operator	Price
....			....		
....			....		
....			....		

RELEASE STATEMENT

A release statement is used for hair tinting, permanent waving or any other treatment that may require the cosmetologist's or salon owner's release from responsibility for accidents or damages.

SAMPLE RELEASE

Patron's Name .... Address ....

Condition of Hair: ....

Hair Coloring: Kind .... Given by ....

I fully understand that the hair coloring treatment which I have requested and am about to receive is ordinarily harmless to normal hair, but may damage my hair because of its present condition.

In view of this, I accept full responsibility for any possible damage that may result, directly or indirectly, to my hair.

Signature of Patron ....

Witnessed by .... Date ....

TEMPORARY COLOR RINSES

Introduction

The most important of the temporary hair colorings are color rinses that contain certified colors. They can be used as follows:

1. To bring out highlights in hair of any shade
2. To temporarily restore faded hair to its natural shade
3. To neutralize the yellowish tinge of white or grey hair
4. To tone down over-lightened hair

For patrons who want to highlight the color of their hair or add beauty to grey hair, rinses containing certified colors are satisfactory. Color rinses wash out with soap and water, but as a rule remain color-true from shampoo to shampoo. They come in various color shades: blonde, brown, black, red, silver and slate. These rinses are applied easily and quickly and are valuable as an introduction to hair coloring.

Procedure

After shampooing, rinsing and towel drying the hair, apply **prepared color rinse** with brush or plastic applicator bottle.

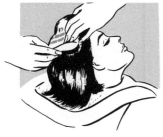

1. Apply around the front hairline.

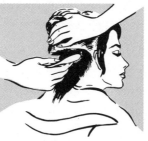

2. Apply around the nape hairline.

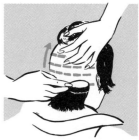

3. Apply up to crown area in layers.

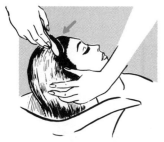

4. Apply to crown area in layers.

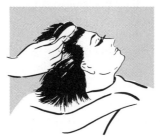

5. Check for complete coverage.

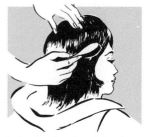

6. Brush color rinse through the hair.

7. Leave rinse on from two to five minutes, depending upon shade desired.
8. Rinse thoroughly with warm water until the water runs clear.
9. Set, dry and style hair in the usual manner.

For any variations in this procedure, follow manufacturer's directions, or be guided by your instructor.

Clean-Up

1. Discard all disposable supplies and materials.
2. Close containers; wipe off and put them in their proper places.
3. Clean and sanitize implements.
4. Tidy up station.
5. Wash and sanitize hands.

SEMI-PERMANENT TINTS

Semi-permanent tints offer a form of hair coloring suitable for the patron who has previously been reluctant to have her hair color changed.

The semi-permanent tint is a formulated coloring material which fills a gap between a temporary color rinse and a permanent hair color tint, without in any way taking the place of either.

Natural hair, which is drab or dull, may be improved in color tone by the use of semi-permanent tints, since there is no lightening action on the hair.

There is available a wide range of colors, and the results obtained will depend mainly on the original color, to a lesser degree on the texture of the patron's hair, and on the length of development time.

The various shades may be blended to create individual color tones.

There are blue-grey or silver-grey shades specifically designed for hair ranging from 10% to 100% grey.

Semi-permanent hair colorings are formulated to last from four to six weeks. No peroxide is required. The hair fades naturally, provided a **mild non-stripping shampoo** is used. These tints require no retouching.

Advantages

1. The color is self-penetrating.
2. The color is applied the same way each time.
3. Retouching is eliminated.
4. Color does not rub off because it has penetrated the hair shaft.
5. Hair will return close to its natural color in four to six weeks.

Semi-permanent tints require a 24-hour patch test. Some semi-permanent hair colorings require pre-shampooing; others do not. Read manufacturer's directions.

Types

1. Semi-permanent tints which cover grey completely but do not affect the remaining pigmented hair
2. Semi-permanent tints which make grey hair more beautifully grey without changing the natural pigment
3. Semi-permanent tints which add color and highlights to hair that is not grey

Materials and Supplies

Towels	Cotton	Clips
Tint cape for patron	Neutral shampoo	Record card
Protective gloves	Selected color tint	Talcum powder
Comb	Color chart	Plastic cap
Applicators	Neutral rinse	Timer

Preliminary Steps

1. Give preliminary patch test 24 hours before tinting.
2. If the patch test is negative, proceed with the tinting treatment.
3. Assemble all necessary supplies.
4. Prepare patron. Protect her clothing with towel and tint cape. Remove her jewelry and glasses.
5. Examine patron's scalp for irritation or abrasions.
6. Select the desired shade of color.

Procedure

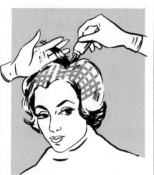

Apply tint to scalp area.

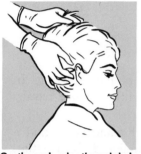

Gently work color through hair.

The semi-permanent tint is applied by using the nozzle of an applicator bottle to sectioned hair, or applied at the shampoo bowl with either a brush or applicator bottle.

Since manufacturers' directions vary, be guided by their instructions, or by your instructor.

The following is the procedure for applying semi-permanent tints:

1. Give a mild shampoo, if required.
2. Towel dry hair (follow manufacturer's directions).
3. Put on protective gloves.
4. Apply tint to the hair throughout the scalp area.
5. Gently work color through the hair with fingers until hair is thoroughly saturated. (Do not massage into scalp.)
6. Pile hair loosely on top of the head.
7. Be guided by manufacturer whether to use or omit a plastic cap covering.
8. Strand test for color.
9. When color has developed, wet hair with warm water and work up a lather.
10. Rinse with warm water until water runs clear.
11. Give neutral rinse.

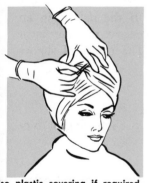

Use plastic covering if required.

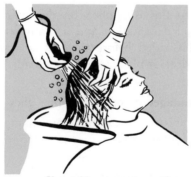

Rinse with warm water until water runs clear.

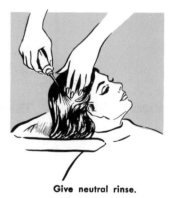

Give neutral rinse.

12. Towel blot hair; set, dry and style.
13. Fill out record card.

Clean-Up

1. Discard all disposable supplies and materials.
2. Close containers; wipe off and put them in their proper places.
3. Clean and sanitize implements.
4. Remove stains from tint cape.
5. Tidy up station.
6. Wash and sanitize hands.

Penetrating tints. Oxidizing-penetrating tints containing an aniline derivative are tints that penetrate through the cuticle of the hair into the cortical layer. Here they are oxidized by the peroxide, which has been added, into color pigments which are distributed throughout the hair in much the same manner as the natural pigment.

Penetrating tints may be referred to as:

1. Single application tints, also called one-process or one-step tints.
2. Double application tints, also called two-process or two-step tints.

One-Step Tint

One-step application tints (cream or liquid) perform two actions: they lighten and add color to the hair in a single application.

Two-Step Tint

Two-step application tints (cream or liquid) perform only one action at a time. They require two separate and distinct applications to the hair:

1. The application of a softener or lightener
2. The application of a tint or toner

**ONE-STEP TINTS
(Cream Or Liquid)**

One-step tints represent a simplified method of hair coloring. In one application, the hair can be colored permanently **without** requiring pre-shampooing, pre-softening or pre-lightening.

In most instances, one-step tints contain a lightening agent and a shampoo with an oil base, combined with an aniline derivative tint. When ready for use, 20 volume hydrogen peroxide is added in fixed proportions, according to manufacturer's directions. .

A one-step tint is applied on **dry hair only.** If the hair is in an extremely soiled condition and a shampoo is necessary, the hair must be thoroughly dried before the tint is applied. The choice of shades varies from deepest black to lightest blonde.

Advantages

The advantages of one-step tints: they . . .

1. Eliminate time consuming pre-shampooing, pre-softening or pre-lightening processes.
2. Leave no line of demarcation.
3. Color the hair lighter or darker than the patron's natural color.
4. Blend in grey or white hair to match patron's natural hair shade.
5. Tone down streaks, off-shades, discolorations and faded hair ends.

Color Selection

General Rules for One-Step Color Selection

1. To match the natural color of hair and to cover grey hair, select the color closest to the natural shade.
2. To brighten or lighten the hair, and to cover grey hair, select a shade lighter than the natural color. The selected tint must contain enough color to produce the desired shade on grey hair.
3. To darken the hair and cover grey hair, select a color darker than the natural hair color.
4. Study the manufacturer's color chart to learn how to make correct color selections.

HELPFUL SUGGESTIONS
SECTIONING, OUTLINING AND SUB-DIVIDING

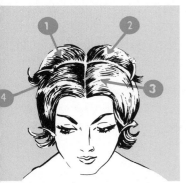

Sectioning the hair in four quarters

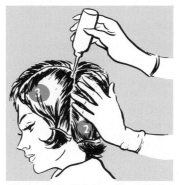

(Optional) Outlining parting with tint

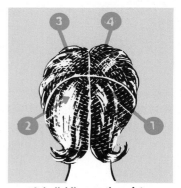

Sub-dividing sections into ¼-inch strands

USING PLASTIC BOTTLE APPLICATOR

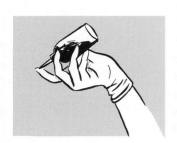

Preparing mixture — shake gently back and forth

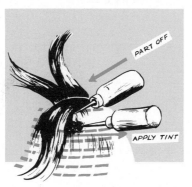

Use plastic bottle with nozzle to part hair and apply tint to ¼'' strand

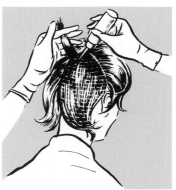

Applying tint to ¼-inch strands

USING BRUSH AS APPLICATOR

STRAND TESTING

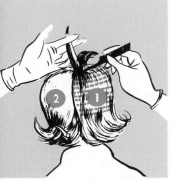

Part each strand with rat-tail comb

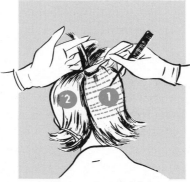

Apply to each strand first on top-side and then the under-side

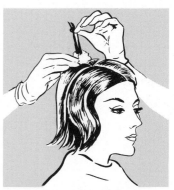

Strand test for color development

TINTING VIRGIN HAIR
One-Step Method

Virgin hair is hair which has neither been lightened nor tinted. **Note:** The cosmetologist should note whether the hair has been permanently waved or chemically straightened and what, if any, damage resulted thereby.

The procedure given here for a one-step tint application is in general use today. However, if your instructor's routine varies, follow his or her procedure.

Materials And Supplies

Towels	Applicators:	Selected color tint
Tint cape for patron	Tint brushes	Hydrogen peroxide
Protective gloves	Swab sticks	(20 volume)
Comb	Plastic bottles	Color chart
Glass or plastic bowls	Timer	Neutral rinse
Record card	Cotton	Clips
Talcum powder	Neutral shampoo	

Conditioners and Color Fillers

If the hair is damaged, pre-conditioning treatments should be given.

To assure even color, it is advisable to apply color filler to damaged hair and hair ends before tint application. (See Fillers, page 228.)

SAFETY PRECAUTION

A **skin** or **patch test** must be given before tinting the hair. The cosmetologist wears protective gloves during the application.

Preliminary Steps

1. Give preliminary patch test 24 hours before tinting.
2. If the patch test is negative, proceed with the tinting treatment.
3. Examine patron's scalp for irritation or abrasions.
4. Tint may be applied with nozzle applicator or brush.

Preparation

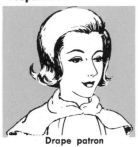
Drape patron

1. Assemble all necessary supplies.
2. Prepare patron. Protect her clothing with a towel and tint cape, and remove her jewelry and glasses.
3. Re-examine patron's scalp.
4. Select the desired shade of color.
5. Put on protective gloves.
6. Make color strand test. (See page 202.)
7. Prepare formula.

Procedure

1. Section hair into four quarters; (optional) outline partings with tint. The primary purpose for outlining the partings is to clearly define the area covered by each section. Outlining prevents straying from one section to another and to assure complete and even coverage.
2. Select section where grey hair is most prevalent. Where no grey hair is present, select area where the hair is most resistant, usually the crown area.
3. Subdivide section into ¼-inch strands.

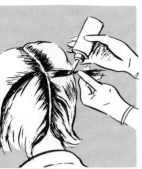

Apply tint one inch from the scalp to hair ends.

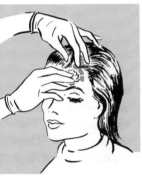

Removing tint stains

4. Pick up a strand of hair and hold it away from the head at the proper angle to expose the scalp area.

5. Apply color mixture to the hair strand, start 1 inch from the scalp and distribute evenly to hair ends. (Follow manufacturer's directions.) Since body heat causes the hair nearest the scalp to process faster, provision must be made to assure even color. For this reason the area nearest the scalp receives the tint last.

6. Tint mixture is permitted to develop for about 15 minutes.

7. Take strand tests often, for color development, until hair has lightened to approximately one-half of the desired shade.

8. Apply tint mixture to scalp area. Be sure that all hair is thoroughly saturated.

9. Leave tint on hair until a strand test indicates that the desired color has been developed evenly from the scalp to the ends.

10. Rinse hair with lukewarm water to remove excess color.

11. Remove stains from around hairline, ears and neck by working in a circular movement with a cotton pledget dipped in left-over tint diluted with shampoo, commercial stain remover, or warm water and a little shampoo.

12. Give a mild, acid balanced (non-strip) shampoo and rinse thoroughly with lukewarm water. Towel dry.

13. Apply a neutral or slightly acid rinse or conditioner to return hair to a more normal condition.

14. Set, dry and style hair.

15. Fill out record card and file.

Clean-Up

1. Discard all disposable supplies and materials.
2. Close containers tightly; wipe off and put them in their proper places.
3. Clean and sanitize implements.
4. Remove stains from tint cape.
5. Tidy up station.
6. Wash and sanitize hands.

TINTING TO DARKER SHADE

When tinting close to or darker than natural hair color, follow the same preparation and procedure as for a one-step tint to a lighter shade, with the following exceptions:

1. Select color close to or darker than patron's natural hair color.
2. Apply the tint from the scalp area to hair ends.
3. When color has developed evenly from scalp area to hair ends, shampoo and rinse in the usual manner.

TINTING LONG HAIR

The procedure followed for **tinting long hair** is usually the same as that for shorter hair. Care must be taken to have additional materials on hand to provide for the extra length of hair.

212

ONE-STEP TINT RETOUCH

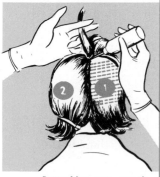

Retouching new growth.

HIGHLIGHTING SHAMPOO TINTS

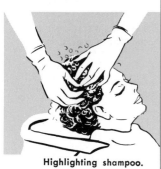

Highlighting shampoo.

PRE-LIGHTEN OR PRE-SOFTEN

To retouch the new growth, follow the same procedure as you would for coloring virgin hair, with the following differences:

1. Apply tint to the new growth only, DO NOT OVERLAP. Check frequently for color development.
2. When you have finished the application, check back to make sure that you have not missed any spots.
3. When the color has almost developed, dilute the remaining tint by adding a mild shampoo, conditioner or water, as directed by the manufacturer.
4. In order to assure complete and even coverage and color, apply this diluted mixture to the entire head. Gently distribute evenly with the fingertips. Retain for a few minutes.
5. Rinse with warm water to remove excess color.
6. Remove stains from hairline, ears and neck areas in the same manner as for "Tinting Virgin Hair".
7. Use a mild shampoo and rinse thoroughly.
8. Finish in the same manner as for virgin hair.

Highlighting shampoo tints: preparations that combine aniline derivative tints, hydrogen peroxide and a neutral shampoo base. They are used when a **very slight change** in hair shade is desired. These tints serve to cleanse the hair and highlight its natural color in a single application. (Patron requires patch test.)

Lightening agent. There are some highlighting shampoos that contain just hydrogen peroxide and shampoo base. By omitting the tint and including only the lightener, color pigment is slightly removed from the hair. (No patch test is required.)

Method of application for both of the above. Distribute the mixture evenly over the entire head at the shampoo bowl. Retain from 8 to 15 minutes. Rinse thoroughly.

Pre-lighten. If the patron desires a drastic color change, lighter than her natural color, and wants to completely cover her grey hair, the hair should first be pre-lightened. The pre-lightener is applied in the same manner as for a regular hair lightening treatment.

Select shade from manufacturer's color chart.

After the pre-lightening has reached the desired shade, the hair is lightly shampooed and towel dried. Then the tint is applied in the usual manner.

Pre-soften. If patron's hair is resistant, the hair should be pre-softened in order for it to readily absorb the tint.

Apply the softener from the scalp to the hair ends as in regular lightening and retain it for a few minutes. During this time, little color change takes place, but the hair becomes more receptive to the tint. Do not rinse out the softener. Towel dry and apply tint, as directed by manufacturer.

SAFETY MEASURES

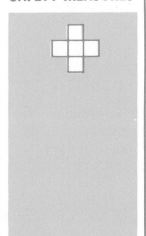

1. Give a 24-hour patch test before the application of a tint.
2. Do not apply tint if abrasions are present on the scalp.
3. Use clean applicator bottles, brushes, combs and towels.
4. Do not brush the hair prior to a tint.
5. Do not apply a tint without reading manufacturer's directions.
6. Take a strand test for color, breakage and/or hair discoloration.
7. Choose a shade of tint which harmonizes with the patron's general complexion.
8. Use an applicator bottle or bowl (plastic or glass) for mixing the tint.
9. Do not mix tint before ready to use; discard left-over tint.
10. If required, use the correct shade of color filler.
11. Suggest reconditioning treatments for tinted hair.
12. Do not apply tint if metallic or compound dye is present.
13. Do not apply tint if a patch test is positive.
14. Take a strand test for correct color shade before applying tint.
15. Use a mild shampoo. If an alkaline or harsh shampoo is used it will strip the color.
16. Do not use water that is too hot; use lukewarm water for removing free color.
17. Protect the patron's clothing by proper draping.
18. Do not permit tint to come in contact with the patron's eyes.
19. Do not overlap during a tint retouch.
20. Fill out a tint record card for each application.
21. Always wash hands before and after serving a patron.
22. Wear gloves to protect the hands.

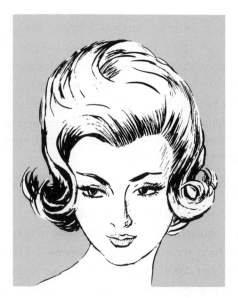

HAIR LIGHTENING

INTRODUCTION

Lightening the hair color, or blonding, is one of the most important and glamorizing services the beauty salon has to offer. Cosmetologists prefer to use the professional term **lighteners** rather than **bleaches** for the products which are designed to remove pigment from the hair. You will find that using the term "lightener" when talking to your patrons has a softer, more pleasing connotation than the harsher term "bleach."

How Lighteners Are Used

Lighteners may be used for two purposes:

1. **As a color treatment,** to lighten the hair to the final shade desired.
2. **As a preliminary treatment,** to prepare the hair for the application of a toner or tint. (This is referred to as Double Application tints, also called Two-Process or Two-Step tints.)
   a) **Toner**—A lightener is always necessary before applying one of the delicate toner shades.
   b) **Tint**—If the patron desires a drastic change to a much lighter than her natural shade, the lightener must be used to remove pigment before a tint is applied.

Effects Of Lighteners

A lightening product is used to lighten the hair to some desired shade. The hair pigment goes through different changing stages of color as it lightens. The amount of change depends on pigmentation of the hair and the length of time the lightening agent is left on. For example: A natural head of black hair will go from black to brown, to red, to red-gold, to gold, to yellow, and finally to pale yellow (almost white) stages. The seven stages of lightening are illustrated on the following page.

The hair also becomes more porous during the lightening treatment, a necessary condition to permit penetration of a toner.

Even natural **light hair** or **grey hair must go through the lightening process in order to achieve the necessary degree of porosity for the acceptance of a toner or tint.**

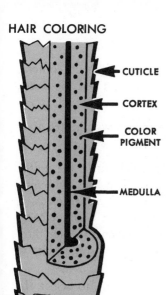

- CUTICLE
- CORTEX
- COLOR PIGMENT
- MEDULLA

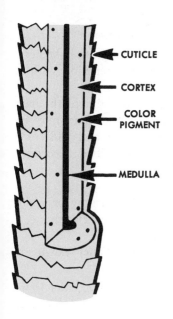

- CUTICLE
- CORTEX
- COLOR PIGMENT
- MEDULLA

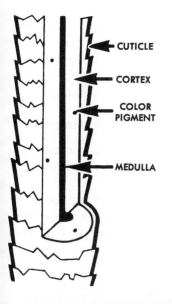

- CUTICLE
- CORTEX
- COLOR PIGMENT
- MEDULLA

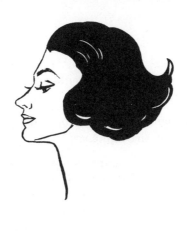

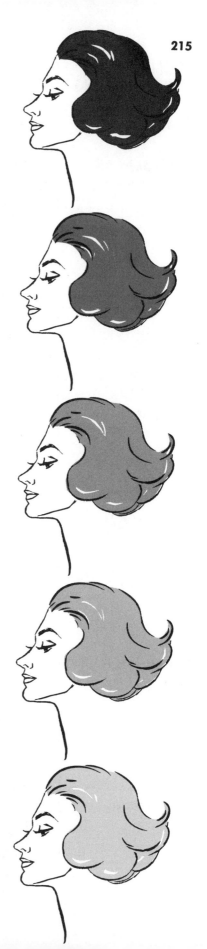

SEVEN STAGES IN LIGHTENING FROM DARK HAIR TO ALMOST WHITE
(Pale Yellow)

A virgin head of dark hair passes through seven stages before it arrives at the almost white stage.

The change in the color depends upon the type of lightener chosen and the length of time that it remains on the hair.

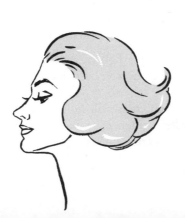

PROBLEMS IN HAIR LIGHTENING

The natural color of hair is determined by its pigment content. Natural hair coloring has either brown, or yellow and red pigments, or a mixture of both.

Brown Pigment

Brown pigment changes to a lighter shade in a few minutes after application of the lightener.

Yellow And Red Pigments

Yellow and red pigments are present in diffused form in the cortex of the hair. The diffused **red** pigment creates "problems" in lightening and tinting treatments. The **diffusion** of the **red** pigment makes it difficult or impossible to completely lighten the pigment without causing great damage to the hair. **Do not promise** a patron that her dark hair can be lightened to the very pale blonde shade if she desires to have silver, or extremely pale toners applied.

Whatever the reason for lightening, it is important to select the right lightener and the **best mixture** for the degree of color change desired. To make an **intelligent choice,** follow manufacturer's **literature** and **color charts.**

TYPES OF LIGHTENERS
Oil Lighteners

Lighteners are classified as oil, cream, and powder or paste lighteners. **Oil lighteners** are usually mixtures of hydrogen peroxide with a sulfonated oil.

1. **Colored oil lighteners** add temporary color and highlight the hair as they lighten. The colors contained are **certified** and may be used without a **patch** test. They **remove** pigment and **add** color tones at the same time. Basically, they are **classified** according to their **action** on the hair, namely:
   a) **Gold**—lightens and adds gold highlights.
   b) **Silver**—lightens and adds silvery highlights to grey or white hair and minimizes red and gold tones on other shades.
   c) **Red**—lightens and adds red highlights.
   d) **Drab**—lightens and adds ash highlights. Tones down or reduces red and gold tones.
2. **Neutral oil lightener** removes pigment without adding color tone. It may be used to pre-soften or pre-lighten hair for tint application.

Cream Lighteners

Cream lighteners are the most popular types of lighteners. They are easy to apply, will not run, drip or dry out. They are easy to control and contain conditioning agents, bluing and thickener, which provide the following benefits:
1. The **conditioning agents** give some protection to the hair.
2. The **bluing agent** helps to drab red and gold tones.
3. The **thickener** gives more control when applying lightener.

Powder Or Paste Lighteners

Powder or paste lighteners, also called quick lighteners, contain an oxygen-releasing booster and inert substances for quicker and stronger action.
1. **Paste lighteners** will hold and not run, but will dry out quickly.
2. **Powder lighteners,** mixed into a smooth creamy paste, do not contain conditioning agents and may dry the hair and irritate the scalp.

CAUTION. A patch test is required **only** if followed by a toner or tint application. If the scalp shows any sensitivity or abrasions, lighteners are not to be used.

ACTION OF HAIR LIGHTENERS

Hair lighteners, depending on manufacturer's directions, can be used as follows:

1. To lighten the entire head of hair for toner application
2. To lighten the hair to a particular shade
3. To brighten and lighten the existing shade
4. To tip, streak, or frost certain parts of the hair
5. To lighten hair that has already been tinted
6. To remove undesirable casts and off-shades
7. To correct dark streaks or spots in hair that has already been lightened or tinted

CHOICE OF HAIR LIGHTENERS

Together with manufacturer's directions, be guided by the following general rules:

1. Choose a cream lightener (blue base) when pre-lightening for pastel toners, such as blonde, silver, platinum or beige.
2. Choose a neutral oil lightener for the purpose of lightening the hair without adding color.
3. Choose an oil lightener (drab series) to avoid red and gold highlights in the natural color of the hair.
4. Choose an oil lightener (red and gold series) to obtain red or gold highlights in the natural color of the hair.
5. Choose a powder lightener for tipping, streaking and frosting **extremely** resistant hair.

HYDROGEN PEROXIDE

The lightening agent for removing pigment from the hair shaft is **hydrogen peroxide.** The **active** ingredient of hydrogen peroxide is oxygen gas. To speed the liberation of the oxygen gas, a small amount of **28% ammonia water** is added. However, this leaves the hair with a straw-like appearance, containing reddish or brassy tones. Commercial lightening products now contain substances which modify or prevent these effects.

For the purpose of hair lightening, hydrogen peroxide is used as a 6% solution, capable of producing 20 volumes of oxygen gas. A weaker strength of peroxide is not suitable for lightening and tinting. A higher strength peroxide, even though it may speed up the lightening action, may be harmful to the hair.

Forms Of Hydrogen Peroxide

Hydrogen peroxide is available in the form of a liquid, cream, powder or tablet. The liquid peroxide should be purchased in pint sizes, kept closed when not in use, and stored in a cool, dark, dry place.

Do not permit peroxide to come in contact with **metal.** Liquid peroxide will weaken in strength when it is kept too long, exposed to air or stored in a warm place. When using hydrogen peroxide in tablets, powder or cream form, follow manufacturer's directions.

**Uses Of
Hydrogen Peroxide**

As a **lightening agent,** hydrogen peroxide solution softens the cuticle of the hair shaft and lightens the shade of the coloring pigment in the cortical layer of the hair.

Lightening makes the hair porous and lighter in color. However, continued use of lighteners will make some hair over-dry and brittle.

As a **softening agent,** hydrogen peroxide softens the cuticle of the hair and makes it more receptive to the penetrating action of an aniline derivative tint. Care must be taken to control the softening process so that the hair is not lightened.

As an **oxidizing agent,** hydrogen peroxide solution is used in all aniline derivative (penetrating) hair tints. It acts as a developer by liberating oxygen gas, which changes para-phenylene-diamine into a dark-colored compound capable of tinting the hair.

LIGHTENING VIRGIN HAIR

A preliminary lightening strand test is necessary to ascertain the length of time a lightening mixture is to be left on the hair. It is also used to help diagnose the condition of the hair.

Patch Test For Toners

A patch test must be made 24 hours prior to the application of a **toner.** To save the patron's time, the strand test for lightening should be made the day she has the patch test.

**Implements
And Supplies**

To produce the best results in hair lightening, the cosmetologist should have available the following:

Towels	Peroxide (20 volume)
Tint cape	Lightening agent
Shampoo	Applicator bottle
Cotton	(plastic, with measurements listed)
Neutral rinse	Protective gloves
Comb, clips	Glass or plastic bowls
Record card	Measuring glass or cup
Talcum powder	Timer

If a paste type lightener is to be used, the brush applicator will be needed.

Procedure

The following general instructions in applying lighteners may be changed by your instructor to conform with manufacturer's directions.
1. **Prepare patron.** Adjust towel and tint cape to cover and protect patron's clothing.
2. **Examine scalp and hair.** Do not give a lightening treatment to a patron with eruptions or abrasions on the scalp. Do not brush or shampoo hair.
3. **Section hair** into four quarters.
4. **Prepare** lightening formula and use immediately to prevent deterioration. Follow manufacturer's directions.
5. **Put on protective gloves.**
6. **Apply lightener.** The order of applying the lightener around the head is immaterial. If the hair seems resistant or especially dark around the crown, then it is advisable to start at the back of the head, so that this region will get more lightening action.

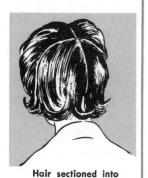

Hair sectioned into
four quarters

Apply lightener in ⅛-inch partings. Start about one-half to one inch from the scalp and extend lightener to a point where the hair shaft shows signs of damage. Apply lightener to both top and underside of hair strand.

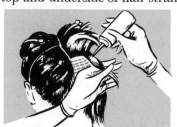

Apply lightener to top side about
½ - 1 inch from scalp.
See steps 6 and 7.

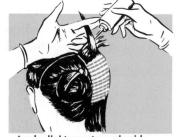

Apply lightener to underside
of strand.
See steps 6 and 7.

7. Continue to apply lightener on both sides of the strand until the entire head is completed. Work mixture into hair with fingers. The hair is more fragile at this point, so **do not comb the lightener through the hair.**

Keep hair moist with lightener during development. (Preliminary strand test will determine whether or not lightener is brought through the hair ends.)

8. **Test for color.** Make first strand test about 15 minutes before whatever time preliminary strand test had indicated to be necessary. Remove mixture from strand with wet towel or cotton. Dry the strand. If the shade is not light enough, reapply mixture and continue testing frequently until desired shade has nearly been developed.

9. **Scalp area and hair ends.** Towel blot excess lightener. If necessary, prepare a fresh mixture of lightener. Use ⅛-inch partings, and continue as follows:

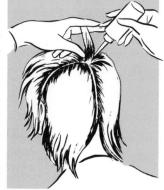

a) Apply lightener over the entire scalp area and on previously lightened hair. Retain lightener for required length of time.

b) When hair has lightened sufficiently, apply lightener to the hair ends and work through with fingertips.

Apply lightener to scalp area.
See step 9.

c) Pile the hair loosely on top of the head.

10. **Remove lightener.** When desired shade has been reached, rinse and shampoo hair lightly with cool water. Use a mild shampoo.

11. Dry hair either with towel or under a cool dryer.

12. Examine scalp for abrasions and hair for breakage. If scalp is normal the hair is ready for toner or tint application.

13. Fill out a complete record card.

14. Clean shampoo bowl, sanitize implements, discard used supplies and put station in order.

LIGHTENER RETOUCH

A lightener retouch is the term commonly used when a lightener is applied to the **new growth only** to match the rest of the lightened hair.

As a general rule, black or dark brown hair would require retouch applications more frequently than the lighter shades.

In retouching, the lightener is applied to the **new growth only,** with the following exceptions:

1. If another color is desired
2. If a lighter shade is desired
3. If color has become heavy or dull from several applications

For each of these conditions, wait until the new growth is almost light enough or has developed fully. Then bring the **remainder** of the lightener through the hair shaft. One to five minutes is ample time to correct any one of these conditions.

Procedure

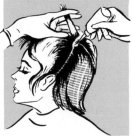

Apply lightener to new growth.

The patron's record card should be consulted by the cosmetologist as a guide to the lightener to be used and time required for the shade to develop.

Cream lightener is generally used for a lightener retouch because its ·adhesive quality prevents the overlapping of the previously lightened hair.

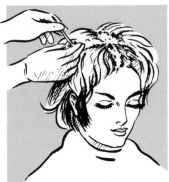

Strand test.

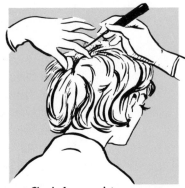

Check for complete coverage.

The **procedure for a lightener retouch** is the same as that for lightening a virgin head, except that the mixture is applied only to the new growth of hair.

CAUTION. Care should be taken not to **overlap** the lightener on to the previously lightened or tinted hair.

SAFETY MEASURES IN HAIR LIGHTENING

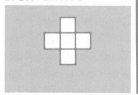

1. Give a 24-hour patch test before the lightener application, if a toner is to follow.
2. Drape patron properly to protect her clothing.
3. Examine the scalp for abrasions before applying a lightener.
4. Do not apply a lightener if irritation or abrasions are present.
5. Use only clean applicator bottles, brushes, sanitized combs and towels.
6. Wear gloves to protect the hands.

7. Analyze the condition of the hair and suggest reconditioning treatments, if required.

8. Test for color, breakage or hair discoloration by giving a strand test prior to hair lightening.

9. Cream or paste lightener must be the thickness of whipped cream to avoid dripping or running, causing overlapping.

10. Apply lightener to resistant areas first. To insure complete coverage, pick up 1/8-inch sections.

11. Work as rapidly as possible when applying the lightener, to produce a uniform shade without streaking.

12. Make frequent strand tests until the desired shade is reached.

13. After completing the lightener application, check the skin and remove any lightener from these areas.

14. Check and, if necessary, change the towel around the patron's neck. Lightener on the towel which is allowed to come in contact with the skin will cause irritation.

15. Lightened hair is fragile and requires special care. Use only a very mild shampoo, and rinse with cool water.

16. If a preliminary shampoo is required, do not brush the hair. Avoid irritating the scalp during the shampoo.

17. Do not allow lightener to stand; use it immediately. Discard leftover lightener.

18. Cap all bottles to avoid loss of strength.

19. Be sure to read manufacturer's directions before mixing a lightener.

20. Fill out record card after each hair lightening treatment.

TONERS

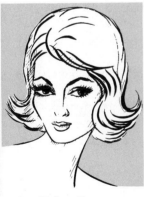

**Pre-Lightening
For Toners**

Toners are aniline derivative tints, and are a permanent, penetrating type of hair coloring, requiring a 24-hour skin or patch test. They consist primarily of pale, delicate colors.

Toners require double applications, and are also known as Two-Step or Two-Process tints.

1. The first application is the lightener.

2. The second application is the toner.

To achieve the desired toner color, **pre-lightening** is required. Hair should be pre-lightened to gold or pale yellow, depending on the toner color to be used.

Toners penetrate the cuticle and deposit color in the same manner as other tints. They depend on the preliminary lightening to leave the hair both light in color and porous. Some toners (the extreme pale shades) require more pre-lightening than others. The lightener must be left on long enough to achieve the necessary porosity. Coarse, resistant or dark hair require longer lightening time than naturally blonde hair.

Although naturally blonde hair may reach the pale yellow stage very quickly, it may **not be porous** enough to permit penetration of the toner. If the required porosity has not been developed, allow for additional lightening time.

White Or Grey Hair

White or grey hair requires a certain amount of pre-lightening to make the hair porous enough to receive a toner. White or grey hair, being almost decolorized, needs pre-lightening before the application of a blonde, silver, or pastel shade toner. Pre-lightening is very important when grey hair is a mixture of light and dark strands. Lengthy lightening will not be necessary; but a certain amount of lightening is required to make the hair porous enough to accept the toner.

Selecting Toner Shades

The pastel colors, such as silver, ash, platinum and beige, are glamour colors which appeal to many women.

For the patron desiring **extremely** pale toner shades of the **very light** hair, the blonde colors are the perfect color tones.

For the patron with grey hair and skin tone changes which accompany the advancing years, the lighter silver tones are flattering.

For the patron desiring extremely pale toner shades of the **very light** silver, platinum or beige colors, the hair must be pre-lightened to the **pale yellow**, or almost **white stage.**

Color selection is frequently left to the cosmetologist's judgment. Other important factors to be considered are patron's age and complexion.

REMINDERS

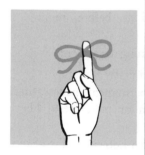

Toners are completely dependent upon a proper preliminary lightening treatment, which must leave the hair light and porous enough to receive pale toner shades. A strand test must first be made, and a complete explanation of the possible outcome should be given to the patron.

The possibility may exist that her hair cannot be decolorized enough to achieve the color of her choice without seriously damaging the hair shaft.

If the red and gold pigments have not been eliminated during the lightening process, the patron's choice of toner color might result in a shade with a greenish cast, or the color might not take at all. When this happens, the toner used must be deeper and not as pale or silvery as the patron may have requested.

During the application and development period, toners have quite a different color than the final shade (related to their basic color). However, when the color has fully developed, the anticipated color will have been achieved. (Example: Ash blonde will have a brownish cast; silver blonde, a bluish cast; and platinum, a violet cast.)

**TONER
APPLICATION**
Preliminary

1. Give 24-hour patch test before toner application.
2. To determine the final color, make strand test when you give a patch test.
3. If the patch test is negative and the scalp is normal and without irritation, proceed with the toner treatment.

Strand Test

1. Mix a small amount of toner with an equal amount of developer. (Be sure to recap bottles immediately.)

2. Apply the mixture to a full strand of lightened hair. Allow color to develop for 15 minutes. Rinse, towel dry, and check color. If color has not developed to desired shade, reapply mixture and check again in 5 minutes. Continue checking until desired shade has been reached.

3. Wash and towel dry. Write down the time it took for color to develop, and use this as a guide for giving a toner treatment.

Supplies

In addition to the toner, use the same implements and supplies as used for lightening virgin hair.

Preparation

1. Arrange all necessary supplies.
2. Prepare patron.
3. Lighten hair to pale yellow (almost white). Then, shampoo hair lightly, rinse thoroughly and towel dry.
4. Select the desired toner shade.

Preparing Formula

Prepare formula at room temperature. Pour bottle of toner into applicator or bowl. Add equal amount of developer. If you use applicator, cover top with gloved hand and turn it over four or five times. Do not shake. When using bowl, stir mixture gently for just a few seconds.

Application Of Toner

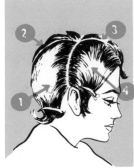

Sectioning the hair into four quarters.

Wear rubber gloves throughout the entire application.

Be sure hair is pre-lightened to the stage necessary for the toner shade to be used.

1. Section hair into four quarters, using comb or tip of applicator.
2. Starting at the crown of the back right quarter, apply mixture to the scalp area. Make small 1/4-inch partings. Continue to apply mixture to the other three sections.
3. When application to the scalp area has been completed, use comb to distribute and blend mixture through entire strand, applying additional mixture to saturate hair.

   Caution. Do not comb toner mixture through over-porous hair ends until the last few minutes of developing time. If the ends absorb too much color, dilute remaining mixture with equal amount of shampoo, conditioner or water before applying to ends.

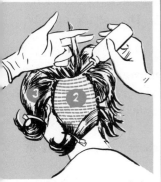

Applying toner to the hair.

4. Pour additional mixture on hair and blend throughout. Leave hair loose to permit circulation of air, insuring better color development.
5. After 15 minutes, dry a strand of hair and test for color If desired color has not been reached, recomb more mixture into tested strand. Repeat test frequently with different strands until you reach desired shade.
6. When treatment is complete, rinse out excess toner thoroughly and shampoo according to manufacturer's recommendations.
7. Towel dry hair.
8. Remove all toner stains from the skin, hairline, ears and neck.
9. Set, dry and style hair.
10. Fill out record card and clean up in the usual manner.

Give a **toner retouch** the same careful consideration as you would give a tint retouch. The new growth must be pre-lightened to the same degree of lightness as was the first toner application. **Caution: Overlapping** the lightener may cause hair damage.

After the lightening process has been completed, the toner is applied as outlined below.

Preliminary

1. Give patch test before application of toner. Also give strand test.
2. Prelighten new growth to stage required for toner.
3. Towel dry hair after lightener has been thoroughly rinsed and shampooed from hair.

Procedure

1. Part hair into 4 sections. Start application at the back of head.
2. Making ¼-inch partings throughout, use a plastic applicator bottle or tinting brush to apply the toner mixture to the new growth area only.
3. If hair shaft is holding color from previous treatment, allow the roots to develop to the same degree of color shown by a strand test. Then, using a comb, distribute and blend color through the hair to about one inch from the hair ends.
4. Strand test frequently. Reapply mixture to tested strands.
5. When strand test shows color has reached close to the desired shade, work the balance of the mixture through the ends. Should the ends absorb too much color, dilute the toner mixture with an equal amount of shampoo, conditioner or water, as directed by manufacturer.
6. When color is evenly developed, as shown by strand test, thoroughly rinse and shampoo, as recommended by manufacturer.
7. Towel dry hair.
8. Remove toner stains from the skin of hairline, ears and neck.
9. Set, dry and style hair.
10. Fill out record card.
11. Clean up in the usual manner.

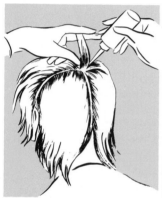

Apply lightener to new growth.

1. Give 24-hour patch test prior to toner application.
2. Do not apply toner if scalp has any irritation, sores or abrasions.
3. Use only glass, porcelain or plastic utensils. **Do not use metallic bowls or dishes.**
4. Always wear rubber gloves to protect hands.
5. For best results, mix ingredients at room temperature immediately before application.
6. Apply toner as rapidly as possible for even results.
7. Discard left-over toner mixture.
8. Remove toner stains from skin with absorbent cotton soaked in mild shampoo and water. **Do not rub.**
9. After a toner application, use a shampoo as directed by manufacturer.
10. Do not give a permanent wave on the same day of toner application.

FROSTING, TIPPING AND STREAKING

For **partial lightening**, such as in achieving frosting, tipping and streaking effects, quick lighteners are often advisable.

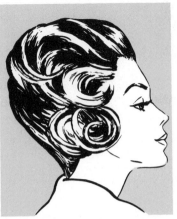

Marbelized streaking

1. **Frosting.** Strands of hair are lightened over various parts of the head. The strands of hair to be lightened are pulled through the holes of a perforated cap. This procedure is followed to protect the scalp when the lightener is applied. The **effect** achieved will depend on how many strands of hair are treated and their location

2. **Tipping** is similar to frosting. Wisps of hair are lightened in various areas, usually across the front of the head. This produces a contrast with the darker shade of hair. Strands of hair are drawn through holes in a perforated cap and lightened.

3. **Streaking.** This is a lightened strand, usually at the front hairline. The width and placement of the lightened strand depend on the "feather" effect to be achieved.

Cap Technique For Frosting And Tipping

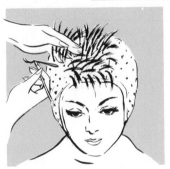

Draw strands through holes with crochet hook.

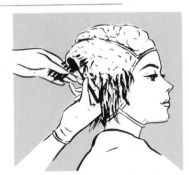

Apply lightener with brush.

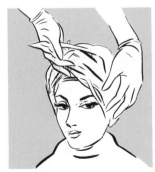

To hasten process, cover the head with aluminum foil or plastic cap.

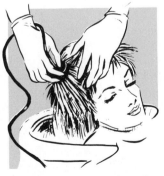

After hair has sufficiently lightened, remove covering. While cap is still on, shampoo or rinse off lightener and towel dry.

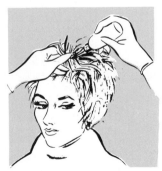

Apply toner in the usual manner.

Frosting All Over

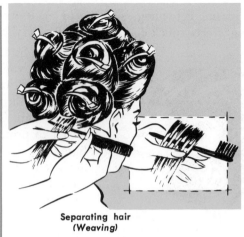

Separating hair
(Weaving)

1. Separate hair (weave).
2. Place aluminum foil underneath hair to be lightened.
3. Apply lightener on both sides of strand.
4. Wrap hair in aluminum foil. Continue this procedure over entire head. Leave one-half inch parting around front hairline.
5. Complete frosting as for cap technique.

Streaking

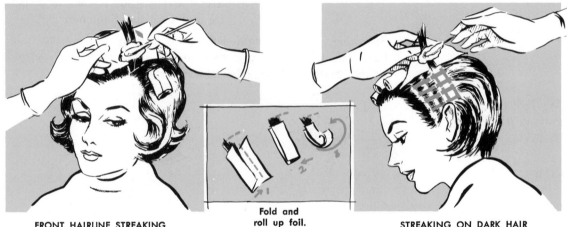

FRONT HAIRLINE STREAKING
Select 3 or 4 sections to be streaked. Comb other hair out of way. Apply lightener ½-inch from scalp. Fold and roll foil. Process and finish the treatment as explained on previous page.

Fold and roll up foil.

STREAKING ON DARK HAIR
Section hair to be streaked. Apply lightener ½-inch from scalp. Fold and roll foil. Process and finish the treatment in the usual manner.

Blonde-On-Blonde Effect

The hair to be treated should be light blonde. Section the hair into a checkerboard pattern, as in Fig. 1. Wrap every other section with aluminum foil by folding and rolling up each one. Thirty to forty sections should be sufficient. (Fig. 2.)

Apply deepest blonde toner to all unwrapped hair, as in Fig 3. After the hair has been sufficiently processed, and before removing foils from rolled strands, rinse thoroughly.

Remove foils; towel dry hair; then, apply the lightest toner to the entire head.

Shampoo, set, dry and style hair in the usual manner.

HAIR COLORING

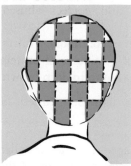

1. Checkerboard pattern.

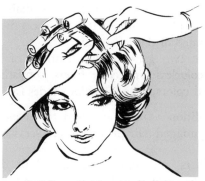

2. Roll up strands not to be lightened with aluminum foil.

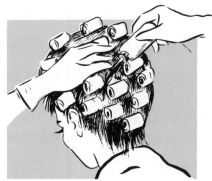

3. Apply toner to unwrapped hair.

SPECIAL PROBLEMS

Damaged Hair

The frequent use of lacquers and hair sprays coats and damages the hair. Hair in this state must be **reconditioned** before it can **successfully** be tinted, lightened, or permanent waved.

Careless application of tints, lighteners and permanent waving solutions to the hair may result in breakage or dry, brittle hair.

The use of either **highly alkaline shampoos or soapless oil shampoos**, the improper use of water temperature and hair dryer, and extreme exposure to the elements, all may cause hair to become damaged.

Hair may need reconditioning treatments for reasons other than damage resulting from the use of harmful products. Sometimes hair is naturally brittle, thin and lifeless. Both **neglect** and the **patron's physical condition** may be contributing factors to these conditions.

Hair is considered damaged when it is in the following condition:

1. Over-porous
2. Brittle and dry
3. Breaks easily
4. No elasticity
5. Rough and harsh to the touch
6. Over-lightened hair that is coarse, spongy and mats easily when wetted
7. Rejects color or absorbs too much color during a tinting process

Any of these hair conditions may create trouble during a tinting, lightening or permanent waving treatment. Therefore, damaged hair should receive reconditioning treatments **previous to and after the application of these chemical agents.**

Reconditioning Procedure

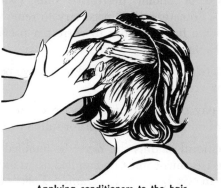

Applying conditioners to the hair

To restore damaged hair to a more normal condition, commercial products containing lanolin or protein substances should be used.

The reconditioning agent is applied to the hair. If heat is applied, use either heating cap, steamer or heating lamp according to manufacturer's directions. As to frequency and length of time for each treatment, be guided by your instructor.

FILLERS

Fillers are preparations which are available in liquid or cream form. They are employed to revitalize, **recondition** and correct abused, lightened, tinted or damaged hair.

There are two general classifications of fillers: **conditioner fillers**, which are colorless; and color fillers, consisting of a mixture of protein and certified colors, range in color shades from platinum to deep brown.

Conditioner Fillers

The **conditioner fillers** are used to recondition lightened, tinted, or otherwise damaged hair prior to a hair service.

Color Fillers

Color fillers are applied to abused or damaged hair to equalize porosity and to deposit a base color prior to a tinting treatment. If the hair is in a damaged condition, and if there is any doubt that the finished color will not be an even shade, a color filler is recommended.

When To Use

A color filler is applied after hair has been pre-lightened and before the application of a toner or tint. A filler is also used for the patron who has been tinting or lightening her hair and desires to return to her natural color.

Advantages

The following are the advantages of color fillers:
1. They deposit color to faded hair shafts and ends.
2. They help hair to hold color.
3. They help to insure a uniform color from the scalp to hair ends.
4. They prevent color streaking.
5. They prevent off-color results.
6. They prevent a dull color appearance.
7. They give more uniform color in a tint back to natural shade.

How To Use

Color fillers may be applied **directly** from their containers to **damaged hair** prior to tinting. Color fillers may be **added** to the **remainder** of the tint or toner and applied to **damaged hair ends**. In all instances, be guided by your instructor.

Selecting Color Fillers

To obtain satisfactory results, select the color filler to match the same basic shade as the toner or tint to be used.

Note—Since manufacturers' directions regarding fillers vary from one another as to color selection, their use and application, be guided by the directions of manufacturer, or by your instructor.

REMOVING PENETRATING TINTS

Removal of aniline derivative tints (**with prepared commercial products**). Sometimes it is necessary to remove or partially remove the tint from the hair in order to correct a previous tinting treatment or to apply a new shade.

Commercial products designed to remove penetrating tints are known as tint or color removers.

They may contain hydrogen peroxide, acids, sodium hydrosulfite, a mixture of mineral and vegetable or sulfonated oils.

The removal of tints can never be handled mechanically. Each color removing treatment must be handled as an **individual problem** in which nothing can ever be taken for granted. **Follow manufacturer's directions.**

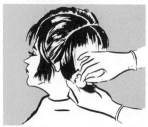
1. Apply mixture to darkest area.

Procedure

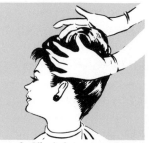

2. Pile hair on top of head.

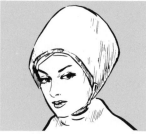

3. If hastening the process is required, put on a heating cap.

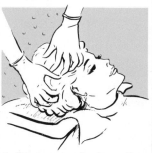

4. Shampoo and rinse thoroughly with cool water.

REMOVING COATING DYES

TINT BACK TO NATURAL COLOR

Chemicals that are sold for the purpose of removing tints should always be used with caution. Follow **manufacturer's directions**.

1. Prepare patron.
2. Follow manufacturer's directions about whether or not to shampoo.
3. Section hair into four quarters.
4. Put on protective gloves.
5. Mix preparation in a glass dish. Follow manufacturer's directions for mixing.
6. Start application immediately where the hair is the darkest. (Fig. 1.)
7. Apply the mixture with a cotton pledget or brush. Saturate the hair thoroughly.
8. After completely covering the hair, strand test immediately, and frequently thereafter.
9. Pile the hair on top of the head. (Fig. 2.)
10. If required by manufacturer, apply a warm, damp towel around the head, or place patron under a steamer or heating cap. (Fig. 3.) **Be guided by your instructor.**
11. When the color has been removed, shampoo thoroughly, using shampoo and cool water. (Fig. 4.) Rinse thoroughly with cool water.

  CAUTION. The tint remover must be rinsed thoroughly from the hair; otherwise, its chemical action will continue.
12. Towel dry or thoroughly dry hair under dryer, as required by manufacturer.
13. If color is to be added, proceed with the application of desired shade of tint.
14. If no color is to be applied, set, dry and style hair in the usual manner.

If the product requires a waiting period before applying tint or other services, be guided by your instructor.

Coating dyes, such as metallic dyes and compound dyes, are coloring agents that do not penetrate, but coat the hair shaft. In removing coating dyes, never guarantee the results, because complete success is not certain. For removing coating dyes be guided by your instructor.

Each tint back to natural color must be handled as an individual problem.

Check the natural shade of the hair next to the scalp.

The determining factors in the selection of the tint shade are:
1. The present condition and color of the hair,
2. The final result desired, which is the original color.

Select an appropriate shade of filler to correspond with the tint to be used. Without the use of an appropriate filler, it would be difficult to obtain a uniform color from the scalp to hair ends, since the hair porosity will vary in degree and area of the head.

Such hair coloring problems require two or more strand tests and guidance by the instructor in color selection and procedure.

Procedure

1. Assemble materials.
2. Prepare patron in the usual manner.
3. Select appropriate tint and color filler, as shown by the strand test.
4. Shampoo and towel dry the hair, or be guided by your instructor.
5. Section hair into four quarters.
6. If a color filler is required, proceed as directed by your instructor.
7. Resection hair into four quarters.
8. Subdivide sections into about ¼-inch partings. Apply the tint **as rapidly as possible** to both sides of the hair strand, from scalp to hair ends.
9. Check for complete coverage.
10. Strand test immediately and frequently until desired shade has developed.
11. Give a mild or non-strip shampoo and use a non-strip rinse. Set, dry and style hair in the usual manner.
12. Fill out a record card and clean up work station.

LIGHTENING STREAKED HAIR

Streaks of discoloration often appear on the hair, caused in part by unsuccessful or unskilled lightener applications.

To correct streaked hair:

1. Prepare lightening formula as for virgin hair.
2. Apply mixture only to the darker streaks.
3. Work one strand at a time.
4. Allow mixture to remain on hair until all streaks are removed.
5. Shampoo hair.

SPOT LIGHTENING

Because the natural pigmentation of the hair is not distributed evenly, hair is often not lightened evenly from scalp to ends. **Uneven** lightening may also be due to **careless** application of the lightener. When this happens, gold bands or darker streaks may appear. This means that these areas have not been lightened enough. Spot lightening then becomes necessary to insure an even color. Reapply the lightener to these particular areas. Let it remain until it is lightened sufficiently to even out the entire head of hair.

LASH AND BROW TINT

An aniline derivative tint should **never** be used for coloring eyebrows or eyelashes; to do so may cause **blindness.** Instead, a harmless coloring agent, such as mascara, should be used.

The choice of color is limited to either brown or black. While black is favored in most cases, brown is recommended for very light blonde complexions. Follow the specific directions of manufacturer when applying the coloring agent.

**Implements
And Supplies**

Petroleum jelly (Vaseline)
Lash and brow tinting solutions
   (Solutions No. 1 and No. 2)
Stain remover
Dish of soapy water

Dish of clear water
Towels
Cotton
Shields
Applicator sticks

Preparation

1. Follow sanitary measures.
2. Place patron in partially reclining position in facial or shampoo chair at approximately a 45-degree angle. **Do not** permit her to lie in a straight position. Such a position would permit the tinting solution to enter the eyes more easily.
3. Place a clean towel across her chest.

Procedure

1. Wash lashes and brows with warm, soapy water, using a cotton pledget. Remove all traces of cosmetic makeup from lashes and brows.
2. Apply petroleum jelly around eyes and on paper shields.
3. Adjust eyeshields. Ask patron to look up, adjust shield and close eye gently. Do the same with the other eye.
4. Apply No. 1 solution to lashes. Moisten cotton-tipped applicator. Touch tip to towel to remove excess moisture. Apply over and under lashes close to skin. Moisten lashes several times. **Break applicator stick, and discard. Use a fresh applicator stick each time solution is required.**
5. Apply No. 1 solution to brows, following natural brow line. Reapply against natural growth, working solution in thoroughly. **Replace cap on No. 1 solution bottle.** (If bottle caps are interchanged, oxidation starts and the liquids lose their value.)

Moisten fresh applicator with stain remover and place on edge of towel for future use. Replace cap on stain remover bottle.

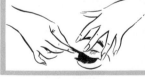 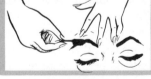 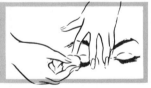

Apply No. 1 solution   Apply No. 1 solution   Wash lashes and brows
to lashes.   to brows.   with cool water.

6. Apply No. 2 solution to lashes and brows in same manner as No. 1 solution. If stain gets on skin, use stain remover immediately. Replace cap on No. 2 bottle.
7. Remove eyeshields and wash lashes and brows with cool water, using cotton pledgets.
8. Place moist eyepads over eyelids. Rewash brows with soap and water. Remove eyepads. Place small roll of cotton under lashes and wash them from above with cool water.
9. Remove stains with stain remover. Replace bottle cap.
10. Soothe skin with lotion or cream. Wash the eyes with boric acid solution.
11. Clean up in the usual manner.

DEFINITIONS

Virgin hair is hair which has neither been lightened nor tinted. **Note:** The cosmetologist should know whether the hair has been permanently waved or chemically straightened, and what, if any, damage resulted thereby.

A **touch-up or retouch** is the application of coloring or lightener to the new growth of hair.

Blending is the process of making the color uniform throughout the hair during hair coloring applications or during retouches.

Coating is the accumulation of residue on the outside of the hair.

Certified color is a temporary coloring which coats the hair and lasts from one shampoo to another.

Pre-softening or softening is the application of a lightener to soften resistant hair and make it more receptive to the tint.

Powder or paste lightener is a strong, fast-acting product used for special effects and to save time in hair lightening.

Pre-lightening is the process of removing partial or total color from the hair before a tinting or toner application.

Decolorization is the removal of natural or artificial color pigment from the hair.

Tint back is the coloring of the hair back to its natural shade.

Toner is an aniline derivative tint, delicate in shade, which is applied to lightened hair to produce blonde, silver and pastel shades.

Tint removal is the removal of an unsatisfactory shade of tint from the hair by the use of a dye solvent, lightener, or softening treatment.

Color testing is a method of determining the action of a selected tint on a small strand of hair by washing and drying in order to observe its progress.

Strand test is a preliminary test given on a small strand of hair before a coloring or lightening treatment. It is used to predetermine the mixture and development time required for the treatment. Color development for color testing is also known as **strand testing.**

Development time is the time needed to develop the color or the lightener.

Semi-permanent hair coloring is hair coloring that lasts from 4 to 6 shampoos. Penetrates hair shaft slightly. Contains no peroxide and needs no peroxide to develop color.

Oxidation is a chemical reaction which takes place when peroxide and tinting solution are mixed and applied to the hair.

A **developer** is an oxidizing agent, such as 20 volume hydrogen peroxide solution; when mixed with a tint, it releases the necessary oxygen gas.

Sensitivity is a condition in which the skin is highly reactive to a specific chemical. Skin reddens or becomes irritated shortly after contact with the chemical. On removal of the chemical the reaction usually subsides.

Allergy is a skin sensitivity to cosmetics, tints, foods or other substances. In hair coloring, a very small number of patrons may be allergic to aniline derivative tints.

Susceptible means capable of being allergic.

Idiosyncrasy is an individual peculiarity which makes one susceptible to chemical substances in cosmetics, drugs and foods.

Skin or patch test is a procedure for determining whether or not a person is allergic to an aniline derivative tint.

Color filler is a preparation containing a certified color used to equalize porosity in over-porous hair so it can take and hold color evenly.

Highlighting refers to the brightening effect on the hair accomplished by the application of a tint or the application of a lightener.

Overlapping is a condition caused in a retouch by having a tint or a lightener overlap any part of the previously tinted or lightened hair.

Line of demarcation is a streak caused by overlapping on previously tinted hair.

Peroxometer is an instrument used primarily by chemists to measure the strength of hydrogen peroxide.

Porosity is the extent to which hair is able to absorb moisture or liquid preparations.

Soap cap is the application of a tint diluted with a shampoo. It is worked through the hair like a shampoo.

Plastic cap is a cap made of plastic, used to hasten the hair coloring process.

Heating cap is used to hasten the coloring process.

Stripping is a term used to indicate the removal of natural hair pigment, coating or penetrating tint from the hair.

Resistant hair is hair with poor porosity.

Conditioner is a cosmetic applied to hair to restore oils, sheen, elasticity and manageability.

Spot lightening is applying a lightener only to dark areas to even out color.

Spot tinting is applying tint to areas insufficiently colored, in order to produce even results throughout.

Frosting, tipping, streaking are techniques for partial lightening of small sections of hair in various parts of the head.

Record card is a written record of the patron's hair structure, condition, lightening and tinting color used, plus other pertinent information concerning the hair.

Lift refers to the degree of lightening. Hair lifted two shades means hair was made two shades lighter.

Accelerating (processing) machine is used to shorten the processing time of a lightening or tinting treatment.

REVIEW QUESTIONS

Hair Coloring

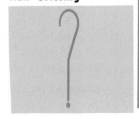

1. Define hair tinting.
2. Give three reasons why a patron may wish to have her hair tinted.
3. What knowledge should a cosmetologist have to be successful in the technique of hair coloring?
4. What are the three main groups of hair coloring?
5. What is meant by a virgin head of hair?
6. What do color rinses contain and how long do they remain on the hair?
7. What is meant by semi-permanent hair coloring?
8. Which tints are the penetrating type?
9. Name three types of hair coloring that coat the hair.
10. What type of dyes are never used professionally?

11. What are aniline derivative tints?
12. Briefly describe the action of aniline derivative tints.
13. State two reasons why aniline derivative tints require a 24-hour patch test.
14. In what two areas is a skin test given?
15. What are two important factors to consider when selecting a color shade?
16. Why should a preliminary strand test be given before the application of a tint?
17. List four conditions which would prohibit the application of an aniline derivative tint.
18. Why is the hair not brushed previous to a tinting treatment?
19. What type of tint can be used to lighten and deposit color in the hair in one application?
20. By what other terms are single application tints known?
21. To which part of the hair is a tint retouch applied?
22. When is pre-softening required for a one-step tint?
23. When is a double application tint recommended?
24. By what other terms are double application tints known?
25. What are two purposes of highlighting shampoo tints?
26. List three precautionary measures to follow when tinting hair back to its natural shade.
27. **List two methods by which unwanted tint may be removed from the hair.**
28. How should each color removing treatment be handled?
29. How are tint stains removed from the skin and scalp?
30. What may be used to prevent porous areas of the hair shaft from absorbing too much tint?
31. When is a color filler recommended?
32. What purposes are served by conditioner fillers?
33. What is meant by a coating dye?
34. Define dye removal.
35. What kind of tint should never be used to colo. eyebrows and eyelashes?

REVIEW QUESTIONS

Hair Lightening

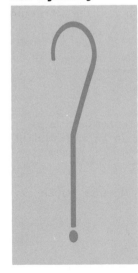

1. Define hair lightening.
2. Lightening the hair is usually a preparatory process for which other hair treatment?
3. What two types of applications are generally used to apply a lightener to the hair?
4. List three types of commercial lighteners.
5. On what parts of the hair shaft are frosting, tipping and streaking usually applied?
6. What is most important in the choice of a lightening product?
7. What strength hydrogen peroxide is commonly used?
8. Why do lightening products contain small quantities of 28% ammonia water?
9. What conditions of the hair require reconditioning treatments?
10. What are toners?
11. To which part of the hair is a lightener retouch applied?
12. What are three causes for over-lightening of the hair?
13. What effect does lightening have on the hair?
14. Why should lightened hair receive corrective treatments?
15. What reaction does hydrogen peroxide have on the hair when used as a softening agent?
16. Why does white or grey hair require some pre-lightening prior to the application of a toner?
17. Why should cold water be used during the shampoo following a hair lightening treatment?

CHAPTER 16

CHEMICAL HAIR RELAXING

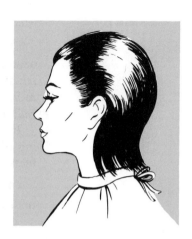

INTRODUCTION

Chemical hair relaxing is the process of permanently rearranging the basic structure of over-curly hair into a straight form. When done professionally, it usually leaves the hair straight and in satisfactory condition, ready to be dressed into almost any style.

To attain proficiency in chemical hair relaxing, the cosmetologist must acquire thorough technical knowledge and expert manipulative skills in this specialized branch of cosmetology.

There are two basic products that are used in chemical hair relaxing: a chemical hair relaxer and a neutralizer.

CHEMICAL HAIR RELAXERS

Sodium Hydroxide

The two general types of hair relaxers are sodium hydroxide, which does not require pre-shampooing, and ammonium thioglycolate, which requires pre-shampooing.

1. **Sodium Hydroxide** (caustic type relaxer) has both a softening and a swelling action on hair fibers. As the relaxing solution penetrates into the cortical layer, the cross-bonds (sulfur and hydrogen) are unlocked and broken. The action of the comb, or the hands, in smoothing the hair and distributing the relaxer, straightens the softened hair.

Manufacturers vary the sodium hydroxide content of the solution from 5% to 10%, and the pH factor from 10 and higher. In general, the more sodium hydroxide used and the higher the pH, the quicker the chemical reaction will take place on the hair, and the greater the danger will be of hair damage.

When using sodium hydroxide, the cosmetologist must soften the hair within a maximum period of eight minutes. If the product is left on the hair longer than the required time (as indicated by a strand test), the hair may turn a reddish color, or it may become brittle with resulting breakage. If the solution is left on the hair longer than ten minutes, the possibility develops of complete hair dissolution. **Because of the extreme action of sodium hydroxide, great care must be exercised in its use.**

2. **Ammonium Thioglycolate** (thio type relaxer). Although this type of relaxer is less drastic in its actions than sodium hydroxide, ammonium thioglycolate softens and relaxes over-curly hair in somewhat the same manner.

NEUTRALIZERS

The neutralizer is also called a "stabilizer" or "fixative." The neutralizer serves to stop the action of any chemical relaxer which may remain in the hair after rinsing. At the same time, the neutralizer re-forms the cystine (sulfur) cross-bonds in their new position and re-hardens the hair.

It is important that the cosmetologist have a thorough understanding of the product being used and its action on the hair. The manufacturer's directions should be followed explicitly.

BASIC STEPS

Chemical hair relaxing involves three basic steps: **processing, neutralizing** and **conditioning**.

Processing

As soon as the chemical relaxer is applied, the hair begins to soften and lose its tight curl.

Neutralizing

As soon as the hair has been sufficiently processed, the chemical relaxer is thoroughly **rinsed out** with warm water, and followed by either a combination mild shampoo and neutralizer, or a prescribed mild shampoo and a neutralizer.

Conditioning

Depending upon the patron's needs, the conditioner may be part of a series of hair treatments, or it may be applied to the hair before or after the relaxing treatment.

Most over-curly hair, except **virgin hair,** is in a damaged condition due to hot comb, hot iron, tinting or lightening treatments. Therefore, conditioning is often necessary before a chemical relaxing treatment, in order to give strength and body to the damaged hair, and to protect it against possible breakage.

Precautions

Hair that has had recent tinting, lightening, hot comb or hot iron services should **not receive a chemical hair relaxing treatment.** A series of reconditioning treatments should be given first, to restore the hair to a nearly normal condition. Then, if the results of strand tests are favorable, a chemical hair relaxing treatment may be given.

Metallic dye. Hair treated with metallic dyes must not be given a hair relaxing treatment; to do so would damage or destroy the hair.

Fine, wooly hair. It is not advisable to use a **strong** relaxer on fine, wooly hair, as it is too weak and fragile to withstand the softening agent in the relaxer. However, the application of **a weak** or **mild** relaxer is permissible.

ANALYSIS OF PATRON'S HAIR

It is essential that the cosmetologist have a working knowledge of human hair, particularly in the case of over-curly hair. Recognition of the qualities of hair is made possible by means of visible inspection, feel and special tests. Before attempting to give a relaxing treatment to over-curly hair, the cosmetologist must judge its texture, porosity, elasticity and the extent, if any, of damage to the hair. (For more complete information on hair analysis, refer to the chapter on **Permanent Waving.**)

PATRON'S HAIR HISTORY

To help assure satisfactory results, records should be kept of each chemical hair relaxing treatment. These records should include the patron's hair history and her release statement.

A release statement is used to protect the cosmetologist, to some extent, from liability for accidents or damages. (For a sample of a patron's record card and release statement, refer to chapter on **Permanent Waving.**

Before starting to process the hair, the cosmetologist must be certain of how the patron will react to the relaxer. Therefore, the patron must receive the following tests:

1. A thorough scalp examination
2. A hair strand test

Scalp Examination

Inspect the scalp carefully for the presence or absence of eruptions, scratches or abrasions. To obtain a clearer view of the scalp, part the hair into half-inch sections. Hair parting may be done with the index and middle fingers. The cosmetologist must exercise great care not to injure the scalp. **Such injuries may become seriously infected when aggravated by the chemicals in the relaxer.**

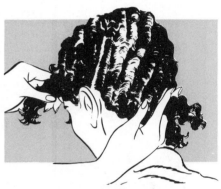

Examining the scalp

If any scalp eruptions or abrasions are present, **do not apply the chemical hair relaxer** until the scalp is again in a healthy condition.

Strand Test

Three strand tests are employed, as follows:

1. **Finger test** determines the degree of porosity in the hair. Hold a strand of hair with thumb and index finger and "run" it between thumb and index finger of the other hand, from the end toward the scalp. If the hair ruffles, it **is** porous and can absorb moisture.

2. **Pull test** (tensile strength) determines the degree of elasticity in the hair. Normally, curly dry hair will stretch about 1/5th its normal length without breaking. Grasp half a dozen strands from the crown area and pull them **gently.** If the hair appears to stretch or pull, it has elasticity and can withstand the relaxer. If not, conditioning treatments are recommended prior to a chemical relaxing treatment.

3. **Relaxer test.** Application of the relaxer to a **hair strand** will indicate the ultimate results of the complete treatment. Take a small section of hair and thread through a hole cut in a piece of wax paper or aluminum foil. Apply relaxer to the hair. Allow it to remain on the hair for two or three minutes, and then remove with a piece of dry cotton. If the hair has been changed to a straight form and a definite processing time has been established, proceed with the treatment. If the hair has not processed sufficiently, repeat the test on another strand and allow a minute or two longer for processing.

CHEMICAL HAIR RELAXING PROCESS

Implements And Supplies

1. Chemical relaxer
2. Stabilizer or neutralizer
3. Shampoo
4. Shampoo cape
5. Protective base
6. Hair conditioner
7. Protective gloves
8. Towels
9. Rollers
10. Comb and brush
11. Spatula
12. Timer
13. Absorbent cotton
14. Neck strip
15. Clips and picks
16. Hair net
17. End papers
18. Creme rinse

Note—The procedure outlined below is based primarily on the use of products containing **sodium hydroxide. Follow manufacturer's directions and be guided by your instructor.**

Preparation

1. Select and arrange the required implements and supplies.
2. Wash and sanitize your hands.
3. Prepare and drape the patron as for a shampoo.
4. Examine scalp and evaluate strand test results.
5. If necessary, trim damaged hair ends. **Do not shampoo.**

PROCEDURE FOR SODIUM HYDROXIDE RELAXER

Section Hair

Part hair into four or five sections, as recommended by your instructor.

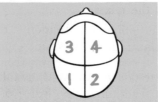

FOUR SECTIONS: Part hair down center from forehead to nape. Part across, starting behind ear. Extend part from ear to ear.

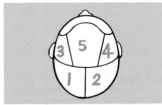

FIVE SECTIONS: Part across, starting behind the ear. Extend part from ear to ear. Divide front area into 3 sections. Divide back area into 2 sections.

Dry Hair

If moisture or perspiration is present on scalp, place patron under a cool dryer for several minutes.

Apply Protective Base

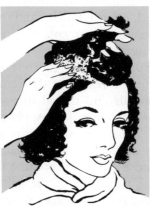

Applying base protective cream

Most relaxers require the use of a protective base to protect the scalp from the active agents in the relaxer. To apply it properly, the hair should first be parted into four or five distinct sections. Then, each section is subdivided into one-half to one-inch partings to permit thorough scalp coverage.

The base is applied freely with the fingers to the entire scalp. The hairline around the forehead, nape of the neck, over and around the ears must be completely covered. The base is actually "laid" on the scalp; it must not be spread or rubbed on; body heat will help to insure complete distribution. Good coverage is important to protect the scalp and hairline from irritation.

Conditioner

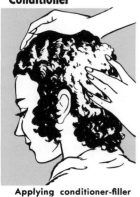

Applying conditioner-filler

In many cases a conditioner-filler is required before the chemical relaxer can be used. The conditioner-filler, usually a protein product, is applied to dry hair over the entire head. It protects over-porous or slightly damaged hair from being over processed in any part of the hair shaft. It evens out porosity of the hair shaft and permits uniform distribution and action of the chemical relaxer.

To receive complete benefits of the conditioner-filler, it should be gently rubbed into the hair from the scalp to the hair ends, by either the hands or a comb. The hair is then towel dried. A cool drier is used until the hair is completely dry. CAUTION. Avoid the use of any heat, which would open the pores of the scalp and skin and cause irritation or injury when the relaxer is applied.

Applying The Relaxer

Divide the head into four or five sections, in the same manner followed as for the application of the base cream.

CAUTION. **It is important to protect the patron's eyes with protective pads when applying the chemical hair relaxer, and protective gloves must be worn by the cosmetologist.**

The processing cream is applied last to the scalp area and hair ends. At the scalp, the body heat will speed up the processing action. At the ends, the hair is in a more porous condition and may be damaged. In both these areas, less processing time is required, and, therefore, the relaxer is applied last.

There are two methods in general use for the application of the chemical hair relaxer:

1. The Comb Method   2. The Finger Method

COMB METHOD

With a comb, remove a quantity of relaxing cream from the jar. Begin with the back right section of the head. Apply the relaxer, starting one-half to one inch from the scalp, and comb to within one-half inch of the hair ends.

First apply the relaxer to the top side of the strand. Then, raise the hair in one-inch sub-sections and apply the relaxer underneath. Flip completed strand up out of the way.

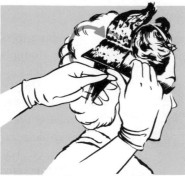

Applying relaxer on top of strand

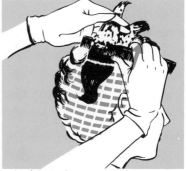

Applying relaxer underneath strand

Complete the right back area, and moving in a clockwise direction, cover each section of the head in the same manner. Then, go back over the head in the same order, applying additional relaxing cream, if necessary, and combing the relaxer down to the scalp and up to the hair ends.

Combing the cream through the hair serves not only to spread the cream, but also to stretch the hair gently into a straight position.

Strand Testing

While spreading the relaxer, the cosmetologist should inspect its action by stretching the strands to see how fast the natural curls are being removed. If the action is too fast in any area, the patron should be taken immediately to the shampoo bowl and the relaxer rinsed from that particular section. The spreading process can be continued over the rest of the head, and finally to the hair ends.

Rinsing Relaxer

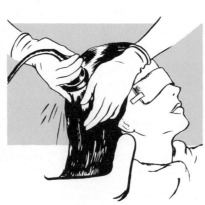

Rinsing out relaxer

When the hair has been sufficiently straightened, the relaxer must be **rinsed out rapidly and thoroughly.** The water must be warm, not hot. If the water is too hot, it may burn the patron, or cause the relaxed hair to revert to its original form. If the water is too cold, it will not stop the processing action. The direct force of the rinse water should be employed to remove the relaxer and avoid tangling of the hair. Unless the relaxer is completely removed, its chemical action continues on the hair. The stream of water should **be directed from the scalp to the hair ends.**

CAUTION. Do not get relaxer or rinse water into the eyes or on unprotected skin. If the relaxer or rinse water accidentally gets into the patron's eyes, it should be washed out immediately with large quantities of warm water and the patron should be taken to the doctor without delay. Continue wearing protective gloves until all relaxer has been removed.

Shampooing

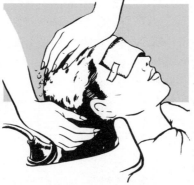

Shampooing the hair

Shampooing the hair. Gently work the shampoo (cream shampoo recommended) into the hair. The hair is very fragile at this point and tangled ends can be broken easily. Use **tepid** water and **avoid firm manipulations,** rubbing or tangling the hair. Most relaxed hair requires at least three shampooings.

Applying Neutralizer

After shampooing the hair, apply a neutralizer. This helps to keep the hair in a relaxed state.

Completely saturate the hair with the neutralizer, then comb with a wide-tooth comb, beginning at the nape and working upward toward

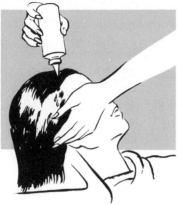

Applying neutralizer

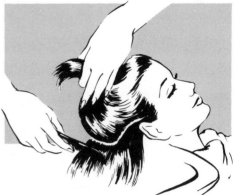

Combing neutralizer through hair

the forehead. Use the comb to:

a) Keep the hair straight.

b) Completely saturate the hair with the neutralizer.

c) Remove any tangles without too much pulling.

After five minutes, rinse out neutralizer thoroughly with warm water and towel blot.

Style hair in the usual manner.

a) Discard used supplies.

b) Cleanse and sanitize equipment.

c) Wash and sanitize hands.

d) Complete hair relaxing record card.

Caution: Different products used for relaxing the hair necessitate different methods of handling the hair during the processing and neutralizing period. Always follow manufacturer's directions and be guided by your instructor.

To avoid hair breakage, a lapse of at least four to six weeks should be allowed (depending on the length, texture and thickness of the hair) before hot irons are again used on the chemically relaxed hair.

Applying Conditioner

Many manufacturers recommend that you apply a conditioner before setting the hair to offset the harshness of the relaxer and to help restore some of the natural oils to the scalp and hair.

Two general types of conditioners are available:

1. **Cream conditioners,** usually lanolin or cholesterol, are applied to the scalp and hair, then carefully rinsed out and towel dried. Setting lotion is applied; the hair is set on rollers, dried, and styled in the usual manner.

2. **Protein (liquid) conditioners** are applied to the scalp and hair prior to hair setting and allowed to remain in the hair to serve as a setting lotion. The hair is set on rollers, dried, and styled in the usual manner.

In applying the conditioners, be guided by your instructor.

CAUTION. Because of the fragile condition of the hair, it is advisable that the hair be wound on larger rollers, without tension.

FINGER METHOD

**Must Wear
Protective Gloves**

The finger method of applying the relaxer to the hair is the same as the **comb method,** except that the fingers and palms are used instead of the comb. Everything else is the same.

Using your fingers, remove a small quantity of relaxing cream from the jar and lay it on the hair, about one-half to one inch from the scalp. Gently work the cream through the entire section of hair to about one-half inch from the ends. Make certain that all hair has been covered.

Working in a clockwise direction, repeat the process with the next section until every section has been treated.

Then, starting with the first section, repeat the procedure, adding relaxer where needed, and also applying relaxer on the hair down to the scalp, but not to the hair ends.

Spreading out the relaxer. Smooth hair out gently, as shown in illustration. The spreading out procedure follows the same pattern which was used in applying the relaxer. There are three specific reasons for this procedure:

1) To be sure the hair is completely covered from the scalp
2) To be sure the hair is completely relaxed from the scalp
3) To be able to determine how fast the hair is being relaxed

After spreading out the relaxer over the entire scalp area and hair shaft, apply the relaxer to the ends and front hairline.

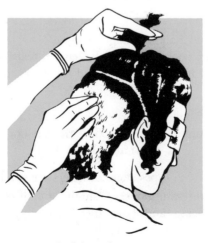 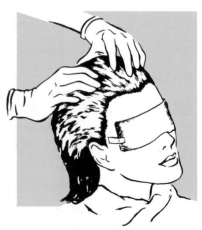

Applying relaxer   Spreading out relaxer

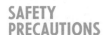

RETOUCH

Follow all steps for a regular chemical hair relaxing treatment, with one exception; you apply the **relaxer only** to the **new growth.** In order to avoid breakage of previously treated hair, it is advisable that you apply a protective cream over the hair which received the earlier treatment, thus avoiding overlapping and damage.

SAFETY PRECAUTIONS

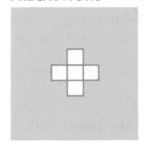

1. Examine the scalp for abrasions; if any are present, do not give a hair relaxing treatment.
2. To be sure a hair relaxing treatment can be given safely, analyze and give patron's hair a strand test.
3. Test the elasticity of the hair for its ability to stretch and return to its normal length without breaking. Also, check the porosity of the hair and its ability to absorb moisture.
4. Do not apply a caustic (sodium hydroxide) relaxer over a thio type relaxer.
5. Do not apply a thio type relaxer over a sodium hydroxide type relaxer.
6. Have a thorough understanding of the product being used and its action on the hair. Follow manufacturer's directions carefully.
7. Never use a strong relaxer on fine, wooly hair, as it may cause breakage.
8. Never give a chemical hair relaxing treatment to hair which has **recently** been straightened by a hot pressing comb.
9. Do not relax damaged hair. Suggest a series of reconditioning treatments. If hair ends are in a damaged condition, trim the hair **before giving a relaxing treatment.**
10. Apply protective base to avoid possible burning or irritation of the scalp by the sodium hydroxide relaxer.
11. After the application of the protective base, check carefully to see that the scalp has been completely and thoroughly covered. Failure to cover the scalp carefully can result in a burn by the chemicals being used.
12. The cosmetologist must wear protective gloves.
13. Protect patron's eyes with protective pads; avoid getting chemicals or rinse water in her eyes.
14. Place the relaxer on the hair shaft; do not rub it into the hair.
15. Use extreme care when applying the relaxer, to avoid accidentally spreading it on the ears, scalp or skin.
16. Test the action of the relaxer frequently to determine how fast the natural curl is being removed.
17. When rinsing the relaxer from the hair, take great care that the water is not too hot. If hot water is used, the hair will revert to its natural curly shape and the entire process will be in vain.
18. Be sure to thoroughly remove the relaxer from the hair. Failure to do so will cause the relaxer to continue to process, resulting in hair damage. Direct stream of water from scalp to hair ends.

19. Use a mild shampoo with warm water, and gently work it into the hair. Do not give vigorous manipulations.

20. Wear protective gloves until all the relaxer has been removed. When rinsing the shampoo from the hair, always work the fingers from the scalp to the ends, following the water stream, to prevent tangling the hair.

21. The application of a neutralizer following the shampoo is an important step; it keeps the hair in a relaxed or straightened form.

22. Use a wide-tooth comb and avoid pulling when combing the hair. Avoid scratching the scalp with comb or fingernails.

23. Apply a conditioner to the scalp and hair before setting, to help restore some of the natural oils which have been removed from the scalp and hair by the relaxer.

24. When retouching the new growth, do not allow the relaxer to overlap onto the hair already relaxed.

25. Do not use hot irons on chemically relaxed hair.

26. Do not give a hair relaxing treatment to hair treated with a metallic dye.

27. Always fill out a record card at the completion of each treatment.

28. Always have patron sign a release statement to protect the cosmetologist and the beauty salon.

PROCEDURE FOR AMMONIUM THIOGLYCOLATE RELAXER

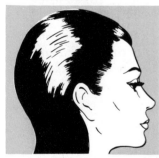

Procedure

Ammonium thioglycolate (also called thio relaxer) is the same type of product used in cold waving, but a heavy cream base is added to the formula to keep the hair in a straightened position.

As in cold waving, the relaxer breaks down sulfur and hydrogen bonds, which softens and swells the hair. By the mechanical action of the hands and/or comb, the hair is smoothed and held in a straightened position.

When the hair is straightened, the neutralizer is applied to it (serving the same purpose as does the neutralizer in cold waving). It re-forms the sulfur and hydrogen bonds and rehardens the hair in its newly straightened position.

Manufacturers vary their products according to the texture and condition of the hair. Tinted and lightened hair require a weaker formula.

The same precautions must be observed in the use of thio relaxers as for the application of sodium hydroxide products.

1. Prepare the patron in the same manner as previously described.

2. Shampoo the hair with a neutral shampoo. (Be careful not to irritate the scalp.)

3. Towel dry the hair, leaving it slightly damp.

4. Apply scalp conditioner to the scalp only.

5. Prepare neutralizer before applying relaxer.

6. Use protective gloves or cream on the hands. Apply relaxer as previously described for sodium hydroxide relaxer.

7. The spreading out and testing procedure is the same as that followed for sodium hydroxide products.

8. When the hair has been sufficiently processed, the relaxer is rinsed out in a three-step process.
   a) Rinse about 50% of the relaxer from the hair with warm water.
   b) Comb the hair smooth and straight with the remaining relaxer left in the hair; continue combing for about five minutes to rearrange the cystine cross-bonds leaving the hair in a straight position.
   c) Rinse the remaining relaxer thoroughly from the hair with warm water, keeping the hair smooth and straight while rinsing.

9. After the relaxer has been thoroughly rinsed from the hair, apply the neutralizer as follows:
   a) Pour the prepared neutralizer through the hair and catch it in a plastic bowl.
   b) Re-pour the neutralizer through the hair and catch it again in a plastic bowl. Repeat this process six or seven times.
   c) Comb the hair smooth and straight to assure complete neutralizing.
   d) Allow the neutralizer to remain on the hair. (Do not rinse with water.)
   e) Set the hair with the neutralizer left on the hair.

Note: Manufacturers may have different procedures for the final steps. Be guided by your instructor.

CAUTION. Because of the fragile condition of the hair, wind the hair on the larger rollers, without tension.

Retouching

Follow all steps for a regular chemical hair relaxing treatment, with the exception of the **relaxer**, which is applied **only** to the **new growth.**

REVIEW QUESTIONS

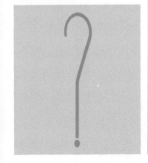

1. What is chemical hair relaxing?
2. What is the action of a chemical hair relaxer?
3. What is the purpose of an analysis of the patron's hair prior to applying a chemical relaxer?
4. List four items to consider in a hair analysis.
5. What are the two methods of chemical hair relaxing in general use?
6. What chemical compound is required in addition to the chemical relaxing agent?
7. **By what other term is the neutralizer known?**
8. What test should be given the patron before she receives a chemical hair relaxing treatment?

9. What is the purpose of the strand test in the chemical relaxing procedure?

10. Why is a scalp examination especially important prior to a chemical hair relaxing treatment?

11. What is the purpose of the patron's record card?

12. Why is it necessary to have the patron sign a release?

13. What hair conditions should prevent treatment with a chemical hair relaxer?

14. Why should hair having good porosity require less processing time than hair with poor porosity?

15. **What is the purpose of the base which is applied to the entire scalp and surrounding areas when a sodium hydroxide relaxer is used?**

16. Why use protective gloves when applying the sodium hydroxide chemical relaxer?

17. After the hair has been treated with a sodium hydroxide relaxer, why should the hair be thoroughly rinsed prior to the application of a shampoo?

18. **Why should the hair not be brushed before applying the chemical hair relaxer?**

19. Why is a cream shampoo preferred for shampooing chemically relaxed hair?

20. Why is it important to keep chemically relaxed hair from tangling during a shampoo?

21. Why should the hair have at least three shampoo applications after being treated with a sodium hydroxide hair relaxer?

22. Why is the neutralizer necessary in the chemical hair relaxing process?

23. When should the hair be combed after a chemical relaxing treatment?

24. **Why is a scalp and hair conditioner applied after a hair relaxing treatment?**

25. **How are large rollers used in styling chemically relaxed hair?**

26. Why should chemically treated hair not be given hot comb treatments?

27. How is a chemical relaxer retouch given?

28. Is the hair shampooed prior to the application of:
    a) a caustic type relaxer?
    b) a thio type relaxer?

29. Give the three-step procedure for removing the thio relaxing cream from the hair.

CHAPTER 17

THERMAL HAIR STRAIGHTENING

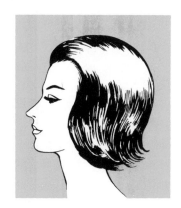

Hair pressing is a profitable service and has a wide popularity in the beauty salon. When properly done, hair pressing straightens over-curly or kinky hair for a limited period of time.

Hair pressing prepares the hair for further treatments, such as thermal roller curling and croquignole thermal curling. A good hair pressing treatment is not harmful to the hair, but leaves it in a natural and lustrous condition.

There are two basic methods of hair pressing:

1. **Soft press method** is accomplished with a pressing comb.
2. **Hard press method** is accomplished with thermal (marcel) irons over the comb press. A **hard press** may also be accomplished by a double comb press.

HAIR CHARACTERISTICS

To perform the hair pressing service successfully, the cosmetologist must be able to recognize the individual differences in hair texture, porosity, elasticity and scalp flexibility. Guided by these observations, the cosmetologist can determine the right temperature for the pressing comb and the degree of pressure the hair and scalp can tolerate without causing breakage, hair loss or burning of the hair or scalp.

Hair texture refers to the degree of coarseness or fineness of the hair. Variations in individual hair texture are traceable to the following factors:

1. **Diameter of the hair** (either coarse, medium or fine).
   Coarse hair has the greatest diameter. Fine hair has the smallest diameter.
2. **Feel of the hair** (either wiry, soft, silky or wooly).

Coarse, over-curly hair has qualities which make it comparatively difficult to press. Coarse hair has the greatest diameter, and during the pressing treatment, it can tolerate more heat and pressure than medium or fine hair. A microscopic analysis of coarse hair reveals that it contains the following layers: cuticle, cortex and medulla.

Medium, curly hair is the normal type of hair met in the beauty salon. No special problem is presented by this type of hair and it is the least resistant to hair pressing.

Fine hair requires special care because it is the most fragile type to press. To avoid hair breakage, apply less heat and pressure than for other hair textures. Only two layers, the cortex and the cuticle, are usually present in fine hair.

Wiry, curly hair may be either coarse, medium or fine. It is recognized by its stiff, hard, glassy feeling. Because of the compact construction of the cuticle cells it is most resistant to hair pressing treatments. Therefore, it requires more heat and pressure than other types of hair.

Elasticity is the ability of the hair to stretch and return to its normal length without breaking. Normal hair has its limitations as to the amount of pull or pressure it can withstand. Under normal conditions, dry hair can be safely stretched about one-fifth its length.

Hair that has normal elasticity presents a healthy and lustrous appearance. A deficiency in the elasticity of hair causes it to become lifeless and limp. Very little elasticity is left in hair that has been abused by lightening or tinting chemicals. Therefore, hair of this type needs special care during hair pressing.

Hair porosity is the ability of the hair to absorb moisture regardless of whether it is coarse, medium or fine. After a hair pressing treatment, hair with good porosity, which comes into contact with water or moisture, returns to its normal, curly appearance.

SCALP CHARACTERISTICS

The condition of the patron's scalp may be classified as follows:

1. **Normal scalp.** The cosmetologist should proceed with an analysis of the texture and elasticity of the hair.
2. **Tight scalp.** If the scalp is tight and the hair coarse, press the hair in the direction in which it grows, to avoid injury to the scalp.
3. **Flexible scalp.** The main difficulty with a flexible scalp is that the cosmetologist may not apply enough pressure to press the hair satisfactorily.

HAIR AND SCALP EXAMINATION

Before the cosmetologist undertakes to press the patron's hair, she should carefully examine the condition of the hair and scalp in order to evaluate the patron's particular needs.

Note: Under no circumstances should hair pressing be given to a patron who has an abrasion, a contagious condition or a scalp injury.

After examining the patron's hair and scalp, if they are not normal, the cosmetologist may give appropriate advice concerning preliminary corrective treatments. If the hair shows signs of neglect or abuse caused by faulty pressing, lightening or tinting, she should recommend a series of reconditioning treatments. Failure to correct dry and brittle hair may result in hair breakage during hair pressing. **Burnt hair strands cannot be reconditioned.**

RECORD CARD

The patron's hair and scalp record is useful for future hair pressing treatments. It is also advisable to question the patron about any lighteners, tints, color restorers or other chemical treatments which may have been given to her hair. When such information is taken into consideration during hair pressing, better results can be expected.

A record card should include the following:

1. Texture of hair: ☐ Coarse   ☐ Medium   ☐ Fine   ☐ Very fine
2. Condition of hair: ☐ Normal   ☐ Dry and brittle   ☐ Lightened   ☐ Tinted   ☐ Damaged.
3. History: Chemical process used ☐ Yes   ☐ No; Color restorer (metallic) ☐ Yes   ☐ No
4. Treatment: ☐ Soft press   ☐ Hard press   ☐ Roller curls
5. Heat: ☐ High   ☐ Medium   ☐ Low
6. Recondition: ☐ Yes   ☐ No   Name of product ....
7. Date ....   Price ....

CORRECTIVE TREATMENTS

Effective **reconditioning treatments** require the application of special hair and scalp preparations, and thorough brushing (with or without the application of a therapeutic light and scalp massage). Hair that has received these treatments usually obtains better results from hair pressing.

Treating A Tight Scalp

A tight scalp can be rendered more flexible by the systematic use of scalp massage, hair brushing and direct high frequency current. The patron will benefit by having a better circulation of blood to the scalp and strengthened holding power of the hair muscles.

PRESSING OIL OR CREAM

The application of pressing oil or cream prior to a hair pressing treatment helps to prepare the hair for pressing. Both these products have the following beneficial effects:

1. They make the hair softer.
2. They prepare and condition the hair for pressing.
3. They help to prevent hair burning or scorching.
4. They help to prevent hair breakage.
5. They help to recondition the hair after pressing.
6. They add sheen to pressed hair.

EFFECTS OF HAIR STRAIGHTENING

Temporary hair straightening. Hair pressing is a temporary treatment; it will not change the inner structure of the hair. Therefore, it will revert back to its natural curly form when it comes in contact with water, either in shampooing, high humidity, or scalp perspiration.

Permanent hair straightening. When chemically straightened (relaxed), over-curly hair will not revert back to its natural curly form because the internal structure of the hair is **permanently changed** into a new, straightened form. This subject is discussed thoroughly in the chapter on **Chemical Hair Relaxing.**

HAIR SECTIONING

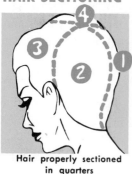

Hair properly sectioned in quarters

The head is divided into four main sections. These sections are subdivided into 1″ to 1½″ partings. The size of sub-sections depends upon the texture and density of the hair.

1. For medium textured hair of average density, the sub-sections should be of average size.
2. For coarse hair with greater density, smaller sections are used in order to assure complete heat penetration and effectiveness.
3. For thin or fine hair with sparse density, larger sections are employed.

PRESSING COMBS

Pressing combs come in two types, regular and electric.

They are constructed of either good quality steel or brass. The handle is usually made of wood, which does not readily absorb heat.

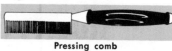

Pressing comb

Teeth. The space between the teeth of the comb varies with the size and style of the comb. Some combs have more space between the teeth, while others have less space.

Size. Pressing combs vary in size; some are short, while others are long.

Heat. Depending upon their composition, combs vary in their ability to accept and retain heat.

Stoves. Pressing combs may be heated on gas stoves or electric heaters.

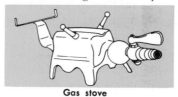
Gas stove

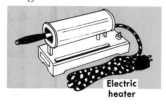
Electric heater

Heating Comb

While the comb is being heated, its teeth should face upward and the handle should be kept away from the fire. After heating the comb to the proper temperature, test it on a piece of light paper. If the paper becomes scorched, allow the comb to cool slightly before applying it to the hair.

Electric pressing combs are now available in two forms. These combs come either with an "ON" and "OFF" switch, or are equipped with a thermostat, which has a control switch, indicating high or low degrees of heat.

Electric pressing comb with on/off switch

Cleaning Comb

For efficient service, the pressing comb should be kept clean and free of carbon.

The comb must be wiped clean of loose hair, grease and dust before and after every use. The intense heat will keep the comb sterile if all loose hair or clinging dirt is removed.

The carbon may be removed from the comb by rubbing its outside surface and between its teeth with any one of the following:

    1. Emery board   2. Fine steel wool pad   3. Fine sandpaper

Following any of these cleaning methods, immerse the metal portion of the comb in a hot soda solution for about one hour; then rinse and dry. It will have acquired a smooth, shiny and sanitary appearance.

PRESSING PROCEDURE

Required Implements

1. Pressing comb
2. Heating appliance
   (gas or electric heater)
3. Pressing oil or cream
4. Hair brush and comb
5. Brilliantine or pomade
6. Shampoo
7. Towels and cape
8. Spatula
9. Neck strip
10. Thermal irons

> **IMPORTANT**
>
> The following preparation and technique serve as one of several ways to give a hair pressing treatment. The procedure and technique may be changed to conform with your instructor's routine.

Preparation For Hair Pressing

1. Select and arrange required materials.
2. Wash and sanitize hands.
3. Drape patron.
4. Shampoo, rinse and towel dry patron's hair
5. Apply pressing oil or cream.
   (*Some cosmetologists prefer to apply pressing oil or cream to the hair after it has been completely dried.*)
6. Dry hair thoroughly with either a hand blow dryer or hood dryer, as directed by your instructor.
7. Comb and divide hair into four main sections. Pin up three sections. Leave right back section for sub-dividing and pressing.
8. Place pressing comb in heater.

Procedure

1. Sub-divide right back section into small hair partings, working from the back towards the front.
   (*Some cosmetologists prefer to start at the front of the head and work towards the back.*)

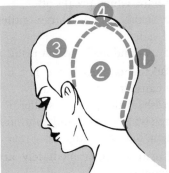

Hair properly sectioned
in quarters

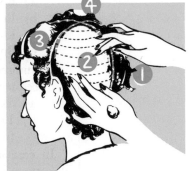

Applying pressing oil
to Section 2.

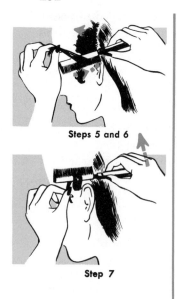

Steps 5 and 6

Step 7

Completion

TOUCH-UPS

SAFETY PRECAUTIONS

2. If necessary, apply additional pressing oil or cream evenly and sparingly over the small hair sections.
3. Test the temperature of the heated pressing comb.
4. Take the end of a small hair section with the index finger and thumb of the left hand and hold it up and away from the scalp.
5. Take the pressing comb in the right hand and insert the teeth of the comb into the top side of the hair section.
6. Draw out the pressing comb slightly and make a quick turn of the pressing comb so that the hair strands wrap themselves partly around the comb. Press the comb slowly through the hair strand until the ends of the hair pass through the teeth of the comb. **The back rod of the comb actually does the pressing.**
7. Press twice on top; reverse the comb and press once on the bottom side.
8. Bring each completed hair section over to the opposite side of the head.
9. Continue steps 4 to 8 on both sections of the right side of the head. Then begin at the back of the left side and work towards the front.

---

1. Apply a little brilliantine or pomade to the hair near the scalp and brush it through the hair.
2. If desired, thermal roller or croquignole curling may be given at this time. The procedures and techniques are found in the chapter on **Thermal Waving and Curling.**
3. Comb and style the hair according to the patron's wishes.
4. Place supplies in their proper places.
5. Sanitize implements and clean equipment.

Touch-ups are sometimes necessary when the hair has regained its curliness due to perspiration, dampness or other conditions. They are usually given up to about five days after the pressing treatment. The process is the same as the regular pressing treatment, with the shampoo omitted.

There are two types of accidents that may occur in hair pressing:
1. **Direct accidents,** which follow immediately after a careless hair pressing and cause injuries, such as:
   a) Burnt hair, which breaks off.
   b) Burnt scalp, which causes either temporary or permanent loss of hair.
   c) Burnt ears and neck, which result in scars.
2. **Indirect accidents,** which are not immediately evident, but subsequently cause injuries, such as:
   a) Skin rash, if the patron is allergic to pressing oil.
   b) Progressive breaking and shortening of the hair because of too frequent hair pressing.

In case of burnt scalp, immediately apply 1% gentian violet jelly directly to the wound.

To avoid damage, the hair should not be pressed more than necessary. Good judgment should be used, with consideration always given to the texture and condition of the hair and scalp. The patron's safety is assured only when the cosmetologist observes every precaution and is especially careful during the actual hair pressing. The cosmetologist **should avoid using** the following:

1. Excessive heat or pressure on the hair and scalp
2. Too much pressing oil on the hair
3. Perfumed pressing oil near the scalp if the patron is allergic to it

---

REMINDERS AND HINTS

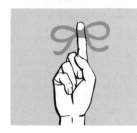

1. Keep the comb clean and free from carbon at all times.
2. Avoid overheating the pressing comb.
3. Test the temperature of the heated comb before applying it to the hair.
4. Adjust the temperature of the pressing comb to the patron's hair texture and condition.
5. Use heated comb carefully to avoid burning the skin, scalp or hair.
6. Prevent the smoking or burning of the hair during the pressing treatment by:
   a) Drying the hair completely after it is shampooed.
   b) Avoiding the excessive application of pressing oil over the hair.
7. Use a moderately warm comb to press short hair on the temples and back of the neck.

PROCEDURE FOR DOUBLE COMB PRESS

A double comb press is recommended when a comb press is not satisfactorily completed. The entire comb press procedure is repeated. However, additional pressing oil or cream is applied to hair strands only if necessary.

To many cosmetologists, a double comb press is also known as a **hard press.**

SPECIAL PROBLEMS
Pressing Fine Hair

When pressing fine or wooly hair, follow the same procedure as for normal hair, being careful not to use a hot pressing comb or too much pressure. To avoid hair breakage, apply less pressure to the hair near the ends. After the hair has been completely pressed, style the hair.

Pressing Short, Fine Hair

In pressing short, fine hair, extra care must be taken at the hairline.

Where the hair is extra short and fine, the pressing comb should not be too hot because the hair will burn easily; besides, a hot comb may cause accidental burns which are very painful and may cause scars. In the event of an accidental burn, immediately apply 1% gentian violet jelly to the wound.

Pressing Coarse Hair

When pressing coarse hair, care must be taken that enough pressure is given, in order that the hair will remain in a straightened condition.

Pressing Tinted, Lightened Or Grey Hair

These types of hair may require special care in hair pressing.

Sometimes **lightened or tinted hair** require reconditioning treatments. This depends on the extent to which it has been damaged. To obtain good results in hair pressing, use a moderately heated pressing comb, applied with light pressure.

Excess heat is to be avoided on **grey, tinted or lightened hair,** as the heat may discolor the hair.

A RELEASE STATEMENT

A release statement is used for hair pressing, permanent waving, hair tinting, or any other treatment that may require the cosmetologist's release from responsibility for accidents or damages.

Sample Release

SAMPLE RELEASE

I fully understand that the treatment I have requested, ----------------------------------, while harmless to normal hair, may be harmful to mine because of its condition as a result of

--.

Therefore, I hereby express my willingness to assume all responsibility and risk for any damage that may result, directly or indirectly, as a result of this requested service.

Signature ....

Witness .... Date ....

REVIEW QUESTIONS

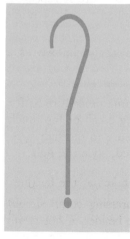

1. What is accomplished by hair pressing?
2. What is a soft press?
3. What is a hard press?
4. Name the layers of a coarse hair, starting from the outer layer.
5. What type of hair is the most resistant to hair pressing?
6. What kind of hair has poor elasticity?
7. What should the cosmetologist look for when examining the patron's hair and scalp?
8. When should the hair not be pressed?
9. Which procedure is followed in a reconditioning treatment for the hair and scalp?
10. What is the proper way to heat the pressing comb?
11. What supplies are needed for hair pressing?
12. What are the main steps in pressing the hair?
13. What important steps follow the hair pressing treatment?
14. Which accidents should be avoided by the cosmetologist?
15. In case of accidental scalp burn, how is it treated?

CHAPTER 18

THERMAL CURLING AND WAVING

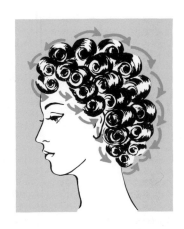

THERMAL CURLING

Thermal Curling is the art of creating curls in the hair with the aid of thermal irons and a comb. Thermal iron curling has become once again very popular after a lapse of about 30 years.

Since thermal curling requires no setting or styling creams or lotions, it may be used to great advantage for the following:

1. **Straight hair**—permits quick styling. Thermal curling eliminates working with wet hair, use of rollers and a long hair-drying process.
2. **Pressed hair**—permits styling the hair without the danger of reversion to its former over-curly condition. Thermal curling prepares the hair for any desired style.

CAUTION. Thermal irons must not be used on "chemically" treated hair; to do so could result in severe breakage of the hair.

3. **Wigs and hairpieces.** Thermal curling presents a quick and effective method for the styling of wigs and hairpieces.

Thermal Irons

Thermal irons should be made of the best quality steel so that they can hold an even temperature. The portion of the irons used to produce the wave is constructed in two sections: one section, known as the **prong**, is solid, perfectly round, with a tapered point; the other section, known as the **shell** (**bowl** or **groove**), is perfectly round, with the inside grooved so that the prong can rest in it when the irons are closed. The edge of the shell nearest the cosmetologist is called the **inner edge**; the one farthest from the cosmetologist is called the **outer edge.**

Thermal irons come in a variety of styles, sizes and weights. Sizes range from small to large jumbo. They come in three different classifications:

1. Conventional (regular) stove-heated
2. Electric self-heated
3. Electric self-heated, vaporizing

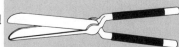

Thermal (marcel) irons

CAUTION. Electric vaporizing thermal irons must not be used on pressed hair because the moisture from the irons could cause the hair to revert to its natural over-curly form.

IMPORTANT. It is advisable that the beginning student learn and become adept in the use of the conventional type irons before attempting the use of the various electric irons. Always be guided by your instructor.

Temperature Of Irons

There is no set temperature for the irons when giving a thermal curl or wave. It all depends on the texture of the hair, whether it is fine or coarse, or whether it has been lightened or tinted. Hair that has been lightened or tinted (also white hair) should be curled or waved with lukewarm irons. Coarse hair, as a rule, can stand more heat than fine hair.

Testing Of Irons

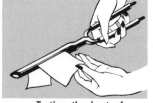

Testing the heat of
the thermal irons

After heating the irons to the desired temperature, test them on a piece of white paper or tissue. If the paper becomes scorched, allow the irons to cool slightly before being applied to the hair.

Care Of Irons

Thermal irons should be kept clean and free from rust and carbon. To remove dirt or grease, wash irons in a soap solution containing a few drops of ammonia. This cuts the oil and grease that usually adhere to the irons. The use of fine sandpaper, or steel wool, with a little oil helps to remove rust and carbon, besides giving the irons a polish. Oil the joints in thermal irons to permit greater facility in movement.

Tempering. New thermal irons are tempered at the factory in order to hold heat uniformly.

Overheated irons usually lose their temper, and in most cases are ruined.

Thermal Comb

The **thermal comb** should be about seven inches long, made of hard rubber, or another non-inflammable substance, and preferably have all fine teeth; fine teeth hold the hair more firmly than coarse teeth.

Holding The Irons

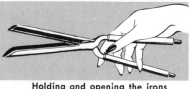

Holding and opening the irons

The irons should be held in the position which is most suitable and comfortable to the cosmetologist, yet permitting complete control and mastery of the irons.

The handle of the irons should be grasped in the right hand, far enough away from the joint to avoid the heat. The three middle fingers are placed in back of the lower handle, with the little finger poised in front of the handle, and the thumb placed over the upper handle.

Rolling The Irons

Practice rolling the thermal irons in the hand, first forward, then backward. The rolling movement should be done without any sway or motion in the arm; only the fingers are used to roll the handles in either direction.

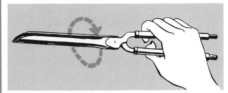
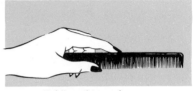

Rolling the irons   Holding the comb

Holding The Comb

The comb should be held between the thumb and all four fingers of the left hand, with one end of the comb resting against the outer edge of the palm. This position assures a strong hold and a firm stroke.

Practicing With Cold Irons

Thermal curling and waving, being a somewhat difficult operation, and employing the use of heated irons, should be practiced with **cold** irons on a mannequin, or hairpiece, pinned to a block until the technique is thoroughly mastered.

To become proficient in thermal curling, you should learn the correct procedure and practice it regularly until mastered.

THERMAL IRON CURLING METHODS

Today's thermal iron curling methods have improved over the older techniques. The following methods may be changed to conform with your instructor's procedures, which are equally correct.

Method 1. Short Hair   Method 3. Longer Hair
Method 2. Medium Length Hair   Method 4. Spiral Curling

Preparation

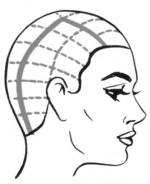

Hair sectioned and subdivided

1. Comb hair thoroughly, removing all tangles.
2. Divide head into five sections.
   a) First section, about $2\frac{1}{2}$ inches wide, extends from center of forehead to nape.
   b) Divide two side panels in half, from top parting to neck, to provide four additional sections.
3. Heat thermal irons (jumbo or large size).
4. Subdivide sections into sub-sections—each approximately $\frac{3}{4}''$ by $2\frac{1}{2}''$ wide.

METHOD 1: SHORT HAIR

Thermal curling short hair is the simplest thermal curling procedure.

1. After the irons have been heated to the desired temperature, pick up a strand of hair and comb up and smooth. **With the groove on top,** insert the irons about one inch from the scalp and hold for a few seconds to form a base. Fig. 1.

2. At the same time, hold the hair ends in the left hand in a firm, taut manner. Begin to rotate the irons under. Fig. 2.

3. Be sure to open and close the irons rapidly to avoid scorching the hair. Continue to rotate the irons as you guide the hair ends into the center of the curl. Fig. 3.

4. Hold for a few seconds. Protect the scalp with the comb by placing the teeth of the comb under the curl and next to the scalp. Fig. 4.

5. With the aid of a comb, remove the curl from the irons by drawing the curl from the irons. Fig. 4.

6. Another way in which the curl can be removed is to place the comb on top of the curl. Fig. 5.

7. The finished curl is shown in Fig. 6.

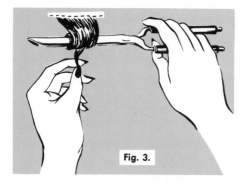

Fig. 1.

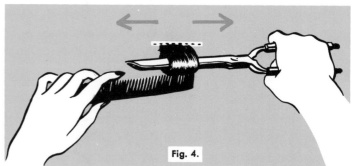

Fig. 2.

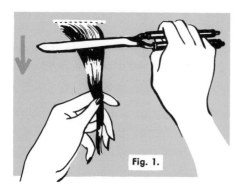

Fig. 3.

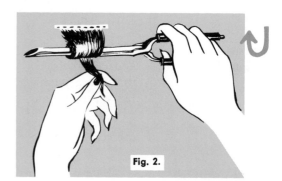

Fig. 4.

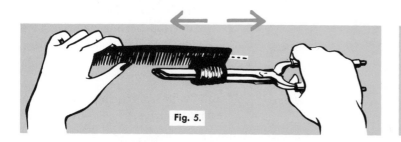

Fig. 5.

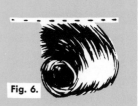

Fig. 6.

METHOD 2: MEDIUM LENGTH HAIR

Thermal curling medium length hair is a little different from curling short hair, which is accomplished by the use of one loop.

1. Comb hair up and smooth. With the groove on top, insert irons about one inch from the scalp. Hold strand for a few seconds. Fig. 1.

2. Slide irons out to about two inches from the scalp. Rotate the irons under, until the strand comes up, as in Fig. 2. Hold strand with left hand.

3. Continue rotating the irons, opening and closing them to keep the curl from binding. Fig. 3.

4. Continue rotating the irons while opening and closing them, until the hair ends disappear into the irons. Fig. 4.

5. Roll the irons slowly to the scalp. Protect the scalp with the teeth of the comb. Hold for a few seconds. Fig. 5. Remove curl from the irons with the aid of the comb. Fig. 6.

6. The curl may also be removed from the irons with the aid of the comb placed on top of the curl.

This procedure is followed over the entire head. Then, the hair is combed and brushed into waves and curls, as desired.

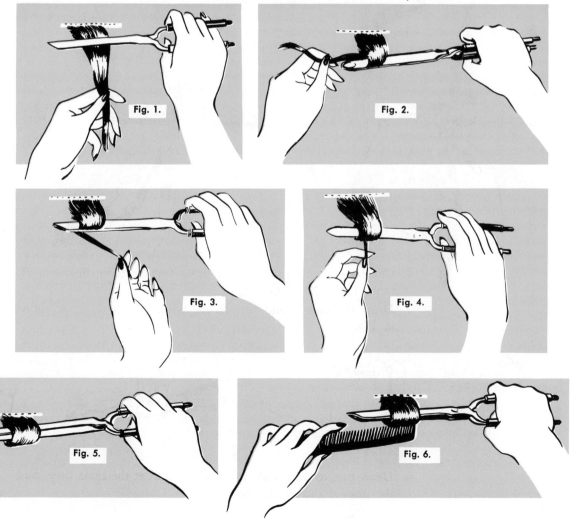

Fig. 1.

Fig. 2.

Fig. 3.

Fig. 4.

Fig. 5.

Fig. 6.

METHOD 3: LONG HAIR

Thermal curling long hair is accomplished by using the figure 8 (two loops) method.

1. With the groove on top, insert the irons on a section of hair at about one inch from the scalp. Close the irons. Fig. 1.

   The thickness of the hair strand depends upon the texture of the hair, whether it is fine or coarse, and the length of the hair.

   The average thickness of the strand is usually about ¾ of an inch. Fine hair requires larger strands, while coarse hair requires smaller strands. Longer hair also requires smaller strands.

2. Roll the irons under. Click and roll the irons until the groove is facing you. Fig. 2.

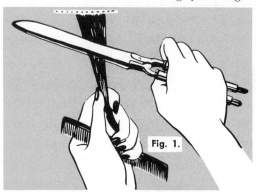
Fig. 1.

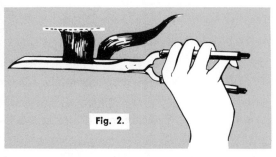
Fig. 2.

3. With the left hand, pick up the ends of the hair. Fig. 3.

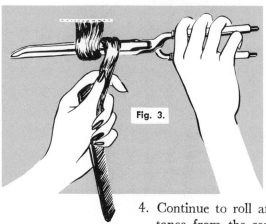
Fig. 3.

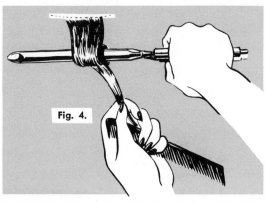
Fig. 4.

4. Continue to roll and click the irons, keeping them the same distance from the scalp. Fig. 4.

5. Draw the hair strand toward the points of the irons, as shown in Fig. 5.

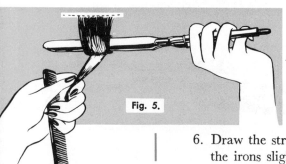
Fig. 5.

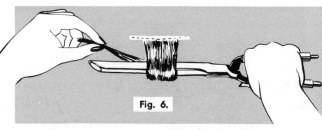
Fig. 6.

6. Draw the strand a little to the right, and at the same time, push the irons slightly to the left. Fig. 6.

7. By pushing the irons forward and pushing the hair with the left hand, you form two loops around the closed irons, with the ends of the strand extending out between the loops. Fig. 7.

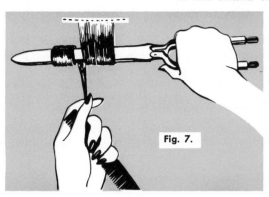

Fig. 7.

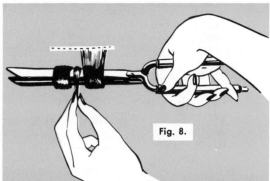

Fig. 8.

8. Roll and click the irons under until the ends of the hair disappear. Fig. 8.
9. Then, roll the irons to the scalp. Protect scalp with the comb.
10. Two ways to remove curl from irons:
   a) Use comb to protect scalp. Hold curl for a few moments to allow heat to penetrate. Push curl off irons with comb; at same time, draw irons out. Fig. 9.

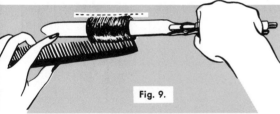

Fig. 9.

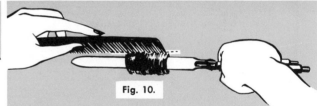

Fig. 10.

   b) To remove curl, use comb on top of curl to draw curl off irons. Fig. 10.

THERMAL CURL VOLUME BASES

There are three bases usually used to achieve the amount of lift (volume) or closeness to the head desired for a hairstyle.

When **fullness** or **maximum lift** is desired, the curl should be placed on its **full base.**

When a **moderate lift** is desired, the curl should be placed **one-half off base.**

When a **slight lift** is desired, the curl should be placed **off base.** The areas where a slight lift is usually desired are around the nape, sides or bangs on the forehead, or wherever the hairstyle calls for a small amount of lift.

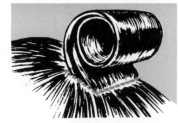

Full Base

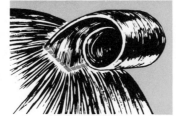

One-Half Off Base

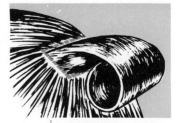

Off Base

METHOD 4: THERMAL SPIRAL CURLING

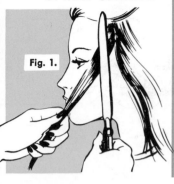

Fig. 1.

Spiral curls are hanging curls and are in great favor with women and girls with long hair.

Part the hair into as many sections as there will be curls, and comb smooth.

1. Heat irons to desired temperature. Comb strand smooth. Insert irons, at an angle, with the groove on top near the base of the strand. Hold strand with left hand. Fig. 1.
2. Rotate irons under and wrap strand around rod. The irons are not moved from their position near the base of the strand. Fig. 2.
3. Keep rotating the irons, and at the same time, open and close them to enlarge the curl and allow more freedom to the irons. Fig. 3.
4. Continue rotating. Fig. 4.

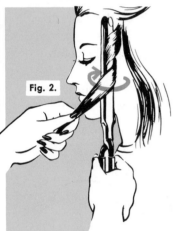

Fig. 2.

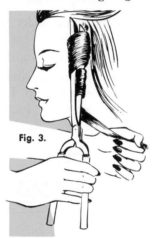

Fig. 3.

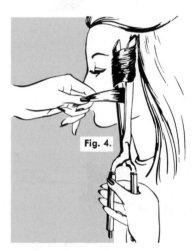

Fig. 4.

5. Completely wrap the entire strand. Fig. 5.
6. Support curl with left hand for a few seconds; then rotate irons, and gently remove them from the curl with the fingers of the left hand. Fig. 6.
7. In order to produce a long-lasting, springy curl, do not disturb the curl until it has cooled. Make as many curls as necessary to produce the desired hairstyle. Fig. 7.

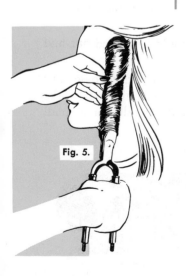

Fig. 5.

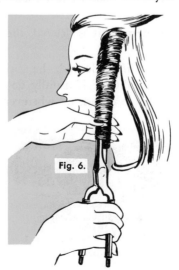

Fig. 6.

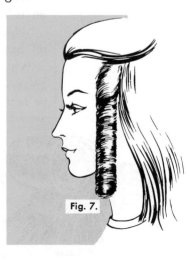

Fig. 7.

HELPFUL HINTS ON THERMAL CURL STYLING

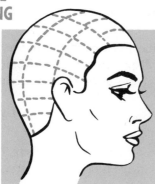

Hair sectioned and subdivided

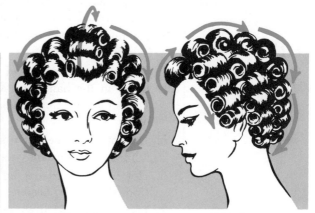

Front view   Side view

Head completely curled with thermal roller curls, also called "style" curls.

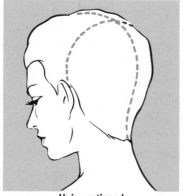

Hair sectioned in quarters.

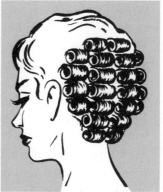

Back of head completely curled.

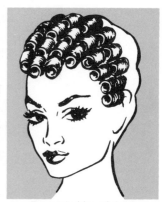

Top and sides of head completely curled.

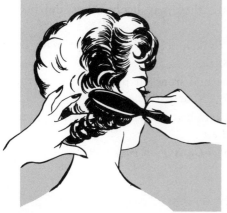

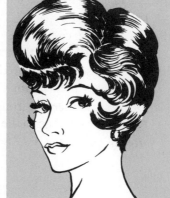

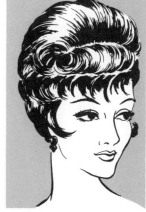

ARRANGING THE HAIR IN A SUITABLE HAIRSTYLE

To style the hair into a suitable hairstyle, brush the hair, working up from the neckline. Push the waves and curls into place as you progress over the entire head.

If the hairstyle is to be finished with curls, do the bottom curls last.

THERMAL CURLING AND WAVING

SAFETY MEASURES

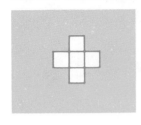

1. Keep thermal irons clean, free from dirt; and oil the joints.
2. Use thermal irons only after receiving instruction in their use.
3. Do not overheat the irons, as this may cause the metal to lose its temper.
4. Test the temperature of the irons on tissue paper before placing them on the hair. This will prevent the hair from being burned. Do not inhale the fumes of the irons as they are injurious to the lungs.
5. Do not place the hot irons near the face to test for temperature; a burn of the face may result.
6. Hot irons should not be cooled by twirling them. They may slip from the hands, become damaged, or cause injury.
7. Handle thermal irons carefully to avoid burning yourself or the patron.
8. Place hot irons in a safe place to cool. Do not leave them where someone may accidently come in contact with them and be burned.
9. When heating irons, do not place handles too close to the heater, as the hand may be burned when removing the irons.
10. Make sure that the irons are properly balanced in heater, or they may fall and be damaged, or injure someone.
11. Use hard rubber or non-inflammable combs only. Celluloid combs must not be used in thermal curling. They are flammable.
12. Place comb between scalp and thermal irons when curling or waving hair, to prevent burning the scalp.
13. To insure a good thermal curl or wave, the hair must be clean.
14. If the hair is thick and bulky, thin and taper the hair first.
15. Never use hot pressing or thermal irons on lightened or tinted hair.
16. Do not allow the hair ends to protrude over the irons; to do so will cause fish hooks and may cause damage to the hair ends.
17. A first aid kit must be available in case of an accident.
18. Do not use metallic combs; they may become hot and burn the patron.
19. Do not use combs with broken teeth. They may break or split the hair, or injure the scalp.
20. Do not use vaporizing thermal irons on pressed hair, as the hair will revert to its original over-curly state.
21. Do not use thermal irons on chemically straightened hair, as they may cause damage to the hair.

Revue questions for Thermal Curling on page 268.

THERMAL WAVING

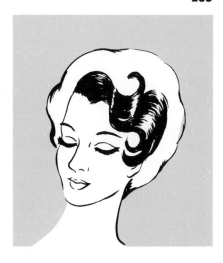

INTRODUCTION

The waving technique known as **Marcel Waving** (Thermal Waving) was developed in 1875 by a Frenchman, Marcel Grateau.

The method of creating waves in hair with heated irons was introduced by Monsieur Marcel after many years of experimentation.

In recognition of his outstanding contribution to hairdressing, this method of hair waving is still referred to as Marcel Waving.

Thermal waving, formerly called **marcel waving,** is the art of imparting waves to straight or pressed hair by means of heated irons and a special manipulative technique. Modern tools, such as thermal irons and combs, contribute to the successful waving of the hair. Correct habits and skills in holding and using these implements can only be acquired by patient practice on wefts, mannequins and live models.

To master thermal waving, it is essential that you practice the movements as illustrated, using cold irons on a strand of hair.

(Turn irons away from cosmetologist.)

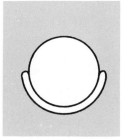
1. Starting position

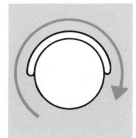
2. One-half turn

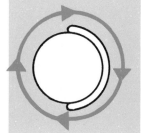
3. Full turn

Exercise

1. Insert hair in irons with rod on top (groove facing upward).
2. Turn irons forward for half turn (from operator).
3. Turn backward to position.
4. Open slightly and slide down one inch, then clamp.
5. Turn irons backward for full turn (from operator).
6. Turn forward to position.
7. Release.

Combing Preparation

Comb the hair thoroughly, following its directional growth. The natural growth will determine whether or not the first wave to be

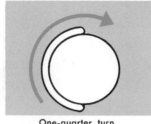

One-quarter turn
of irons

formed will be a "left-going" wave or a "right-going" wave. The procedure given here is for a left-going wave.

Before the wave is begun, comb the hair in a semi-shaping.

1. With the comb, pick up a strand of hair about two inches in width. Insert the irons in the hair with the groove facing upward.

2. Close irons and turn them about one-quarter turn forward. At the same time, draw the hair with the irons about one-quarter inch to the left, and direct the hair one-quarter inch to the right with the comb.

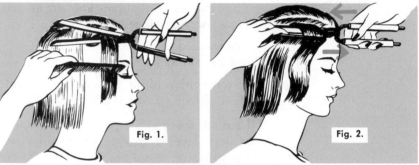

Fig. 1.   Fig. 2.

3. Now, roll the irons one full turn forward (away from you).

   (*In doing this, keep the hair uniform with the comb. You will find that the hair has rolled on a slight slant on the prong of the irons.*)

   Keep position No. 3 for a few seconds in order to allow the hair to become sufficiently heated throughout.

4. Now, reverse movement No. 3 by simply unrolling the hair from the irons, bringing it back into its first resting position. (See movement No. 2.)

   (*When this movement is completed, you will find the comb resting a trifle away from the irons.*)

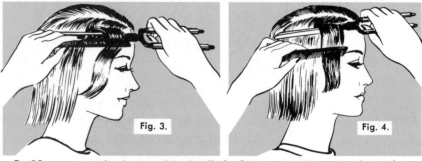

Fig. 3.   Fig. 4.

5. Now, open the irons with the little finger and place the irons just below the ridge, or crest, by swinging the rod of the irons toward you, and then closing them.

   (*The outer edge of the groove should be directly underneath the ridge just produced by the inner edge.*)

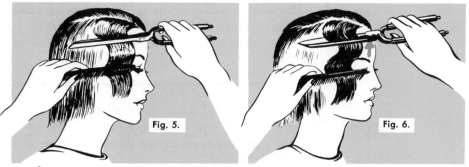

Fig. 5.   Fig. 6.

6. Keep the irons perfectly still and direct the hair with the comb toward the left about one inch, thus forming the hair into a half circle.

(You must remember that in order to perform movement No. 6 properly, you do not move the comb from position explained in footnote of movement No. 4)

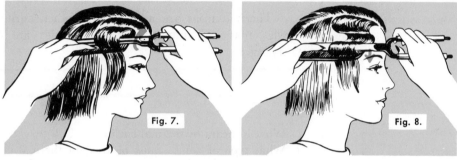

Fig. 7.   Fig. 8.

7. Without opening the irons, roll them one-half turn forward (away from you).

(In this movement, keep comb perfectly still and unchanged.)

8. Now, slide the irons down about one inch.

(This movement is done by opening the irons slightly (loose grip) and then sliding the irons down the strand of hair.)

Right-Going Wave

After completing movement No. 8, you will find the irons and comb in a position to make the second ridge and the beginning of the right-going wave. For a right-going wave, however, the hair is directed opposite to that of a left-going wave.

Joining Or Matching The Waves

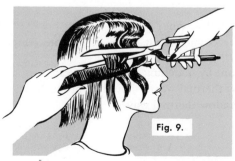

Fig. 9.

After one strand of hair is completely waved, the next strand is waved to match. While picking up the unwaved hair in the comb, a small section of the waved strand is included as a guide to the formation of the new wave.

In waving the second strand of hair, be sure that the comb and iron movements are the same as in the first strand of hair; otherwise, the waves will not match.

DROPPING A WAVE

Dropping a wave means to discontinue it, instead of carrying the wave around the entire head. This is done when the hair is parted on the side, and there are more waves on one side of the head than on the other.

SHADOW THERMAL WAVING

Shadow thermal waves are shallow waves with ridges that are not too sharp. This type of waving includes only the amount of hair one can pick up and wave at one time. The layers of underneath hair are not firmly waved.

Shadow waves are desirable for those patrons who wish to dress their hair close to the head.

CURLING AND WAVING WIGS AND HAIRPIECES

IMPORTANT REMINDER

Thermal irons are a great asset when curling and waving wigs made of human hair. (The wigs are cleaned before styling.)

REVIEW QUESTIONS

Thermal Curling

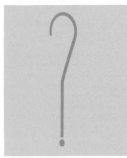

1. What is meant by thermal curling?
2. What type of combs must be used in thermal curling and waving?
3. Define volume in a curl.
4. When is full volume curl given?
5. In order to achieve a slight lift to the hairstyle, on what part of the base is the curl placed?
6. What causes the appearance of a "fish hook" on the hair ends in end curling?
7. What can the cosmetologist do if the hair is burned in iron curling or waving?
8. What would happen if a vaporizing thermal iron were used on pressed hair?
9. Why is it inadvisable to use thermal irons on chemically straightened hair?

REVIEW QUESTIONS

Thermal Waving

1. What is thermal waving?
2. How can the cosmetologist judge the proper temperature of thermal irons for each patron?
3. What is meant by matching thermal waves?
4. Explain how thermal waves should be properly matched.
5. What are shadow thermal waves?

CHAPTER 19

MANICURING

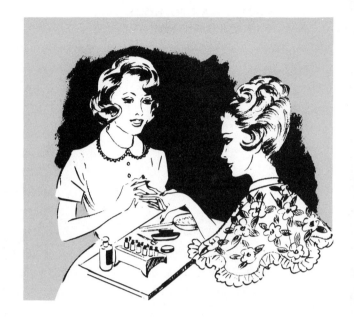

The ancients regarded long, polished and colored fingernails as a mark of distinction between the aristocrat and the common laborer. Manicuring, once considered a luxury for the few, is now within reach of the general public. In fact, every well-groomed person resorts to regular manicures.

Manicuring is not limited to the hands of women. More and more men request the services of a manicurist when they visit a men's hairstyling salon or barber shop for their hair care and other grooming needs.

The word **manicuring** is derived from the Latin "manus" (hand) and "cura" (care), and means the care of the hands and nails. The purpose of a manicure is to improve the appearance of the hands and nails.

If the patron is pleased by a professional manicure, she is more likely to become a regular patron for manicuring, as well as other beauty treatments.

A manicurist should have the following qualifications:

1. Knowledge of the structure of hands, arms and nails
2. Knowledge of the composition of the various cosmetics used in manicuring
3. Ability to give a good manicure in a systematic and efficient manner
4. Ability to care for the patron's manicuring problems
5. Ability to recognize nail disorders which may be treated in the beauty salon, and diseases which should be referred to a physician
6. Ability to please and satisfy patrons

PROPER WAY TO HOLD MANICURE IMPLEMENTS

MANICURING IMPLEMENTS

STEEL FILE
Hold the file firmly in the right hand, with the thumb underneath it for support and the other four fingers on its upper surface.

EMERY BOARD
It is held in the same manner as the steel file.

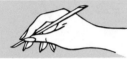

ORANGEWOOD STICK
It is held in the same manner as in writing with a pencil.

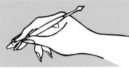

STEEL PUSHER
It is held in the same manner as in writing with a pencil. The dull spade side is used to push back and loosen the cuticle.

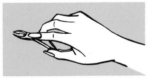

NIPPERS
Pick up the nippers by the handles and turn the cutting edges toward you; place the bent tip of the index finger over the top of the shank. Place the thumb on the side of the handle and the remaining fingers over the opposite handle.

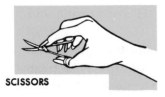

SCISSORS

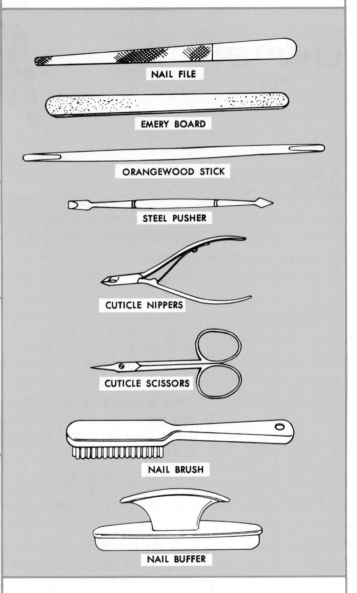

NAIL FILE

EMERY BOARD

ORANGEWOOD STICK

STEEL PUSHER

CUTICLE NIPPERS

CUTICLE SCISSORS

NAIL BRUSH

NAIL BUFFER

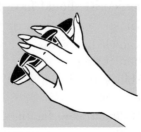
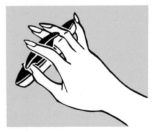

BUFFER
Two ways of holding buffer

**EQUIPMENT,
IMPLEMENTS
AND MATERIALS**

The articles used in manicuring, which are more or less durable or permanent, are referred to as equipment and implements or tools. Materials refer to cosmetics and other supplies that are consumed and, therefore, must be replaced from time to time.

Equipment

The equipment needed in giving a manicure includes:
1. **Manicure table** and **adjustable lamp.**
2. **Patron's chair** and **manicurist's chair** or **stool.**
3. **Cushion** (8 by 12 inches) covered with washable slipcover or sanitized towel on which patron rests arm. A Turkish towel, folded and covered with a small sanitized towel, may be used instead of the cushion.
4. **Supply tray** for holding cosmetics.
5. **Finger bowl** (plastic, china or glass) with removable paper cup for holding warm, soapy water.
6. **Container** for clean absorbent cotton.
7. **Electric heater** for heating oil when giving a hot oil manicure.
8. **Container** for sanitizing solution.
9. **Glass containers** for cosmetics and accessories.

Implements

Implements include:
1. **Orangewood sticks** (2)—to loosen cuticle, work around nail and to apply oil, cream, bleach or solvent to the nail and cuticle.
2. **Nail file** (7 or 8 inches long, thin and flexible)—to shape and smooth the free-edge of the nail.
3. **Cuticle pusher**—to push back and loosen the cuticle.
4. **Cuticle nippers,** or **scissors**—to trim the cuticle around the nails.
5. **Nail brush**—to cleanse the nails and fingertips.
6. **Emery boards** (2)—to shape the free edge of the nail with the coarse side and to bevel the nail with the finer side.
7. **Nail buffer**—to buff and polish the nails. (Some states do not permit the use of a nail buffer.)
8. **Fine camel's hair brush**—to apply lacquer or liquid nail polish. (The brush is usually attached to top of nail polish bottle.)
9. **Tweezers**—to gently lift small bits of cuticle.

Cosmetics

Nail and hand cosmetics vary in their composition and usage according to the purpose they serve.
1. **Nail cleansers** consist of some form of soap, either flaked, beaded or caked.
2. **Cuticle creams** are mixtures of fats and waxes (lanolin, cocoa butter, beeswax) which are intended to prevent or correct brittle nails and dry cuticle.
3. **Cuticle oil** softens and lubricates the skin around the nails.
4. **Cuticle removers** or **solvents** may contain 2-5% of sodium, or potassium hydroxide plus glycerine. After the cuticle is softened with this liquid, it can be easily removed.
5. **Nail bleaches** contain hydrogen peroxide, or diluted organic acids in a liquid form, or mixed with other ingredients to form a white paste. When applied over nails, under the free edge and on fingertips, they remove stains.

6. **Abrasive** is available as a pumice powder, and is used to smooth irregular nail ridges with a buffer.

7. **Pumice stone** is used to smooth the edge of the cuticle around the nails, and to remove light skin stains.

8. **Nail whiteners** are applied as a paste, cream or coated string. They consist mainly of white pigments (zinc oxide or titanium dioxide). When applied under the free edge of the nail, they keep the tips looking white.

9. **Nail polish removers** contain organic solvents and are used to dissolve the old polish present on the nail. To offset the drying action of the solvent, oil may be present in the nail polish remover.

10. **Hand creams** and **lotions** keep the skin soft by replacing the natural oils lost from the skin. They are recommended for overcoming a dry, chapped or irritated condition of the skin.
    Hand creams are similar in composition to vanishing creams. Other ingredients which may be present are glycerine, cocoa butter, lecithin or gums.
    Hand lotions are dilute emulsions of stearic acid and water, to which may be added mucilage of quince seed, gum, lanolin or glycerine.

11. **Dry nail polish** is usually prepared in the form of paste or powder. The main ingredient is a mild abrasive, such as tin oxide talc, silica or kaolin. It smooths the nail and also imparts a sheen to the nail during buffing.

12. A **base coat** is a liquid product applied before the liquid nail polish. With this application, the nail polish adheres readily to the nail surface. It also forms a hard gloss which prevents the color in the nail polish from staining the nail tissue.

13. **Nail polish thinner**, containing acetone or other solvent, is used to thin out the nail polish when it has thickened.

14. **Liquid nail polish** or **lacquer** is used to color or gloss the nail. It is a solution of nitrocellulose in volatile solvents, such as **amyl acetate**, together with a **plasticiser** (castor oil), which prevents too rapid drying. Also present are resin and color.

15. **Nail strengtheners** are products designed to prevent the nails from splitting or peeling. These are applied to the tips of the nails only. **They are never applied over polish.** The nails must be thoroughly clean, free of oils or creams, and dry. The application is used before the base coat is applied. The product usually contains formaldehyde. **Cuticle shields** are used during the application to prevent the product from touching the skin or cuticle.

16. A **nail dryer** is a fine spray which protects the nail polish against stickiness and dulling. It can be used either as a spray over the top coat or directly on the nail polish.

17. A **top coat** or **sealer** is a liquid applied over the nail polish. This product protects the polish and minimizes chipping or cracking of the colored polish. Some manufacturers combine a base coat and a top coat or sealer in a one-bottle product.

Materials

Materials include the following:

1. **Absorbent cotton**—to apply cosmetics to the nails
2. **Soap** (liquid or any form)—for finger bath
3. **Warm water**—for finger bath
4. **Individual sanitized towel**—for each patron
5. **Cleansing tissue**—to use whenever necessary
6. **Chamois**—to replace soiled chamois on buffer
7. **Paper cups**—to replace used paper cups in finger bowl
8. **Antiseptic**—to apply on minor cuts.
9. **Disinfectant**—to sanitize implements, and sponge manicure table
10. **Spatula**—to remove creams from jars
11. **Mending tissue paper** and **mending liquid**—to repair or cover broken, split or torn nails
12. **Perforated adhesive tape**—to hold compresses on injured nails or tissues, or to cover broken nails
13. **Scotch tape**—to repair or cover broken, split or torn nails
14. **70% Alcohol**—to use in jar wet sanitizer. Also used to sanitize patron's fingers before giving a manicure.

SHAPE OF NAILS

Nails naturally vary greatly in shape, but are usually classified into four general shapes: **square, round, oval,** and **pointed.**

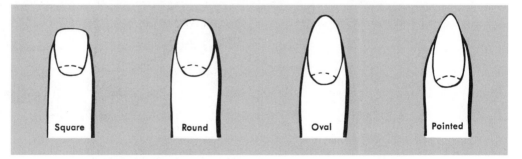

Square   Round   Oval   Pointed

In selecting the nail shape best suited for the patron, consult her wishes and give consideration to the type of fingers she has.

The shape of the nail should conform to that of the fingertips for a more natural effect. In general, the oval-shaped nail, nicely rounded at the base, and slightly pointed at the tips, fits most hands. Only a beautiful hand can afford to direct attention to itself by exaggeration of shape and color. Women who perform work with their hands usually require shorter, more round-shaped nails in order to avoid nail breakage and injury.

PROFESSIONAL MANICURE

It is of great importance to both the cosmetologist and the salon for the cosmetologist to be able to give a professional manicure. A patron who is satisfied with the manicure will most likely return for other services.

PREPARATION OF THE MANICURE TABLE

To give a professional manicure, all rules of sanitation must be followed. The table and the hands of the manicurist must be perfectly clean. Everything, including containers, bowls, implements, and materials, must be in perfect order. Do not ask the patron to sit at the table with the remains of the previous manicure in sight. Always clean the table immediately upon completion of a manicure, so that it will be ready for the next patron. This will make the manicure more pleasing to the patron and will put her in a more receptive mood for your advice and suggestions.

Procedure

1. Sponge the manicure tabletop with disinfectant.
2. Place a clean towel over the armrest or cushion.
3. Place bowl of warm, soapy water to the left of the patron.

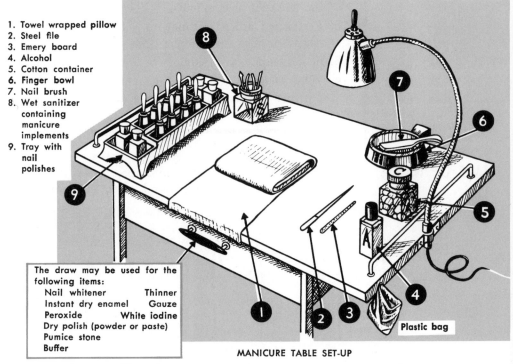

1. Towel wrapped pillow
2. Steel file
3. Emery board
4. Alcohol
5. Cotton container
6. Finger bowl
7. Nail brush
8. Wet sanitizer containing manicure implements
9. Tray with nail polishes

The draw may be used for the following items:
Nail whitener	Thinner
Instant dry enamel	Gauze
Peroxide	White iodine
Dry polish (powder or paste)	
Pumice stone	
Buffer	

MANICURE TABLE SET-UP

(*Your instructor's manicure table set-up is equally correct.*)

4. Place the metal implements and orangewood sticks in a jar **wet sanitizer containing cotton saturated with alcohol.**
5. Arrange cream jars, lotion bottles and nail polishes to the left of the manicurist in the order to be used.
6. Place the nail file (which has been sponged with alcohol) and fresh emery boards to the right of the manicurist.
7. Attach a small plastic bag to the table with scotch tape, on either the right or left side, in which to place soiled materials.

The manicure table drawer should be used to store supplies and must always be kept clean and neat. Use closed container or plastic bag for waste materials.

PLAIN MANICURE

Preparation

Procedure

1. **Prepare manicure table.** Arrange required sanitized implements, cosmetics and materials.
2. Seat patron.
3. Wash your hands.
4. Examine patron's hands.
5. Sanitize patron's fingers with 70% alcohol.

The routine outlined in this text is one of several ways to give a manicure. Whatever routine your instructor outlines for you is equally correct.

1. **Remove old polish.** (Start with the little finger.) Moisten a piece of cotton with the nail polish remover and press over the nail for a few moments to soften the polish. With a firm movement, bring the cotton from the base of the nail to the tip. Do not smear the old polish into the cuticle or surrounding tissues.

Alternate method of removing nail polish is to moisten small pieces of cotton with nail polish remover and press over old polish on each nail. Then moisten another pledget of cotton with nail polish remover and use for removing the small pledgets on the nails. This acts as a blotter and does not leave a polish smear on cuticle.

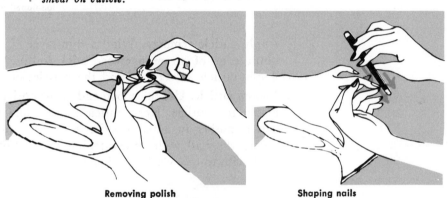

Removing polish   Shaping nails

2. **Shape nails.** Discuss with patron the nail shape best suited for her. File the nails of the **left hand,** from the little finger towards the thumb, in the following manner:
   a) Hold the patron's finger between the thumb and the first two fingers of the left hand.
   b) Hold the file in the right hand and tilt it slightly so that filing is confined mainly to the underside of the free edge.
   c) Shape nails into graceful oval tips, never extreme points. Use the file or emery board to shape the nail. File each nail from corner to center, going from right to left and then from left to right. On each side of the nail, use two short, quick strokes and one long, sweeping stroke.

Caution: Never file deep into the corners of the nail. If the nails are permitted to grow out at the sides, they will look longer and wear better.

3. **Soften cuticle.** After completing the left hand, file two nails of the right hand. Then immerse fingers of the left hand into soap bath to permit softening of the cuticle. Finish filing nails of right hand. Remove left hand from finger bowl.

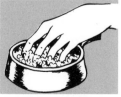

Soften cuticle

4. **Dry fingertips.** Holding a towel with both hands, carefully dry the left hand, including the area between the fingers. At the same time, gently loosen and push back the cuticle and adhering skin on each nail, using the cushion of the fingertips over the towel.

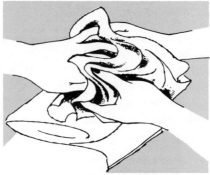

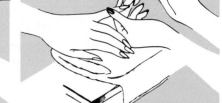

Towel drying fingertips

Applying cuticle remover with cotton-tipped orangewood stick

5. **Apply cuticle remover.** Wind a thin layer of cotton around the blunt edge of an orangewood stick for use as an applicator. Apply cuticle solvent around the cuticles of left hand.

6. **Loosen cuticle.** Use the spoon end of the cuticle pusher to gently loosen the cuticle. Keep cuticle moist while working. Use the cuticle pusher in a flat position to remove dead cuticle adhering to the nail without scratching the nail plate. Push cuticle back with towel over index finger.

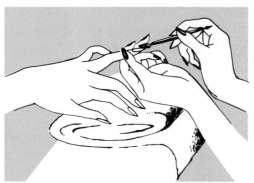

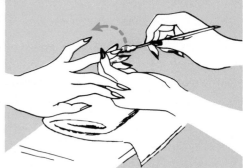

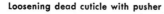

Loosening dead cuticle with pusher

Cleaning under free-edge with cotton-tipped orangewood stick

7. **Clean under free edge.** Use cotton-tipped orangewood stick, dipped in soapy water, and clean under free edge, from the center toward each side, with gentle pressure.

CAUTION. In using both the cuticle pusher and orangewood stick, avoid too much pressure so that live tissue at the root of the nail will not be injured.

8. **Trim cuticle.** If necessary, use cuticle nippers to remove dead cuticle, hangnails or uneven cuticle. In cutting the cuticle, be careful to remove it as a single segment.

9. **Bleach under free edges** with cotton - tipped orangewood stick. Apply hydrogen peroxide or other bleaching preparation under free edge of each nail of left hand.

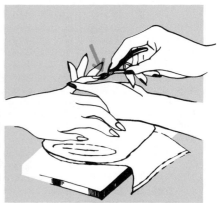

Trimming cuticle with nippers

Apply nail whitening (optional). Use orangewood stick as applicator to apply chalk paste, or use a string treated with nail whitening under free edge of nails.

10. **Apply cuticle oil or cream** around the sides and base of the nail and massage with the thumb in a rotary movement.

11. **Soften cuticle of right hand.** Immerse right hand into finger bowl (soap bath), while continuing to treat the left hand.

12. **Remove right hand from soap bath.** Treat nails and cuticle of right hand as described in Steps 4 to 11.

13. **Cleanse nails.** Brush nails over soap bath with a downward movement to clean nails and fingers of both hands.

14. **Dry hands and nails thoroughly**

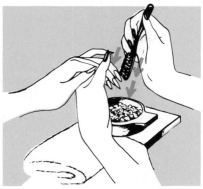

Cleaning nails, using brush in downward movement

Completion

1. **Bevel nails.** Carefully re-examine the nails for defects. Use fine side of emery board like a nail file to give the nails a smooth beveled edge.

Buff nails if buffing is required. Consult Men's Manicure on page 281

2. **Apply base coat.** Apply base coat with long strokes to the left hand, starting with the little finger and working toward the thumb. Allow to dry until "slick to a light touch." (Your teacher's routine in applying base coat, polish and top coat is equally correct.)

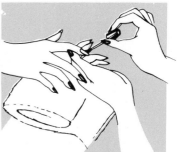

Applying base coat

3. **Apply liquid polish.** Dip the camel's hair brush into the polish and wipe off excess by pressing it gently against the sides of the bottle. Apply the polish lightly and quickly, using sweeping strokes from the base of the free edge of the nail, as outlined in the illustrations.

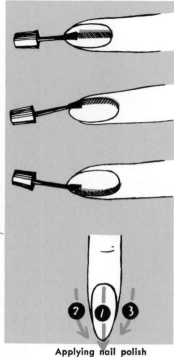

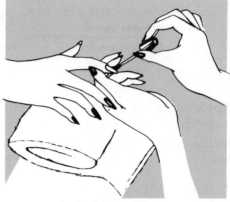

Applying nail polish

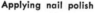

Applying nail polish

To minimize chipping, remove nail polish at hairline tip of nail after each coat of polish. Dip the brush in the polish each time before applying to the next nail.

Always keep the polish thin enough to flow freely. If the polish is thick, add a little polish solvent and then shake well.

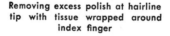

Removing excess polish at hairline tip with tissue wrapped around index finger

4. **Remove excess polish.** Dip a cotton-tipped orangewood stick into nail polish remover. Apply it carefully around cuticle and nail edges to remove excess polish.

5. **Apply top or seal coat.** Apply top coat with long strokes, first to the left hand and then to the right, in the same manner as the base coat. Brush around and under tips of nails for added support and protection.

6. **Apply hand lotion.** After the top coat is completely dry, as an extra service, apply hand lotion with light manipulations over the hands from wrists to fingertips.

INDIVIDUAL NAIL STYLING

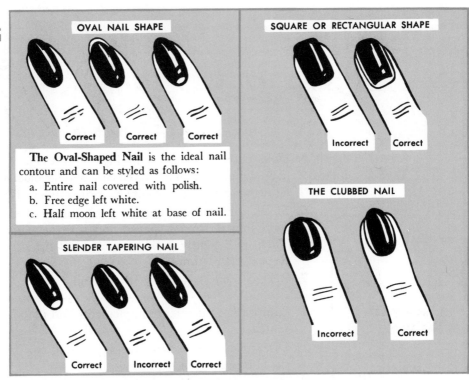

OVAL NAIL SHAPE

Correct   Correct   Correct

The Oval-Shaped Nail is the ideal nail contour and can be styled as follows:

a. Entire nail covered with polish.
b. Free edge left white.
c. Half moon left white at base of nail.

SLENDER TAPERING NAIL

Correct   Incorrect   Correct

SQUARE OR RECTANGULAR SHAPE

Incorrect   Correct

THE CLUBBED NAIL

Incorrect   Correct

HAND MASSAGE

Procedure

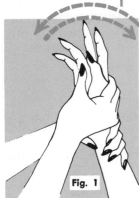

Fig. 1

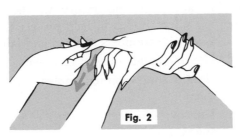

Fig. 2

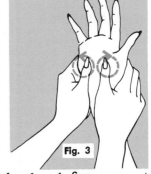

Fig. 3

A **hand massage** should be included with each manicure. It keeps the hands flexible and well-groomed, and the skin smooth.

1. Hold the patron's hand firmly, as in Fig. 1. Bend hand slowly with a forward and backward movement to limber the wrist. Repeat three times.

2. Grasp each finger, as in Fig. 2. Gently bend each finger, one at a time, to limber the top of the hand and finger joints. As the fingers and thumbs are bent, slide your thumb down towards fingertips.

3. With patron's elbow on table, hold the hand upright, as in Fig. 3. Massage palm of hand with cushions of your thumbs. Use a circular movement in alternate directions. This movement will completely relax patron's hand.

4. Rest patron's arm on table. Grasp each finger at the base and rotate gently in large circles, ending with a gentle squeeze of fingertips, as in Fig. 4. Repeat three times.

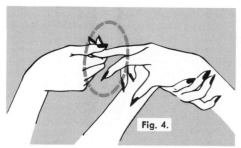
Fig. 4.

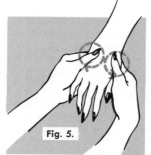
Fig. 5.

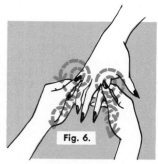
Fig. 6.

5. Hold patron's hand, as in Fig. 5. Massage wrist, then top of hand with a circular movement. Sliding back with both hands, wring wrist in opposite direction three times. Repeat three times.

6. Finish massage by tapering each finger. Begin at the base of each finger. Rotate, pause and squeeze with gentle pressure. Then, pull lightly with pressure until tip is reached. (Fig. 6.) Repeat three times.

7. Repeat Steps 1 to 6 on other hand.

Final Sanitary Care For Manicuring

1. Sanitize used manicure implements and place them in a cabinet sanitizer.

2. Discard used materials (tissues, cotton, emery board, etc.) into closed containers or plastic bag.

3. Wipe top of manicure table with disinfectant, and place everything in order.

4. Clean the tops of nail polish bottles with polish remover.

5. Inspect the manicure drawer for cleanliness and order.

6. Wash and dry your hands.

SAFETY RULES IN MANICURING

Observing safety rules in manicuring can be of great help in preventing accidents and injury to the patron or manicurist. The following safety rules will help protect the patron:

1. Keep all containers covered and labeled.

2. Use dry hands to hold or move containers.

3. Handle sharp-pointed implements carefully and avoid dropping them.

4. Dull over-sharpened cutting edges of sharp implements with an emery board.

5. Smooth sharp nail edges with an emery board.

6. Do not file too deeply into nail corners.

7. Do not use a sharp, pointed implement to cleanse under the nail.

8. Avoid excessive friction in nail buffing.

9. Apply an antiseptic immediately if the skin is accidentally cut.

10. Apply styptic powder to stop the bleeding from a small cut. Never use a styptic pencil.

11. Avoid pushing the cuticle back too far.

12. Avoid too much pressure at the base of the nail.

13. Do not work on a nail whose surrounding skin is inflamed or contains pus.

OIL MANICURE
Procedure

An oil manicure is beneficial for ridged and brittle nails and dry cuticles. It also improves the hands by leaving the skin soft and pliable.

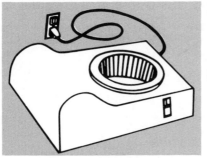

Hot oil manicure heater

1. Heat vegetable (olive) oil or commercial preparation to a comfortable temperature in an electric heater.
2. Proceed with the manicure to the point where you place the hand in the finger bowl; at that point, have patron place her fingers in the heated oil.
3. Massage the hands and wrists with the oil; then treat the cuticles in the usual manner. Cuticle remover, cuticle oil or cream is not needed.
4. Remove oil from the hands with warm, damp towel.
5. Apply skin freshener.
6. Wipe each nail carefully with polish remover, to remove all traces of the oil before applying the base coat.
7. Complete as for a plain manicure.

MEN'S MANICURE

Men usually prefer a conservative manicure. The nails are filed either round or square. A dry polish is applied instead of a liquid polish.

Implements, materials and supplies are the same as those used for a regular manicure. Follow procedure for a general manicure up to the application of base coat.

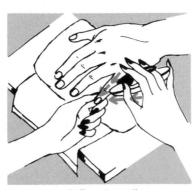

Buffing the nails

Buff nails. Apply a small dab of paste polish over the buffer. Then buff the nails with downward strokes, from the base to the free edge of each nail, until a smooth, clear gloss has been obtained. To prevent heating or burning sensation, lift the buffer from the nail after each stroke. Buffing the nails increases the circulation of the blood to the fingertips, smooths the nails and gives them a natural gloss or sheen.

Remove all particles or residue from the nails by washing and drying the fingertips.

If a clear liquid enamel is used, buffing is not required. Apply enamel in the same manner as for a regular manicure.

ELECTRIC OR MACHINE MANICURE

The electric or machine manicure is a portable device operated by a small motor. It employs a variety of tools which are attached to the machine as needed to perform the various operations.

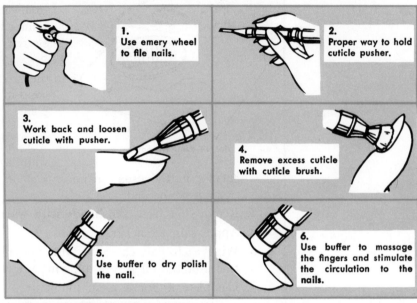

1. Use emery wheel to file nails.

2. Proper way to hold cuticle pusher.

3. Work back and loosen cuticle with pusher.

4. Remove excess cuticle with cuticle brush.

5. Use buffer to dry polish the nail.

6. Use buffer to massage the fingers and stimulate the circulation to the nails.

Before using an electric manicure machine, observe manufacturer's demonstration and follow instructions carefully.

SPECIAL PROBLEMS

Special problems include unusual nail conditions which should be corrected by the manicurist in order to please the patron.

Nails Broken At Sides

Nails broken at sides occur when the manicurist removes the corner of the nail out of the nail groove. As a result, the free edge is weakened, and the nail cracks and splits at the slightest pressure. Do not file deep into the corners of the nail. Nails will appear longer and will wear better when the sides of nails are allowed to grow. Permitting this natural line of nail growth gives a more tapered look to the finger and a longer, slimmer look to the hand.

NAIL REPAIR

Nail repair falls into **three** general groups:
1. Capping of fragile tips
2. Repairing of partially broken or split nails
3. Reattaching tips that are broken off completely

To Cap A Fragile Tip

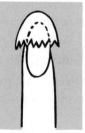

Capping a fragile tip

1. Tear a wedge-shaped piece of mending tissue the width of the nail at one end and a bit wider at the other.
2. Trim the wide end to fit the nail tip.
3. Saturate the patch with mending fluid and lay flat on nail. The rounded tip should extend about 1/8 inch around the free edge of the nail.
4. Smooth patch very lightly with fingertip, moistened in polish remover.
5. Have patron turn her palm upward and apply additional mend-

ing tissue to exposed edges of tissue. Dip a **very small** orange-wood stick in polish remover. Turn the tissue inward over nail edge, pressing firmly to inner surface of nail.

6. Let the cap dry thoroughly before applying the base coat, polish and top coat.

To Repair A Split Nail

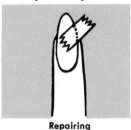

Repairing
a split nail

1. Tear a small piece of mending tissue and saturate with mending liquid until tissue is transparent.
2. Place saturated tissue over the split area.
3. Tuck the tissue under the nail with orangewood stick. The surface of the patch must be smoothed **away** from nail edge with cushion of finger moistened in polish remover.
4. If the split is deep, add a second patch for reinforcement.
5. Dry patch thoroughly before applying the base coat, polish and top coat.

To Reattach A Broken Nail Tip

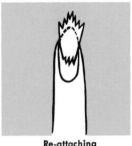

Re-attaching
a broken
nail tip

1. Use a thin, flat wisp of cotton saturated with mending liquid. Lay it flat on the nail, extending beyond the broken edge.
2. Fit the broken nail tip in place **over saturated cotton.**
3. Dip the orangewood stick in polish remover, turn ends of cotton back over the nail tip, covering edges of break. Use a very light touch when doing this.
4. Saturate a strip of tissue with mending liquid. Apply diagonally across the nail. If possible, tuck it in at corner beneath stub of nail.
5. Smooth surface **away** from nail-edge with fingertip moistened in remover.
6. Allow to dry thoroughly before applying base coat, polish and top coat.

> CAUTION. Unless the nail repair job dries thoroughly before the application of liquid material, it will slip or be rough and uneven.

OTHER NAIL PROBLEMS

Loose Skin Around Nail

A fringe of loose skin left around the nail after a manicure is caused by trimming the cuticle closer than necessary and then rolling back the epidermis. To prevent the occurrence of such loose skin, trim the cuticle only enough to allow a tiny margin of cuticle to remain.

ARTIFICIAL NAILS

Clean, attractive hands and nails are an admirable part of a woman's top-to-toe grooming. When a woman cannot grow natural nails of the desired strength and length, she may solve the problem by the application of artificial nails. These may be of the press-on type, or made of a mixture that builds the nail as it is brushed on. When properly applied and manicured, artificial nails look natural.

Artificial nails may be used for the following purposes:

1. To conceal broken or damaged nails
2. To improve the appearance of very short or badly shaped nails
3. To help overcome the habit of nail biting
4. To protect a nail or nails against splitting or breakage

Build-On Artificial Nails

When one or more nails are to be lengthened, the manicurist should build the type of nail which best conforms to the shape of the patron's fingers and hands.

Implements And Supplies

1. Regular implements used in manicuring
2. Instant nail lengthener kit
   a) Nail forms
   b) Measuring spoon
   c) Cup
   d) Nail lengthener powder
   e) Special liquid to dilute powder
   f) Brushes for application

Procedure

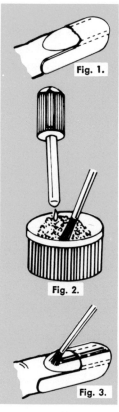

Fig. 1.

Fig. 2.

Fig. 3.

1. Give manicure up to, but not including, application of base coat.
2. Roughen nail surface slightly with emery board.
3. Lightly moisten glue on inside of nail form with brush and place under nail. Then press firmly around finger. Fig. 1.
4. Prepare smooth-flowing mixture as directed by manufacturer. Fig. 2.
5. Brush the mixture on the nail. Start at the base of the nail and continue brushing towards and over the free-edge and nail form until desired length is obtained, adding an extra amount to the nail form. Apply it the the same way as with nail polish. Fig. 3.
6. Allow the nails to dry and then apply second coat, being careful not to disturb previous coat. Apply third coat if necessary.
7. Wipe off excess mixture on sides of nail form; clean cuticle or sides of nail with orangestick dipped in polish remover.
8. Allow nail to dry thoroughly for 10-15 min.

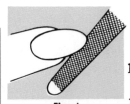

Fig. 4

9. Gently remove nail forms from nail. File new nail to shape. Fig. 4.
10. Wash the nail or nails thoroughly. Allow to dry.
11. Apply base coat, polish and top coat or sealer.

Repairing Broken Nail

Procedure for repairing a broken nail:

Prepare mixture. If required, adjust nail form. Apply three coats to existing nail, with each application extending the tip slightly beyond the previous application. Allow a little drying time between each application.

Let nails dry thoroughly for 10-15 minutes before shaping, and then apply polish.

To Remove Build-On Artificial Nails

Remove nail polish; saturate cotton pledget with polish remover. Apply to the artificial nail. Continue application until the artificial nail has loosened around the cuticle, the tip and sides of the nail. Continue to loosen very gently with the aid of a metal pusher, thus removing the artificial nail completely.

Safety Precautions

1. Clean the brush by dipping into polish remover and wiping.
2. Clean the mixing dish by lifting hardened content out with a metal pusher.
3. Make sure bottles are tightly capped when not in use.
4. Do not store product near heat or use near open flame.
5. Do not apply to injured or inflamed skin.

PRESS-ON ARTIFICIAL NAILS

Models, actresses, saleswomen and others, whose hands are on display, may wear a complete set of press-on artificial nails every day, while women who do other types of work may wish to wear artificial nails only for special occasions.

Artificial nails are constructed of either **plastic** or **nylon,** so the manufacturer's instructions must be followed carefully. Manufacturers advise against wearing artificial nails for more than forty-eight hours to allow for natural nail growth.

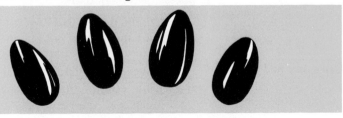

Implements And Supplies

Regular implements and supplies used in manicuring:
Artificial nails   Nail adhesive   Adhesive remover

Preparation

1. Remove polish from patron's nails and give manicure up to, but not including, the application of polish.
2. Roughen the patron's nails by going over the surface with an emery board.

3. Select the proper nail size for each finger. With a sharp manicure scissors, trim and then file the artificial nail at the cuticle end so that it fits to the shape of the natural nail. The artificial nails can be flattened by being firmly pressed down before application. They can also be reshaped by being held in warm water for a few seconds and molded to the desired shape.

Procedure

1. Apply a small amount of adhesive evenly on the edges of the patron's nails. Do not apply adhesive on the center of the nails.
2. Apply adhesive on the inside of the artificial nail, excluding the tip.
3. Allow the adhesive to dry thoroughly (about two minutes).
4. Press artificial nail gently onto the natural nail with the base touching the cuticle, or under it. As each nail is applied, hold firmly in place for about a minute.
5. Carefully wipe away any excess adhesive from the tips and around the nails.
6. Allow the artificial nails to dry thoroughly. Advise the patron to avoid disturbing the nails while they are drying.
7. Finish the manicure. Apply base coat, polish and top coat or sealer.

To Remove Press-On Artificial Nails

Apply a few drops of oily nail polish remover around the edge of the nail; then gently lift from the side with an orangewood stick. Do not attempt to pull or twist off the nail as this could damage or injure the natural nail. Adhesive remover can be used to assist nail remover. It can also be used to remove any surplus adhesive from the natural nails and from the artificial nails. These should be dried carefully and stored in a box. With proper care, artificial nails can be reused.

To Remove Polish

To remove nail polish from nails constructed of **plastic,** use only nail polish remover which has an oily base and does not contain acetone. CAUTION: Polish remover containing acetone will damage plastic artificial nails.

If **nylon**-constructed fingernails have been used, an acetone type of polish remover will not affect them.

Reminders And Hints

1. Never apply artificial nails over sore or infected areas.
2. Most manufacturers suggest that artificial nails not be worn for longer than forty-eight hours at a time, in order to allow for natural growth of the nail.
3. Most artificial nail adhesives are flammable, so be cautious with cigarettes, matches, and lighters.
4. When wearing artificial nails, do not subject them to a long period of immersion in water as they might tend to loosen.
5. Do not contaminate the adhesive with oil, cream or powder.

MANICURE WITH HAND AND ARM MASSAGE

The procedure used is similar to manicure with hand massage. All applications, including massage, are extended to the forearm, including the elbow.

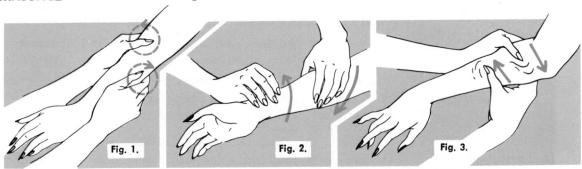

Fig. 1.   Fig. 2.   Fig. 3.

Procedure

Complete hand massage as outlined on page 279.

1. Place patron's arm on table, palm turned downward, as in Fig. 1. Massage arms from wrists to elbows. Use a slow, circular motion in alternate directions. Repeat three times. Turn patron's arm upward and repeat same movements three times.

2. Place your fingers as in Fig. 2. Massage firmly underpart of arm to the elbow, using fingers of each hand in alternate cross-wise directions. Repeat three times.

3. Place your hands as in Fig. 3. Massage top of arm from the wrist to the elbow. Apply thumbs in opposite directions with a squeezing motion. Repeat three times.

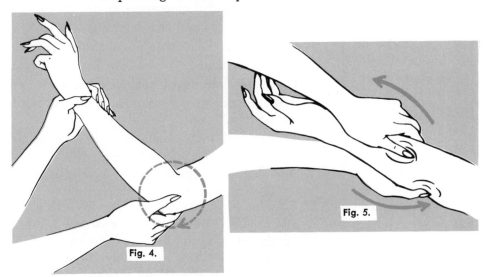

Fig. 4.   Fig. 5.

4. Cup your hand into elbow joint, as in Fig. 4. Massage elbow with a circular motion. Repeat three times.

5. Turn patron's palm upward, as in Fig. 5. Stroke arm firmly in opposite directions from the elbow to wrist. Finally, stroke each finger, ending with a gentle squeeze of the fingertips.

6. Repeat Steps 1 to 5 on other arm.

Note—The above massage manipulations may be extended to and including the shoulders.

PEDICURING

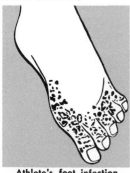

Athlete's foot infection

Equipment, Implements And Supplies

Preparation

Procedure

Pedicuring is the care of the feet, legs and toenails. It is a part of the patron's well-groomed look. The feet and heels in today's shoe fashions are more or less exposed. **Neglected toenails** and rough, harsh heels detract from the loveliest of footwear. Foot care not only improves **personal appearance, but also adds to the comfort of the body.**

Abnormal foot conditions, such as corns, callouses and ingrown nails, are best treated by a qualified chiropodist or podiatrist.

CAUTION. Patrons having athlete's foot (watery blisters and thick white skin between the toes), or other foot infections, should not be given a pedicure. They should be referred to a physician for medical help.

The equipment, implements and materials required for pedicuring are the same as those for manicuring, with the following additions:

1. Low stool for cosmetologist or manicurist
2. Ottoman on which to rest patron's foot
3. Two basins of warm water, large enough for foot bath
4. Waterproof apron, or an extra Turkish towel, placed over the lap to protect the uniform
5. Two Turkish towels for drying patron's feet
6. Special toenail nippers   7. Witch hazel or astringent
8. Antiseptic solution   9. Cotton pledgets and foot powder
10. Paper towels

1. Arrange required equipment, implements and materials.
2. Seat patron in facial chair; have patron remove shoes and hose.
3. Have patron place her feet on a clean paper towel on foot rest.
4. Wash your hands.
5. Fill the two basins with enough warm water to cover her ankles.
6. Add antiseptic to one basin. Have patron place both feet in bath for 3-5 minutes.
7. Remove feet from basin; rinse feet in the second basin, and wipe dry.
8. Add soap to the second basin for the pedicure.

1. Remove old polish from the nails of both feet, as in Fig. 1.
2. File nails of left foot with file or rough side of emery board, working from the little toe toward the big toe. Shape the nails straight across. Do not cut or file corners of nails. Smooth rough edges with fine side of emery board, as in Fig. 2.
3. Place left foot in warm, soapy water, as in Fig. 3.

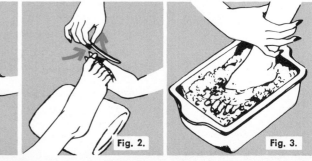

Fig. 1.   Fig. 2.   Fig. 3.

4. Shape nails of right foot.
5. Remove left foot from basin and dry, as in Fig. 4.
6. With a cotton-tipped orangewood stick, apply cuticle solvent to the cuticle and under the free edge of each toenail, as in Fig. 5.

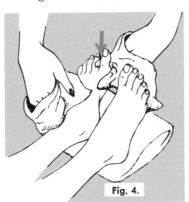

Fig. 4.

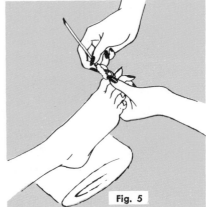

Fig. 5

7. Place right foot in bath.
8. Gently loosen cuticle on left foot. Keep it moist with cuticle solvent. Loosen with the cotton-tipped orangewood stick. Do not use too much pressure. Avoid the use of the metal pusher.
9. Do not cut the cuticle. Only remove a large ragged hangnail.
10. Rinse the left foot and dry. Massage the side groove of each toenail in a circular movement, using cuticle cream or oil.
11. Repeat Steps 5 to 10 on right foot.
12. Scrub toes of both feet in warm, soapy water and dry thoroughly.

FOOT MASSAGE

1. Apply emollient cream over the feet.
2. Start at instep of left foot and apply firm, rotary movements down to the center of the toes, as in Fig. 1.
3. Slide thumbs firmly back **to instep** and repeat same movement.
4. Slide thumbs back to hollow **of heel** and repeat same movement.
5. Slide thumbs back to base **of foot** and repeat same movement.
6. Start at heel and work down to the center of the toes, as in Fig. 2.

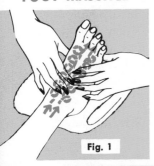

Fig. 1

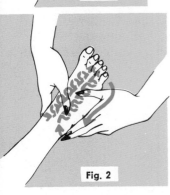

Fig. 2

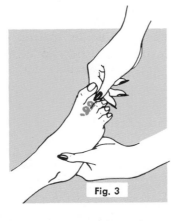

Fig. 3

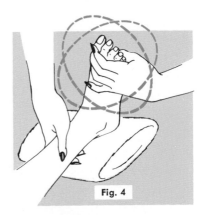

Fig. 4

7. Slide firmly back to heel, and repeat same movement up each side of the foot.

8. Hold small toe in one hand and the big toe in the other hand, and apply three rotary movements; do the same with the other toes, as in Fig. 3.

9. Slide right hand to the ankle and the heel of your left hand to the ball of the foot, apply six firm, rotary movements, as in Fig. 4.

10. Change to right foot and repeat Steps 2 to 9.

Completion

1. Remove cream from both feet with warm towel.
2. Apply witch hazel or astringent to feet with a large cotton pledget.
3. Dust lightly with talcum powder.
4. Wipe each toenail with polish remover to remove all traces of cream.

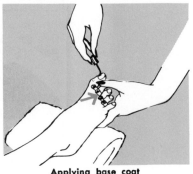

Applying base coat

Note—Inserting cotton between the toes before application of liquid materials will prevent polish smear.

5. Apply base coat, polish and top coat in the same manner as for a manicure.

6. **Clean-up.** Clean and **sanitize implements** — place in dry sanitizer. Discard used materials. Clean up booth. Wash your hands.

LEG MASSAGE

Foot massage may be extended up to and beyond the knee.

CAUTION. When massaging from the ankle to the knee, **do not massage over the shinbone or over the knee.** It is advisable to keep the pressure to the muscular tissue on either side of the shinbone. On the calf area of the leg, you may use kneading upward movement up to the underpart of the knee.

Removing Hair From Legs

For complete instructions, see chapter on **Removal of Superfluous Hair.**

Hiding Varicose Veins

Besides recommending the patron to a doctor for bad cases of varicose veins, the pedicurist can suggest the use of "Cover Mark," waterproof commercial product for concealing varicose veins disfiguration.

REVIEW
QUESTIONS

Manicuring

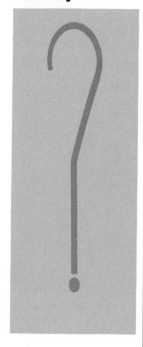

1. What is meant by manicuring?
2. In what manner does a manicurist prepare the table for a manicure?
3. When does the manicurist wash her hands for a manicure?
4. When are manicuring implements sanitized?
5. List five essential implements used in manicuring.
6. List the most commonly used cosmetics in manicuring.
7. List the important steps in giving a plain manicure.
8. How often should a manicure be given?
9. Why should filing be done from the corners to the center of the nail?
10. After an accidental cut in manicuring, what do you apply to avoid an infection?
11. For what purpose is styptic powder used in manicuring?
12. What is the action of a soap bath?
13. What is the action of a cuticle solvent?
14. Why is a base coat applied before the nail polish?
15. What is the purpose and effect of top coat or sealer?
16. For what nail and cuticle conditions are oil manicures recommended?
17. List the three general classifications of nail repair.
18. For whom are press-on artificial nails recommended?
19. For what length of time can press-on artificial nails be worn?
20. What is the purpose of hand and arm massage?
21. Why is it important to follow safety rules in manicuring?
22. List three important sanitary rules for the manicurist to follow to protect the patron's welfare.

Pedicuring

1. What is meant by pedicuring?
2. Which foot conditions should not be treated by the cosmetologist?
3. What are the signs of athlete's foot?
4. Why should athlete's foot not be treated in a beauty salon or school?
5. How can ingrown toenails be prevented in pedicuring?
6. What does the professional weekly pedicure and foot and leg massage do for the patron?

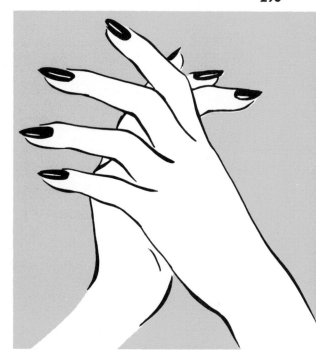

CHAPTER 20

THE NAIL AND DISORDERS OF THE NAIL

INTRODUCTION

The condition of the nail, like that of the skin, reflects the general health of the body. The normal, healthy nail is firm and flexible and exhibits a slightly pinkish color. Its surface should be smooth, curved and unspotted, without any hollows or wavy ridges.

The **nail,** an appendage of the skin, is a horny translucent plate which serves to protect the tips of the fingers and toes. **Onyx** (on′iks) is the technical term for nail.

Nail Composition

The nail is composed mainly of **keratin** (ker′ah-tin), a protein substance which forms the base of all horny tissue. The nail is whitish in appearance. The pinkish color of the nail bed can be seen through the nail. The horny nail plate contains no nerves or blood vessels.

NAIL STRUCTURE

The nails consist of three parts: the nail body, the nail root, and the free edge.

The **nail body,** or **plate,** is the visible portion of the nail which rests upon, and is attached to, the **nail bed.** The nail body extends from the root to the **free edge.**

Although the nail plate seems to be made of one piece, it is actually constructed in layers. The readiness with which nails split, in both their length and thickness, clearly demonstrates this form of structure.

The **nail root** is at the base of the nail and is imbedded **underneath** the skin. The nail root originates from an actively growing tissue known as the **matrix.**

The **free edge** is the end portion of the nail plate which reaches over the fingertips.

**STRUCTURES
ADJOINING
THE NAIL**

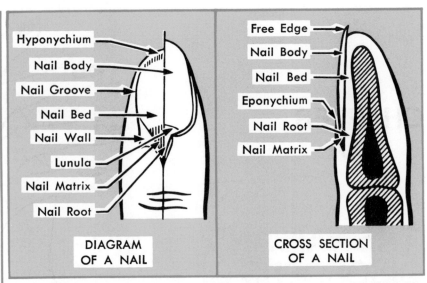

DIAGRAM
OF A NAIL

CROSS SECTION
OF A NAIL

Nail Bed

The **nail bed** is the portion of the skin upon which the **nail body** rests. It is supplied with many blood vessels which provide the nourishment necessary for the continued growth of the nail. The nail bed is also abundantly supplied with nerves.

Matrix

The **matrix** (ma'triks) is that part of the nail bed that extends beneath the nail root, and contains nerves, lymph and blood vessels. The matrix produces the nail as its cells undergo a reproducing and hardening process. The matrix will continue to grow as long as it receives nutrition and remains in a healthy condition.

However, the growth of the nails may be retarded if an individual is in poor health, if a nail disorder or disease is present, or if there is an injury to the nail matrix.

Lunula

The **lunula** (lu'nu-lah), or **half-moon,** is located at the base of the nail. The area underneath the lunula is the matrix. The light color of the lunula may be due to the reflection of light where the matrix and the connective tissue of the nail bed join.

Parts Surrounding Nail

The **cuticle** (ku'ti-kl) is the overlapping epidermis around the nail. A normal cuticle around the nail should be loose and pliable.

The **eponychium** (ep-o-nik'e-um) is the extension of the cuticle at the base of the nail body which partly overlaps the lunula.

The **hyponychium** (hi-po-nik'e-um) is that portion of the epidermis under the free edge of the nail.

The **perionychium** (per-i-o-nik'e-um) is that portion of the cuticle surrounding the entire nail border.

The **nail walls** are the folds of skin overlapping the sides of the nail.

The **nail grooves** are slits, or tracks, on the sides of the nail upon which the nail moves as it grows.

The **mantle** (man'tl) is the deep fold of skin in which the nail root is imbedded.

NAIL GROWTH

The growth of the nail is influenced by nutrition, health and disease. The nail grows forward, starting at the **matrix** and extending over the tip of the finger.

The average rate of growth in the normal adult is about one-eighth of an inch per month, being faster in the summer than in the winter. The nails of children grow more rapidly, whereas those of elderly persons grow more slowly. The nail grows fastest on the middle finger and slowest on the thumb. Although toenails grow more slowly than fingernails, they are thicker and harder.

NAIL MALFORMATION

If the nail is separated from the nail bed through injury, it becomes distorted or discolored. Should the nail bed be injured after the loss of a nail, a badly formed nail will result.

The nails are neither shed automatically nor periodically, as hairs are. If the nail is torn off accidentally, or lost through an infection or disease, it will be replaced **only** as long as the matrix remains in **good** condition. Nails lost under such conditions are, on regrowth, frequently badly shaped, due to interference at the base of the nail. Ordinarily, replacement of the nail takes about four months.

VARIOUS SHAPED NAILS

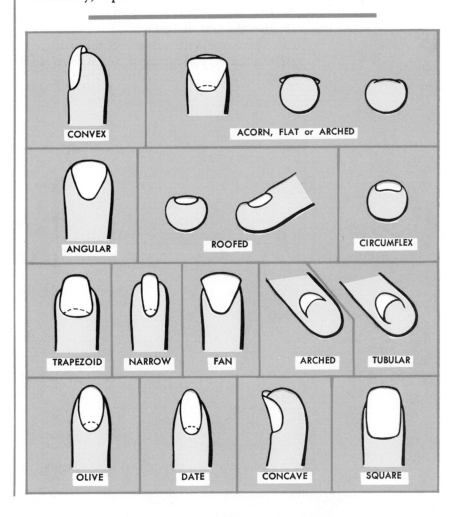

CONVEX

ACORN, FLAT or ARCHED

ANGULAR

ROOFED

CIRCUMFLEX

TRAPEZOID

NARROW

FAN

ARCHED

TUBULAR

OLIVE

DATE

CONCAVE

SQUARE

REVIEW
QUESTIONS

THE NAIL

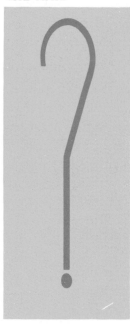

1. What are nails?
2. Describe the appearance of a healthy nail.
3. Of what is the nail composed?
4. What is the technical term for nail?
5. What is the main function of the nails?
6. Of what main substance is the nail composed?
7. Locate the following:
    a) nail root   c) free edge
    b) nail body   d) nail bed
8. Where is the lunula located?
9. What two factors promote the growth of the nails?
10. What three factors retard the growth of the nail?
11. What part of the nail contains the nerve and blood supply?
12. Where does the formation of the nail occur?
13. What gives lunula the half-moon whitish appearance?
14. Define the following:
    a) cuticle
    b) mantle
    c) nail grooves
15. What is the hyponychium?
16. Where is the eponychium found?
17. Define perionychium.
18. How does the nail receive its nourishment?
19. How does the nail grow?
20. What is the average growth of the nail?
21. If a healthy nail is torn off, will it be replaced by a new one?

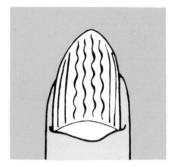

CORRUGATIONS or
WAVY RIDGES

NAIL DISORDERS

NAIL IRREGULARITIES

Diseases of the nail should never be treated by manicurists. However, they should recognize normal and abnormal nail conditions, and understand the reasons for these conditions. Simple nail irregularities and blemishes come within the province of cosmetology and can be treated by the manicurist. A patron having a nail condition where infection, soreness or irritation is present should be referred to a physician.

Corrugations, or **wavy ridges,** are caused by uneven growth of the nails, usually the result of illness or injury. When manicuring a patron with this condition, carefully buff the nails slightly with pumice powder. This will help to remove or minimize the ridges.

Furrows (depressions) in the nails may run either lengthwise or across the nail. These are usually the result of illness or an injury to the nail cells in or near the matrix. Since these nails are exceedingly fragile great care must be exercised in giving a manicure. Avoid the use of the metal pusher, use a cotton-tipped orangewood stick around the cuticle.

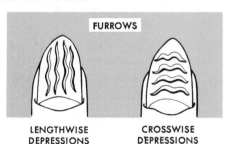

FURROWS

LENGTHWISE
DEPRESSIONS

CROSSWISE
DEPRESSIONS

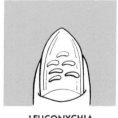

LEUCONYCHIA
(lu-kō nĭk'ē-ah)

Leuconychia, or **white spots,** appear frequently in the nails but do not indicate disease. They may be caused by injury to the base of the nail. As the nail continues to grow, these white spots eventually disappear.

Onychauxis, or **hypertrophy,** is an overgrowth of the nail, usually in thickness rather than length. It is usually caused by an internal disturbance, such as a local infection. If infection is present, the nail is not to be manicured. If infection is not present, the nail may be included in the manicure. File it smooth and buff with pumice powder.

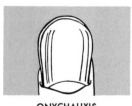

ONYCHAUXIS
(on-ē-kawk'sis)

or

HYPERTROPHY
(hī-per'trō-fi)

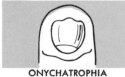

ONYCHATROPHIA
(ō-nik-ah-trō'fē-ah)

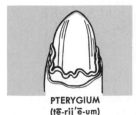

PTERYGIUM
(tē-rij'ē-um)

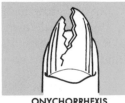

ONYCHOPHAGY
(on-ē-kō-fa'jē)

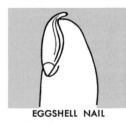

ONYCHORRHEXIS
(on-ē-kō-rek'sis)

Onychatrophia, atrophy or **wasting away** of the nail, causes the nail to lose its luster, become smaller and sometimes shed entirely. Injury or disease may account for this nail irregularity. File the nail smooth with the fine side of the emery board. Advise the patron to protect it from further injury, or from exposure to strong soaps and washing powders.

Pterygium is a forward growth of the cuticle which adheres to the base of the nail. Use the cuticle nippers carefully to remove the growth. Suggest oil manicures.

Onychophagy, or **bitten nails,** is a result of an acquired nervous habit that prompts the individual to chew the nail or the hardened cuticle. Advise the patron that frequent manicures and care of hardened cuticle often help to overcome this habit.

Onychorrhexis refers to **split** or **brittle nails.** Among the causes of split nails are injury to the finger, careless filing of the nails, excessive use of cuticle solvents and nail polish removers. Suggest oil manicures.

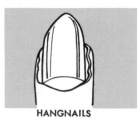

HANGNAILS

EGGSHELL NAIL

BLUE NAIL

Hangnail (agnail) is a condition in which the cuticle splits around the nail. Dryness of the cuticle, cutting off too much cuticle, or carelessness in removing the cuticle may result in hangnails. Advise the patron that proper nail care, such as hot oil manicures, will aid in correcting such condition. If not properly cared for, a hangnail may become infected.

Eggshell nails are recognized by the nail plate being noticeably thin, white and much more flexible than in the normal nails. The nail plate separates from the nail bed and curves at the free edge. This disorder may be caused by a chronic illness of systemic or nervous origin.

Blue nails may be attributed to poor blood circulation, or a heart disorder. The patron may receive the regular manicure treatment.

A **bruised nail** will show dark, purplish (almost black or brown) spots in the nail. These are usually due to injury and bleeding in the nail bed. The dried blood attaches itself to the nail and grows out with it. In manicuring, treat this injured nail gently. Avoid pressure.

Treating cuts. If a cut is accidently inflicted on a patron during a manicure, **apply an antiseptic immediately.** Do not buff or apply nail polish to the injured finger. To protect against infection, apply a **sterile band-aid.**

Infected finger. In the case of an infected finger, the patron should be referred to a physician.

NAIL DISEASES

There are several nail diseases that may be met during cosmetology practice. However, **any nail disease** which shows signs of infection or inflammation (redness, pain, swelling or pus) must not be treated in a beauty salon. **Medical treatment is required** for all nail diseases.

Occupation plays an important role in the cause of many nail infections. Infections develop more readily in those who constantly immerse their hands in alkaline solutions. Natural oils are removed from the skin by frequent exposure to soaps, solvents and other substances. The hands of the cosmetologist are daily exposed to chemical materials. Many of these are harmless, but others have potential dangers. The cosmetologist should safeguard her hands and nails by wearing protective gloves when working with chemicals.

Onychosis (onychonosus) is a technical term applied to any nail disease.

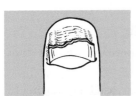

ONYCHOMYCOSIS
(on-ē-kō-mī-kō′sis)

Onychomycosis, tinea unguium or **ringworm of the nails,** is an infectious disease caused by a **vegetable** parasite. A **common form** consists of whitish patches that can be scraped off the surface. **Another form** appears as long yellowish streaks within the nail substance. The disease invades the free edge and spreads toward the root. The infected portion is thick and discolored. In a **third form,** the deeper layers of the nail are invaded, causing the superficial layers to appear irregularly thinned. These infected layers peel off and expose the diseased parts of the nail bed.

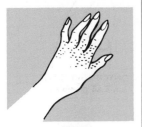

TINEA
(tin′ē-ah)
UNGUIUM
(ung′gwē-um)

Ringworm (tinea) of the hands. A highly contagious disease caused by a fungus (vegetable parasite). The principal symptoms are papular, red lesions occurring in patches or rings over the hands. Itching may be slight or severe.

Most cases of dermatitis of the hands resemble tinea, but are actually a contact dermatitis, plus a staphylococcic infection. Only a physician can determine this condition.

Ringworm of the feet (athlete's foot). In acute conditions, deep, itchy, colorless vesicles appear. These appear singly and in groups and sometimes on only one foot. They spread over the sole and between the toes, perhaps involving the nail fold and infecting the nail. When the vesicles rupture, the skin becomes red and oozes. The lesions dry as they heal. Fungus infection of the feet is likely to become chronic.

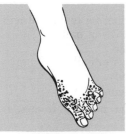

ATHLETE'S FOOT

Both the prevention of infection and beneficial treatment are accomplished by keeping the skin cool, dry, and clean.

Paronychia, or **felon,** is an infectious and inflammatory condition of the tissues surrounding the nails. This condition is traceable to bacterial infection.

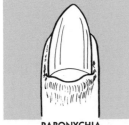

PARONYCHIA
(par-ō-nǐk′ē-ah)

Onychia is an inflammation of the nail matrix, accompanied by pus formation. Improper sanitization of nail implements and bacterial infection may cause this disease.

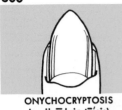

ONYCHOCRYPTOSIS
(on-ik-ō-krip-tō′sis)

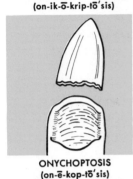

ONYCHOPTOSIS
(on-ē-kop-tō′sis)

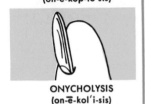

ONYCHOLYSIS
(on-ē-kol′i-sis)

Onychocryptosis, or **ingrown nails,** may affect either the finger or toe. In this condition, the nail grows into the sides of the flesh and may cause an infection. Filing the nails too much in the corners and failing to correct hangnails are often responsible for ingrown nails.

Onychoptosis is the periodic shedding of one or more nails, either in whole or in part. This condition may follow certain diseases, such as syphilis.

Onycholysis is a loosening of the nail, without shedding. It is frequently associated with an internal disorder.

Onychophyma denotes a swelling of the nails.

Onychophosis refers to a growth of horny epithelium in the nail bed.

Onychogryposis pertains to enlarged and increased curvature of the nails.

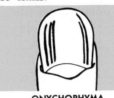

ONYCHOPHYMA
(on-ē-kō-fī′mah)

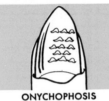

ONYCHOPHOSIS
(on-ē-kō-fō′sis)

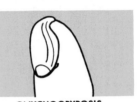

ONYCHOGRYPOSIS
(on-ē-kō-grī-pō′sis)

1. Should an infected nail of finger be given a manicure?
2. What are hangnails? Give their cause.
3. How are hangnails treated?
4. What may cause wavy ridges?
5. Match the following:
   - a) leuconychia
   - b) onychauxis
   - c) onychophagy
   - d) atrophy
   - e) pterygium

   1) cuticle adhering to base of nail
   2) wasting away of nail
   3) bitten nails
   4) white spots in nail
   5) hypertrophy
6. How is an accidental cut treated during a manicure?
7. **List 12 abnormal conditions of the nails that may be treated by a manicurist.**
8. What is the technical name for split or brittle nails?
9. What treatment would you recommend for brittle nails?
10. Define onychosis.
11. What is the technical term for ingrown nails?
12. What causes a paronychia condition?
13. Define onychia.
14. What parasite causes ringworm of the nails?
15. What parasite causes ringworm of the hands?
16. Match the following:
    - a) onycholysis
    - b) onychophyma
    - c) onychoptosis

    1) swelling of nail
    2) periodic shedding of nail
    3) loosening of nail
17. Which foot conditions should not be treated by the cosmetologist?
18. What are the signs of athlete's foot (ringworm of the feet)?
19. Why should athlete's foot not be treated in a beauty salon or school?

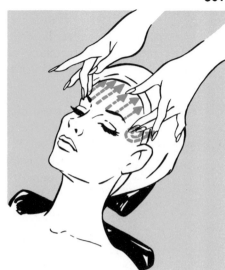

CHAPTER 21

THEORY OF MASSAGE

INTRODUCTION

Massage is one of the oldest and most useful methods of physical treatment. In cosmetology, it is also employed for reasons of health and beauty. When used properly, it helps the skin become more pliable and attractive. To master massage techniques, a knowledge of anatomy and physiology is required, and considerable practice in performing the various movements is necessary.

Massage involves the application of external manipulations to the body. This is accomplished by means of the hands, or with the aid of mechanical or electrical appliances, such as therapeutic lamps (dermal light and infra-red rays), high-frequency current, facial steamers, heating caps, scalp steamers, and vibrators.

Area Of Massage

The cosmetologist is limited to massage only certain areas of the body, mainly:

1. The scalp
2. The face, neck and shoulders
3. The upper chest and back
4. The hands and arms
5. The foot and leg

Massage must always be applied upon the skin. First, apply cream, ointment, or oil. This application permits better hand movements and prevents drag or damage to tissues.

CAUTION. Massage should not be used when certain conditions exist, such as a heart condition, high blood pressure, inflamed and swollen joints, and glandular swelling. Nor should it be employed when abrasions of the skin, diseases of the skin and broken capillaries are evident.

Qualifications

Massage calls for a firm, sure touch, which inspires confidence in the patron. Therefore, the cosmetologist must develop:

1. Strong, flexible hands
2. A quiet temperament
3. Self-control
4. The use of psychology

Hands for massaging should be kept soft by the use of creams, oils and lotions. The nails should be beveled smooth to prevent any scratching of the skin. The wrist and fingers should be flexible, and the palms firm, warm and dry.

How Manipulative Movements Are Accomplished

Every massage treatment combines one or more of the basic movements. Each manipulation is applied in a definite way, for a particular purpose. It is used according to the patron's condition and the desired results. The result of a massage treatment will depend on the amount of pressure, direction of movement, and the duration of each type of manipulation. **Direction of movement is from the insertion of a muscle toward its origin.**

BASIC MANIPULATIONS USED IN MASSAGE

Effleurage (ef-loo-rahzh'). This is a light, continuous movement applied to the skin with the fingers and palms in a slow and rhythmic manner. No pressure is employed. **Over large surfaces,** the palm is used,

Effleurage (Stroking Movement)

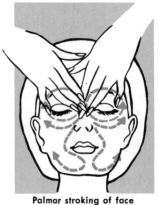

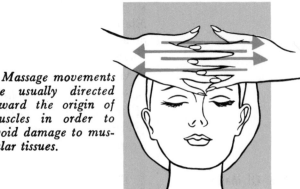

Massage movements are usually directed toward the origin of muscles in order to avoid damage to muscular tissues.

Palmar stroking of face

Digital stroking of forehead

while **over small surfaces,** the cushions of the fingertips are employed. Effleurage is frequently applied to the forehead, face, scalp, back, shoulders, neck, chest, arms and hands for its soothing and relaxing effects.

Position Of Fingers

For the correct **position for stroking,** the fingers should be slightly curved, with just the **cushions of the fingertips** touching the skin. Do not use the end of the fingertips for massage movements. Fingertips cannot control the degree of pressure. Besides, the free edges of the fingernails are likely to scratch the skin.

Position Of Palms

For the correct **position of the palms for stroking,** hold the whole hand loosely; keep the wrist and fingers flexible, and slightly curve the fingers to conform to the shape of the area being massaged.

Petrissage (Kneading Movement)

Petrissage (pe'tre-sahzh). In this movement, grasp the skin and flesh between the fingers and palm of the hand. As the tissues are lifted from their underlying structures, they are squeezed, rolled or pinched with a **light, firm pressure.** This movement invigorates the part being treated, and is usually limited to back, shoulder and arm massage.

Purpose Of Kneading

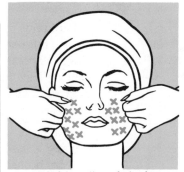

Digital kneading of cheeks

Purpose of kneading. The pressure should be light but firm. When grasping and releasing the fleshy parts, you must be in rhythm, never jerky. Kneading movements give **deeper stimulation** and improve the circulation.

Digital Kneading

Digital kneading of cheeks can be achieved by light pinching movements.

Fulling

Fulling, a form of petrissage, is used mainly in massage of the arms. With the fingers of both hands grasping the arm, a kneading movement is applied over the flesh. The kneading movement must be used with light pressure on the underside of the patron's forearm, **and on the upper arm.**

Friction (Deep Rubbing Movement)

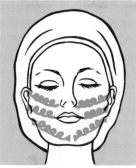

Circular friction of face

This movement requires pressure on the skin while it is being moved over the underlying structures. **The fingers or palms are** employed in this movement. Friction has a marked influence on the circulation and glandular activity of the skin.

Circular friction movements are usually employed on the scalp, arms and hands. **Light** circular friction movements are generally used on the face and neck.

Chucking, rolling and wringing are variations of friction which are employed principally to massage the arms.

Chucking

The **chucking movement** is accomplished by grasping the flesh firmly in one hand and moving the hand up and down along the bone, while the other hand keeps the arm in a steady position.

Rolling

The **rolling movement** requires that the tissues be compressed firmly against the bone and twisted around the arm. Both hands of the cosmetologist are active as the flesh is twisted down the arm in the same direction.

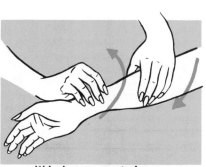

Wringing movement of arm

Wringing

Wringing is a vigorous movement in which the cosmetologist's hands are placed a little distance apart on both sides of the arm. While the hands are worked downward, the flesh is twisted against the bones in opposite directions.

**Percussion Or
Tapotement**

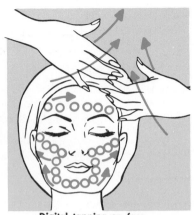

Percussion (per-kush'un) **or tapotement** (tah-pot-man') consists of tapping, slapping and hacking movements. This form of massage is the
most stimulating. It should be applied
with care and discretion.

**Tapping
Movements**

In facial massage, only **light digital
tapping** is used. In **tapping**, the fingertips are brought down against the skin
in rapid succession. The fingers must
be flexible to create an even force over
the area being treated.

Digital tapping on face

**Slapping And
Hacking Movements**

Hacking and **slapping movements** are used mainly to massage the
back, shoulders and arms.

In slapping movements, flexible wrists permit the palms to come in
contact with the skin in light, firm, and rapid slapping movements.
One hand follows the other. With each slapping stroke (which must
be nothing more than a firm, light and quick contact with the skin)
the flesh is slightly lifted.

Hacking movements employ the wrists and outer edges of the
hands. Both the wrists and fingers must move in fast, light, firm,
flexible motions against the skin in alternate succession.

**Vibration
(Shaking Movement)**

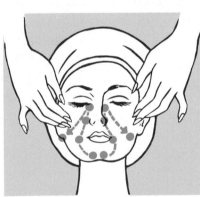

Vibration. This movement is
accomplished by rapid muscular
contractions in the arms of the cosmetologist, while the balls of the
fingertips are pressed firmly on the
point of application. It is a highly
stimulating movement. Use sparingly and never exceed a few
seconds duration on any one spot.
Muscular contractions can also be
produced by the use of a mechanical vibrator.

Vibratory movement of face

Joint Movements

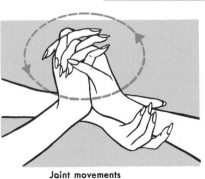

Joint movements are restricted
to the massage of the arm and
hand. These movements are applied either with or without resistance. For information on joint
movement, consult chapter on
Manicuring.

Joint movements

MOTOR NERVE POINTS OF THE FACE AND NECK

In order to obtain the maximum benefits from a facial massage, the cosmetologist must consider the motor nerve points which affect the underlying muscles of the face and neck.

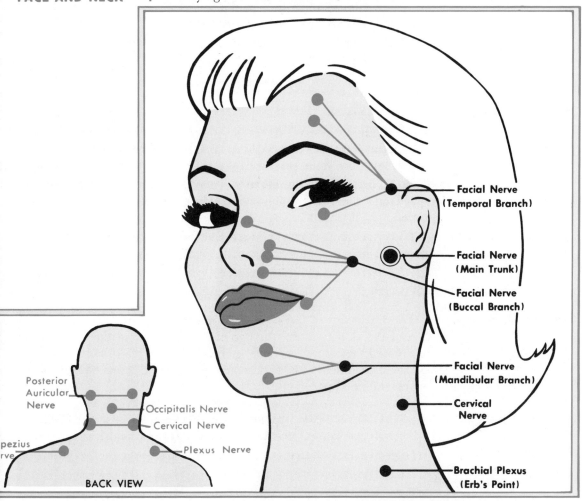

Facial Nerve (Temporal Branch)

Facial Nerve (Main Trunk)

Facial Nerve (Buccal Branch)

Facial Nerve (Mandibular Branch)

Cervical Nerve

Brachial Plexus (Erb's Point)

Posterior Auricular Nerve

Occipitalis Nerve

Cervical Nerve

pezius rve

Plexus Nerve

BACK VIEW

PHYSIOLOGICAL EFFECTS OF MASSAGE

To obtain proper results from a scalp or facial massage, the cosmetologist must have a thorough knowledge of all the structures involved: the muscles, nerves and blood vessels.

Almost every muscle and nerve has a **motor point.** The position of motor points will vary in location on individuals, due to differences in body structure. However, a few manipulations on the right motor points will readily induce relaxation at the beginning of the massage treatment.

Skillfully applied massage influences the structures and functions of the body, either directly or indirectly. The immediate effects of massage are **first noticed on the skin.** The part being massaged responds by a more active circulation, secretion, nutrition and excretion.

The following beneficial results may be obtained by proper facial and scalp massage:

1. The skin and all its structures are nourished.

2. Fat cells in the subcutaneous tissue are reduced.
3. The skin is rendered soft and pliable.
4. The circulation of the blood is increased.
5. The activity of the skin glands is stimulated.
6. The muscle fiber is stimulated and strengthened.
7. The nerves are soothed and rested.
8. Pain is sometimes relieved.

Theory Of Massage

Rest and relaxation are brought about by giving light but firm, slow, rhythmic movements, or very slow, light hand vibrations over the motor points for a very short time. Another technique is to pause briefly and use light pressure over the motor points.

Body tissues are stimulated by movements of moderate pressure, speed and time, or by light hand vibrations of moderate speed and time.

Body contours or fatty tissues are reduced by firm kneading, or fast, firm, but light slapping movements, over a fairly long period of time. Moderately fast hand vibrations with firm pressure will also accomplish this reduction.

Frequency Of Massage

The frequency of facial or scalp massage depends upon the condition of the skin or scalp, the age of the patron, and the condition to be treated. As a general rule, normal skin or scalp can be kept in excellent condition with a massage once a week, accompanied by the proper home care.

Electrical Appliances For Facial And Scalp Massage

The following electrical appliances may be used for facial massage:
Therapeutic lamps (dermal light and infra-red lamp)
High-frequency current
Facial steamers

For a scalp massage, therapeutic lamps, high-frequency current, scalp steamers, heating caps and a vibrator may be used.

REVIEW QUESTIONS

Theory Of Massage

1. What is meant by massage?
2. Why is massage employed?
3. What four qualifications should a cosmetologist possess?
4. List three skin conditions when massage should not be given.
5. Give the technical and common names for five kinds of massage movements.
6. What are the massage effects on skin?
7. How does massage affect:
   a) muscle fibers   c) blood circulation   e) pain
   b) fat cells   d) nerves
8. Which electrical appliances are used with: a) facial massage; b) scalp massage?
9. What kind of massage movements produce a soothing effect?
10. What kind of massage movements produce a stimulating effect?
11. What kind of massage movements help to reduce fatty tissues?

CHAPTER 22

FACIAL TREATMENTS

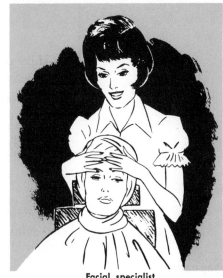

Facial specialist

INTRODUCTION

Giving a facial is one of the most restful treatments the beauty salon has to offer. The patron enjoys the relaxation and stimulation from massage, the soothing effects of creams and lotions, and the finished application of an attractive makeup. Facials may be given as often as once a week, except where otherwise indicated.

Facial treatments can be developed into a profitable service. The patron's hairstyle may be beautiful, but if the face it frames is covered with an unattractive skin, the effect of the hairstyle will be lost.

The cosmetologist does not treat skin diseases. She should be able, however, to recognize various skin ailments in order to leave them alone, and to know when to refer the patron to her doctor for treatment.

Facial treatments fall under **two categories:**

1. **Preservative**—to maintain the health of the facial skin by correct cleansing methods, increased circulation, relaxation of the nerves, and activation of the skin glands and metabolism through massage.

2. **Corrective**—to correct some facial skin conditions, such as dryness, oiliness, blackheads, aging lines and minor conditions of acne.

BENEFITS OF TREATMENTS

Facial treatments are beneficial for:

1. Cleansing the skin
2. Increasing circulation
3. Activating glandular activity
4. Relaxing the nerves
5. Maintaining muscle tone
6. Strengthening weak muscle tissue
7. Correcting certain skin disorders
8. Helping to prevent the formation of wrinkles and aging lines
9. Softening and improving skin texture and complexion
10. Giving a youthful feeling

POINTS TO REMEMBER IN FACIAL MASSAGE

1. Have patron thoroughly relaxed.
2. Provide quiet atmosphere; speak softly.
3. Maintain a clean, orderly arrangement of supplies.
4. Follow systematic procedure.
5. If hands are cold, warm them before touching patron.
6. Make sure fingernails are not too long or pointed.

PLAIN FACIAL

The facial booth should be located in the most quiet area in the school or salon. From the moment the patron enters the booth, help her to relax by talking to her quietly and gently. Perform all work as **noiselessly** as possible.

Preparation

All creams and packs should be removed from their containers with a spatula; **never,** under any circumstances, should the fingers be dipped into any of the products used.

Everything that is to be used for the facial should be set out and arranged in an orderly manner.

Implements And Supplies

1. Cleansing lotion
2. Cleansing cream
3. Massage cream
4. Witch hazel
5. Antiseptic solution
6. Infra-red lamp
7. Cleansing tissues
8. Absorbent cotton
9. Two safety pins
10. Head covering or headband
11. Cotton pads
12. Clean sheet or drape
13. Towels
14. Spatulas
15. Facial steamer
16. Talcum powder
17. Tissue strips
18. High frequency machine

Procedure For A Plain Facial

The information given here may be changed to conform with your instructor's routine.

Prepare Patron

1. **Prepare patron.**
   a) Ask the patron to remove neck and ear jewelry and to **place** same in purse.
   b) Help patron remove outer garments and carefully hang them up.
   c) Place a clean towel over the headrest of the facial chair. Later on, use this towel to drape head.
   d) Place another towel across the upper part of facial chair to protect the patron's shoulders from touching the chair.
   e) Place a clean towel, lengthwise, across the footrest.
   f) Tilt the facial chair back slightly and seat patron.

Drape Patron's Body

2. **Drape body of patron.**

   There are several ways in which the patron may be draped. Be guided by your instructor.

   a) Place two folded towels over the front and back of the patron. Pin the towels together about four inches from the top, at the shoulders. Fig. 1.

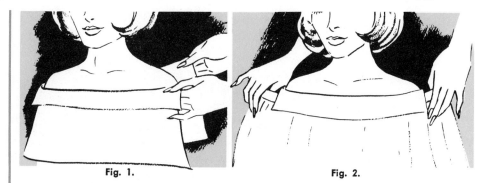

Fig. 1.   Fig. 2.

b) Place the drape loosely over the front and sides of the patron, while she removes her blouse and drops her lingerie straps. Tuck the drape under the front towel, draw the ends, and hold. Fig. 2.

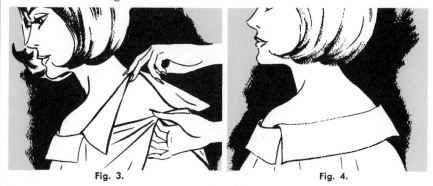

Fig. 3.   Fig. 4.

c) Lift the folded towel in the back and pin the drape under the towel; then, let the towel down over the drape. Fig. 3.
d) Towels and drape properly pinned securely. Fig. 4.

Drape Patron's Head

3. **Drape the head of the patron.**
   a) Place a tissue strip around the patron's hairline to hold back her hair. Fig. 1.
   b) Take a towel lengthwise, drape from nape to top front. Fig. 2.
   c) Pin it with a small safety pin, but leave it open, as in Fig. 3.

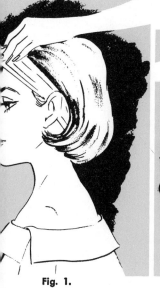

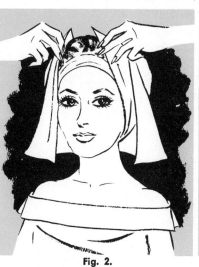

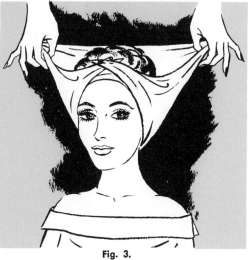

Fig. 1.   Fig. 2.   Fig. 3.

d) Bring the two other ends of the towel up across the back of the head; bring the center part of the towel up to the first pinning and double pin them together. Fig. 4.

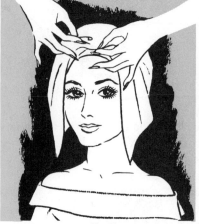 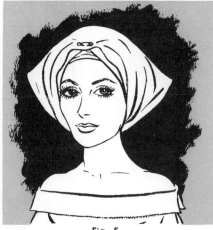

Fig. 4.   Fig. 5.

e) After the towel has been double pinned, take both corner ends of the towel and bring them back to the nape. Finish head draping by folding evenly and pinning at nape. Fig. 5.

f) **Prepared turban types and head bands.**
    These are available and are fastened with magnetic, self-attaching patches. They may be either the laundered or disposable type. Fig. 6.

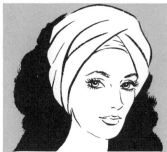

Fig. 6.
Optional—Prepared head bands

Drape Patron's Feet

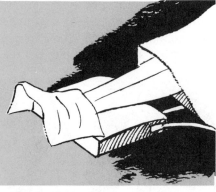

4. **Drape the feet of the patron.**
    a) Recline patron to a comfortable position.
    b) Remove her shoes and place them under the footstool.
    c) Cover her feet with towel and tuck the edges in.
    Sanitize your hands before proceeding with the facial.

Analyze Skin

5. **Analyze skin.**
    a) Remove makeup to determine:
        1. If the skin is dry
        2. If the skin is oily
        3. If comedones or acne are present
        4. If broken capillaries are visible
        5. If the skin texture is soft and velvety, or harsh and rough
        6. The skin's color and fine lines

b) This analysis will determine:
1. The choice of cream to be used in massage
2. The amount of pressure to use in massage movements
3. The areas that need extra attention
4. The type of astringent to use
5. The color of makeup to apply

The procedure given here may be changed to conform with your instructor's routine, as she may have developed a routine which is equally correct.

Apply Cleansing Cream

6. **Apply cleansing cream.**
   a) Remove a little cleansing cream from the jar with a spatula. Blend it with the fingers to soften the cream. (Remove lipstick and eye makeup very carefully.)

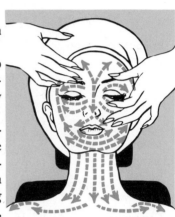

Spreading cream over face, neck, chest and back

   b) Apply cream over the face, using both hands. Start at the chin and with a sweeping movement slide to end of jaw; from base of nose to temples; along side of nose up over the bridge, between the brows, across forehead to temples.
   c) Take additional cream and blend. In long, even strokes, smooth down the neck, chest and back.
   d) Start at center of forehead: Go lightly around eyes to temples and back to center of forehead.
   e) Slide down nose to upper lip; smooth to temples and forehead; lightly down to chin; then firmly up the jawline to temples and forehead.

Remove Cleansing Cream

7. **Remove cleansing cream.**
   a) Remove cream with tissue mitts, or warm, moist towel. Start at forehead and follow the contour of the face. Remove all the cream from one area before proceeding to the next. Finish with neck, chest and back.
   (If the eyebrows are to be arched, it should be done at this time.)

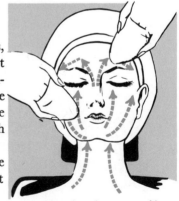

Removing cleansing cream with tissues or warm, moist towel

Steam Face (Optional)

8. **Steam face** (optional).
   a) Steam face mildly with warm, moist towels or facial steamer.

Apply Massage Cream

9. **Apply cream.**
   a) Select the appropriate cream for the skin type. Apply it in the same manner as the cleansing cream, to face, neck, shoulders and chest.
   Use a lanolin or hormone cream for dry skin, but a cold cream will do for normal or oily skin.

312

Give Facial Manipulations

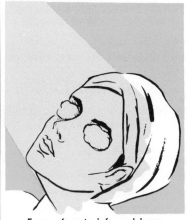

Expose face to infra-red lamp

Remove Massage Cream

Apply Astringent Lotion

Apply Foundation And Makeup

Complete Procedure

Clean Up

10. **Give facial manipulations** (either before or during exposure to infra-red lamp).
    a) Cover patron's eyes with cotton pads moistened with witch hazel.
    b) Place lamp at a comfortable distance.
    c) Apply lamp for 3-5 minutes.
    d) Massage face as described on next page.

11. **Remove massage cream.**
    a) Remove cream with tissues or warm moist towel in the same manner as done with cleansing cream.

12. **Apply astringent lotion.**
    a) Sponge face with cotton pledgets moistened with astringent lotion.

13. **Apply foundation and makeup.**

14. **Complete.**
    a) Return facial chair to upright position.
    b) Remove protective head covering from head.
    c) Remove protective towels and body covering.
    d) Assist patron with her garments and shoes.

15. **Cleanup.**
    a) Discard all disposable supplies and materials.
    b) Close containers tightly, clean them and put them in their proper places.
    c) Tidy up booth. Return used articles to be sanitized, or unused cosmetics to the dispensary.
    d) Wash and sanitize your hands.

TWELVE REASONS WHY A PATRON MAY FIND FAULT WHEN RECEIVING A FACIAL

1. Offensive body odor, foul breath or tobacco odor
2. Harming or scratching the skin
3. Excessive or rough massage
4. Getting facial creams into eyes
5. Using towels that are too hot
6. Breathing into the patron's face
7. Not being careful or sanitary
8. Not showing interest in the patron's skin problems
9. Careless in removing cream, leaving a greasy film behind the ears, under the chin or in other areas
10. Not permitting the patron to relax, either by talking or being tense while giving facial manipulations
11. Jumping up and down for materials or supplies
12. Heavy, rough or cold hands

In giving facial manipulations, you must remember that an even tempo or rhythm induces relaxation. Do not remove the hands from the face once the manipulations have been started. Should it become necessary to remove the hands, feather them off, and then very gently replace them with feather-like movements.

> Each instructor may have developed her own routine in giving manipulations. The following illustrations merely show the different movements that may be used on the various parts of the face, chest and back. Follow your instructor's routine.

Massage movements are usually directed towards the **origin** of muscles in order to avoid damage to muscular tissues.

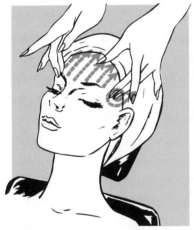

1. LINEAR MOVEMENT OVER FORE-HEAD. Slide to temples, rotate with pressure on upward stroke, slide to left eyebrow; then stroke to hairline across forehead and back.

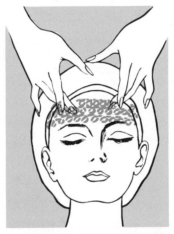

2. CIRCULAR MOVEMENT OVER FOREHEAD. Start at eyebrowline, **work across middle of forehead, and then towards the hairline.**

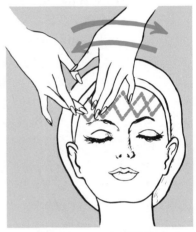

3. CRISS-CROSS MOVEMENT. Start **at one side of forehead and work back.**

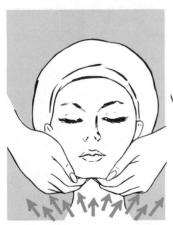

4. CHIN MOVEMENT. Lift chin, using a slight pressure.

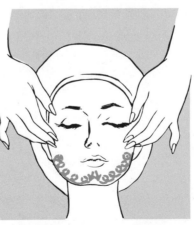

5. LOWER CHEEK. Use circular movement from chin to ear and rotate.

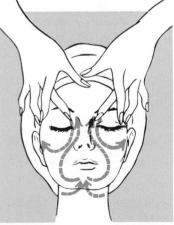

6. Mouth, nose and cheek movements.

Note: Many facial specialists prefer to start massage manipulations on the forehead; while others prefer to start at the chin. Both are correct. Be guided by your instructor.

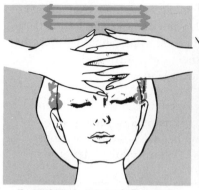

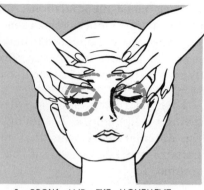

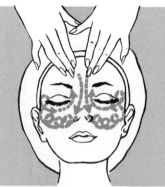

7. STROKING (HEADACHE) MOVE-MENT. Slide fingers to center of **forehead,** then draw fingers, with slight pressure, toward temples, and rotate.

8. BROW AND EYE MOVEMENT. Place middle finger at inner corner of eyes and index fingers over brows. Slide to outer corners of eyes, under eyes and back.

9. NOSE AND UPPER CHEEKS. **Slide fingers down nose. Apply rotary movement across cheeks to temples, and rotate gently. Slide fingers under eyes and back to bridge of nose.**

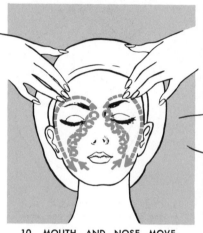

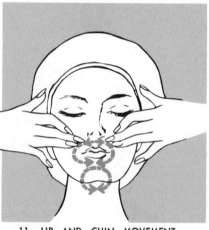

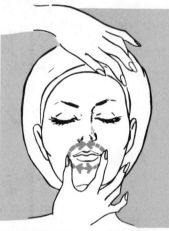

10. MOUTH AND NOSE MOVE-MENT. Apply circular movement from corner of mouth up sides of **nose. Slide fingers over brows and down to corners of mouth.**

11. LIP AND CHIN MOVEMENT. Draw fingers from center of upper lip, around mouth, going under lower lip and the chin.

12. (OPTIONAL MOVEMENT.) Hold head with left hand; draw fingers of right hand from under the lower **lip, around mouth, to center of upper lip.**

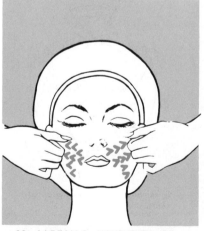

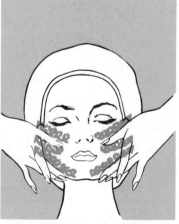

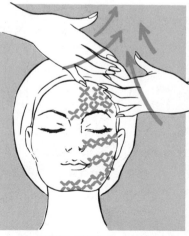

13. LIFTING MOVEMENTS OF CHEEKS. Proceed from the mouth to ears, and then from nose to top part of ears.

14. THE ROTARY MOVEMENT OF CHEEKS. Massage from chin to ear lobes, mouth to middle of ears, and from nose to top of ears.

15. LIGHT TAPPING MOVEMENT, from chin to ear lobe, mouth to ear, nose to top of ear, and then across forehead. Repeat on other side.

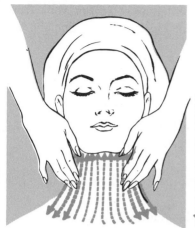

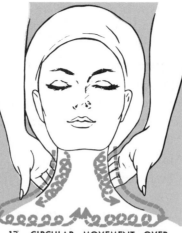

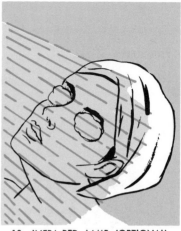

16. STROKING MOVEMENT OF NECK. Apply light upward strokes over front of neck. Use heavier pressure on sides of neck in downward strokes.

17. CIRCULAR MOVEMENT OVER NECK AND CHEST. Starting at back of ears, apply circular movement down side of neck, over shoulders and across chest.

18. INFRA-RED LAMP (OPTIONAL). Protect eyes with eye pads; adjust lamp over patron's face; leave on for about 5 minutes.

CHEST, BACK AND NECK MANIPULATIONS (OPTIONAL)

Some instructors prefer to treat these areas first before starting the regular facial. A suggested procedure is as follows:

1. Apply and remove cleansing cream.
2. Apply emollient cream.
3. Give manipulations as outlined below.
4. Remove cream with tissues or warm, moist towel.
5. Dust the back lightly with talcum powder and smooth.

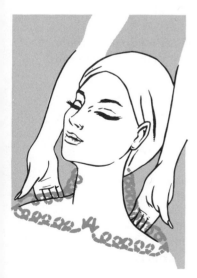

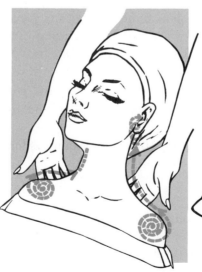

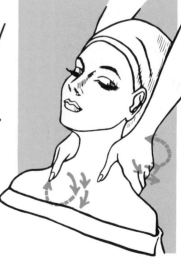

1. CHEST AND BACK MOVEMENTS. Use rotary movements across chest and shoulders, then to spine. Slide **fingers to base of neck. Rotate 3 times.**

2. SHOULDERS AND BACK MOVEMENTS. Rotate shoulders 3 times. **Glide fingers to spine, then to base of neck. Apply circular movements up to back of ear and then slide fingers to front of ear lobe. Rotate 3 times.**

3. BACK MASSAGE (OPTIONAL). To stimulate and relax patron use thumbs and bent index fingers to grasp the tissue at the back of the neck. Rotate 6 times. Repeat over shoulders and back to the spine.

FACIAL FOR DRY SKIN

Procedure

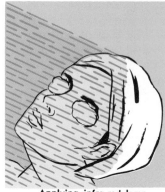

Applying infra-red lamp

A dry skin is caused by an insufficient flow of sebum (oil) from the sebaceous glands. This type of facial assists in correcting the dry condition of the skin.

1. Prepare patron as for plain facial.
2. Apply cleansing cream; remove with tissues or warm, moist towel.
3. Sponge face with cleansing lotion (for dry skin).
4. Apply massage cream suitable for dry skin.
5. Apply muscle oil, or eye cream, over and under the eyes.
6. Apply muscle oil over the neck.
7. Cover patron's eyes with cotton pads moistened with witch hazel or boric acid solution.
8. Expose face and neck to infra-red lamp for not more than five minutes.
9. Give manipulations three to five times.
10. Remove cream with tissues or warm, moist towel.
11. Apply skin lotion suitable for dry skin.
12. Blot face with tissues or towel.
13. Apply base foundation and makeup suitable for the patron's skin tones.
14. Complete and clean up as for plain facial.

> **CAUTION.** For dry skin, avoid using lotions which contain a large percentage of alcohol. Read manufacturer's directions.

DRY SCALY SKIN FACIAL WITH HIGH-FREQUENCY CURRENT

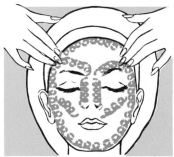

High-frequency indirect method
Patron holds electrode

1. Follow Steps 1 to 8 as in **facial for dry skin.**
2. Give manipulations, using the **indirect method** of applying the **high-frequency current,** for not more than seven minutes.
3. Apply two or three cold towels to the face and neck.
4. Sponge the face and neck with skin freshener.
5. Apply base foundation and makeup suitable for patron's skin tones.
6. Completion and clean up as for plain facial.

FACIAL FOR OILY SKIN AND BLACKHEADS (COMEDONES)

Procedure

An oily skin and/or blackheads are mostly due to improper diet consisting of too much starchy and oily foods. **Comedones** are caused by a hardened mass of sebum, found in the ducts of sebaceous glands.

1. Prepare patron as for plain facial.
2. Apply cleansing cream. Remove cleansing cream with warm, moist towel. If skin is extremely oily, it may be washed with warm water and a medicated soap.
3. Apply cleansing lotion for oily skin.

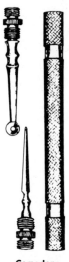

Comedone extractor

4. a) Re-apply cleansing cream and steam the face with three or four warm towels, **or**

 b) Steam the face with the facial steamer to open the pores.

5. Cover the fingertips with tissue and gently press out blackheads. **Do not** press hard enough to bruise skin tissue. Blackheads may also be removed with a sanitized comedone extractor.

6. Sponge the face with an antiseptic.

7. Cover the patron's eyes with cotton pledgets moistened with boric acid solution.

8. Apply the blue light over the bare skin for not more than 3-5 minutes.

9. Apply massage cream suitable for this condition.

10. Give manipulations.

11. Remove cream with warm, moist towel.

12. Prepare a pledget of cotton moistened with an astringent lotion. Apply it to the face and neck with upward and outward movements to close the pores.

13. Blot excess moisture with tissues.

14. Apply base foundation and suitable makeup.

15. Complete and clean up as for plain facial.

TREATMENT FOR ACNE

Acne, being a disorder of the sebaceous glands, requires medical direction. If the patron is under medical care, the role of the cosmetologist is to work closely with the patron's physician and carry out his instructions as to the kind and frequency of treatment.

Under medical direction, the cosmetologist must limit the cosmetic treatment of acne to measures designed to be helpful, such as:

1. Reducing the oiliness of the skin by local applications

2. Removing blackheads with a sanitized comedone extractor

3. Cleansing the skin

4. Using special medicated preparations

5. Suggesting a regulated diet

Implements And Supplies

1. Acne cream or ointment

2. Acne lotion

3. Antiseptic

4. Cleansing cream

5. Medicated cleansing lotion
6. Towels
7. Astringent lotion for oily skin
8. High frequency facial glass electrode
9. Medicated soap
10. Skin toner
11. Cotton or mask
12. Other supplies used in a plain facial

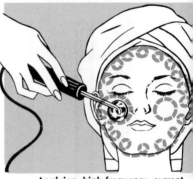

Applying high-frequency current
with facial electrode

**Procedure For
Acne Treatment**

1. Prepare patron as for plain facial.
2. Cleanse face with medicated soap and warm water, using a small towel wrung out of water.
3. Apply acne cream or ointment over face and neck.
4. Apply the high-frequency current with **direct** application over the affected parts for not more than five minutes.
5. Remove the acne cream or ointment with tissues or warm, moist towel.
6. Saturate a thin cotton mask with acne lotion. Apply cotton mask to face and affected parts and re-saturate with acne lotion, if necessary. Retain for ten minutes.
7. Remove mask and blot residue with **cool,** wet towel.
8. Saturate cotton pledgets with astringent lotion and apply with a light blotting movement.
9. Moisten a piece of cotton with an antiseptic lotion and touch each pimple (acne).
10. Apply lipstick only, unless a medicated foundation lotion is used.
11. Complete and clean up as for plain facial.

> **CAUTION.** Avoid the use of regular facial makeup.

Diet For Acne

A faulty diet is one of the common causes of acne. Foods high **in** fats, starches and sugars tend to make acne worse. The patron should consult her physician and follow a prescribed diet.

The patron should **avoid:** all sweets, creams, fried foods, rich salad dressings, butter, white bread, potatoes (unless baked and without butter), potato chips, whole milk, ice cream, chocolate, and fatty meats.

Her diet should **include:** all fruits, fresh and cooked vegetables, lean meats, broiled fish, chicken, fowl, gluten and whole wheat bread.

It would be advisable for her to drink about eight glasses of water daily, and get plenty of exercise and fresh air.

PACKS AND MASKS

Face packs and masks are popular in the beauty salon. They can be used as part of a facial or applied as a separate treatment.

Face packs and masks differ in their composition and usage. **Packs** are usually applied directly to the skin. On the other hand, **masks** are applied directly to the skin with the aid of gauze layers.

Good quality packs and masks, when applied to the skin, should feel comfortable and produce slight tingling and tightening effects. Whatever product is used, follow manufacturer's direction as to preparation, application and removal from the skin.

Depending on their composition, packs can cleanse, soften, smooth, stimulate and refresh the facial skin. The results obtained are temporary in nature. The skin must be cleansed before applying a pack or mask.

PACK FACIALS

A bleach pack can be used to reduce the visibility of freckles. It may take as much as five applications before any improvement is noticed.

Clay and lemon packs are usually recommended for normal or oily type skins.

Implements And Supplies

All items needed for a plain facial, plus witch hazel, boric acid solution and facial packs.

Procedure

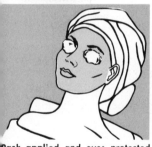

1. Give plain facial, including removal of massage cream.
2. Apply chosen pack. Keep away from nose, eyes and mouth.
3. Place cotton pads moistened with boric acid solution over eyes.
4. Apply and allow pack to remain on skin until dry, as directed by manufacturer.
5. Remove pack carefully with warm steam towel.
6. Apply astringent and pat dry.   7. Apply makeup.

Pack applied and eyes protected

There are various commercial packs available. Follow manufacturer's directions as to their preparation and application.

MASK FACIALS

A hot oil mask is usually recommended for a **dry skin** and for skin inclined to **wrinkle.**

Implements And Supplies

All items needed for a plain facial, plus the following:
1. Two layers of 8-inch gauze with openings for nose and eyes
2. Two layers of 8-inch gauze for neck covering

Procedure

1. Give plain facial, including removal of emollient cream.
2. Cover eyes with eye pads.
3. Moisten gauze with warm oil and place on face, starting at throat.
4. Apply red dermal lamp or infrared rays for 5 to 10 minutes.

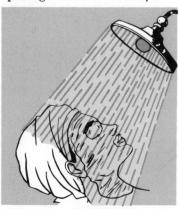

Dermal lamp

5. Remove gauze.

6. Apply additional emollient cream.

7. Give facial manipulations.

8. Remove cream with warm steam towel.

9. Apply astringent lotion and then apply makeup.

Various commercial masks are now available. Follow manufacturer's directions as to their preparation and application.

REVIEW QUESTIONS

Facial Treatments

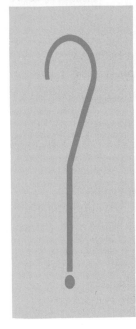

1. Facial treatments help to: (Choose the correct statements)—a) increase the circulation; b) relax the nerves; c) decrease the circulation; d) cleanse the skin; e) correct certain skin conditions.

2. Facial treatments help to correct: (Choose the correct statements) —a) dry skin; b) blackheads; c) oily skin; d) warts; e) scars; f) acne; g) aging lines.

3. About how often should a facial be given for a normal skin?

4. Why must the cosmetologist analyze the patron's skin before giving her a facial?

5. What conditions are revealed by an analysis of the skin?

6. In facial massage, the patron should be thoroughly ....

7. In facial massage, the patron will object to heavy, rough or .... hands.

8. An emollient cream is used to overcome a .... condition of the skin.

9. An astringent lotion is used to correct an .... condition of the skin.

10. What is the main cause of a dry skin?

11. What is the main cause of excessively oily skin?

12. Use a sanitized .... extractor to gently press out blackheads.

13. The skin must be in a .... condition before receiving a facial treatment.

Masks And Packs

1. When may a facial mask or pack be given?

2. In what condition must the skin be prior to the application of a mask or pack?

3. For what types of skin are facial packs recommended?

4. For what type of skin is a hot oil mask recommended?

5. When is a lemon pack usually recommended?

6. When is a bleach pack recommended?

CHAPTER 23

FACIAL MAKEUP

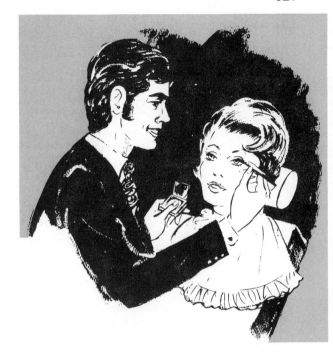

PART I
FACIAL
MAKEUP

Makeup is applied to the face for the purpose of improving its appearance. The main objectives of makeup application are to emphasize the good points and to make defects less conspicuous. There is no fixed pattern for applying makeup. In practicing this art, the cosmetologist must observe the patron carefully and treat her as an individual. A beautifully made-up face is never overdone. Cosmetics should be chosen that will harmonize with, and enhance, the natural coloring of the skin.

**Implements
And Supplies**

Everything that is to be used should be set out and arranged in an orderly manner.

1. Crepe or tissue strips and clips
2. Towels
3. Facial tissues and lintless blotting tissue
4. Sterile gauze, cotton wool and cotton pledgets
5. Cotton and suede-tipped swabs
6. Disposable sponges and puffs
7. Sheets, towels and/or protective capes for draping
8. Headbands, turbans, or other protective hair covering
9. Spatulas for removing products from containers
10. Containers for sterilized items
11. Containers for used items
12. Liquid sanitizer
13. Cleansing creams and lotions
14. Astringent and skin freshener lotions
15. Moisture creams, colorless bases and corrective color bases
16. Cream, liquid and cake foundations

17. Special sticks or creams for covering imperfections and for high-lighting or shadowing facial features
18. Liquid, cream and powdered cheekcolor (rouge)
19. Loose and pressed face powder
20. Tweezers and assorted pencils for eyebrows
21. Eyecolor shades
22. Lashline colors with pencils and brushes
23. Mascara (dry and creamy type) with applicators
24. Assorted artificial eyelashes and small scissors for trimming to size
25. Lash applicators and special eyelash adhesives
26. Lipcolors, gloss, or moisturizer finishes
27. Pencils and brushes for lipcolor application
28. Glosses and sprays for a final glamour touch (optional)

Preparing The Patron

Usually, makeup is applied after a facial massage. However, if it is applied just before a comb-out is given, the rollers and clips should be removed.

The draping procedure is as follows:
1. Sanitize hands.
2. Place paper towel on headrest of facial chair.
3. Seat patron in a slightly reclining position.
4. Place tissue strip around patron's hairline to keep hair out of the way. Place towel on patron's head and pin at napeline.
5. Place tissue strip around patron's neck; put protective cape over tissue and secure cape at nape. Turn neck tissue strip down to form a band over cape.

Procedure In Applying Makeup

The procedure given here may be changed to conform with your instructor's routine, which is equally correct.

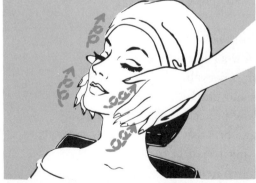

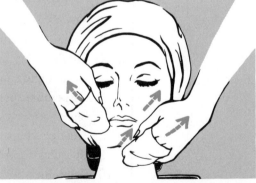

1. Apply cleansing cream. Remove a small quantity of cleansing cream from the jar with a spatula and place it in the palm of the left hand. With the fingertips of the right hand, place a dab of cream on the forehead, nose, cheeks, chin and neck. Spread cream over the face and neck with light, upward and outward circular movements.

2. Remove cleansing cream with tissue mitts, using an upward and outward motion. Clean in and around corners of the mouth with a swab. Clean gently across the eyelashes and tear ducts with clean swabs.

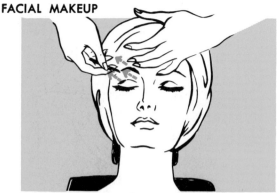

3. **Arching the eyebrows.** Arching is a complete service in itself. The procedure for arching is given in another section of this chapter. However, a few straggling hairs may be removed during a facial makeup by tweezing the hair in the same direction in which it grows.

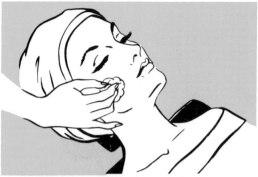

4. **Apply astringent lotion or skin toner.** For oily skin, apply astringent lotion; for a dry skin, apply a skin toner. Moisten cotton pad with the lotion; pat it lightly over the entire face and under chin and neck. Blot off excess moisture with tissues.

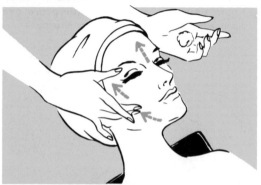

5. **Apply foundation.** Place amount needed on palm of hand. Choose kind of foundation and shade best suited to patron's skin. Apply sparingly and evenly over the entire face and around neckline with a gentle upward motion. Blend carefully near the hairline. Remove excess foundation and smooth with cosmetic sponge.

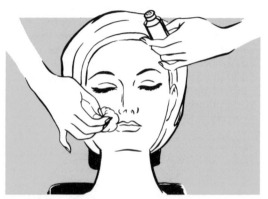

6. **Apply powder.** With a puff, cotton pledget (pressed square of cotton) or sanitized cotton, lightly powder the entire face and neck. Cosmetic sponge may also be used. Powdering the eyelids will prevent eye makeup from smearing. Remove excess powder.

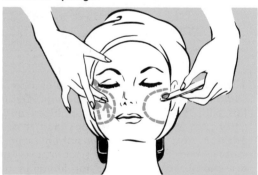

7. **Apply cheekcolor (rouge).** Apply liquid or cream cheekcolor on cheekbones with a sanitized applicator. Blend carefully upward and outward with fingers or cosmetic sponge. (*Cream or liquid cheekcolor may be applied before face powder; dry cake or powdered cheekcolor is usually applied after face powder.*)

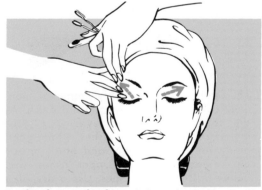

8. **Apply eyeshadow.** Select shade to match eyes, or to complement them. Apply lightly on upper lid and softly blend outward with fingertips. Use a sanitized applicator. If artificial lashes are desired without eyelash line, they should be applied at this time. They may be also applied after the lash line.

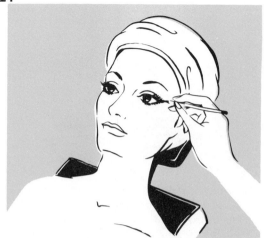

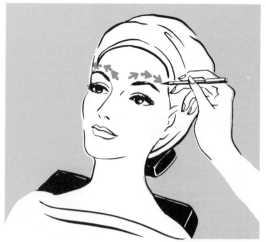

9. Apply eyeliner. Eyeliner can be used to make the eyes look larger and lashes appear thicker. Choose shade of eyeliner to harmonize with mascara. Pull upper eyelids taut and gently draw a very fine line along entire lid, as close to the lashes as possible. If eyebrow pencil is used, be sure the point is sharp so line will be only an illusion. Care should be taken to avoid injury or discomfort to the patron.

10. Use eyebrow pencil. Brush the brows in place. With light, feathery strokes, sketch on brows with fine, pointed pencil. Cream, liquid and cake eyebrow coloring are available and are applied with a brush.

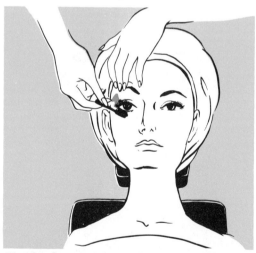

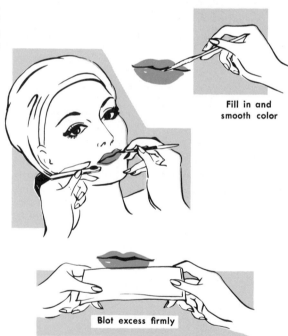

Fill in and
smooth color

Blot excess firmly

11. Apply mascara. Apply cream or moistened cake mascara to a sanitized brush. Ask the patron to open her eyes wide. Brush the mascara onto the lashes while gently lifting the eyelid. Apply and brush upward on the underside of the upper lashes. Then, gently tip the lower lashes. Use a dry, clean brush to remove any excess mascara and to separate the lashes. Apply according to manufacturer's directions.

12. Apply lipcolor. Remove lipcolor from its container with a sanitized spatula. Outline lips with the fine point of a sanitized applicator. Ask patron to close lips in a relaxed position. Rest ring finger on patron's chin to steady hand. Fill in lips. For smooth coverage, ask patron to stretch lips for filling in any crevices.

Completion

a) Remove the head drape and tissue strip.

b) Remove the cape and tissue strip from neck.

c) Check the patron's hairline and neck area so there is no line of demarcation.

d) Brush the hairline and do a final blending if necessary.

e) Assist the patron in dressing and in rearranging her hair.

Cleansing. Follow the basic principles for cleansing the face.

MAKEUP FOR DARK COMPLEXIONED WOMEN

Brow shaping. Tweeze out all unnecessary hair beneath the brow lines and shape brows correctly.

Skin conditioning. If skin is dry, apply a moisturizer; if oily, an astringent.

Foundation. If skin is of a darker hue, select two foundation shades, one light and one darker. With a facial sponge, apply the lighter shade first; then, the darker shade. With the facial sponge, lightly blend together to create a highlight effect. Where skin appears to be darker in some areas, blend in makeup a little heavier.

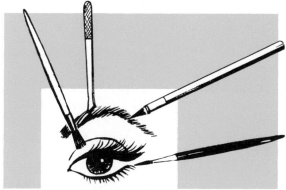
Eye makeup

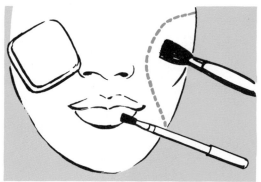
Face makeup

Rouge (cheekcolor). Brush on cheekcolor in area, as shown in illustration.

Powder well to set the foundation. Avoid leaving shiny spots.

Eyeshadow and eyecolor. Select eyeshadow or eyecolor and apply with appropriate brush or swab, as shown in the illustration. A slightly heavier shade or color may be applied on the lid near the lashes.

(*Eyeshadow is the term used when a definite shadowing is desired. Eyecolor may shadow or highlight, depending on the density of the color. For example, pale blue would highlight the area; dark blue would shadow the area.*)

Eyeliner: Using a brush as shown in the illustration, draw the eyeliner pattern along the edge of the lashes. If desired, the outer corners may be made heavier and turned slightly upward. (The patron may prefer not to have a line on the lower lid.)

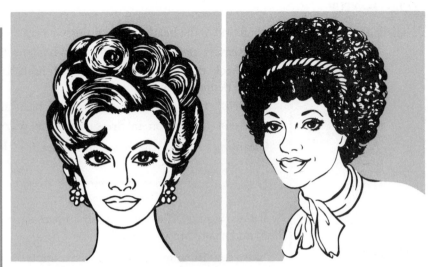

Eyebrow pencil. With a pointed eyebrow pencil, sketch in with light strokes the desired height of the arch.

Lips. Outline lips with the lipcolor brush or pencil, using the appropriate color to form a well-defined shape. Use the brush to fill in with a soft shade of lipcolor.

FALSE EYELASHES

To apply false eyelashes, you will need tweezers, scissors, a set of lashes and lash adhesive.

1. **Start with the upper lash.** If the lash is too long to fit the curve of the upper lid, the outside edges should be trimmed. With your fingers, bend the lashes into a horseshoe shape. This makes them more flexible so they will fit the contour of the eyelid. Fig. 1.

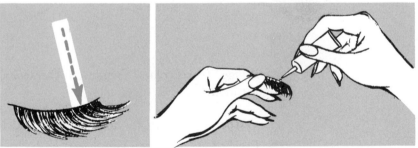

Fig. 1.   **Fig. 2.**

2. **Feather the lashes.** This is done by nipping into them with the points of your scissors. This creates a more natural look.
3. **Apply a thin strip of lash adhesive** to the base of the lashes and allow a few seconds for setting. Fig. 2.
4. **Apply the lashes.** Start with the shorter, or inside, part of the lashes and place them in a position midway between the inside corner of the eye and where the curve of the iris begins. Position the rest of the lashes as close to the patron's own lashes as

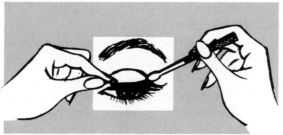

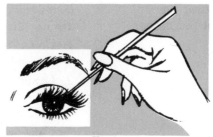

Fig. 3.   Fig. 4

possible. The rounded end of a lashliner brush may be used to press the lashes on. Fig. 3. (The line is usually drawn on before the application of the lashes and retouched after the lashes are in place. Fig. 4.)

5. **Apply bottom lashes.** Lash adhesive is used in the same manner as in the application of the upper lashes. The lashes are placed on top of the lower lashes. Shorter lashes should be placed toward the center of the eye, and longer ones, toward the outer edge.

Removing False Eyelashes

There are commercial preparations, such as pads saturated with specially prepared lotions, to facilitate the removal of artificial eyelashes. The lash base may also be softened by the application of a face cloth saturated in warm water and a gentle face soap or cleanser. Hold the pad or cloth over the eyes for a few seconds to soften the adhesive. Starting from the inner corner of the lashline, gently pull the lash. Cotton tipped swabs may be used to remove the makeup and adhesive remaining on the lid.

COSMETICS USED IN FACIAL MAKEUP

Probably no single item of makeup is as important as the foundation (makeup base). Its proper application creates a pleasing contour of the face, provides a base for color harmony, conceals blemishes and protects the skin from soil, wind and weather.

Foundation Or Makeup Base

Skin tones determine the color of the foundation. Skin tones are generally classified as—from lightest to darkest—white, creamy, beige, pink, florid, olive, sallow, tan, brown and ebony.

Choice of foundation shade. Generally, the shade or color of the foundation should closely match or coordinate with the patron's natural skin color. A shade slightly darker than the skin color may also be suitable.

For either a sallow or pale skin tone, use a rosy foundation and powder to give it glow.

For a florid skin tone, use a beige foundation and powder to soften the reddish tones.

For all other skin tones (fair, medium or dark), select the depth of foundation and powder to blend with the lightness or darkness of the skin tone.

Reminder. Too light a foundation makes the face look pale and artificial. A little foundation goes a long way. Using too much foundation is undesirable as it gives the skin a pasty appearance.

Selecting The Right Foundation

Foundation makeup tends to give a matt, or a non-oily finish. There are three types of foundations:

1. **Cream foundation** gives the most natural look and a longer lasting makeup. It is formulated for both **dry** and **oily** type skin.
2. **Liquid (lotion) foundation** has a color suspended in an emulsion of delicate light oil. For quick and effective blending, apply it on one skin area at a time, using long, smooth strokes.
3. **Cake foundation** adds color, gives a smooth and velvety look, and helps conceal minor skin discoloration. It is generally quite harmless. Cake foundation is applied with a moistened pad. Cake foundation is very effective for an **oily skin.**

Concealing Skin Blemishes

Skin **blemishes** can be concealed with the aid of:

1. **Stick foundation.** Makeup in stick form is particularly useful in the covering or masking of minor skin blemishes. The advantage of a stick is that it can easily be applied to a small blemish and can give a relatively thick film coverage.
2. **Blemish masking creams** are similar to the pigmented foundation creams.

Face Powders

Face powders improve the overall attractiveness of the skin by concealing skin blemishes, by toning down excessive coloring, gloss or shine, by enhancing the natural skin coloring and by adding delicate scent. Modern powders make the skin soft and velvety to the touch.

Face powders are available in cake or powdered form, in a wide variety of shades, and in different weights. Light and medium weights may be used on dry and normal skin. A heavyweight powder is better on oily skin. Face powder should be selected to blend with the color tone of the skin.

For Oily Skin

An **oily skin.** A powder of marked covering power is required to hide the excessive shine. Such a powder requires an absorbent base to take up the excessive perspiration and sebaceous secretion.

For Dry Skin

A **dry skin** has less shine than an oily skin. In some cases, it may be more lined and wrinkled, in which case a face powder with less absorbent power is required.

Powder Shades

The shade of face powder should either match the foundation or be a shade lighter. The powder, however, may be a coordinating shade, or it may be slightly darker, in order to achieve the desired color balance.

**Cheekcolor
And Lipcolor**

The purpose of rouge (cheekcolor) is to give a soft glow of color to the face, help create better contours and minimize imperfect features.

There are four types of cheekcolor: liquid, cream, dry and brush-on. For ordinary street makeup, any one of these may be used. Cheekcolor should be carefully applied and blended to look natural.

1. **Liquid rouge** (cheekcolor) blends well and is suitable for all skin types.
2. **Cream rouge** (cheekcolor) closely resembles pigmented foundation creams. It is applied before the face powder and blends well when the skin is not excessively oily.
3. **Dry (compact) rouge** imparts a matt finish. Usually applied after face powder, it blends harmoniously with the facial makeup.
4. **Brushed-on rouge** is usually applied after face powder. It is blended smoothly with a cosmetic brush.

Lipcolor adds color to the lips, corrects the shape of the mouth and enhances the beauty of the face. Artistry and a keen sense of fashion are essential in selecting the appropriate color shade.

The basic shades of lipcolor are **blue-red, yellow-red, orange and true-red.** All other shades originate from these basic colors.

Lipcolor is available in **stick, cream** and **liquid** form. **Caution:** It is unsanitary to use the same lipcolor applicator on more than one patron.

Eye Makeup

Eyeshadow and **eyecolor** are available in stick, cream and cake form.

Shades of eyecolor are produced in pastel-blue, pastel-turquoise, lavender-mauve, grey, blue, pastel-green, metallic-silver, metallic-blue, and other currently fashionable shades. (Eyeshadow refers to the darker colors that create shadow.)

Eyecolor, when applied to the upper lids, complements the eyes by making them look brighter and more expressive. As a general rule, the eyecolor should match the eye color, or be a shade lighter than the eyes. The daytime shade of eyecolor should be more subtle, whereas the nighttime shade can be a bit more daring.

Eyelid liners are intended for application to the eyelids, close to the lashes. They are made in shading tones and may either be in stick or liquid form, packaged with a small semi-stiff applicator brush. Black, brown and dark blue are the basic shades, but shades may correspond with eyeshadow or eyecolor. The eyeliner may be the same shade as the mascara.

Eyebrow pencils are used to modify the natural outline of the eyebrows, usually after tweezing. They may be used to darken the eyebrows, to fill in where the brow is thin or devoid of hair, and to correct misshapened brows. Eyebrow pencils cannot be sanitized. The mechanical pencil with a fine lead is the most sanitary type of eyebrow pencil. A new lead should be inserted for each patron.

Mascara is available in liquid, cake and cream form. Colors come in black, brown and a variety of other shades. When applied to the eyelashes, it makes them look fuller and longer. It can also be used to darken the eyebrows. The color of mascara should match or coordinate with the color used on the eyebrows. Generally, the lashes are darker, not lighter, than the eyebrows.

MAKEUP FOR FACIAL TYPES

The **oval face** is generally accepted as the perfect face. The contours and proportions of this type face form the basis for modifying all other facial types. In the oval face, the length is one and a half times larger than the width.

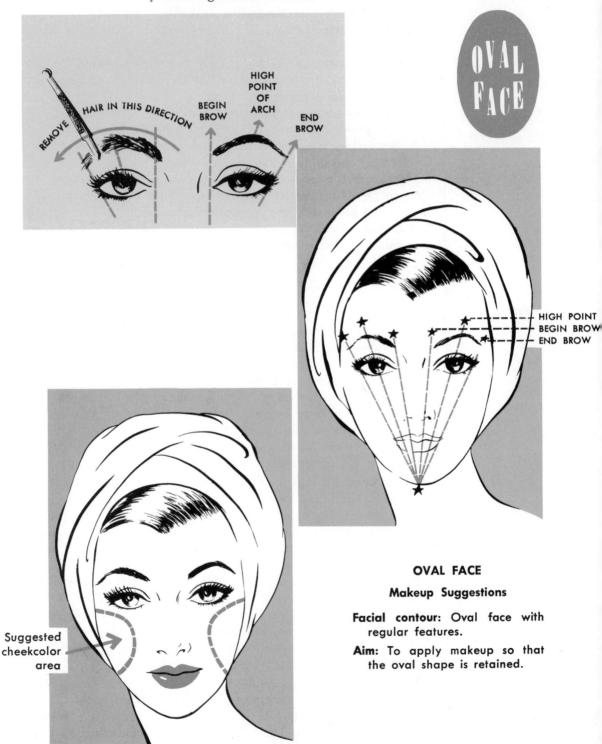

OVAL FACE

Makeup Suggestions

Facial contour: Oval face with regular features.

Aim: To apply makeup so that the oval shape is retained.

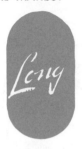

Long

Facial contour: Long, narrow face with hollow cheeks.

Aim: To shorten the length of the face and create the illusion of width.

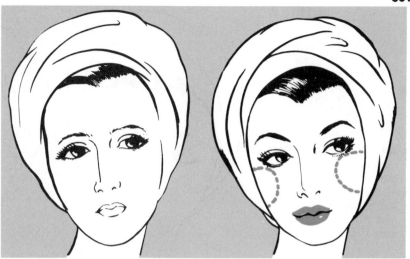

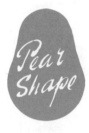

Pear Shape

Facial contour: Narrow forehead, wide jawline and chin.

Aim: To create the illusion of width across the forehead and length in the face.

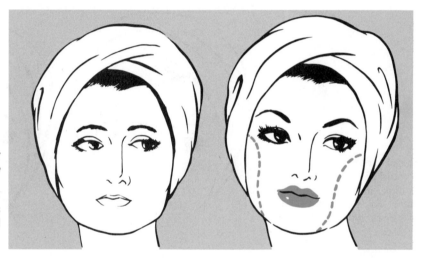

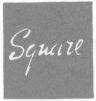

Square

Facial contour: Straight forehead hairline and square jawline.

Aim: To slenderize the appearance of the face and offset the squareness of the features.

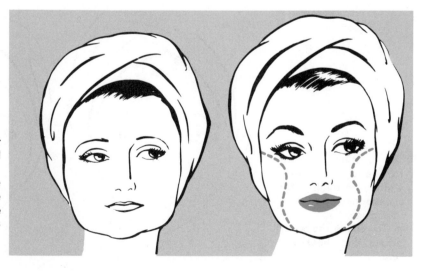

332

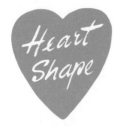

Heart Shape

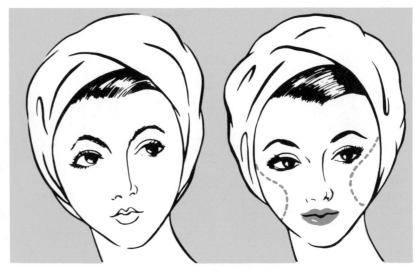

Facial contour: Wide forehead and narrow chin line.

Aim: To minimize the width across forehead and increase width across jawbone line.

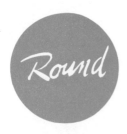

Round

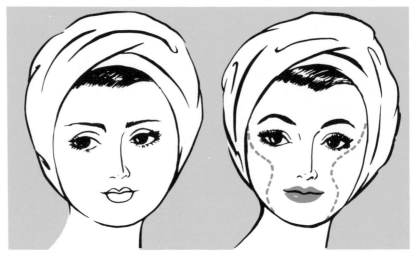

Facial contour: Round hairline and round chin line.

Aim: To slenderize the appearance of the face.

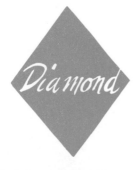

Diamond

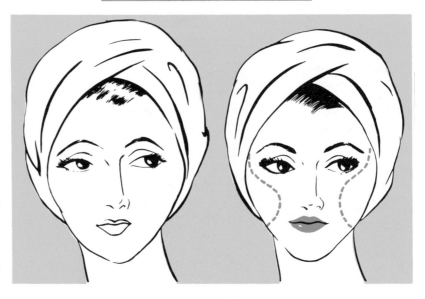

Facial contour: Narrow forehead, extreme width through the cheekbones, and narrow chin.

Aim: To reduce the width across the cheekbone line.

CORRECTIVE MAKEUP

Corrective facial makeup helps to play up the good features and tone down the bad ones. Facial features can be **accented** with proper **highlighting, subdued** with the correct **shadowing** or **shading,** and **balanced** with the proper hairstyle.

Highlight

A **highlight** is produced when a shade lighter than the original foundation is used on a particular part of the face. The proper use of highlights brings out the parts of the facial features to be **emphasized.**

Shadow

A **shadow** is formed when the foundation used is darker than the original one. The use of shadows (dark colors and shades) **minimizes** or **subdues** prominent features and makes them less noticeable.

When **two tones** of foundations are used, care must be taken to blend them properly, so that there will be no line of demarcation.

Color Harmony

Color harmony can be achieved when the makeup tones flatter the color combination of the eyes, hair and skin. To determine what is best for each patron, the makeup artist must:

1. Analyze the color of the patron's skin, hair and eyes.
2. Examine the front and profile views of her facial features.
3. Select and apply those makeup highlights and/or shades which will produce the desired corrective results.

Concealing Wrinkles With Foundation Cream

Age lines and crevices, due to dryness of the skin, can be concealed with foundation cream. Foundation cream should be used sparingly. It should be applied evenly in a light, outward, circular motion over the entire surface of the face. Care should be taken to remove any heavy distribution of foundation cream in lines and crevices of the face.

Corrective Makeup For Forehead

Low forehead. Applying a **lighter** foundation cream to the forehead gives it a **higher** appearance between the brows and hairline.

Bulging forehead. To minimize a bulging forehead, apply a darker foundation to the prominent part of the forehead and blend downward on the temples.

With a suitable hairstyle, attention can be drawn away from the forehead.

Corrective Makeup For Nose And Chin

Large or protruding nose. Avoid placing cheekcolor close to the nose. A **lighter** foundation applied in a straight line down the center of the nose will make it appear straighter. A **darker** shade of foundation may be placed on the sides and tip of the nose to make it appear shorter and smaller. The foundation must be carefully blended so there is no visible line.

When blending darker foundation on the nose, avoid carrying the dark tone into laugh lines, as it will accentuate them.

To minimize a **prominent chin**, shadow with a darker foundation. To make a small nose appear larger, highlight the nose with a lighter foundation.

To make a **small chin** more prominent, **highlight** chin with a **lighter** foundation.

Use a **darker** foundation to **minimize** the drooping or sagging areas of the chin and jawline.

Corrective Makeup For Jawline And Neck

The neck and the jaws are just as important as the eyes, cheeks and lips. When applying makeup, blend the foundation below the neckline of the dress, to prevent a line of demarcation or contrast.

Broad jaws. Starting at the temple, use a **darker** shade of foundation down the side of the face. This will **minimize** the lower part of the face and create an illusion of **width** to the upper part of the face.

Narrow jawline. Highlight the jawline by using a **lighter** foundation cream than the one used on the face.

Round, square or triangular face. To minimize width at the jawline, and to create the illusion of ovalness, blend a darker foundation beneath the cheekbone on the heavy areas of the jawline.

Small face—neck short and thick. Use a **darker** foundation on the neck than the one used on the face. This will make the neck appear thinner.

Long, thin neck. Use a **lighter** foundation on the neck than the one used on the face. This will create fullness and counteract the long, thin appearance of the neck.

Corrective Makeup For Lips

(For corrective makeup for the brows and eyes, consult Part 2 of this chapter.)

Thin Lower Lip

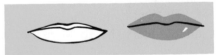

1. **Thin lower lip.** Extend curve of lower lip to balance.

Thin Upper Lip

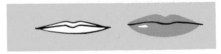

2. **Thin upper lip.** Build up curve of upper lip to balance.

Thin Lips

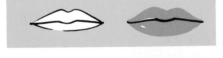

3. **Thin lips.** Increase size of both upper and lower lips with a gentle, curving line.

Small Mouth

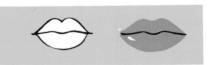

4. **Small mouth.** Build outsides of upper and lower lips and extend the corners of the mouth.

Drooping Corners

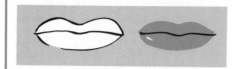

5. **Drooping corners.** Build up the upper lip at corners of the mouth.

Large Lips

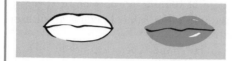

6. **Large, full lips.** Outline the lips, keeping the color inside of the lipline. Blend color carefully within the lipline.

Mouth Too Oval

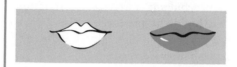

7. **Mouth too oval.** Color the center upper lips into a slight Cupid's bow.

Sharp Cupid's Bow

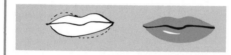

8. **Sharp Cupid's bow.** Use pencil or lip brush to apply color on the upper lip. Round off the sharp peaks and widen the curve of the upper lip. Fill in lower lip with color.

Uneven Lips

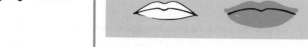

9. **Uneven lips.** Fill in areas as shown on the illustration.

FASHION EFFECTS

Eyes And Brows Makeup

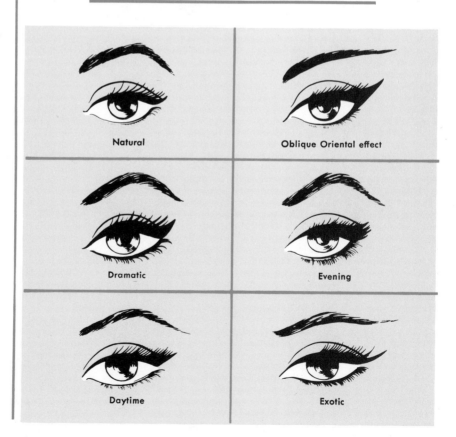

Natural

Oblique Oriental effect

Dramatic

Evening

Daytime

Exotic

1. What is the purpose of facial makeup?
2. Name three types of foundations.
3. Why is the foundation or base makeup important in facial makeup?
4. To which parts of the eye is the following makeup applied: a) eyeshadow; b) mascara; c) eyebrow pencil?
5. What effect is created when using: a) eyecolor; b) mascara; c) eyebrow pencil?
6. Name four types of cheekcolor (rouge).
7. When is the best time to apply: a) cream rouge; b) dry (cake) rouge?
8. What type of foundation may be used for: a) oily skin; b) dry skin?
9. Why shouldn't the same lipcolor applicator be used on more than one patron?
10. Which facial shape type is generally accepted as the perfect face?
11. How are age lines concealed?
12. How may a low forehead be made to appear higher?
13. How can a bulging forehead be minimized?
14. How is a highlight produced?
15. For what purpose is a highlight effect used?
16. How is a shadow formed?
17. For what purpose is a shadow effect used?
18. What does color harmony mean in relation to makeup?

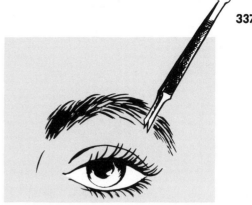

PART II EYEBROW ARCHING

The correct shaping of the eyebrows has a marked effect on the beauty and contour of the face.

The natural arch or growth of the eyebrow follows the bony structure, or the curved line of the orbit (eye socket). Most people have a disorderly growth of hairs both above and below the natural line. These hairs should be removed, to give a clean-cut and attractive appearance.

Because of the sensitivity of the skin around the eyes, some patrons cannot tolerate tweezing. For these, shaving, or a wax depilatory, may be used. How to apply a wax depilatory will be found in the chapter on **Removal of Superfluous Hair.**

Implements, Supplies And Cosmetics

1. Emollient cream
2. Absorbent cotton
3. Cleansing tissue
4. Eyebrow brush
5. Tweezers
6. Astringent lotion
7. Antiseptic lotion
8. Eyebrow pencil

Procedure

1. **Prepare patron.** Seat patron in facial chair in reclining position, as for a facial massage. Or, patron may be seated in half-upright position and the cosmetologist works from the side.
2. **Select type of arch.** Discuss with patron the type of eyebrows suitable for her facial characteristics.
3. **Cover patron's eyes** with cotton pledgets moistened with witch hazel or boric acid.
4. **Brush eyebrows** with a small brush, to remove powder and scaliness.
5. **Soften brows.** Saturate two pledgets of cotton, or towel, with hot water and place over brows. Allow to remain on brows long enough to soften and relax eyebrow tissue sufficiently.

    Brows and surrounding skin may also be softened by rubbing emollient cream into them.
6. **Remove hairs between brows.**

    Tweezing. When tweezing, stretch the skin taut with index finger and thumb (or index and middle finger) of left hand. Grasp each hair individually with tweezers and pull with a quick motion in the direction in which the hair grows.

(If left-handed, reverse the procedure.)

Sponge tweezed area frequently, using cotton moistened with an antiseptic lotion, to avoid infection. Remoisten cotton with antiseptic as necessary.

Hairs between the brows and above brow line are tweezed first, as the area under the brow line is much more sensitive.

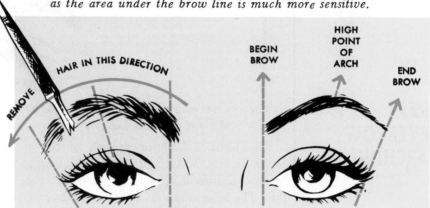

7. **Remove hairs from above eyebrow line.** Brush hairs downward. Shape the upper section of one eyebrow, then shape the other. Sponge area with antiseptic frequently.

8. **Remove hairs from under eyebrow line.** Brush hairs upward. Shape the lower section of one eyebrow, then shape the other. Sponge area with an antiseptic.

(*Optional: Apply emollient cream and massage brows. Remove with tissues.*)

9. **Apply an astringent.** After the tweezing has been completed, sponge the brows and surrounding skin with an astringent to contract the area.

10. **Apply brow makeup.** Brush brows, placing the hair in its normal position. Use eyebrow pencil where necessary.

The eyebrows should be treated about once a week.

CORRECTIVE PLACING AND SHAPING OF THE EYEBROWS

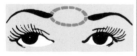

The perfect eyebrow

High Forehead

Low Forehead

Should a patron desire to correct misshaped eyebrows, remove all unnecessary hairs; then instruct her in the proper use of the eyebrow pencil to correct the defects.

Where the hairs have been pulled out leaving little white spots in the brow, darken them with the pencil, using the eyebrow brush over it to soften the pencil mark.

Where the arch is too high, remove the superfluous hairs from the top of the brow and fill in the lower part with eyebrow pencil.

Where the arch is too low, remove the superfluous hair from the lower part of the brow and build up the shape of the brow by using an eyebrow pencil.

The eyebrow arch is slightly elevated to detract from a high forehead.

A low arch gives more height to the very low forehead.

Wide-Set Eyes	The eyes can be made to appear closer together by extending the eyebrow line to the inside corner of the eyes.
Close-Set Eyes	To make the eyes appear farther apart, space brows farther apart by widening the distance between them; also slightly extend the brows outward.
Round Face	Arch the eyebrows high to make the face seem narrower. Start on a line directly in line with the inner corner of the eye, and extend slightly beyond the outer corner of the eye.
Long Face	The illusion of a shorter face can be created by making the eyebrows almost straight. Do not extend the eyebrow line farther than the ends of the eyes.
Narrow Forehead	To offset a narrow forehead, arch the eyebrows slightly on the ends only. Start the line directly above the inside corners of the eye and continue to the ends of the cheekbones.
To Make The Face Oval	The face will appear more oval if there is a high arch on the ends of the eyebrows. Begin the line directly above the inner corner of the eye and extend slightly beyond the outer corner of the eye, but not too far out on the cheekbone.
Corrective Makeup For Eyes	Eyes can be made to appear larger or smaller through the use of eyeshadow.

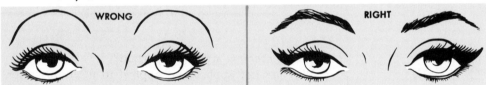

Round Eyes	Round eyes can be lengthened by extending the shadow beyond the outer corner of the eyes.

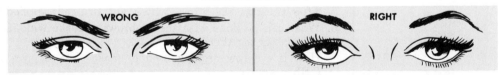

Closed-Set Eyes	For eyes that are set too close together, apply shadow lightly up from the outer edge of the eyes.

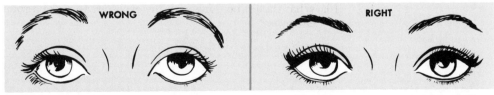

Bulging Eyes	**Bulging** eyes can be minimized by blending the shadow carefully over the prominent part of the upper lid, carrying it lightly to the line of the brow. Use **dark** shadow as in illustration.

Wide-Set Eyes

For eyes that are set too far apart, use the shadow on the upper inner side of the eyelid.

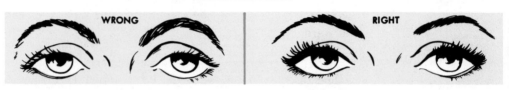

WRONG   RIGHT

Heavy Lidded Eyes

Shadow evenly and lightly across the lid from the edge of the eyelash line to the small crease in the side of the eyes.

Small Eyes

Small eyes can be made to appear larger by extending the eyeliner and shadow, or eyecolor, slightly above and beyond the outer corners of the eye.

Deep-Sunken Eyes

For **deep-sunken eyes**, use very little shadow on the lids nearest the temples and leave untouched the part next to the nose and inner corner of the eyes.

Dark Circles Under Eyes

For **dark circles under eyes**, apply a **lighter** foundation cream, blending it into the dark area.

Puffy Eyes

For **puffy eyes**, apply a **darker** shade of foundation cream to the area.

REVIEW QUESTIONS

Eyebrow Arching

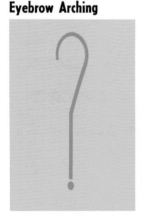

1. Why is eyebrow arching important?
2. Why are hot applications applied to the brows prior to arching or shaping?
3. What is the correct way to tweeze the hair when arching?
4. While arching the brows, why is an antiseptic applied to tweezed areas?
5. After tweezing the brows, why is an astringent applied?
6. What can be done with the eyebrows to make wide-set eyes appear to be closer together?
7. How is eyebrow arching used to make close-set eyes appear to be farther apart?
8. How are eyebrows of a long face arched in order to create the illusion of a shorter face?
9. How can the eyebrows be shaped to give the appearance of reducing a high forehead?
10. What should be done with the eyebrows to make a round face appear narrower?

CHAPTER 24

ELECTROLYSIS SUPERFLUOUS HAIR REMOVAL

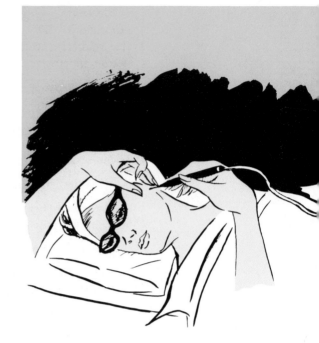

INTRODUCTION

Superfluous hair is not a new problem. It has plagued women from time immemorial, and throughout the ages they have sought ways and means to disguise or get rid of it. Unwanted hair on the face is a problem of great concern to many women. Intelligent electrologists recognize this and prepare themselves to solve the problem of unwanted hair.

Today there are two types of hair removal:

1. Temporary
2. Permanent

PERMANENT HAIR REMOVAL

ELECTROLYSIS

There are several methods of temporary hair removal which will be discussed in another section of this chapter. This section will concern itself only with permanent hair removal, which is accomplished by **electrolysis** (e-lek-trol'i-sis).

No one dreamed that unwanted hair could be removed permanently until 1875, when Dr. Charles E. Michel, an ophthalmologist, used an electric current directed through a thin wire to remove ingrowing eyelashes. When he found that the lashes did not grow back, he suggested that this method could be valuable in removing unwanted hair from the face.

A few dermatologists tried Dr. Michel's method, but the process was so slow and tedious that it could not be used to any great extent.

In 1916, the multiple needle machine was developed, and electrolysis became a practical aid to beauty. The demand for treatments grew —slowly at first, and then more rapidly when the shortwave method was introduced. This newer method was much faster, requiring less time to clear an area. Thus, permanent removal of heavy growths on large areas, such as arms and legs, became practical.

DEFINITIONS

Electrolysis is the process of removing hair permanently by means of electricity. The term "electrolysis" has become synonymous with both the multiple needle galvanic method and the more modern single needle shortwave method.

Electrologist is a person trained to give electrolysis treatments for permanent hair removal.

Hypertrichosis (hi-per-trik-o'sis) is a growth of hair in excess of the normal. It is a Greek word, combining **hyper** (meaning "over") and **tricho** (meaning "hair").

Hirsuties (her-su'she-ez) is excessive hairiness.

Hirsutism (her'sut-izm) is the presence of excess hair on areas where it is not normally expected.

The following terms are synonymous with shortwave electrolysis:

Thermolysis (ther-mol'i-sis)

Diathermy (di'ah-ther-me)

High-frequency (hi-fre'quen-se)

METHODS OF PERMANENT HAIR REMOVAL

There are two methods of permanent hair removal: the **galvanic multiple needle,** and the newer, more advanced **shortwave** method.

1. The galvanic method destroys the hair by decomposing the papilla (the source of nourishment for the hair).
2. The shortwave method destroys the hair by coagulating the papilla, such coagulation being caused by heat.

SHORTWAVE METHOD

Note. Since the shortwave method is the one extensively used, the procedure for this method is given here.

The **shortwave** is the newer, more rapid method of permanent hair removal, and the one most generally used today. In fact, the overwhelming majority of all permanent hair removal treatments today are performed by the shortwave method. Only **one** needle is used, but it is a much finer needle than the one used in the galvanic method.

Equipment And Supplies

Everything needed for a shortwave treatment should be ready and at hand. Here is a checklist of essential equipment and supplies:

A shortwave machine	Antiseptic lotion
A fluorescent magnifying light	Sunglasses to protect patron's eyes
Treatment chair and ottoman for patron	After-treatment lotion
Cotton pads	Antiseptic powder

Preparation Of Patron

Seat the patron comfortably in a reclining position. Place a clean towel or facial tissue under her head and have another tissue handy for disposal of hairs as you remove them.

Adjust the position of the operating arm of the machine to approximately 6 to 8 inches above the area to be worked on.

Sanitize the area to be treated, using a cotton pad saturated with a good antiseptic. Use only **sanitized tweezers** and **needle.**

Preparing Machine

Procedure for giving a shortwave treatment is as follows:

Turn machine to "ON."

Adjust machine according to manufacturer's instructions.

Turn **Timer Control** to "automatic." (See chart provided with machine.)

Turn **Time and Intensity Control** knobs to "O," as a starting point.

Plug in foot pedal and make sure it is placed in a comfortable position.

Adjust operator's stool to desired height.

The quicker the current is shut off, the less sensation the patron will feel. Therefore, the timer should be set at the shortest time interval, usually "O" for **fine hair,** "½" for **medium hair** and "1" for **heavy hair.** When need arises to use more current, increase the intensity up to 10 before increasing time to ½.

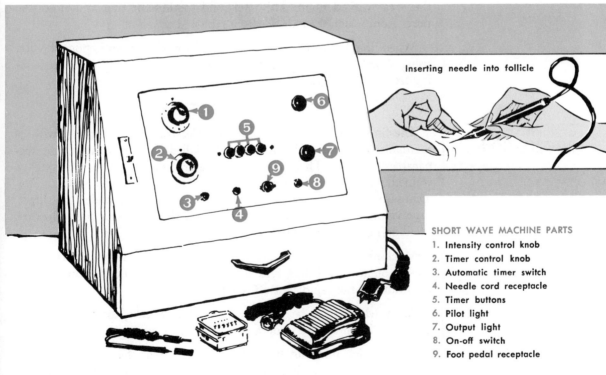

Inserting needle into follicle

SHORT WAVE MACHINE PARTS
1. Intensity control knob
2. Timer control knob
3. Automatic timer switch
4. Needle cord receptacle
5. Timer buttons
6. Pilot light
7. Output light
8. On-off switch
9. Foot pedal receptacle

A good shortwave machine is F.C.C. (Federal Communications Commission) approved.

It is automatically timed, thus eliminating human failure, or the necessity for the electrologist to keep close watch on the time.

The depth of insertion will vary according to the coarseness of the hair, usually from one-eighth of an inch to one-quarter of an inch.

**Inserting Needle
Into Follicle**

Most hair grows at an angle to the surface of the skin. The electrologist must insert the needle on the underside of the hair and slide it slowly into the follicle alongside the hair root.

After you have inserted the needle, depress the foot pedal. The current goes on and shuts off **automatically. Never depress the foot pedal** while you are inserting the needle. Remove the needle and lift the hair out gently with tweezers. If it does not glide out easily, reinsert the needle a second time, repeating the procedure outlined above. If the hair still does not glide out easily, remove it forcibly with tweezers and treat again during subsequent treatments.

In making insertions, it is important to observe carefully the angle or slant of the hair follicle before you insert the needle. The slant of follicles varies from 15 to 90 degrees. Hairs that have been tweezed, grow in all directions. Some follicles are curved, and for this reason the needle point is rounded. No force should ever be used because the side or wall of the follicle might be pierced and the current would not reach the papilla.

**After-Treatment
Procedure**

After the treatment is completed, turn machine off. Saturate a pad of cotton with a special after-treatment lotion and press gently on the area worked upon. This cools and soothes the skin and closes the pores from which the hair has been removed.

When the lotion has dried, gently press on an antiseptic powder, using a piece of sterile cotton. The patron is then ready to leave, looking fresh and well-groomed.

**GENERAL
INFORMATION**

The importance of training. The electrologist is dealing with a woman's skin, and an inefficient or unskilled operator could cause irreparable damage. Therefore, every electrologist must be thoroughly trained, both in the theory and in the practice of electrolysis. This means that she must use live models to practice on, under the direct supervision of a licensed instructor, until she has been properly certified and is confident of her skill.

Machines. Shortwave machines embody many safety factors. They are automatically timed and F.C.C.-approved. Pain is reduced to a minimum by the rapid shut-off of current.

Areas which may be treated. Lips, chin, cheeks, arms, legs, body, eyebrows, hairlines and underarms.

Areas which may not be treated. Do not treat the eyelids, inside of the ears, nostrils or moles. Do not treat **diabetic** patrons or those getting **hormone** treatments without written sanction of a doctor.

Causes of unwanted hair. No one knows the exact cause. Authorities agree, however, that heredity has something to do with it, as unwanted hair often seems to run in families and appears to be more common in certain races. Glandular disturbances are also known to influence hair growth.

Regrowth. It takes from 8 to 13 weeks for the hair to grow from the papilla to the surface of the skin. When a patron has been tweezing regularly, the hair tweezed one week is not the hair she tweezed the preceding week, but hair which she tweezed many weeks before. Due to distorted follicles (sometimes caused by tweezing or waxing, sometimes due to natural causes), it is not always possible to destroy the papilla with the first treatment, and the hair will grow again. Additional treatment will be required for permanent removal. The regrowth will vary; it is usually not more than 10% in virgin hair, but may be as much as 20% or 25% in cases of distorted follicles.

IMPORTANT REMINDERS

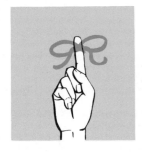

Patrons should be told that sometimes, after a treatment on legs or arms, tiny scabs may appear. These soon drop off, leaving the skin in a normal, healthy condition. Application of a special after-treatment lotion will hasten the **healing** process.

Hands, implements and the area to be treated must be very carefully **sanitized.**

Never remove hairs from areas where the skin shows signs of **eruption, abrasion** or **inflammation.**

Do not remove hairs from warts or moles.

Never use force when inserting the needle.

Do not treat hairs that are too close together. Work checkerboard fashion. Needles placed **too close together** may result in **pitting.**

Do not treat children.

Instructing the patron on how to care for her skin after treatment is very important. See that the patron does not pick or tamper with the skin.

REVIEW QUESTIONS

Electrolysis

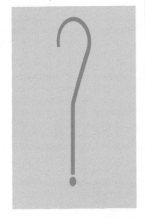

1. What is the technical term for superfluous hair?
2. What are the known causes of superfluous hair?
3. What is electrolysis?
4. What are the two methods by which electrolysis treatments may be given?
5. What is the fundamental difference between the two methods?
6. By what other names is the shortwave method known?
7. Which method of electrolysis is extensively used today?
8. Why are shortwave treatments more popular than galvanic treatments?
9. Does hair ever regrow after an electrolysis treatment? Under what condition?
10. What areas can be treated by electrolysis?
11. Can the electrologist remove hair from moles and warts?

THE TEMPORARY REMOVAL OF SUPERFLUOUS HAIR

Unwanted hair on the body is a problem to many women. It is a remediable defect which can be properly handled in the beauty salon. To render the greatest service to patrons, cosmetologists should be familiar with the problem and how best to care for it.

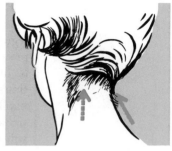

Nape fuzz

Various methods can be employed to cope with superfluous hair. They include both temporary and permanent methods.

1. **Temporary methods.** Repeated treatments at regular intervals are necessary as the new hair grows out.
2. **Permanent methods** actually destroy the hair papilla and prevent any possible regrowth of the hair. (See section on **Electrolysis** in the first part of this chapter.)

TEMPORARY METHODS

Shaving is usually recommended when the annoying hairs cover a large area, such as in the armpits and on the arms and legs. A shaving cream is applied before shaving off the hair.

An electric razor may also be used. The application of a pre-shaving lotion will help to reduce any irritation.

Tweezing is commonly used for shaping the eyebrows and for removing undesirable hairs around the mouth and chin. (The procedure for tweezing the eyebrows will be found in the chapter on **Facial Treatments.**)

Hair Lightening

To lessen the visibility of superfluous hair, you can lighten it by applying an oil bleach mixed with two parts of peroxide.

Procedure

Apply mixture thoroughly to the hair with tint brush or swab. Repeat application to keep the lightener wet until the hair has lightened to desired shade.

Lightening time varies from 15-50 minutes, depending on the color and texture of the hair. Dark, coarse hair takes more time than fine, lanuga hair, which is softer and lighter.

Remove lightener; then apply an emollient cream.

Depilatories

Depilatories also belong to the group of temporary methods for the removal of superfluous hair. There are **physical** (wax) and **chemical** types of depilatories.

Wax-Type

The **wax type of depilatory** may be applied over such parts of the body as the cheeks, chin, upper lip, nape area, arms and legs. The general procedure employed is as follows:

1. Remove clothing from part to be treated and seat patron in a comfortable position.

2. Wash skin area with a mild soap and water. Rinse thoroughly and dry.
3. Spread talcum powder over skin surface.
4. Melt wax in a double boiler on stove.
5. Test temperature and consistency of heated wax by applying a little of it on your arm.

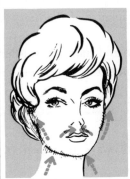 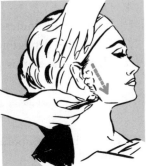 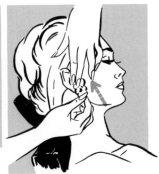

Superfluous hair   Spread wax downward   Pull wax off upward

6. Spread warm wax evenly over the skin surface with spatula or fingertips, following the same direction as the hair growth.
7. Allow wax to cool and harden.
8. Quickly pull off the adhering wax against the direction of hair growth.
9. Gently massage treated area.
10. Dust off remaining powder from skin.
11. Apply an emollient cream or antiseptic lotion to area treated.

Reminders And Hints

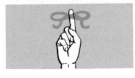

1. To prevent burns, test temperature of heated wax before applying it to patron's skin.
2. Keep wax from running into eyes or over any areas where it is not wanted.
3. Do not use a wax depilatory under the arms, or over warts, moles, abrasions, irritated or inflamed areas.

CHEMICAL DEPILATORIES

The **chemical depilatories**, available as a cream, paste, or powder mixed with water into a paste, are generally used to remove hair from legs.

A **skin test** is advisable to determine whether the individual is sensitive to the action of this type of depilatory.

To give such a test, select a hairless part of the arm, apply a portion of the depilatory according to manufacturer's directions, and leave on skin from 7-10 minutes. If, at the end of this time, there are no signs of redness or swelling, the depilatory can be used with safety over a large area of the skin.

Procedure

The cream or powder depilatory may be used as follows:

1. The cream type is applied directly from the container, while the powder type is mixed, according to the directions of manufacturer, to form a smooth paste.
2. After the skin has been cleansed and dried, a thick layer of the depilatory is applied over the area where the hair is to be removed.
3. The surrounding skin is protected with vaseline.
4. Depending on the thickness of the hair, the depilatory is retained from 5-10 minutes.
5. Then, the depilatory and hair are washed off with warm water.
6. Finally, the skin is patted dry and cold cream is applied.

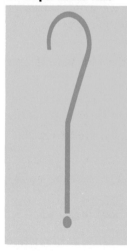

QUESTIONS AND ANSWERS

Temporary Removal Of Superfluous Hair

1. Name three temporary ways in which superfluous hair may be removed.
2. For which parts of the body is shaving most suitable?
3. Which parts of the face are most suitable for hair tweezing?
4. What may be used to minimize the unwanted hair on the face or lips?
5. Name three forms of chemical depilatories.
6. Why should a patron be given a skin test before the application of a chemical depilatory?
7. When using a chemical depilatory, why is 7-10 minutes allowed as the time limit?
8. On what type of skin is a chemical depilatory recommended?
9. What are the advantages of a chemical depilatory?
10. Give the disadvantages of a chemical depilatory.
11. Give three important safety precautions to observe when using wax.
12. Why must wax never be applied over warts, moles, growths or abrasions?
13. Why should the temperature of the heated wax be tested?
14. What are the disadvantages of temporary methods of hair removal?

CHAPTER 25

CELLS

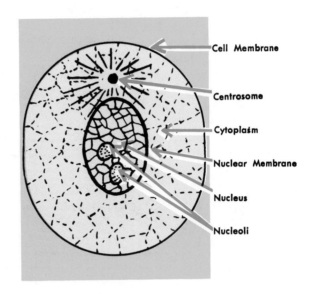

Cell Membrane

Centrosome

Cytoplasm

Nuclear Membrane

Nucleus

Nucleoli

INTRODUCTION

To develop a general knowledge of how to care for the scalp, skin, hair and nails, an individual must have a thorough understanding of the health, growth and repair of these areas, as well as of how they function. It is, therefore, important for cosmetologists to study and understand the major parts of the body upon which they render services or apply treatments.

The body is composed of cells, tissues, organs, and systems. It is made up of one-fourth solid matter and three-fourths liquid.

CELLS

Cells are the basic units of all living things, which include humans, animals, plants and bacteria. Every part of the body is composed of cells, which differ from each other in size, shape, structure and function.

A cell is a minute (mi-nut') portion of living substance containing **protoplasm** (pro'to-plazm), which is a colorless jelly-like substance in which food elements and water are present. The two main parts of the cell are:

1. **Nucleus** (nu'kle-us) (dense protoplasm) is found in the center and plays an important part in the reproduction of the cell.
2. **Cytoplasm** (si'to-plazm) (less dense protoplasm) is found outside the nucleus and contains food materials necessary for the growth, reproduction and self-repair of the cell.

STRUCTURE OF THE CELL

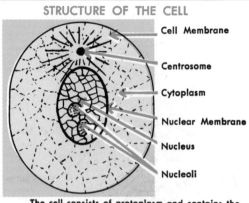

- Cell Membrane
- Centrosome
- Cytoplasm
- Nuclear Membrane
- Nucleus
- Nucleoli

The cell consists of protoplasm and contains the above essential parts.

The protoplasm of the cell contains the following important structures:

Nucleus (nu'kle-us) (dense protoplasm) found in the center, which plays an important part in the reproduction of the cell.

Cytoplasm (si'to-plazm) (less dense protoplasm) is found outside of the nucleus and contains food materials necessary for the growth, reproduction and self-repair of the cell.

Centrosome (sen'tro-som), a small, round body in the cytoplasm, which also affects the reproduction of the cell.

Cell membrane encloses the protoplasm. It permits soluble substances to enter and leave the cell.

Diagrams Illustrating Indirect Division of the Human Cell

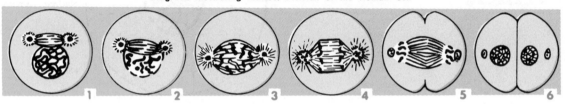

1   2   3   4   5   6

Cell Growth And Production

As long as the cell receives an adequate supply of food, oxygen and water, eliminates waste products, and is favored with proper temperature, it will continue to grow and thrive. However, if these requirements are not fulfilled, and the presence of toxins (poisons) or pressure is evident, then the growth and the health of the cells are impaired. Most body cells are capable of growth and self-repair during their life cycle.

In the human body, when a cell reaches maturity, reproduction takes place by indirect division. This is a process in which a series of changes occur in the nucleus before the entire cell divides in half. Remember that the nucleus is surrounded by a thinner form of protoplasm, called cytoplasm, which supplies the food materials necessary for growth and reproduction.

Metabolism

Metabolism (me-tab'o-lizm) is a complex chemical process whereby the body cells are nourished and supplied with the energy needed to carry on their many activities.

There are two phases to metabolism:

1. **Anabolism** (an-ab'o-lizm)—the building up of cellular tissues. During anabolism, the cells of the body absorb water, food and oxygen for the purpose of growth, reproduction and repair.
2. **Catabolism** (kah-tab'o-lizm)—the breaking down of cellular tissues. During catabolism, the cells consume what they have absorbed in order to perform specialized functions, such as muscular effort, secretions or digestion.

Cells have various duties. They create and renew all parts of the body; they assist in blood circulation by carrying food to the blood and waste matter from the blood, and they control all body functions.

Tissues

Tissues are composed of groups of cells of the same kind. Each tissue has a specific function and can be recognized by its characteristic appearance. Body tissues are classified as follows:

1. **Connective tissue** serves to support, protect and bind together other tissues of the body. Bone, cartilage, ligament, tendon, and fat tissue are examples of connective tissue.
2. **Muscular tissue** contracts and moves various parts of the body.
3. **Nerve tissue** carries messages to and from the brain, and controls and coordinates all body functions.
4. **Epithelial** (ep-i-the'le-al) **tissue** is a protective covering on body surfaces, such as the skin, mucous membranes, linings of the heart, digestive and respiratory organs and glands.
5. **Liquid tissue** carries food, waste products and hormones by means of the blood and lymph.

Organs

Organs are structures containing two or more different tissues which are combined to accomplish a specific function.

The most important organs of the body are: the brain, which controls the body; the heart, which circulates the blood; the lungs, which supply oxygen to the blood; the liver, which removes toxic products of digestion; the kidneys, which excrete water and other waste products; and the stomach and intestines, which digest the food.

Systems

Systems are groups of organs that cooperate for a common purpose, namely the welfare of the entire body. The human body is composed of the following important systems:

Skeletal (skel'e-tal) System—Bones
Muscular (mus'ku-lar) System—Muscles
Nervous (ner'vus) System—Nerves
Circulatory (ser'ku-lah-to-re) System—Blood supply
Endocrine (en'do-krin) System—Ductless glands
Excretory (eks'kre-to-re) System—Organs of elimination
Respiratory (re-spir'ah-to-re) System—Lungs
Digestive (di-jes'tiv) System—Stomach and intestines
Reproductive (re-pro-duk'tiv) System—Reproducing

Skeletal System

This is the physical foundation or framework of the body. The function of the skeletal system is to serve as a means of protection, support and locomotion.

Muscular System

The muscular system covers, shapes and supports the skeleton. Its function is to produce all the movements of the body.

Nervous System

The nervous system controls and coordinates the functions of all the other systems, and makes them work harmoniously and efficiently.

Circulatory System

The circulatory system consists of a closed system of vessels, such as arteries, veins and capillaries, which carry blood from the heart to all parts of the body, and then back to the heart. This system supplies body cells with food materials, and also carries away waste products.

Endocrine System

The endocrine system is composed of a group of specialized glands, which can either benefit or adversely affect the growth, reproduction and health of the body.

Excretory System

The excretory system, which includes the kidneys, liver, skin, intestines and lungs, purifies the body by the elimination of waste products.

Respiratory System

The respiratory system, whose most important organs are the trachea (windpipe), bronchial tubes and lungs, supplies the body with oxygen and removes carbon dioxide.

Digestive System

The digestive system changes food into a soluble form, suitable for use by the cells of the body.

Reproductive System

The reproductive system performs the function of reproducing and perpetuating the human race.

All these systems are closely interrelated and dependent upon each other. While each forms a unit specially designed to perform a specific function, that function cannot be performed without the complete cooperation of some other system or systems.

REVIEW QUESTIONS

Cells

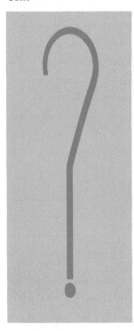

1. What is a cell?
2. In what four ways do cells differ from each other?
3. Of what substance are cells composed?
4. Name the two main structures found in the protoplasm.
5. What is the function of the (a) nucleus? (b) cytoplasm?
6. How does a human cell reproduce?
7. What is metabolism?
8. Name two phases of metabolism.
9. What activities occur during the anabolism or construction process of the cells?
10. What activities occur during the catabolism or destructive process of the cells?
11. What are tissues?
12. List five classifications of body tissues.
13. What is an organ?
14. Which organ circulates the blood in the human body?
15. Which organ supplies oxygen to the blood?
16. What are systems?
17. Name nine body systems.
18. Which system controls and coordinates the functions of all other systems in the body?
19. Which system is the physical framework of the body?
20. Which system covers, shapes and supports the skeleton?
21. To what system do the arteries, veins and capillaries belong?

CHAPTER 26

SKIN AND DISORDERS OF THE SKIN

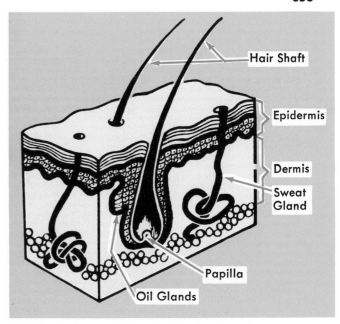

Hair Shaft

Epidermis

Dermis

Sweat Gland

Papilla

Oil Glands

INTRODUCTION

Everyone is concerned with the **health** and **appearance** of her skin. But the scientific study of the **skin and scalp** is of particular importance to cosmetologists. It gives them the basic knowledge they need to offer an effective program of skin care, as well as various cosmetic and scalp treatments.

The skin is the largest organ of the body and performs many vital functions required for health and beauty. The cosmetologist who has a thorough understanding of the skin, its structure and functions, will be in a better position to give patrons professional advice on scalp, facial and hand care.

A **healthy skin** is slightly moist, soft, flexible, and acidic, and is free from any blemish or disease. Its **texture,** as revealed by feel and appearance, should be smooth and fine-grained. A **good complexion** shows itself in the fine texture and healthy color of the skin.

The skin **varies in thickness,** being thinnest on the eyelids and thickest on the palms and soles. Continued pressure or friction over any part of the skin will cause it to thicken, as in a **callous.**

The **scalp** is constructed similar to the skin elsewhere on the human body. However, larger and deeper hair follicles are present on the scalp to accommodate the longer hair of the head.

HISTOLOGY OF THE SKIN

The skin contains two clearly defined divisions: the epidermis and the dermis.

1. The **epidermis** (ep-i-der′mis) is the outermost layer of the skin. This layer is commonly called **cuticle** or **scarf skin.**
2. The **dermis** (der′mis) is the underlying, or inner layer, of the skin. It is also called **derma, corium, cutis** or **true skin.**

354

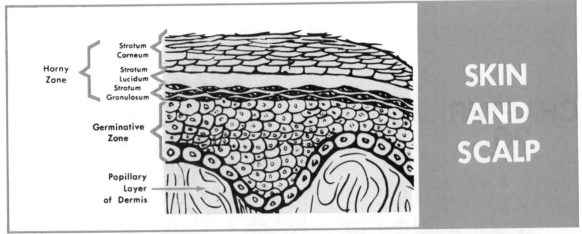

SKIN AND SCALP

Horny Zone
- Stratum Corneum
- Stratum Lucidum
- Stratum Granulosum

Germinative Zone

Papillary Layer of Dermis

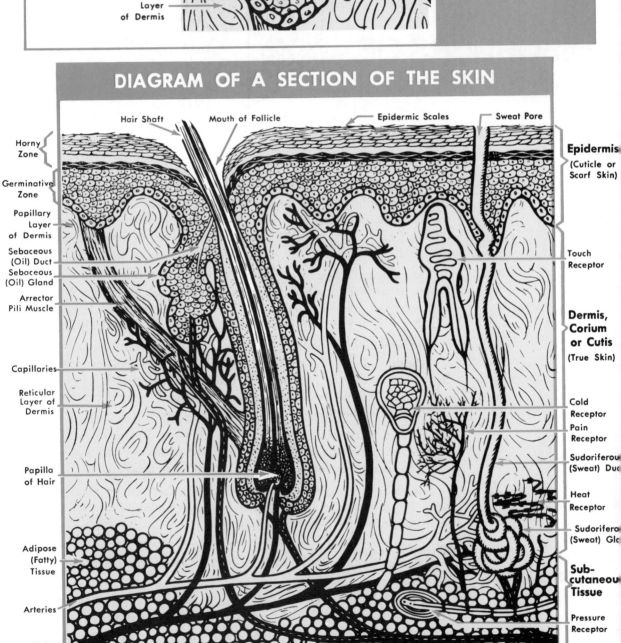

DIAGRAM OF A SECTION OF THE SKIN

Hair Shaft
Mouth of Follicle
Epidermic Scales
Sweat Pore

Horny Zone
Germinative Zone
Papillary Layer of Dermis
Sebaceous (Oil) Duct
Sebaceous (Oil) Gland
Arrector Pili Muscle
Capillaries
Reticular Layer of Dermis
Papilla of Hair
Adipose (Fatty) Tissue
Arteries
Veins

Epidermis (Cuticle or Scarf Skin)
Touch Receptor
Dermis, Corium or Cutis (True Skin)
Cold Receptor
Pain Receptor
Sudoriferous (Sweat) Duct
Heat Receptor
Sudoriferous (Sweat) Gland
Sub-cutaneous Tissue
Pressure Receptor

Epidermis

The **epidermis** forms the outer protective covering of the skin of the body. It contains no blood vessels, but has many small nerve endings. The epidermis contains the following layers:

1. The **stratum corneum** (stra'tum kor'ne-um), or horny layer, consists of tightly packed, scale-like cells which are continually being shed and replaced. As these cells develop from underneath layers, they form **keratin** (ker'ah-tin), a chemical substance which acts as a waterproof covering for the skin.

2. The **stratum lucidum** (lu'si-dum), or clear layer, consists of small, transparent cells through which light can pass.

3. The **stratum granulosum** (gran-u-lo'sum), or granular layer, consists of cells which look like distinct granules. These cells are almost dead and undergo a change into a horny substance.

*4. The **stratum germinativum** (jer'mi-na-tiv-um), formerly known as the stratum mucosum (mu-ko'sum), is composed of several layers of differently shaped cells. The deepest layer is responsible for the growth of the epidermis. It also contains a dark pigment called **melanin** (mel'ah-nin), which protects the sensitive cells below from the destructive effects of excessive ultra-violet rays of the sun or ultra-violet rays from a lamp.

Dermis

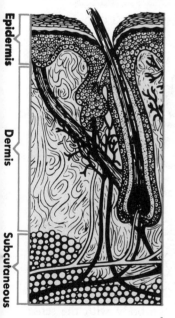

The **dermis** is the true skin. It is a highly sensitive and vascular layer of connective tissue. Within its structure are found numerous blood vessels, lymph vessels, nerves, sweat glands, oil glands, hair follicles, arrector pili muscles and papillae. The dermis consists of two layers: the papillary or superficial layer, and the reticular or deeper layer.

1. The **papillary** (pap'i-la-re) **layer** lies directly beneath the epidermis. It contains small cone-shaped projections of **elastic** tissue that point upward into the epidermis. These projections are called **papillae** (pah-pil'e). Some of these papillae contain looped capillaries, others contain nerve fiber endings called **tactile corpuscles** (tak'til kor'pus-ls). This layer also contains some of the **melanin skin pigment.**

2. The **reticular** (re-tik'u-lar) **layer** contains the following structures within its network:

   a) Fat cells   e) Sweat glands
   b) Blood vessels   f) Hair follicles
   c) Lymph vessels   g) Arrector pili muscles
   d) Oil glands

Subcutaneous Tissue

†**Subcutaneous** (sub-ku-ta'ne-us) tissue is a layer of fatty tissue found below the dermis. This tissue is also called **adipose** (ad'i-pos) tissue or **subcutis.** This fatty tissue varies in thickness according to the age, sex and general health of the individual. It gives smoothness

---

* *Stratum germinativum is also referred to as basal or Malpighian layer.*

† *Some histologists regard the subcutaneous tissue as a continuation of the dermis.*

356

and contour to the body, contains fat for use as energy, and also acts as a protective cushion for the outer skin. Circulation is maintained by a network of arteries and lymphatics.

HOW THE SKIN IS NOURISHED

Blood and lymph supply nourishment to the skin. From 1/2 to 2/3 of the total blood supply of the body is distributed to the skin. The blood and lymph, as they circulate through the skin, contribute essential materials for growth, nourishment and repair of the skin, hair and nails. In the subcutaneous tissue are found networks of arteries and lymphatics, which send their smaller branches to hair papillae, hair follicles and skin glands. The capillaries are quite numerous in the skin.

NERVES OF THE SKIN

The skin contains the surface endings of many nerve fibers classified as:

1. Motor nerve fibers, which are distributed to arrector pili muscles that are attached to the hair follicles
2. Sensory nerve fibers, which react to heat, cold, touch, pressure and pain
3. Secretory nerve fibers, which are distributed to the sweat and oil glands of the skin

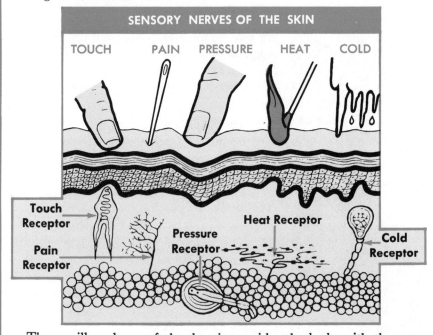

Sense Of Touch

The papillary layer of the dermis provides the body with the sense of touch. Nerves supplying the skin register basic types of sensations: touch, pain, heat, cold, pressure or deep touch. Nerve endings are most abundant in the fingertips. **Complex sensations,** such as the feeling of vibration, seem to depend on a combination of these nerve endings.

SKIN ELASTICITY

Pliability of the skin depends on the elasticity of the fibers of the dermis. For example, expanded healthy skin will regain its former shape almost immediately.

Aging skin. The aging process of the skin is a subject of vital importance to everyone. Perhaps the most outstanding characteristic of the aged skin is its loss of elasticity.

SKIN COLOR

The **color of the skin,** whether fair or dark, depends primarily on the **melanin** or coloring matter that is deposited in the stratum germinativum and the papillary layer of the dermis. To a limited extent, it depends on the blood supply in the skin. The pigment varies in different people. In various races and nationalities, the distinctive color of the skin is an hereditary trait.

THE GLANDS OF THE SKIN

The skin contains two types of duct glands that extract materials from the blood to form different substances.

1. The **sudoriferous** (su-dor-if'er-us), or **sweat glands,** excrete sweat.
2. The **sebaceous** (se-ba'shus), or **oil glands,** secrete sebum.

The **sweat glands** (tubular type) consist of a coiled base, or **fundus** (fun'dus), and a tube-like **duct** which terminates at the skin surface to form the **sweat pore.** Practically all parts of the body are supplied with sweat glands, which are more numerous on the palms, soles, forehead and under the armpits. The sweat glands regulate body temperature and help to eliminate waste products from the body. Their activity is greatly increased by heat, exercise, emotions and certain drugs. The excretion of sweat is under the control of the nervous system. Normally, one to two pints of liquids containing salts are eliminated daily through the sweat pores in the skin.

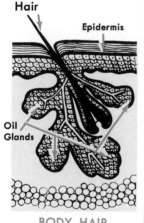

BODY HAIR AND FOLLICLE

Body hair (lanugo) with multiple oil (sebaceous) glands.

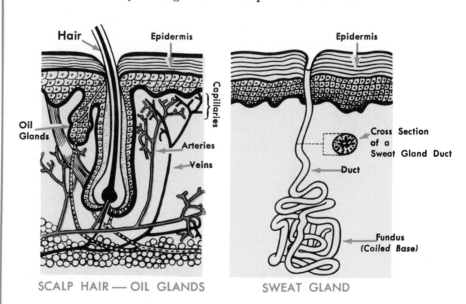

SCALP HAIR — OIL GLANDS

SWEAT GLAND

Oil Glands

The **oil glands** (saccular type) consist of little sacs, whose ducts open into the hair follicle. They secrete **sebum** (se'bum), which lubricates the skin and preserves the softness of the hair. With the exception of the palms and soles, these glands are found in all **parts** of the body, particularly the face.

Sebum is a semi-fluid, oily substance produced by the oil glands. Ordinarily, it flows through the oil **ducts** leading to the **mouths** of the hair follicles. However, when the sebum becomes hardened and the duct becomes blocked, a **blackhead** is formed. Cleanliness is of prime importance in keeping the skin free of blemishes.

FUNCTIONS OF THE SKIN

The principal functions of the skin are: protection, sensation, heat regulation, excretion, secretion and absorption.

1. **Protection.** The skin protects the body from injury and bacterial invasion. The outermost layer of the epidermis is covered with a thin layer of sebum, thus rendering it waterproof. It is resistant to different degrees of temperature, minor injuries, chemically active substances, and many microbes. If germs do invade, the skin becomes inflamed and in the process destroys them.

2. **Sensation.** Through its sensory nerve endings, the skin responds to heat, cold, touch, pressure and pain. **Extreme stimulation** of a sensory nerve ending produces pain. A **minor burn** is very painful, but a **deep burn** that destroys the nerves may be painless.

3. **Heat regulation.** The healthy body maintains a constant internal temperature of about 98.6 degrees Fahrenheit. As changes occur in the outside temperature, the blood and sweat glands of the skin make necessary adjustments in their functions. Heat regulation is a function of the skin, which is an organ that protects the body from environment. **Heat is lost by the evaporation of sweat.**

4. **Excretion.** Perspiration from the sweat glands is excreted from the skin. Water lost by perspiration carries salt and other chemicals with it.

5. **Secretion.** Sebum is secreted by the sebaceous glands. Excessive flow of oil from the oil glands may produce **seborrhea** (seb-o-re'ah). Emotional stress may increase the flow of sebum.

6. **Absorption** is limited, but it does occur. Female hormones applied in a face cream can enter the body through the skin and influence the body to a very minor degree. Fatty materials, such as lanolin creams, are absorbed largely through the hair follicle and sebaceous gland openings.

The skin has an immunity responsiveness to many things that touch it or gain entry into it.

Structures related to the skin are: hair, nails, sweat and oil glands.

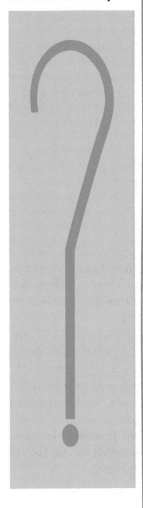

REVIEW QUESTIONS

The Skin And Scalp

1. Briefly describe the skin.
2. What is the appearance of a good complexion?
3. Name the two main divisions of the skin.
4. Locate the epidermis and give its main function.
5. Name the four layers of the epidermis.
6. Which epidermal layer is continually being shed and replaced?
7. Which epidermal layer consists of small, transparent cells?
8. Which epidermal layer starts to undergo a change into a horny substance?
9. Which layer of the epidermis is responsible for its reproduction and growth?
10. Describe the structure of the dermis.
11. Name the two layers of the dermis.
12. Which structures are found in the papillary layer?
13. Which structures are found in the reticular layer?
14. What is the function of the subcutaneous tissue?
15. About how much blood is found in the skin?
16. How is the skin nourished?
17. Name three types of nerve fibers found in the skin.
18. Which part of the body is abundantly supplied with nerve endings?
19. To which structures in the skin are the motor nerve fibers distributed?
20. What renders the skin flexible?
21. Where is the coloring matter of the skin found?
22. To what five things will the sensory nerves of the skin react?
23. What are the functions of the nerve fibers distributed to sweat and oil glands?
24. What is meant by pliability of the skin?
25. What is the characteristic of aged skin?
26. What determines the color of the skin?
27. What are the six important functions of the skin?
28. What regulates the temperature of the body?
29. What is the normal temperature of the human body?
30. Name one cosmetic that the skin can absorb in small amounts.
31. Name four structures related to the skin.

Glands

1. Name two types of duct glands that are found in the skin.
2. Describe the structure of the sweat glands.
3. Where are sweat glands found?
4. What is the function of the sweat glands?
5. Name four things capable of increasing the activity of the sweat glands.
6. Describe the structure of the oil glands.
7. Which substance is secreted by the oil glands?
8. What is the chief function of sebum?
9. Where are the oil glands found?

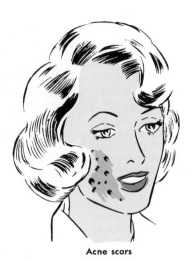

Acne scars

DISORDERS
OF THE SKIN

This information has been compiled to help the cosmetologist become familiar with certain common skin and scalp disorders with which she may come into contact in the beauty salon. There are few disorders of the skin or scalp that logically come within the province of the cosmetologist.

The cosmetologist must be prepared to recognize certain skin conditions and must know how to act properly with relation to them. Some skin and scalp disorders may be treated in cooperation with, and under the supervision of, a physician. Medicinal preparations, issued by prescription for scalp, skin or hair disorders, may be applied as prescribed only with the permission of a physician.

Any condition which the cosmetologist does not positively know to be one of the simple disorders that is rightfully handled in the beauty salon should be **referred** tactfully but firmly to a physician.

The most important thing to know is that a patron who has an inflammatory **skin disorder**, which may or may not be infectious, should not be served in the beauty salon. The cosmetologist should be able to **recognize** these conditions and to **suggest** that proper measures be taken to prevent more serious consequences.

Thus, the cosmetologist **safeguards** her own **health,** as well as the health of the **public.**

Listed below are a number of important terms which should be familiar to the cosmetologist in order that she properly understands the subject of skin, scalp and hair disorders.

Dermatology (der-mah-tol′o-je) is the study of the skin, its nature, structure, functions, diseases and treatment.

Dermatologist (der-mah-tol′o-jist) is a skin specialist.

Pathology (pa-thol′o-je) is the study of disease.

Trichology (tri-kol′o-je) is the study of the hair and its diseases.

Etiology (e-te-ol'o-je) is the study of the causes of disease.

Diagnosis (di-ag-no'sis) is the recognition of a disease from its symptoms.

Prognosis (prog-no'sis) is the foretelling of the probable course of a disease.

LESIONS OF THE SKIN

A lesion is a structural change in the tissues caused by injury or disease. There are three types: primary, secondary and tertiary. The cosmetologist is concerned with primary and secondary lesions only.

Knowing the principal skin lesions helps the cosmetologist to distinguish between conditions that may or conditions that may not be treated in a beauty salon.

Symptom is a sign of disease. The symptoms in diseases of the skin are divided into two groups.

1. **Subjective** refers to symptoms that can be felt, as itching, burning or pains.
2. **Objective** refers to symptoms that can be seen, as pimples pustules or inflammation.

Primary Lesions

1. **Macule** (mak'ul) is a small, discolored spot or patch on the surface of the skin, neither raised nor sunken, as freckles.
2. **Papule** (pap'ul) is a small, elevated pimple in the skin, containing no fluid, but which may develop pus.
3. **Wheal** (whel) is an itchy, swollen lesion that lasts only a few hours. (Examples: hives, or the bite of an insect, such as by a mosquito.)
4. **Tubercle** (tu'ber-kl) is a solid lump larger than a papule. It projects above the surface or lies within or under the skin. It varies in size from a pea to a hickory nut.
5. **Tumor** (tu'mer) is an external swelling, varying in size, shape and color.
6. **Vesicle** (ves'i-kl) is a blister with clear fluid in it. Vesicles lie within or just beneath the epidermis. (Example: Poison ivy produces small vesicles.)
7. **Bulla** (bul'ah) is a blister containing a watery fluid, similar to a vesicle, but larger.
8. **Pustule** (pus'tul) is an elevation of the skin having an inflamed base, containing pus.

Secondary Lesions

The secondary lesions are those in the skin which develop in the later stages of disease. These are:

1. **Scale** is an accumulation of epidermal flakes, dry or greasy. (Example: abnormal or excessive dandruff.)
2. **Crust** (scab) is an accumulation of serum and pus, mixed perhaps with epidermal material. (Example: the scab on a sore.)
3. **Excoriation** (eks-ko're-a'shun) is a skin sore or abrasion produced by scratching or scraping. (Example: a raw surface due to the loss of the superficial skin after an injury.)

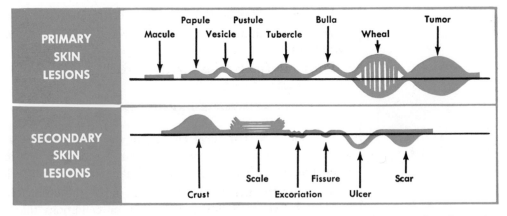

| PRIMARY SKIN LESIONS | Macule · Papule · Vesicle · Pustule · Tubercle · Bulla · Wheal · Tumor |
| SECONDARY SKIN LESIONS | Crust · Scale · Excoriation · Fissure · Ulcer · Scar |

4. **Fissure** (fish'ur) is a crack in the skin penetrating into the derma, as in the case of chapped hands or lips.

5. **Ulcer** (ul'ser) is an open lesion on the skin or mucous membrane of the body, accompanied by pus and loss of skin depth.

6. **Scar (cicatrix)** (si-ka'triks) is likely to form after the healing of an injury or skin condition which has penetrated the dermal layer.

7. **Stain** is an abnormal discoloration remaining after the disappearance of moles, freckles or liver spots, sometimes apparent after certain diseases.

DEFINITIONS OF COMMON TERMS APPLIED TO DISEASE

Before describing the diseases of the skin and scalp so that they will be recognized by the cosmetologist, it is well to understand what is meant by disease.

A **disease** is any departure from a normal state of health.

A **skin disease** is an infection of the skin characterized by an objective lesion (one that can be seen), which may consist of scales, pimples, or pustules.

An **acute disease** is one manifested by symptoms of a more or less violent character and of short duration.

A **chronic disease** is one of long duration, usually mild but recurring.

An **infectious** (in-fek'shus) **disease** is one due to pathogenic germs taken into the body as a result of contact with a contaminated object or lesion.

A **contagious disease** is one that is communicable by contact.

Note:—The terms "infectious disease," "communicable disease," and "contagious disease" are often used interchangeably.

A **congenital disease** is one that is present in the infant at birth.

A **seasonal disease** is one that is influenced by the weather, as prickly heat in the summer, and forms of eczema, which are more prevalent in cold weather.

An **occupational disease**, such as dermatitis, is one that is due to certain kinds of employment, and is caused by coming in contact with cosmetics, chemicals or tints.

A **parasitic disease** is one that is caused by vegetable or animal parasites, such as pediculosis, or ringworm.

A **pathogenic disease** is one produced by disease-producing bacteria, such as staphylococcus and streptococcus, pus-forming bacteria.

A **systemic disease** is due to under- or over-functioning of the internal glands. It may be caused by faulty diet.

A **venereal disease** is a contagious disease commonly acquired by contact with an infected person during sexual intercourse.

An **epidemic** is the manifestation of a disease that attacks simultaneously a large number of persons living in a particular locality. Infantile paralysis, influenza, virus, or smallpox are examples of epidemic-causing diseases.

Allergy is a sensitivity which certain persons develop to normally harmless substances. Skin allergies are quite common. Contact with certain types of cosmetics, medicines and tints, or eating certain foods, all may bring about an itching eruption, accompanied by redness, swelling, blisters, oozing and scaling.

Inflammation is a skin disorder characterized by redness, pain, swelling and heat.

DISORDERS OF THE SEBACEOUS (OIL) GLANDS

There are several common disorders of the sebaceous (oil) glands which the cosmetologist should be able to identify and understand.

Comedones

Comedones (kom-e-donz), or **blackheads**, are a worm-like mass of hardened sebum, appearing most frequently on the face, forehead and nose.

Blackheads accompanied by pimples often occur in youths between the ages of 13 and 20. During the adolescent period, the activity of the sebaceous glands is stimulated, thereby contributing to the formation of blackheads and pimples.

When the hair follicle is filled with an excess of oil from the sebaceous gland, a blackhead forms and creates a blockage at the mouth of the follicle. Should this condition become severe, medical attention is necessary.

The treatment for blackheads is to reduce the skin's oiliness by local applications of cleansers, and the removal of blackheads under sterile conditions. Thorough skin cleansing each night is a very important factor. Cleansing creams and lotions often achieve better results than common soap and water.

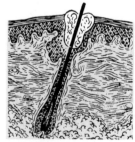

Blackhead (plug of sebaceous matter and dirt) forming around mouth of hair follicle

Milia

Milia (mil'e-ah), or **whiteheads**, is a disorder of the sebaceous (oil) glands caused by the accumulation of sebaceous matter beneath the skin. This may occur on any part of the face, neck and occasionally on the chest and shoulders. Whiteheads are associated with fine-textured, dry types of skin.

364

Acne

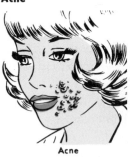

Acne

Acne (ak'ne) is a chronic inflammatory disorder of the sebaceous glands, occurring most frequently on the face, back and chest. The cause of acne is generally held to be microbic, but predisposing factors are adolescence and disturbance of the digestive tract. Acne, or common pimples, is also known as **acne simplex** or **acne vulgaris.**

Acne appears in a variety of different types, ranging from the simple (non-contagious) pimple to serious, deep-seated skin conditions. It is always advisable to have the condition examined and diagnosed by a competent physician before any service is given in the beauty salon.

Seborrhea

Seborrhea (seb-o-re'ah) is a skin condition due to over-activity and excessive secretion of the sebaceous, or oil, glands. An oily or shiny condition of the nose, forehead or scalp indicates the presence of seborrhea. On the scalp, it is readily detected by the unusual amount of oil on the hair.

Rosacea

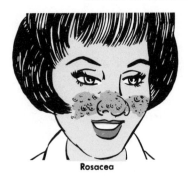

Rosacea

Rosacea, formerly called **acne rosacea,** is a chronic inflammatory congestion of the cheeks and nose. It is characterized by redness, dilation of the blood-vessels, and the formation of papules and pustules. It is usually caused by poor digestion and over-indulgence in alcoholic liquors. It may also be caused by over-exposure to extreme climate, faulty elimination and hyper-acidity. It is usually aggravated by eating and drinking hot, highly spiced, or highly seasoned foods or drinks.

Steatoma

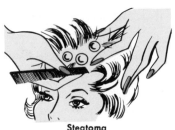

Steatoma

Steatoma (ste-ah-to'mah), or **sebaceous cyst,** is a subcutaneous tumor of the sebaceous glands, the contents consisting of sebum, from a pea to an orange in size; usually occurring on the scalp, neck and back. A steatoma is sometimes called a **wen.**

Asteatosis

Asteatosis (as'te-ah-to'sis) is a condition of dry, scaly skin, characterized by absolute or partial deficiency of sebum, due to senile changes (old age) or some bodily disorders. In local conditions, it may be caused by alkalies, such as those found in soaps and washing powders.

DISORDERS OF SUDORIFEROUS (SWEAT) GLANDS

Bromidrosis (brom-id-ro′sis), or **osmidrosis** (oz-mi-dro′sis), refers to foul-smelling perspiration, usually noticeable in the armpits or on the feet.

Anidrosis (an-i-dro′sis), or lack of perspiration, is often a result of fever or certain skin diseases. It requires medical treatment.

Hyperidrosis (hi-per-i-dro′sis), or excessive perspiration, is caused by excessive heat, or general body weakness. The most commonly affected parts are the armpits, joints and feet. It requires medical treatment.

Miliaria rubra (mil-e-a′re-a roob′ra) (prickly heat) is an acute, inflammatory disorder of sweat glands characterized by an eruption of small red vesicles, accompanied by burning and itching of skin. It is caused by exposure to excessive heat and overweight.

INFLAMMATIONS

Dermatitis (der-mah-ti′tis) is a term used to denote an inflammatory condition of the skin. The lesions come in various forms, such as vesicles or papules.

Eczema (ek′ze-mah) is an inflammation of the skin, of acute or chronic nature, presenting many forms of dry or moist lesions. It is frequently accompanied by itching, burning, and various other unpleasant sensations. All cases of eczema should be referred to a physician for treatment. Its cause is unknown.

Psoriasis (so-ri′ah-sis) is a common, chronic, inflammatory skin disease whose cause is unknown. It is usually found on the scalp, elbows, knees, chest and lower back, rarely on the face. The lesions are round, dry patches covered with coarse, silvery scales. If irritated bleeding points occur. While not contagious, it can be spread by irritating it.

Herpes simplex (hur′pez sim′pleks) is a virus infection of unknown origin, commonly called **fever blisters.** It is characterized by the eruption of a single or group of vesicles on a red swollen base. The blisters usually appear on the lips, nostrils or other part of the face, and rarely last more than a week. Indigestion may be one of the causes.

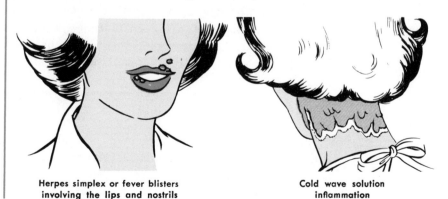

Herpes simplex or fever blisters
involving the lips and nostrils

Cold wave solution
inflammation

Occupational disorders in cosmetology refer to abnormal conditions resulting from contact with chemicals or tints in the course of performing services in the beauty salon. Some individuals may develop allergies to ingredients in cosmetics, antiseptics, cold waving lotions and aniline derivative tints which may cause eruptive skin infections known as **dermatitis venenata** (ven-e-na′tah). It is important that cosmetologists employ protective measures, such as the use of rubber gloves or protective creams whenever possible.

PIGMENTATIONS OF THE SKIN

In abnormal conditions, **pigment** may come from inside or outside the body.

Abnormal colors are seen in every skin disorder and many systemic disorders. Pigmentation is observed when certain drugs are being taken internally.

Tan is caused by excessive exposure to the sun.

Lentigines (len-tij′i-nez) (singular, lentigo), or freckles, are small yellowish to brownish colored spots on parts exposed to sunlight and air.

Stains are abnormal brown skin patches, having a circular and irregular shape. Their permanent color is due to the presence of blood pigment. They occur during aging, after certain diseases and after the disappearance of moles, freckles and liver spots. The cause of these stains is unknown.

Chloasma (klo-az′mah) is characterized by increased deposits of pigment in the skin. It is found mainly on the forehead, nose and cheeks. Chloasma is also called **moth patches** or **liver spots.**

Naevus (ne′vus) is commonly known as birthmark. It is a small or large malformation of the skin due to pigmentation or dilated capillaries.

Leucoderma (lu-ko-der′mah) refers to abnormal whiteness in patches of the skin, due to congenital defective pigmentations. It is classified as:

1. **Vitiligo** (vit-i-li′go)—an acquired condition of leucoderma, affecting the skin or the hair. The only treatment is a matching cosmetic color, making it less conspicuous.
2. **Albinism** (al′bin-izm)—congenital absence of melanin pigment in the body, including the skin, hair and eyes. The silky hair is white. The skin is pinkish white and will not tan.

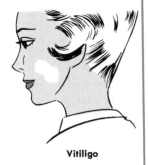

Vitiligo

HYPERTROPHIES (NEW GROWTHS)

Keratoma (ker-ah-to′mah), or callous, is an acquired, superficial, round, thickened patch of epidermis, due to **pressure** friction on the hands and feet.

If the thickening grows inward, it is called a **corn.**

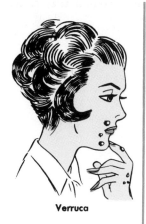

Verruca

A **mole** is a small, brownish spot, or blemish, on the skin. Moles are believed to be inherited. They range in color from pale tan to brown or bluish black. Some moles are small and flat, resembling freckles, while others are more deeply seated and darker in color. Large, dark hairs often occur in moles. Any change in a mole requires medical attention.

CAUTION: Do not treat or remove hair from moles.

Verruca (ve-roo'kah) is the technical term for wart. It is caused by a virus and is infectious. It can spread from one location to another, particularly along a scratch in the skin.

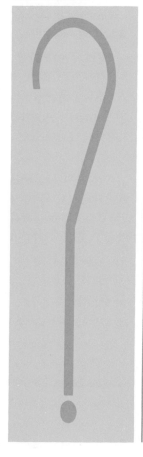

REVIEW QUESTIONS

Skin Disorders

1. Why should the cosmetologist be able to recognize the common skin, scalp and hair disorders?
2. What is the purpose of studying infectious diseases of the skin, scalp and hair?
3. Why should the cosmetologist refuse to treat a patron with an infectious or contagious disease?
4. Define dermatology.
5. What is a dermatologist?
6. What is a lesion?
7. What is the difference between objective and subjective lesions? Give one example of each.
8. Name eight primary lesions of the skin.
9. Name seven secondary lesions of the skin.
10. Define disease.
11. What are the common terms for: a) comedones; b) milia?
12. What causes the formation of comedones?
13. Define acne.
14. Which of the following terms apply to disorders of the sebaceous (oil) glands?
    Milia, acne, bromidrosis, anidrosis, comedones, seborrhea and hyperidrosis
15. Briefly describe: bromidrosis, anidrosis, hyperidrosis, and miliaria rubra.
16. Define dermatitis.
17. Define eczema.
18. What is the characteristic appearance of psoriasis?
19. On which five parts of the body is psoriasis usually found?
20. Define herpes simplex. What is it commonly called?
21. Where do fever blisters usually occur?

22. Define dermatitis venenata. Name two hair services that may cause dermatitis venenata.

23. What are freckles, and what causes them?

24. What are the common names for chloasma?

25. What is the common name for naevus?

26. Define leucoderma, vitiligo.

27. Define albinism.

28. What is the technical term for callous?

29. What is a mole?

30. What is the technical term for a wart?

CHAPTER 27

HAIR AND DISORDERS OF THE SCALP AND HAIR

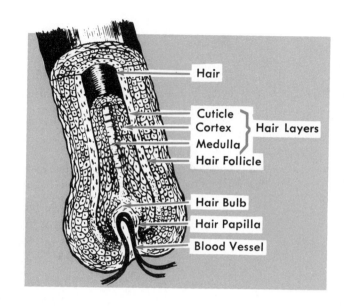

Hair

Cuticle
Cortex } Hair Layers
Medulla
Hair Follicle

Hair Bulb
Hair Papilla
Blood Vessel

THE HAIR

Hair is an **appendage** (ah-pen'daj) of the skin. It is a slender, thread-like outgrowth of the skin of the human body. There is no sense of feeling in hair, due to the complete absence of nerves.

The study of the hair, technically called **trichology** (tri-kol'o-je), is of paramount importance to cosmetologists because hair is what they primarily deal with. The chief purposes of hair are **protection** of the head and body from heat, cold and injury, and **adornment** of the head and face.

To keep the hair healthy and beautiful, proper attention must be given to its care and treatment. **Knowledge** and **analysis** (ah-nal'i-sis) of the patron's hair, tactful suggestions for its improvement, and sincere interest in maintaining its health and beauty, are all part of every cosmetologist's responsibilities.

Abusing the hair by harmful cosmetic applications, or faulty hair treatments, can cause the hair structure to become weakened or damaged.

Composition Of Hair

Hair is chiefly composed of a **protein** (pro'te-in) called **keratin** (ker'ah-tin), which is present in all horny growths, such as nails, claws and hoofs.

The average chemical composition of normal hair has been estimated by chemical analysts to be: carbon, 50.65%; hydrogen, 6.36%; nitrogen, 17.14%; sulfur, 5.0% and oxygen, 20.85%.

(The sulfur content of the hair is particularly important to permanent waving, hair relaxing and hair coloring. For detailed information, consult chapter on chemistry).

Division Of Hair

Full grown human hair is divided into two principal parts: root and shaft.

1. The **hair root** is that portion of the hair structure which is found beneath the skin surface. This is the portion of the hair enclosed within the follicle.
2. The **hair shaft** is that portion of the hair structure extending above the skin surface.

Structures Associated With Hair Root

Structures closely associated with the hair root are the hair follicle, hair bulb and hair papilla.

The **hair follicle** (fol'i-kl) is a tube-like depression or pocket in the skin or scalp, encasing the **hair root.** For every hair there is a follicle which varies in depth, depending on the thickness and location of the skin or scalp.

One or more oil glands are attached to each hair follicle.

The funnel-shaped mouths of hair follicles are favorite **breeding** places for germs and for the **accumulation** of sebum and dirt.

The follicle does not run straight down into the skin or scalp, but is set at an angle so that the hair above the surface has a "natural flow" in a definite direction. This natural flow is sometimes called the "hair-stream" of the scalp. Since the angles run according to areas set by nature, hair emerges from the scalp slanting in a given direction.

The **hair bulb** is a thickened, club-shaped structure forming the lower part of the hair root. The lower part of the hair bulb is hollowed out to fit over and cover the hair papilla.

The **hair papilla** is a small cone-shaped elevation, located at the bottom of the hair follicle, which fits into the hair bulb. Within the hair papilla is a **rich blood and nerve supply,** which contributes to the growth and regeneration of the hair. It is through the papilla that nourishment reaches the hair bulb.

Structures Connected To Hair Follicles

The **arrector pili** (ah-rek'tor pi'li) is a small involuntary muscle attached to the underside of a hair follicle. Fear or cold contracts it, causing the hair **to stand up straight,** and giving the skin the appearance of "goose flesh." Eyelash and eyebrow hairs lack an arrector pili muscle.

Sebaceous (se-ba'shus), or **oil, glands** consist of little sacular structures situated in the dermis. Their ducts are connected to hair follicles. Secretion of an oily substance, **sebum** (se'bum), serves to give luster and pliability to the hair, and keeps the skin surface soft and supple. However, the oil glands frequently become trouble-makers. By over-producing, they bring on a common form of oily dandruff, and can be an important contributing cause of hair loss or baldness.

CROSS SECTION OF HAIR

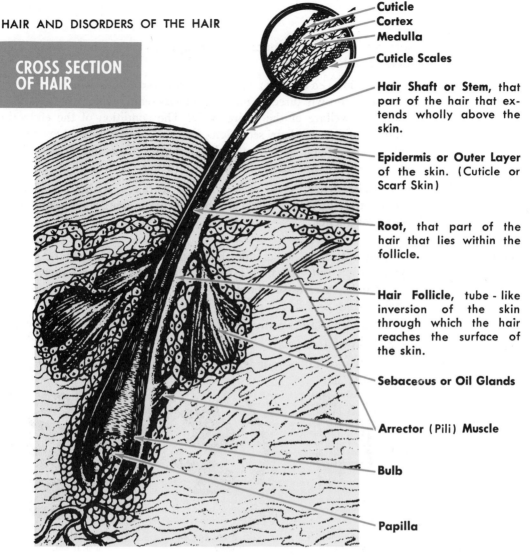

Cuticle
Cortex
Medulla
Cuticle Scales

Hair Shaft or Stem, that part of the hair that extends wholly above the skin.

Epidermis or Outer Layer of the skin. (Cuticle or Scarf Skin)

Root, that part of the hair that lies within the follicle.

Hair Follicle, tube-like inversion of the skin through which the hair reaches the surface of the skin.

Sebaceous or Oil Glands

Arrector (Pili) Muscle

Bulb

Papilla

Sebum

The production of sebum is influenced by five factors, some of which are subject to personal control. They are:

1. Diet
2. Blood circulation
3. Emotional disturbances
4. Stimulation of endocrine glands
5. Drugs

Diet exerts an influence on the general health of the hair. It is most easily corrected. The over-eating of sweet, starchy, and fatty foods may cause the sebaceous glands to become over-active and secrete too much sebum (oil).

Blood circulation. The hair derives its nourishment from the blood supply. The blood, in turn, depends on the foods eaten for many of its elements. In the absence of necessary food elements, the health of the hair may decline.

Emotional disturbances or mental tensions are linked with the condition of hair through the nervous system. The well-being of hair is affected by all the emotions and thoughts. Healthy hair is an indication of a healthy body.

Endocrine (en'do-krin) **glands** are ductless glands which have their secretions thrown directly into the bloodstream, which in turn influences the welfare of the entire body. The condition of the endocrine glands influences their secretion. During adolescence, they become very active. Their activity usually decreases after middle age. Endocrine gland disturbances, however, influence the health of the hair.

Certain drugs, such as hormones, if taken without a doctor's advice, may adversely affect the hair in permanent waving and other hair treatments.

Hair Structure

Shapes of hair. As a rule, hair has one of three general shapes. As it grows out, the hair assumes the shape, size and direction of the follicle. A **cross-sectional view** of the hair under the microscope reveals that usually:

1. Straight hair is round.
2. Wavy hair is oval.
3. Curly or kinky hair is almost flat.

> *There is no strict rule regarding cross-sectional shapes of hair. Oval, straight and curly hair have been found in all shapes.*

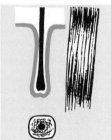
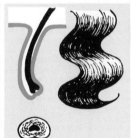
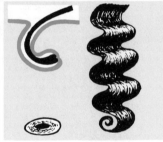

1. Straight hair is usually round.
2. Wavy hair is usually oval.
3. Curly or kinky hair is almost flat.

The structure of the hair is composed of cells arranged in three layers:

1. **Cuticle** (ku'ti-kl), the outside horny layer, is composed of transparent, overlapping, protective scale-like cells, pointing away from the scalp and towards the hair ends. Chemical solutions loosen these scales so that solutions can enter into the hair cortex.

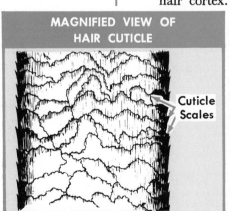

MAGNIFIED VIEW OF HAIR CUTICLE

Cuticle Scales

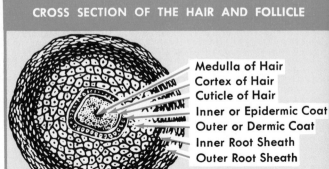

CROSS SECTION OF THE HAIR AND FOLLICLE

Medulla of Hair
Cortex of Hair
Cuticle of Hair
Inner or Epidermic Coat
Outer or Dermic Coat
Inner Root Sheath
Outer Root Sheath

2. **Cortex** (kor'teks), the middle or inner layer, which gives strength and elasticity to the hair, is made up of a fibrous substance formed by elongated cells. This layer contains the pigment which gives the hair its color.

3. **Medulla** (me-dul'ah), the innermost layer, is referred to as the pith or marrow of the hair shaft, and is composed of round cells. The medulla may be absent in fine and very fine hair.

Hair Distribution

Hair is found all over the body, except on the palms, soles, lips, and eyelids.

There are three types of hair on the body:

1. **Long hair,** which grows from the scalp, protects the scalp against the sun's rays and injury, gives adornment to the head, and forms a pleasing frame for the face. **Soft, long hair** also grows in the armpits of both sexes and on the faces of men.

2. **Short, or bristly, hair,** such as the eyebrows and eyelashes, adds beauty and line of color to the face. **Eyebrows** divert sweat from the eyes. The **eyelashes** help protect the eyes from dust particles and strong glare from light or sun.

3. **Lanugo** (la-nu'go) **hair** is the fine, soft, downy hair of the cheeks, forehead and nearly all areas of the body. It helps in the efficient evaporation of perspiration.

Hair Growth

Hair cycle. If the hair is normal and healthy, each individual hair goes through a steady cycle of events: **growth, fall** and **replacement.**

The formation and growth of hair cells depend on proper nourishment and oxygen which only the **bloodstream can supply.** Therefore, the function of blood is indispensable to the health and life of hair.

When the body is healthy, hair flourishes. If the body is ill, hair weakens. When the bloodstream provides the hair papilla with food elements, the hair grows.

Normal hair growth. The average growth of healthy hair on the scalp of an adult is about one-half inch per month. Research indicates that hair may grow faster in the case of younger people, and in some instances, may even grow up to three-quarters of an inch per month.

The rate of growth of human hair will differ on specific parts of the body, between sexes, among races, and with age. Scalp hair will also differ among individuals in **strength, elasticity,** and **waviness.**

Racial factors have a bearing on hair growth. For example, the American Indians and the Chinese have long, thick, straight, black hair. The Negro's hair is usually short and very curly.

The growth of scalp hair occurs more rapidly between the ages of 15 and 30, and declines sharply between 50 and 60. Scalp hair grows faster in women than in men.

Hair growth is also influenced by:

1. Seasons of the year
2. Nutrition and hormones

Climatic conditions will affect the hair in the following ways:

1. Moisture in the air will deepen the natural wave.
2. Cold air will cause the hair to contract.
3. Heat will cause the hair to swell or expand and absorb moisture.

Hair growth is not increased by any of the following:

1. Close clipping, shaving, trimming, cutting or singeing have no effect upon the rate of hair growth.
2. The application of ointments or oils will not increase hair growth. They act as lubricants to the hair shaft but do not feed the hair.
3. Hair does not grow after death. The flesh and skin contract, thus giving the appearance of some growth.

Normal hair shedding. A certain amount of hair is shed daily. This is nature's method of making way for new hair. The average daily shedding is estimated at 50 to 80 hairs. Hair loss beyond this estimated average may indicate scalp or hair trouble.

Replacement Of Hair

Material for the growth of the hair comes from the papilla. As long as the papilla is not destroyed, the hair will grow. If the hair is pulled out from the roots, it will nevertheless grow again. Should the papilla be destroyed, it will **never** grow again.

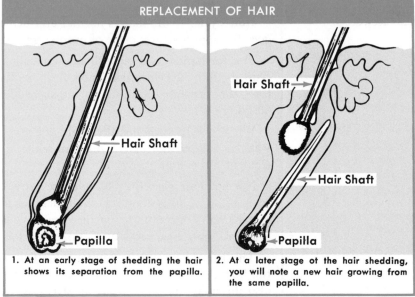

REPLACEMENT OF HAIR

Hair Shaft

Hair Shaft

Papilla

1. At an early stage of shedding the hair shows its separation from the papilla.

Hair Shaft

Hair Shaft

Papilla

2. At a later stage of the hair shedding, you will note a new hair growing from the same papilla.

In human beings, new hair **replaces** old hair in the following ways:

1. The bulb loosens and separates from the papilla.
2. The bulb moves upward in the follicle.
3. The hair moves slowly to the surface, where it is shed.
4. The new hair is formed by cell division that takes place at a point at the root of the hair and around the papilla.

Life And Density Of Hair

The exact life span of hair has not been agreed upon. The average life of hair will range from **two to four years.** Other factors, such as sex, age, type of hair, heredity and health, have a bearing on the duration of hair life.

(While the life span of hair may differ with each individual, the figures two to four years indicate a fair estimated period, considering age, health, climate and other personal factors. Some authorities estimate the life span of hair to range up to 7 years.)

Eyebrow hairs and eyelashes are replaced every four to five months.

The average area of a head is about 120 square inches. There is an average of 1000 hairs to a square inch.

The number of hairs on the head varies with the color of the hair:

Blonde	140,000	Black	108,000
Brown	110,000	Red	90,000

Color Of Hair

The natural color of hair, its strength and texture, depend mainly on hereditary qualities of a physical nature. The color of hair is an inherited characteristic, and is easy to observe and classify. To be successful in giving hair lightening and tinting treatments, the cosmetologist should understand the color and distribution of hair pigmentation. The cosmetologist should also understand hair texture, porosity and elasticity.

The cortex contains coloring matter, minute grains of **melanin** (mel'ah-nin), or pigment. The source of pigment has not been definitely settled. It is probably derived from the color-forming substances in the blood, as is all pigment of the human body. The color and shade of the hair depend on the color and amount of grains of pigment it contains.

Greying Of Hair

Grey hair is due mainly to the absence of hair pigment in the cortical layer of the hair. Grey hair is really mottled hair—spots of white or whitish yellow scattered about in the hair shafts. Normally, grey hair grows out in this condition from the hair bulb. Greying does not take place after the hair has grown.

In most cases, the greying of hair is a result of the natural aging process in humans, but it is not related to the hair's texture or growth. Greying can also happen as a result of some serious illness or nervous shock. An early diminishing of the pigment brought on by emotional tensions may also cause hair to turn grey.

Premature grey hair in a young person is usually the result of a defect in pigment formation occurring at birth. Often it is found that several members of a family are affected with premature greyness.

Hair Definitions And Technical Terms

Hirsuties (her-su'shi-ez), or **hypertrichosis** (hi-per-tri-ko'sis), means hairy, or superfluous hair. It is recognized by the growth of hair in unusual amounts or locations, as on the faces of women.

Technical terms given to hair on the head and face:
Capilli (kah-pil'i)—the head
Cilia (sil'e-ah)—the eyelashes
Supercilia (su-per-sil'e-ah)—the eyebrows
Barba (bar'bah)—the face

Albino (al-bi'no) is a person born with white hair, the result of an absence of coloring matter in the hair shaft, accompanied by a lack of marked pigment coloring in the skin, or iris of the eyes.

Definitions Of
Directional Hair Growth

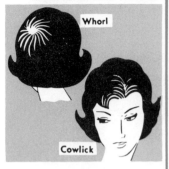

Whorl

Cowlick

HAIR ANALYSIS

The Use Of
The Four Senses

Hair Texture

Hair-stream. Hair in an area sloping in the same direction is known as a hair-stream. This is due to the follicles in the area being arranged in a uniform manner. When two such streams slope in opposite directions, they form a **natural parting** of the hair.

Whorl. Hair which forms in a swirl effect, as in the crown, is called a whorl.

Cowlick. A tuft of hair standing up is known as a cowlick. Areas in which cowlicks are noticeable are usually at the front hairline. This is caused by the follicles pointing straight up. However, cowlicks may be located in other parts of the scalp. In styling, they must be considered and the hair styled accordingly.

Much of the cosmetologist's time is taken up with treating and arranging patrons' hair. For this reason it is important that the cosmetologist be able to recognize and distinguish the various types of human hair.

Hair knowledge and skill can be acquired by constant observation and practice in the use of the senses of sight, touch, hearing and smell.

1. **Sight.** Observing the hair will immediately impart some knowledge. However, sight alone will not enable accurate judgment to be made of hair qualities. Sight contributes approximately 15 percent to hair analysis, but the **sense of touch** is most important in the analysis of hair.
2. **Touch.** Unless cosmetologists develop to their full capacity the **sense of touch** in relation to hair, they cannot give professional hair treatments to patrons. When the sense of touch is fully developed, fewer mistakes are made in judging the hair.
3. **Hearing.** The patron likes to talk about her hair, her health problems, her hair's reaction to applied cosmetics, and its behavior after certain medications have been taken. Since both her health and the application of certain cosmetics to her hair will affect hair treatments, listen carefully to what she tells you.
4. **Smell.** Uncleanliness and certain scalp disorders will create an odor. If the patron has good health, a clean scalp, and shampoos her hair weekly, the hair will be free from odor.

The important qualities by which human hair is judged are porosity, texture, elasticity and condition.

Hair texture refers to the degree of coarseness or fineness of the hair, and may vary on different parts of the head. Variations in hair texture are due to:

1. **Diameter of the hair** indicates whether the hair is coarse, medium, fine or very fine. Coarse hair has the greatest diameter, and very fine hair has the smallest.
2. **Feel of the hair** indicates whether the hair is harsh, soft or wiry.

Coarse hair contains three layers: the medulla, cortex and cuticle. Usually the scales of the outside layer are closely overlapped and raised away from the hair shaft, which is responsible for the hygroscopic (hi-gro-skop'ik) quality (ability to absorb moisture) of coarse hair.

Medium texture of hair is the normal type most commonly met in the beauty salon. The medulla, cortex and cuticle layers are present to a lesser degree than in coarse hair. This type of hair does not present any special problem.

Fine or very fine hair requires special care. Its microscopic structure reveals that only two layers, the cortex and cuticle, are present.

Wiry hair, whether coarse, medium or fine, has a hard, glassy finish due to the cuticle scales lying flat against the hair shaft. It takes longer to give this type of hair a permanent wave, tinting or lightening treatment.

Hair Porosity

Hair porosity is the ability of the hair to absorb moisture regardless of whether the hair is coarse, medium or fine.

Good porosity—hair with the cuticle scales raised from the hair shaft. Hair of this type can absorb a normal amount of moisture or chemicals.

Moderate porosity (normal hair)—the average type of hair found in the beauty salon. It is less porous than hair with good porosity.

Usually hair with good or moderate porosity presents no problem in receiving hair treatments, whether they be permanent waving, hair tinting or lightening.

Poor porosity (resistant hair)—hair with the cuticle scales lying close to the hair shaft. This type of hair usually absorbs the least amount of moisture.

Hair with poor porosity requires thorough analysis and strand tests before the application of any hair cosmetics.

Extreme porosity—poor condition (tinted, lightened, permanently waved, or damaged hair)—hair that has been made extremely porous by continuous or faulty treatments. This hair readily absorbs liquids and requires special care.

Hair Elasticity

Hair elasticity is the ability of the hair to stretch and return to its original form without breaking. Hair with normal elasticity is springy and gives a live and lustrous appearance. Normal, dry hair is capable of being stretched about 20% of its length, and will spring back when released. However, wet hair can be stretched 40% to 50% of its length. Porous hair will stretch more than hair with poor porosity.

Hair may be classified as having good elasticity, normal elasticity, or poor elasticity.

For additional information on hair elasticity, see chapter on **Permanent Waving.**

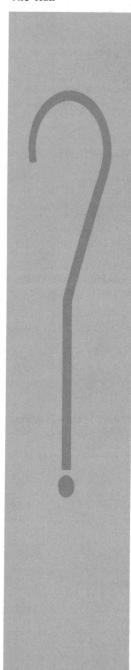

1. Define hair.
2. What is the technical term for the study of hair?
3. Why is the study of hair important to the cosmetologist?
4. What are the main purposes of hair?
5. What kind of treatment may cause the hair structure to become weakened?
6. Give the name of the protein found in hair.
7. Name the two parts into which the length of the hair is divided.
8. How do strongly alkaline solutions harm the hair shaft?
9. What is the hair root?
10. What is the hair shaft?
11. What is the hair follicle?
12. What is meant by hair-stream?
13. What is the hair bulb?
14. What is the hair papilla?
15. What muscle and gland are attached to the hair follicle?
16. How does the hair receive its nourishment?
17. What is the function of the papilla?
18. For what foreign bodies are the mouths of hair follicles favorite breeding places?
19. What causes "goose pimples"?
20. What function is performed by the oil glands for the scalp?
21. List five factors which influence the production of sebum.
22. What determines the size and shape of the hair?
23. Name three general shapes of hair.
24. Name three layers found in hair.
25. Which hair layer serves to protect its inner structure?
26. Which hair layer contains coloring matter?
27. Which layer is sometimes missing in women's hair?
28. Which parts of the body do not contain any hair?
29. Briefly describe the appearance of lanugo hair. Where is it usually found?
30. What is the function of lanugo hair?
31. What is meant by hair cycle?
32. Briefly explain the hair replacement process.
33. What is the average rate of growth of hair on the head?
34. Since the number of hairs on the head usually varies with the color of the hair, about how many hairs are there on the head for:
a) light blonde; b) black; c) brown?
35. List three ways in which climatic conditions will affect the hair.
36. About how many square inches does an average scalp area contain?
37. What is melanin?
38. What is the average number of hairs shed daily?
39. What is the average life span of scalp hair?
40. What causes the hair to turn grey?
41. What is: a) cowlick; b) whorl?
42. What is an albino?
43. Name the four senses used when analyzing the hair.
44. Name the four important qualities by which hair is judged.
45. Which two senses are used to judge these qualities?
46. Define hair texture.
47. Define hair porosity.
48. Define hair elasticity.
49. To what extent can normal hair be stretched: a) when dry; b) when wet?

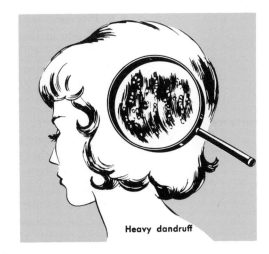
Heavy dandruff

DISORDERS OF THE SCALP AND HAIR

DISORDERS OF THE SCALP

Just as the skin is continually being shed and replaced, the uppermost layer of the scalp is being cast off all the time. Ordinarily, these horny scales are loose and fall off freely. The natural shedding of these horny scales should not be mistaken for dandruff.

DANDRUFF

Dandruff is the small, white scales that usually appear on the scalp and hair. It is also known by the medical term of **pityriasis** (**pit-e-ri′ah-sis**).

Causes Of Dandruff

Long-neglected, excessive dandruff may lead to baldness.

1. A direct cause of dandruff is the excessive shedding of the epithelial cells. Instead of growing to the surface and falling off, the horny scales accumulate on the scalp.
2. Indirect or associated causes of dandruff are a sluggish condition of the scalp, occasioned by poor circulation, infection, injury, lack of nerve stimulation, improper diet and uncleanliness. Contributing causes are the use of strong shampoos and insufficient rinsing of the hair after a shampoo.

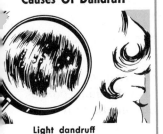
Light dandruff

Types Of Dandruff

The two principal types of dandruff are:

1. **Pityriasis capitis simplex**—dry type
2. **Pityriasis steatoides** (ste-ah-toy′dez)—a greasy or waxy type

Pityriasis capitis simplex (dry dandruff) is characterized by an itchy scalp and small white scales, which are usually attached in masses to the scalp, or scattered loosely in the hair. Occasionally, they are so profuse that they fall to the shoulders. Dry dandruff is often the result of a sluggish scalp caused by poor circulation, lack of nerve stimulation, improper diet, emotional and glandular disturbances or uncleanliness.

Treatment

Frequent scalp treatments and mild shampoos, regular scalp massage, daily use of antiseptic scalp lotions, and applications of scalp ointment will correct this condition.

Pityriasis steatoides (greasy or waxy type of dandruff) is a scaly condition of the epidermis. The scales become mixed with sebum, causing them to stick to the scalp in patches. The associated itchiness causes the person to scratch the scalp. If the greasy scales are torn off, bleeding or oozing of sebum may follow. Medical treatment is advisable.

Summary

The nature of dandruff is not clearly defined by medical authorities. It is generally believed to be of infectious origin. Some authorities hold that it is due to a specific microbe. However, from the cosmetologist's point of view, both forms of dandruff are to be considered contagious and may be spread by the use of common brushes, combs and other articles. Therefore, the cosmetologist must take the necessary precautions to sanitize everything that comes into contact with the patron.

ALOPECIA

Alopecia (al-o-pe'she-ah) is the technical term for any abnormal form of loss of hair.

The natural falling out of the hair should not be confused with alopecia. When hair has grown to its full length, it comes out by itself and is replaced by a new hair. The natural shedding of hair occurs most frequently in spring and fall. On the other hand, the hair lost in alopecia does not come back, unless special treatments are given to encourage hair growth.

Certain hairstyles, such as ponytail and tight braids, may be contributing factors in constant hair loss or baldness.

Alopecia senilis (se-nil'is) is the form of baldness occurring in old age. This loss of hair is permanent.

Alopecia prematura (pre-mah-tu'rah) is the form of baldness, beginning any time before middle age with a slow thinning process. This condition is caused by the first hairs falling out and being replaced by weaker ones.

Alopecia areata (ar-e-a'tah) is the sudden falling out of hair in round patches, or baldness in spots, sometimes caused by anemia, scarlet fever, typhoid fever, or syphilis. Affected areas are slightly depressed, smooth and very pale, due to a decreased blood supply. Patches may be round or irregular in shape, and they may vary in size from one-half inch to two or three inches in diameter. In most conditions of alopecia areata, the nervous system has been subjected to some injury. Since the flow of blood is influenced by the nervous system, the affected area is also poorly nourished.

Alopecia may appear in a variety of different forms, caused by many abnormal conditions. Sometimes an alopecia condition may be improved by proper scalp treatments.

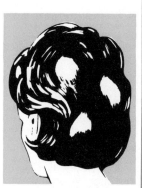

Alopecia areata

CONTAGIOUS DISORDERS

Vegetable Parasitic Infections

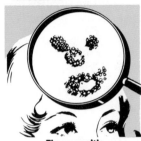

Tinea capitis

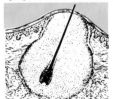

Favus

Animal Parasitic Infections

Staphylococci Infections

Tinea (tin'e-ah) is the medical term for **ringworm**. Ringworm is caused by **vegetable parasites**. All forms are contagious. **Tinea** is transmissible from one person to another. The disease is commonly carried by scales or hairs containing fungi. Shower baths, swimming pools and unsanitized articles are also sources of transmission.

Ringworm starts with a small, reddened patch of little blisters. They spread outward and heal in the middle with scaling. Several such patches may be present. Any ringworm condition should be referred to a physician.

Tinea capitis (ringworm of the scalp) is a contagious, vegetable parasitic disease of the hairy scalp, characterized by red papules, or spots, at the opening of the hair follicles. The patches spread, the hair becomes brittle and lifeless, and breaks off, leaving a stump, or falls from the enlarged open follicles.

Tinea favosa (fa-vo'sah), also called **favus** (fa'vus), or **honeycomb ringworm**, is an infectious growth caused by a vegetable parasite. It is characterized by dry, sulfur-yellowish, cup-like crusts on the scalp, called **scutula** (skut'u-lah), which have a peculiar mousy odor. Scars from favus are bald patches, which may be pink or white and shiny. It is very contagious and should be referred to a physician.

Scabies (the itch) is a highly contagious, animal parasitic skin disease, caused by the itch mite. Vesicles and pustules may form from the irritation of the parasites, or from scratching the affected areas.

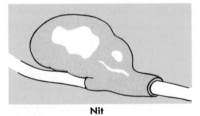

Nit

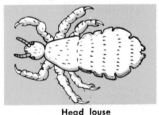

Head louse

Pediculosis (pe-dik-u-lo'sis) **capitis** is a contagious condition caused by the head louse (animal parasite) infesting the hair of the scalp. As the parasites feed on the scalp, itching symptoms are felt and scratching may cause an infection. The head louse is transmitted from one person to another by contact with infested hats, combs, brushes or other personal articles. To **kill head lice**, advise patron to apply larkspur tincture, or other medication, to the entire head before retiring. The next morning, she should shampoo with germicidal soap. Treatment should be repeated as necessary. Never treat in the beauty salon.

Furuncle (fer-un'kl), or **boil**, is an acute staphylococci infection of a hair follicle which produces constant pain. A furuncle is the result of an active inflammatory process, limited to a definite area, and subsequently producing a pustule perforated by a hair.

Carbuncle (kar'bun-kl) is the result of an acute staphylococci infection, and is larger than a furuncle, or boil. It should be referred to a physician.

Furuncle or boil

DISORDERS OF THE HAIR

(Non Contagious)

Canities

Canities (kah-nish´i-ez) is the technical term for grey hair. Its immediate cause is the loss of natural pigment in the hair. It may be either of two types:

1. **Congenital canities** exists at or before birth. It occurs in albinos and occasionally in persons with perfectly normal hair. A patchy type of congenital canities may develop either slowly or rapidly, according to the cause of the condition.

2. **Acquired canities** may be due to old age; it may be premature in early adult life.

Causes of acquired canities may be worry, anxiety, nervous strain, prolonged illness, various wasting diseases and heredity.

Ringed hair. Alternate bands of grey and dark hair.

Hypertrichosis

Hypertrichosis (hi-per-tri-ko´sis), or **hirsuties** (her-su´she-ez), means superfluous hair; an abnormal development of hair on areas of the body normally bearing only downy hair.

Treatments: Tweeze or remove by depilatories, electrolysis, shaving or epilation.
CAUTION. Small pigmented areas—**do not treat.**

Trichoptilosis

Trichoptilosis (trik-op-ti-lo´sis) is the technical name for split hair ends. Treatment: The hair should be well oiled to soften and lubricate the excessively dry ends. The ends may also be removed by cutting.

Trichorrhexis Nodosa

Trichorrhexis nodosa (trik-o-rek´sis no-do´sah), or knotted hair, is a dry, brittle condition with the formation of nodular swellings along the hair shaft. The hair breaks easily and shows a queer brush-like spreading out of the fibers of the broken-off hair. Softening the hair with ointments may prove beneficial.

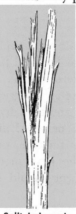
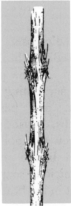
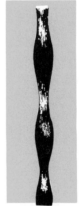

Split hair ends   Knotted hair   Beaded hair

Monilethrix

Monilethrix (mon-il´e-thriks) is the technical term for beaded hair. The hair breaks between the beads or nodes. Scalp and hair treatments may be beneficial.

Fragilitas Crinium

Fragilitas crinium (frah-jil´i-tas krin´e-um) is the technical term for brittle hair. The hairs may split at any part of their length. Hair treatments may be given.

REVIEW QUESTIONS

Disorders Of The Scalp And Hair

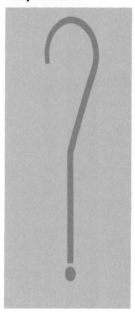

1. How is dandruff recognized?
2. What is a direct cause of dandruff?
3. List six conditions that may be the cause of dandruff.
4. Give the medical term for: a) dandruff; b) dry type of dandruff; c) greasy or waxy type of dandruff.
5. What is meant by alopecia?
6. Is the ordinary falling out of hair considered a disease? Explain.
7. What is alopecia senilis?
8. Define alopecia prematura.
9. At what time of the year is falling out of the hair most noticeable?
10. What is alopecia areata?
11. What is the common term for tinea?
12. What is the cause of tinea?
13. Briefly describe ringworm.
14. What is the common name for pediculosis capitis? Should this condition be treated by the cosmetologist?
15. What is a furuncle?
16. What is the technical term for grey hair?
17. Give several causes for grey hair.
18. Briefly describe the following: a) trichoptilosis; b) hypertrichosis.
19. What is meant by ringed hair?
20. What is another term for hypertrichosis?
21. Give the medical terms for: a) knotted hair; b) beaded hair.
22. What is meant by fragilitas crinium?

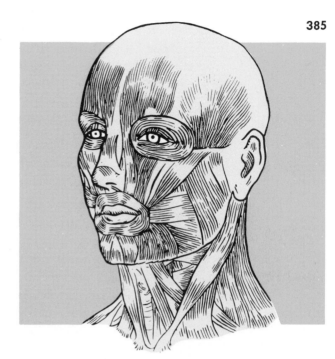

CHAPTER 28

ANATOMY

INTRODUCTION

While the cosmetologist is by no means a physician or an anatomist, it is desirable that she possess a working knowledge of the structure of those areas upon which cosmetic treatments are given.

The names of the bones, principal muscles, arteries and nerves are seldom used in the routine of the beauty salon. However, an understanding of this phase of anatomy is helpful in understanding the reasons for certain steps which are required in giving facial and scalp treatments, as well as in hand and arm massage.

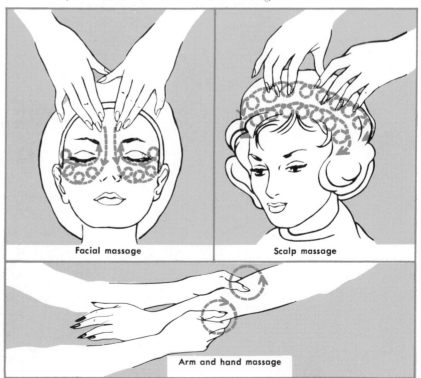

Facial massage

Scalp massage

Arm and hand massage

BONES

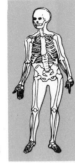

Functions Of Bones

Bones Of The Skull

Eight Bones Of The Cranium

Bone is the hardest structure of the body. It is composed of fibrous tissues firmly bound together, consisting of about one-third animal matter and two-thirds mineral matter.

The **skeletal system** is the physical foundation of the body. It is composed of differently shaped bones united by movable and immovable joints.

The following are the functions of bone:
1. To give shape and strength to the body
2. To protect organs from injury
3. To serve as attachments for muscles
4. To act as levers for all bodily movements

The **skull** is the skeleton of the head. It is an oval, bony case that shapes the head and protects the brain. The skull is divided into two parts: **the cranium, consisting of eight bones, and the skeleton of the face, consisting of fourteen bones.**

The following bones are involved indirectly in connection with scalp and facial manipulations: (*The bones are numbered to correspond with the bones shown on the illustration.*)

1. **Occipital** (ok-sip'i-tal) **bone** forms the lower back part of the cranium.
2. **Two parietal** (pah-ri'e-tal) **bones** form the sides and top (crown) of the cranium.

The following facial bones are affected by massage:
Nasal Bones
Zygomatic Bones
Maxilla Bone
Mandible Bone

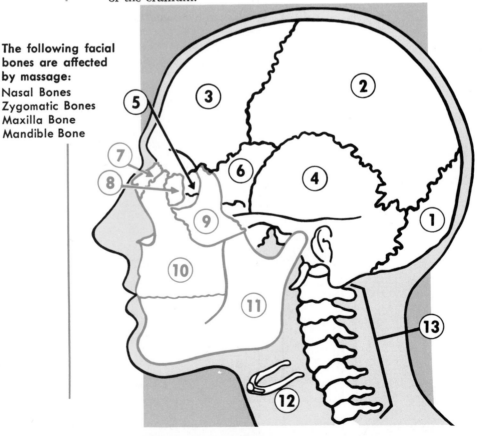

3. **Frontal** (frun'tal) **bone** forms the forehead.

4. **Two temporal** (tem'po-ral) **bones** form the sides of the head in the ear region (below the parietal bones).
(The ethmoid and sphenoid bones are not affected by massage.)

5. **Ethmoid** (eth'moid) **bones** are light and spongy bones between the eyesockets and form part of the nasal cavities.

6. **Sphenoid** (sfe'noid) **bone** joins together all the bones of the cranium.

Fourteen Bones Of The Face

7. **Two nasal** (na'sal) **bones** form the bridge of the nose.

8. **Two lacrimal** (lak'ri-mal) **bones** are small fragile bones located at the front part of the inner wall of the eyesockets.

9. **Two zygomatic** (zi-go-mat'ik), or **malar bones,** form the prominence of the cheeks.

These unnumbered bones do not appear on illustration: Two turbinal (tur'bi-nal) bones are thin layers of spongy bone situated on either of the outer walls of the nasal depression. Vomer (vo'mer) is a single bone that forms part of the dividing wall of the nose. Two palatine (pal'ah-tin) bones form the floor and outer wall of the nose, roof of the mouth, and floor of the orbits.

10. **Two maxillae** (mak-sil'e) are the upper jawbones which join to form the whole upper jaw.

11. **Mandible** (man'di-bl) is the lower jawbone and is the largest and strongest bone of the face. It forms the lower jaw.

Bones Of The Neck

12. **Hyoid** (hi'oid) **bone,** a "U" shaped bone, is located in the front part of the throat, and is referred to as the "Adam's apple."

13. **Cervical vertebrae** (ser'vi-kal ver'te-bre) form the top part of the spinal column located in the neck region.

Bones Of The Chest (Thorax)

Thorax (tho'raks), or **chest,** is an elastic bony cage made up of the breast bone, the spine, the ribs, and connective cartilage. It serves as a protective covering for the heart, lungs, and other delicate internal organs. This framework is held in place by 24 ribs, 12 on each side.

Bones Of The Shoulder, Arm And Hand

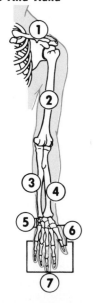

(Corresponding numbers can be found on the illustration.)

1. **Shoulder.** Each side of the shoulder is made up of one clavicle and one scapula, forming the back of the shoulder.

The following are the **bones in the arm:**

2. **Humerus** (hu'mer-us)—the largest bone of the upper arm.

3. **Ulna** (ul'nah)—the large bone on the little finger side of the forearm.

4. **Radius** (ra'de-us)—the small bone on the thumb side of the forearm.

5. The wrist, or **carpus** (kar'pus)—a flexible joint composed of eight small, irregular bones, held together by ligaments.

The hand is divided into two regions:

6. **The palm, or metacarpus (met-ah-kar'pus), consists of five long, slender bones, called metacarpal bones.**

7. The fingers, or **digits** (dij'its), consist of three phalanges (fah-lan'jez) in each finger, and two in the thumb, totaling 14 bones.

388

Bones Of The Skull

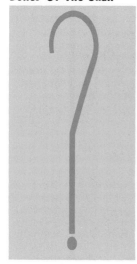

1. What is the hardest structure of the body?
2. List four functions of the bones.
3. Define "skull."
4. Into how many parts is the skull divided? Name them.
5. The cranium consists of how many bones?
6. List the skull bones affected by scalp massage.
7. Locate the occipital bone.
8. Locate the parietal bones.
9. Which bone forms the forehead?
10. What bones are located in the ear region?
11. Which bone joins together all the cranial bones?
12. How many bones are found in the face?
13. List the facial bones affected by facial massage.
14. What is formed by the maxillae?
15. Which bony structure is formed by the mandible?
16. Which bones form the prominence of the cheek?
17. Where is the hyoid bone located?
18. Locate the cervical vertebrae.
19. What is the bony chest cage called?

Bones Of The Arm And Hand

1. Name the two bones found in the shoulder.
2. Name the bones of the a) upper arm; and b) the two bones of the forearm.
3. How many bones are found in the a) wrist; b) palm; and c) fingers of the hand?
4. What is another name for the wrist bones?
5. What are the bones in the palm of the hand called?
6. What is the technical name for the fingers of the hand?
7. Define phalanges.

MUSCLES

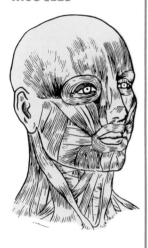

No outward sign of human life is more distinctive than that of **muscular** movement.

The **muscular system** covers, shapes and supports the skeleton. Its function is to produce all movements of the body.

The muscular system consists of over 500 muscles, large and small, comprising 40% to 50% of the weight of the human body.

Muscles are contractile fibrous tissue upon which the various movements of the body depend for their variety and action. The muscular system relies upon the skeletal and nervous systems for its activities.

The following are the three kinds of **muscular tissue: striated,** striped or voluntary, which are controlled by the will, such as those of the face, arms and legs; **non-striated,** smooth or involuntary, which function without the action of the **will,** such as those of the stomach and intestines; and the **cardiac,** or heart muscle, which is the heart itself, and is not duplicated anywhere else in the body.

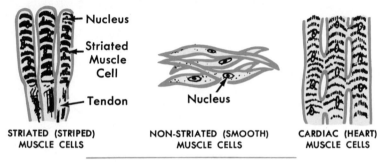

STRIATED (STRIPED) MUSCLE CELLS   NON-STRIATED (SMOOTH) MUSCLE CELLS   CARDIAC (HEART) MUSCLE CELLS

Origin And Insertion Of Muscles

When a muscle contracts and shortens, one of its attachments usually remains **fixed** and the other one **moves.**

Origin of a muscle is the term applied to the more **fixed** attachment, such as muscles attached to bones, or to some other muscle. Muscles attached to bones are usually referred to as **skeletal** muscles.

Insertion of a muscle is the term applied to the more **movable** attachment, such as muscles attached to a movable muscle, to a movable bone, or to the skin.

Stimulation Of Muscles

Muscular tissue may be stimulated by any of the following:
1. **Chemicals**—certain acids and salts
2. **Massage**—hand massage and vibrator
3. **Electric current**—high-frequency
4. **Light rays**—infra-red rays
5. **Heat rays**—heating lamps, and heating caps
6. **Moist heat**—steamers, or moderately warm steam towels
7. **Nerve impulses**—through the nervous system

Muscles Affected By Massage

The cosmetologist is concerned with the **voluntary muscles** of the head, face, neck, arms and hands. It is essential to know where these muscles are located, and what they control. The direction of pressure in massage is usually performed **from the insertion to the origin.**

The muscles are numbered to correspond with the muscles shown on the illustration.

Muscles Of The Scalp

1. **Epicranius** (ep-i-kra'ne-us), or **occipito-frontalis** (ok-sip'i-to fron-ta'lis), is a broad muscle that covers the top of the skull. It consists of two parts: 2. the **occipitalis** (ok-sip-i-ta'lis), or back part; and 3. the **frontalis** (fron-ta'lis), or front part. Both are connected by a tendon 4. **aponeurosis** (ap-o-nu-ro'sis). The frontalis raises the eyebrows, draws the scalp forward and causes wrinkles across the forehead.

Muscles Of The Eyebrows

5. **Orbicularis oculi** (or-bik-u-la'ris ok'u-li) completely surrounds the margin of the eyesocket and closes the eye.

6. **Corrugator** (kor'u-ga-tor) muscle is beneath the **frontalis** and **orbicularis occuli** and draws the eyebrows down and in. It produces vertical lines and causes frowning.

Muscles Of The Nose

7. The **procerus** (pro-se'rus) covers the top of the nose, depresses the eyebrow, and causes wrinkles across the bridge of the nose.

The other nasal muscles are small muscles around the nasal openings which contract and expand the opening of the nostrils.

Diagram Of The Muscles Of The Head, Face and Neck

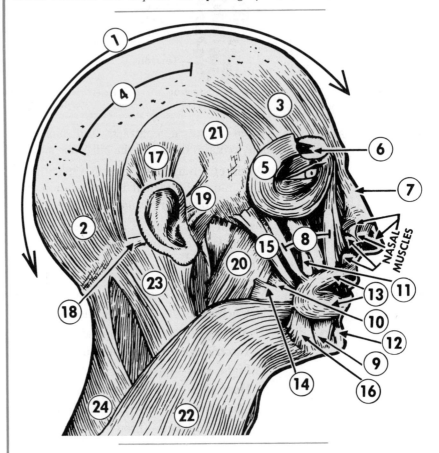

Muscles Of The Mouth

8. **Quadratus labii superioris** (kwod-ra'tus la'be-i su-pe-re-or'is) consists of three parts. It surrounds the upper part of the lip, raises and draws back the upper lip, and elevates the nostrils, as in expressing **distaste.**

9. **Quadratus labii inferioris** (in-fe-re-or'is) surrounds the lower part of the lip. It depresses the lower lip and draws it a little to one side, as in the expression of **sarcasm.**

10. **Buccinator** (buk'se-na-tor) is the muscle between the upper and lower jaws. It compresses the cheeks and expels air between the lips, as in **blowing.**

11. **Caninus** (ka-ni'nus) lies under the quadratus labii superioris. It raises the angle of the mouth, as in **snarling.**

12. **Mentalis** (men-ta'lis) is situated at the tip of the chin. It raises and pushes up the lower lip, causing wrinkling of the chin, as in **doubt** or **displeasure.**

13. **Orbicularis oris** (or-bik-u-la'ris o'ris) forms a flat band around the upper and lower lips. It compresses, contracts, puckers and wrinkles the lips, as in **kissing** or **whistling.**

14. **Risorius** (ri-so're-us) extends from the masseter muscle to the angle of the mouth. It draws the corner of the mouth out and back, as in **grinning.**

15. **Zygomaticus** (zi-go-mat'i-kus) extends from the zygomatic bone to the angle of the mouth. It elevates the lip, as in **laughing.**

16. **Triangularis** (tri-ang-gu-la'ris) extends along the side of the chin. It draws down the corner of the mouth.

Muscles Of The Ear

Three muscles of the ear are practically functionless:

17. **Auricularis** (au-rik-u-la'ris) **superior** is above the ear.

18. **Auricularis posterior** is behind the ear.

19. **Auricularis anterior** is in front of the ear.

Muscles Of Mastication

20. **Masseter** (mas-e'ter) and 21. **temporalis** (tem-po-ra'lis) are muscles that coordinate in opening and closing the mouth, and are referred to as **chewing** muscles.

Muscles Of The Neck

22. **Platysma** (plah-tiz'mah) is a broad muscle that extends from the chest and shoulder muscles to the side of the chin. It depresses the lower jaw and lip, as in the expression of **sadness.**

23. **Sterno-cleido-mastoid** (ster-no-kli'do-mas'toid) extends from the collar and chest bones to the temporal bone in back of the ear. It rotates the head and also bends the head, as in **nodding.**

Muscles That Attach Arm To Body

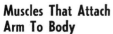

The principal muscles that attach the arms to the body and permit movements of the shoulders and arms are:

24. **Trapezius** (tra-pe'ze-us) and 25. **latissimus dorsi** (la-tis'e-mus dor'si) cover the back of the neck and upper and middle region of the back. They rotate the shoulder blade and control swinging movement of the arm.

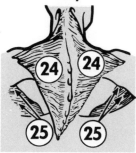

Pectoralis (pek-tor-al'is) **major** and **pectoralis minor** cover the front of the chest. They also assist in swinging movements of the arm.

Serratus anterior (se-ra'tus an-te're-or) assists in breathing and in raising the arm.

Muscles Of The Shoulder, Arm And Hand

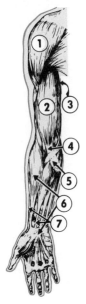

The principal muscles of the shoulder and upper arm are:

1. **Deltoid** (del'toid) is the large, thick, triangular shaped muscle that covers the shoulder, lifts and turns the arm.
2. **Biceps** (bi'seps) is the two-headed and principal muscle on the front of the upper arm. It lifts the forearm, flexes the elbow, and turns the palm downward.
3. **Triceps** (tri'seps) is the three-headed muscle of the arm which covers the entire back of the upper arm and extends the forearm forward.

The forearm is made up of a series of muscles and strong tendons. The cosmetologist is concerned with the following:

4. **Pronators** (pro-na'tors), the most important of the group, turn the hand inward, so that the palm faces downward.
5. **Supinators** (su-pi-na'tors) turn the hand outward and the palm upward.
6. **Flexors** (flek'sors) bend the wrist, draw the hand up, and close fingers toward the forearm.
7. **Extensors** (eks-ten'sors) straighten the wrist, hand and fingers to form a straight line.

The hand has many small muscles overlapping from joint to joint, imparting flexibility and strength. When the hands are properly cared for, these muscles will remain supple and graceful.

REVIEW QUESTIONS

Muscles

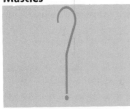

1. Define muscle.
2. What are the important functions of the muscles of the body?
3. Name three kinds of muscular tissue.
4. Distinguish between voluntary and involuntary muscles.
5. On which two systems of the body is the muscular system dependent for its activities?
6. Briefly define: a) origin of muscle; b) insertion of muscle.
7. Name seven sources capable of stimulating muscular tissue.

Muscles Of The Head, Face, Neck And Back

1. Locate the scalp muscle and name its two parts.
2. What is the function of the frontalis?
3. Which muscle surrounds the eye-socket?
4. Name the muscle of the eyebrow.
5. Which muscle forms a flat band around the upper and lower lips?
6. Which muscle covers the bridge of the nose?
7. Which muscles cover the back of the neck?
8. Which muscle depresses the lower jaw and lip?
9. Which muscle draws the head backwards or to one side?

Muscles Of The Arm And Hand

1. Name the three principal muscles of the upper arm and shoulder.
2. Name four types of muscles found in the forearm.
3. Distinguish between the functions of the pronator and supinator muscles.
4. Distinguish between the flexor and extensor muscles.

THE NERVOUS SYSTEM

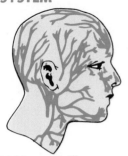

Divisions Of The Nervous System

Cerebro-Spinal Nervous System

Peripheral System

Sympathetic Nervous System

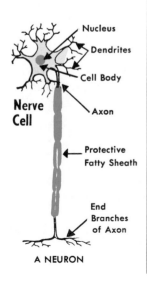

Nerve Cell

Nucleus
Dendrites
Cell Body
Axon
Protective Fatty Sheath
End Branches of Axon

A NEURON

The **nervous** (ner'vus) system is one of the most important systems of the body. It controls and coordinates the functions of all the other systems and makes them work harmoniously and efficiently. Every square inch of the human body is supplied with fine fibers which we know as **nerves.**

The **main purposes** in studying the nervous system are to understand:
1. How the cosmetologist administers scalp and facial services for the patron's benefit.
2. What effects these treatments have on the nerves in the skin and scalp, and on the body as a whole.

The principal parts that compose the nervous system are the brain, spinal cord and their nerves. Generally, the nervous system is composed of three main divisions:
1. The **cerebro-spinal** (ser-e'bro-spi'nal) or **central** nervous system
2. The **peripheral** (pe-rif'er-al) nervous system
3. The **sympathetic** (sym-pa-thet'ik) nervous system

The **cerebro-spinal nervous system** consists of the brain and spinal cord. The following are its functions:
1. Control consciousness and all mental activities
2. Control voluntary functions of the five senses, such as seeing, smelling, tasting, feeling and hearing
3. Control voluntary muscle actions, such as all body movements and facial expressions

The sensory and motor nerve fibers extend from the brain and spinal cord and are distributed to all parts of the body: they are referred to as the **peripheral** system. Their function is to carry messages to and from the central nervous system.

The **sympathetic nervous system** is related structurally to the cerebro-spinal (central) nervous system, but its functions are **independent** of the will. (Sympathetic nervous system is also referred to as the automatic nervous system, meaning self-control, by some anatomists.)

The sympathetic nervous system is **very important** in the operation of the internal body functions, such as breathing, circulation, digestion, and glandular activities. Its main purpose is to regulate these internal operations, keeping them in balance and working properly.

A **neuron** (nu'ron), or **nerve cell,** is the structural unit of the nervous system. It is composed of a **cell body** and long and short fibers called **cell processes** (pros'e-sez). The cell body stores energy and food for the cell processes, which convey the nerve impulses throughout the body. Practically all the nerve cells are contained in the brain and spinal cord.

Nerves are long, white cords made up of fibers (cell processes) that carry messages to and from various parts of the body. Nerves have their origin in the brain and spinal cord, and distribute branches to all parts of the body, which furnish both sensation and motion.

Types Of Nerves

Sensory nerves, called **afferent** (af'er-ent) **nerves,** carry impulses or messages from sense organs **to the brain,** where sensations of touch, cold, heat, sight, hearing, taste, smell and pain are experienced.

Motor nerves, called **efferent** (ef'er-ent) **nerves,** carry impulses **from the brain** to the muscles. The transmitted impulses produce movement.

Sensory nerves are situated **near the surface** of the skin. Motor nerves are **in the muscles.** As impulses pass from the sensory nerves to the brain and back over the motor nerves to the muscles, a complete circuit is established and movement of the muscle results.

Nerve Reflex

Nerve reflex (re'fleks) is the path traveled by a nerve impulse, through the spinal cord and brain, in response to a stimulus. (Example: the quick removal of the hand from a hot object.) A reflex act does not have to be learned.

The Brain

The **brain** is the largest mass of nerve tissue in the body and is contained in the cranium. The weight of the average brain is 44 to 48 ounces. It is considered to be the central power station of the body, sending and receiving telegraphic messages. Twelve pairs of cranial nerves originate in the brain and reach various parts of the head, face and neck.

The Spinal Cord

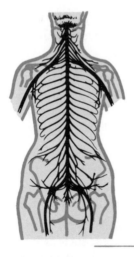

The **spinal cord** is composed of masses of nerve cells with fibers running upward and downward. It originates in the brain and extends down to the lower extremity of the trunk, and is enclosed and protected by the spinal column.

Thirty-one pairs of **spinal nerves,** extending from the spinal cord, are distributed to the muscles and skin of the trunk and limbs.

Some of the spinal nerves supply the internal organs controlled by the sympathetic nervous system.

Nerve Fatigue

Nerve fatigue can be caused by excessive mental or muscular work, resulting in an accumulation of waste products. Weariness, irritability, poor complexion, and dull eyes may be signs of nerve exhaustion.

The supply of **nerve energy** is dependent upon proper food, exercise and oxygen. Rest and relaxation are absolutely necessary to renew nerve energy.

Appropriate **massage manipulations** help to relieve nerve fatigue. When giving manipulations, the cosmetologist should always **pause** over nerve centers.

Nutrition

Nerves are nourished through blood vessels, lymph spaces, and lymphatics found in the connective tissue surrounding **them.**

Nerve Stimulation

Stimulation to the nerves causes muscles to **contract** and **expand**. **Heat** on the skin causes **relaxation; cold** causes **contraction**.

Nerve stimulation may be accomplished by any of the following:
1. Chemicals (certain acids or salts)
2. Massage (hand massage or electric vibrator)
3. Electrical current (high-frequency)
4. Light rays (infra-red)
5. Heat rays (heating lamps, and heating caps)
6. Moist heat (steamers or moderately warm steam towels)

CRANIAL NERVES

There are twelve pairs of cranial nerves, all connected to a part of the brain surface. They emerge through openings on the sides and base of the cranium and reach various parts of the head, face and neck. They are classified as motor, sensory and mixed nerves, containing both motor and sensory fibers.

The cranial nerves are named numerically, according to the order in which they arise from the brain, and also by names which describe their nature or function.

First—Olfactory (ol-fak′to-re) (sensory)—controls the sense of smell.

Second—Optic (op′tik) (sensory)—controls the sense of sight.

Third—Oculomotor (ok-u-lo-mo′tor) (motor)—controls the motion of the eye.

Fourth—Trochlear (trok′le-ar) (motor)—controls the motion of the eye.

Fifth—Trigeminal (tri-jem′i-nal) or **trifacial** (tri-fa′shal) (sensory-motor)—controls the sensations of the face, tongue and teeth.

Sixth—Abducent (ab-du′sent) (motor)—controls the motion of the eye.

Seventh—Facial (fa′shal) (sensory-motor)—controls motion of the face, scalp, neck, ear, and sections of the palate and tongue.

Eighth—Acoustic (ah-koos′tik) or **auditory** (aw′di-to-re) (sensory) —controls the sense of hearing.

Ninth—Glossopharyngeal (glos-o-fah-rin′je-al) (sensory-motor)— controls the sense of taste.

Tenth—Vagas (va′gus) or **pneumogastric** (nu-mo-gas′trik) sensory-motor)—controls motion and sensations of the ear, pharynx, larynx, heart, lungs, esophagus, etc.

Eleventh—Accessory (ak-ses′o-re) (motor)—controls the motion of neck muscles.

Twelfth—Hypoglossal (hi-po-glos′al) (motor)—controls the motion of the tongue.

NERVES OF INTEREST TO THE COSMETOLOGIST

The cranial nerves which are of interest to the cosmetologist in giving facial and scalp treatments are as follows:
Fifth cranial (trigeminal or trifacial)
Seventh cranial (facial)
Eleventh cranial (accessory)

Also of interest to the cosmetologist is the spinal (cervical) nerve, which originates in the spinal cord and is involved in scalp and neck massage.

Fifth Cranial Nerve

Fifth cranial, trifacial or **trigeminal** (tri-jem′i-nal) nerve is the largest of the cranial nerves. It is the chief sensory nerve of the face, and the motor nerve of the muscles of mastication.

The following are the important branches of the fifth cranial nerve that are affected by massage:

1. **Supra-orbital** (su′prah-or′bi-tal) **nerve** affects the skin of the forehead, scalp, eyebrows, and upper eyelids.
2. **Supra-trochlear** (su′prah-trok′le-ar) **nerve** affects the skin between the eyes and upper side of the nose.
3. **Infra-trochlear** (in′fra-trok′le-ar) **nerve** affects the membrane and skin of the nose.

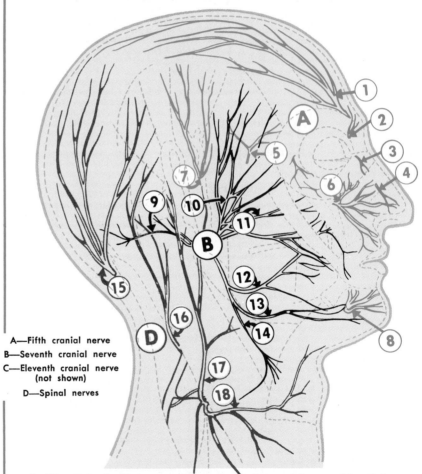

A—Fifth cranial nerve
B—Seventh cranial nerve
C—Eleventh cranial nerve
(not shown)
D—Spinal nerves

4. **Nasal** (na′zal) **nerve** affects the point and lower side of the nose.
5. **Zygomatic** (zi-go-mat′ik) **nerve** affects the skin of the temple, side of the forehead and upper part of the cheek.
6. **Infra-orbital** (in′frah-or′bi-tal) **nerve** affects the skin of the lower eyelid, side of the nose, upper lip and mouth.
7. **Auriculo-temporal** (aw-rik′u-lo tem′po-ral) **nerve** affects the external ear and skin above the temple, up to the top of skull.
8. **Mental** (men′tal) **nerve** affects the skin of the lower lip and chin.

Seventh Cranial Nerve

The **seventh cranial (facial) nerve** is the chief motor nerve of the face. It emerges near the lower part of the ear; its divisions and their branches supply and control all the muscles of facial expression, and extend to the muscles of the neck. Of all the branches of the facial nerve, the following are the most important:

9. **Posterior auricular** (pos-ter′ior aw-rik′u-lar) **nerve** affects the muscles behind the ear at the base of the skull.

10. **Temporal** (tem′po-ral) **nerve** affects the muscles of the temples, side of forehead, eyebrow, eyelid, and upper part of the cheek.

11. **Zygomatic** (zi-go-mat′ik) **nerve** (**upper and lower**) affects the muscles of the upper part of the cheek.

12. **Buccal** (buk′al) **nerve** affects the muscles of the mouth.

13. **Mandibular** (man-dib′ular) **nerve** affects the muscles of the chin and lower lip.

14. **Cervical** (ser′vi-cal) **nerve** (branch of the facial nerve) affects the side of the neck.

Eleventh Cranial Nerve

Eleventh (accessory) **cranial nerve** (spinal branch) affects the muscles of the neck and back (not shown on illustration).

Spinal (Cervical) Nerves

Spinal or cervical (ser′vi-cal) **nerves** originate at the spinal cord, and their branches supply the muscles and scalp at the back of the head and neck, as follows:

15. **Greater occipital** (ok-sip′i-tal) **nerve,** located in the back of the head, affects the scalp as far up as the top of the head.

16. **Smaller (lesser) occipital nerve,** located at base of the skull, affects the scalp and muscles of this region.

17. **Greater auricular** (aw-rik′u-lar) **nerve,** located at side of the neck, affects the external ear, and area in front and back of the ear.

18. **Cutaneous** (ku-ta′ne-us) **colli nerve,** located at side of the neck, affects the front and side of the neck as far down as the breastbone.

Nerves Of The Arm And Hand

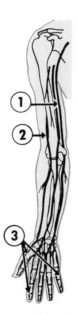

The principal nerves and their branches which supply the superficial parts of the arm and hand are:

1. **The ulnar** (ul′nar) **nerve** and its branches supply the little finger side of the arm, and the palm of the hand.

2. **The radial** (ra′de-al) **nerve** and its branches supply the thumb side of the arm, and the back of the hand.

3. **The digital** (dij′i-tal) **nerve** and its branches supply the fingers of the hand.

REVIEW QUESTIONS

The Nervous System

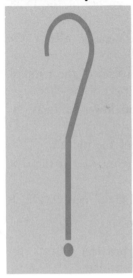

1. Give two reasons why the cosmetologist should study the nervous system.
2. What are the three principal parts that make up the nervous system?
3. Name the three main divisions of the nervous system.
4. Name the three main functions of the cerebro-spinal nervous system.
5. Explain the peripheral system and what its function is.
6. Name the main function of the sympathetic (automatic) nervous system.
7. What is a neuron?
8. What is a neuron, or nerve cell, composed of?
9. Define nerves.
10. Name two kinds of nerves which are found in the body.
11. What is the function of sensory nerves?
12. What is another name for a) sensory nerves; and b) motor nerves?
13. What is the function of motor nerves?
14. Give an example of nerve reflex.
15. What are three causes of nerve fatigue?
16. List six agents by which nerve stimulation may be accomplished.
17. How many pairs of cranial nerves are there? Spinal nerves?
18. Which three cranial nerves are the most important in the massaging of the head, face and neck?

Nerves Of The Head, Face And Neck

19. Which is the largest cranial nerve?
20. What is the function of the fifth or trifacial nerve?
21. Which cranial nerve controls the muscles of facial expression?
22. Which cranial nerve controls the sense of: a) sight; b) smell; c) hearing?
23. Which region of the head is supplied by the greater occipital nerve?
24. Which cranial nerve supplies the neck muscles?
25. Which branches of the trifacial nerve supply the following regions?
    a) forehead
    b) lower side of nose
    c) skin of upper lip
    d) skin of lower lip
    e) skin above temple
    f) skin of upper part of cheek
26. Which branches of the facial nerve supply the following regions or muscles?
    a) muscle of side of forehead
    b) muscle of chin and lower lip
    c) platysma muscle
    d) muscle behind ear
    e) mouth muscle
    f) muscles of upper part of cheek

Nerves Of The Arm And Hand

1. Name and locate the principal nerves of the arm and hand.
2. Which nerves supply the fingers?

THE CIRCULATORY SYSTEM

The **circulatory** (ser'ku-lah-to-re), or **vascular** (vas'ku-lar), **system** is vitally related to the maintenance of good health. Proper circulation is a beauty aid to the entire body, as well as to the skin, hair and nails.

The blood vascular system controls the circulation of the blood through the body in a steady stream by means of the **heart** and the blood vessels (the arteries, veins, and capillaries).

The Heart

The heart is an efficient pump. It keeps the blood moving within the circulatory system.

The heart is a muscular, conical-shaped organ, about the size of a closed fist. It is located in the chest cavity, and enclosed in a membrane, the **pericardium** (per-i-kar'de-um). The **vagus** (va'gus) and nerves from the **sympathetic nervous system** regulate the heartbeat. In a normal adult, the heart beats about 72 to 80 times a minute.

The interior of the heart contains four chambers and four valves. The upper thin-walled chambers are the **right atrium** (a'tre-um) and **left atrium.** The lower thick-walled chambers are the **right ventricle** (ven'tri-kl) and **left ventricle. Valves** allow the blood to flow in only one direction. With each contraction and relaxation of the heart, the blood flows in, travels from the **atria** (a'tre-ah) to the ventricles, and is then driven out, to be distributed all over the body. Atrium is also called **auricle** (aw'ri-kl).

Diagram Of The Heart

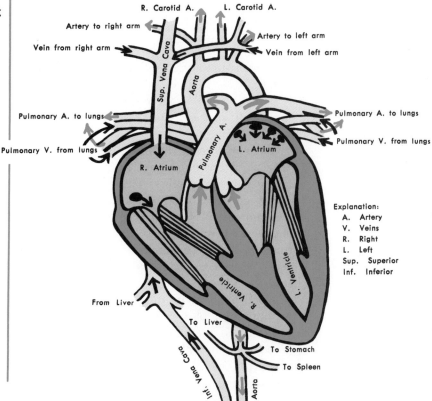

R. Carotid A.   L. Carotid A.

Artery to right arm

Vein from right arm

Sup. Vena Cava

Aorta

Pulmonary A. to lungs

Pulmonary V. from lungs

R. Atrium

Pulmonary A.

L. Atrium

Artery to left arm

Vein from left arm

Pulmonary A. to lungs

Pulmonary V. from lungs

From Liver

R. Ventricle

L. Ventricle

To Liver

To Stomach

To Spleen

Inf. Vena Cava

Aorta

Explanation:
A.   Artery
V.   Veins
R.   Right
L.   Left
Sup.   Superior
Inf.   Inferior

Blood Vessels

The arteries, capillaries and veins are tube-like in construction. They transport blood to and from the heart and to various tissues of the body.

Arteries (ar'ter-ez) are thick-walled muscular and elastic tubes that carry **pure** blood from the heart to the capillaries.

Capillaries (kap'i-la-rez) are minute, thin-walled blood vessels that connect the smaller arteries with the veins. Through their walls, the tissues receive nourishment and eliminate waste products.

Cross Section Of A Vein

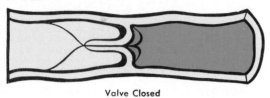

Valve Closed

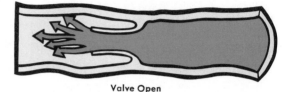

Valve Open

Veins are thin-walled blood vessels that are less elastic than arteries. They contain cup-like valves to prevent back-flow, and carry impure blood from the various capillaries back to the heart. Veins are located closer to the outer surface of the body than the arteries.

The Circulation Of The Blood

The blood is in constant circulation, from the moment it leaves until it returns to the heart. There are two systems that take care of this circulation:

1. **Pulmonary** (pul'mo-na-re) **circulation** is the blood circulation that goes from the heart to the lungs to be purified, and then returns to the heart.
2. **General circulation** is the blood circulation from the heart throughout the body and back again to the heart.

The Blood

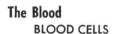

Red Corpuscles

White Corpuscles

Platelets

Blood is the nutritive fluid circulating through the blood circulatory system. It is a sticky, salty fluid, with a normal temperature that remains at 98.6° Fahrenheit, and it makes up about one-twentieth of the weight of the body. From eight to ten pints of blood fill the blood vessels of an adult.

Color of blood. The blood itself is bright red in color in the arteries (except in the pulmonary artery) and dark red in the veins (except in the pulmonary vein). This change in color is due to the gain or loss of oxygen as the blood passes through the lungs.

Composition of blood. The blood is composed of one-third cells (red and white corpuscles and blood platelets) and two-thirds plasma. The function of **red corpuscles** (red blood cells) is to carry oxygen to the cells. **White corpuscles** (white blood cells), or **leucocytes,** perform the function of destroying disease causing germs.

Blood platelets are much smaller than the red blood cells. They play an important part in the **clotting of the blood** over a wound.

Plasma is the fluid part of the blood in which the red and white blood cells and blood platelets flow. It is straw-like in color. About nine-tenths of the plasma is water, and it carries food and secretions to the cells, and carbon dioxide from the cells.

Chief Functions Of The Blood

The following are the primary functions of the blood:

1. Carry water, oxygen, food and secretions to all cells of the body.
2. Carry away carbon dioxide and waste products to be eliminated through the lungs, skin, kidneys and large intestine.
3. Help to equalize the body temperature, thus protecting the body from extreme heat and cold.
4. Aid in protecting the body from harmful bacteria and infections, through the action of the white blood cells.
5. Clot the blood, thereby closing injured minute blood vessels and preventing the loss of blood.

The Lymph-Vascular System

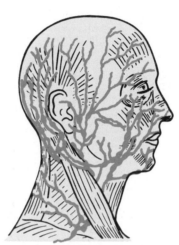

Lymph Nodes of the
Head, Face and Neck

The **lymph-vascular** (limf-vas'ku-lar) system, also called (lymphatic system), acts as an aid to the venous system, and consists of lymph spaces, lymph vessels, lymph glands and lacteals.

Lymph is a colorless, watery fluid that circulates through the lymphatic system and is derived from the plasma of the blood, mainly by filtration.

The lymph acts as a middleman between the blood and the tissues. It carries nourishment from the blood to the cells, and removes waste material from the cells.

ARTERIES OF THE HEAD, FACE AND NECK

The **common carotid** (kah-rot'id) **arteries** are the main sources of blood supply to the head, face and neck. They are located on either side of the neck and divide into internal and external carotid arteries. The **internal division** of the common carotid artery supplies the brain, eyesockets, eyelids and forehead; while the **external division** supplies the superficial parts of the head, face and neck.

The **external carotid artery** subdivides into a number of branches which supply blood to various regions of the head, face and neck. Of particular interest to the cosmetologist are the following arteries:

Facial Artery

A. **Facial artery (external maxillary)** (mak'si-ler-e) supplies the lower region of the face, mouth and nose. Some of its branches are:

1. **Submental** (sub-men'tal) **artery**, which supplies the chin and lower lip.
2. **Inferior labial** (la'be-al) **artery**, which supplies the lower lip.
3. **Angular** (ang'gu-lar) **artery**, which supplies side of nose.
4. **Superior labial artery**, which supplies the upper lip, septum of nose, and wing of nose.

**Diagram Of The
Arteries Of The Head,
Face And Neck**

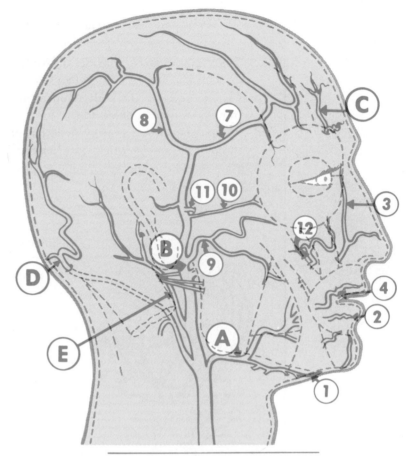

**Superficial Temporal
Artery**

B. **Superficial temporal** (tem′po-ral) **artery** is a continuation of the external carotid artery, which supplies muscles, skin and scalp to front, side and top of head. Some of its important branches are:

7. **Frontal** (frun′tal) **artery** supplies the forehead.

8. **Parietal** (pah-ri′e-tal) **artery** supplies the crown and side of head.

9. **Transverse** (trans-vers′) **facial artery** supplies the masseter.

10. **Middle temporal** (tem′por-al) **artery** supplies the temples.

11. **Anterior auricular** (aw-rik′u-lar) **artery** supplies the anterior part of the ear. (Not shown in illustration.)

Supra-Orbital Artery

C. The **supra-orbital** (su′prah-or′bi-tal) **artery**, branch of the internal carotid artery, supplies part of the forehead, the eyesocket, eyelid and upper muscles of the eye.

Infra-Orbital Artery

12. **Infra-orbital artery** originates from the internal maxillary artery, and it supplies the muscles of the eye.

Occipital Artery

D. **Occipital** (ok-sip′i-tal) **artery** supplies the back of the head, up to the crown.

**Posterior Auricular
Artery**

E. **Posterior auricular** (aw-rik′u-lar) **artery** supplies the scalp, back and above the ear and skin behind the ear.

Veins Of The Head, Face And Neck

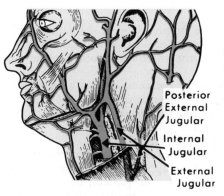

Posterior
External
Jugular

Internal
Jugular

External
Jugular

The blood returning to the heart from the head, face and neck flows on each side of the neck in two principal veins: the **internal jugular** and **external jugular**. The most important veins are parallel to the arteries and take the same names as the arteries.

Blood Supply For The Arm And Hand

The **ulnar** (ul'nar) and **radial** (ra'de-al) **arteries** are the main blood supply for the arm and hand. The **ulnar artery** and its numerous branches supply the little finger side of the arm and the palm of the hand. The **radial artery** and its branches supply the thumb side of the arm and the back of the hand.

Veins

The important veins are located almost parallel with the arteries and take the same names as the arteries. While the arteries are found deep in the tissues, the veins lie nearer to the surface of the arms and hands.

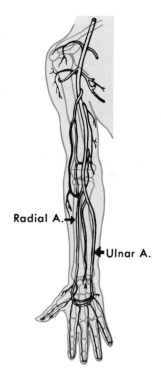

Radial A.→

←Ulnar A.

REVIEW QUESTIONS

Blood Circulation

1. Why is it necessary for the cosmetologist to understand the functions of the circulatory system?
2. What are the five important functions of the blood-vascular system?
3. What is the function of the heart?
4. Name three kinds of vessels found in the blood-vascular system.
5. Which blood vessels carry pure blood from the heart to the body?
6. Which blood vessels are nearest to the skin's surface?
7. What is the function of the veins?
8. Which two systems take care of blood circulation throughout the body?
9. What is the composition of blood?
10. What is the normal temperature of blood?
11. What is the composition of blood plasma?
12. What is the most important function of the red blood cells?
13. What is a function of the white blood cells?
14. What is lymph?
15. List the important functions of lymph.
16. From what source is the lymph derived?

Blood Vessels Of The Head, Face And Neck

1. Which main arteries supply blood to the entire head, face and neck?
2. Name two main divisions of the common carotid arteries.
3. Which branches of the common carotid arteries supply the cranial cavity?
4. Which branches of the common carotid arteries supply blood to the skin and muscles of the head and face?
5. Give the common name for the external maxillary artery.
6. Name the artery that supplies the chin.
7. Which artery supplies the forehead?
8. What part of the head does the occipital artery supply?
9. Name the arteries that supply the: a) upper lip; b) lower lip.
10. What part of the head does the parietal artery supply? Frontal artery?
11. Name two main branches of the superficial temporal artery.
12. What artery supplies that part of the scalp that is in back of and above the ear?
13. Name the artery that supplies the eye muscles.
14. Name the principal veins by which the blood from the head, face and neck is returned to the heart.

Blood Circulation Of Arms, Hands

1. Name the principal arteries supplying the arm and hand.
2. Which artery supplies the little finger side of the arm and palm of the hand?
3. Which artery supplies the thumb side of the arm?

GLANDS

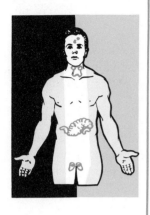

Glands are specialized organs which vary in size and function. The blood and nerves are intimately connected with the glands. The nervous system controls the functional activities of the glands. The glands have the ability to remove certain constituents from the blood and to convert them into new compounds.

There are two main sets of glands:

1. One group is called the **duct glands,** possessing canals which lead from the gland to a particular part of the body. Sweat and oil glands of the skin and intestinal glands belong to this group. Information on sweat and oil glands can be found in the chapter on **The Skin.**

2. The other group, known as **ductless glands,** has its secretions thrown directly into the bloodstream, which in turn influences the welfare of the entire body.

THE EXCRETORY SYSTEM

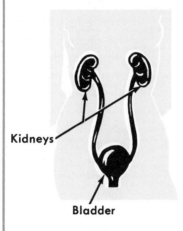

Kidneys

Bladder

The **excretory** (eks'kre-to-re) **system,** including the kidneys, liver, skin, intestines and lungs, purifies the body by the elimination of waste matter.

Each plays the following part in the excretory system:

1. The **kidneys** excrete urine.
2. The **liver** discharges bile pigments.
3. The **skin** eliminates perspiration.
4. The **large intestine** (in-tes'tin) evacuates decomposed and undigested food.
5. The **lungs** exhale carbon dioxide (di-ok'sid).

Metabolism of the cells of the body forms various toxic substances which, if retained, would have a tendency to poison the body.

THE RESPIRATORY SYSTEM

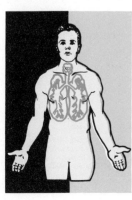

The **respiratory** (re-spir'ah-to-re) **system** is situated within the chest cavity, which is protected on both sides by the ribs. The diaphragm (di'ah-fram), a muscular partition which controls breathing, separates the chest from the abdominal (ab-dom'i-nal) regions.

The **lungs** are spongy tissues composed of microscopic cells into which the inhaled air penetrates. These tiny air cells are enclosed in a skin-like tissue. Behind this, the fine capillaries of the blood vascular system are found.

With each **respiratory** cycle, an exchange of gases takes place. During inhalation (in-ha-la'shun), oxygen is absorbed into the blood, while carbon dioxide is expelled during exhalation (eks-ha-la'shun). Oxygen is required to change food into energy.

Oxygen is more essential than either food or water. Although a man or woman may live more than sixty days without food, and a few days without water, if air is excluded for a few minutes, death ensues.

Nose breathing is healthier than mouth breathing because the air is warmed by the surface capillaries, and the bacteria in the air are caught by the hairs which line the mucous (mu'cus) membranes of the nasal passages.

Breathing is necessary to carry on the life functions. The rate of breathing depends upon the activity of the individual. Muscular activities and energy expenditures increase the body's demands for oxygen. As a result, the rate of breathing is increased. A person requires about three times as much oxygen when walking than when standing.

Abdominal breathing is of value in building health. **Costal breathing** involves light, or shallow, breathing of the lungs, without action of the diaphragm. Abdominal breathing means deep breathing, which brings the diaphragm into action. The greatest exchange of gases is accomplished with abdominal breathing.

THE DIGESTIVE SYSTEM

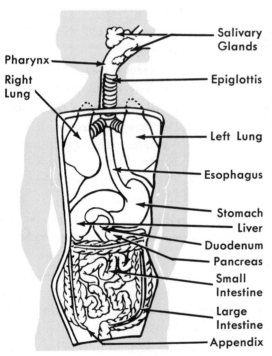

Pharynx

Right Lung

Salivary Glands

Epiglottis

Left Lung

Esophagus

Stomach
Liver
Duodenum
Pancreas
Small Intestine
Large Intestine
Appendix

Diagram illustrating the Human Alimentary Canal with its Principal Digestive Glands.

The **digestive** (di-ges'tiv) **system** changes food into soluble (sol'yu-bl) form, suitable for use by the cells of the body. Digestion is started in the mouth and completed in the small intestine (in-testin). From the mouth, the food passes down the pharynx (far'inks) and the esophagus (e-sof'ah-gus), or food pipe, and into the stomach. The food is completely digested in the small intestine. The large intestine (colon) stores the refuse for elimination through the rectum. The complete digestive process of food takes about nine hours.

Digestion is the process of converting food into a form which can be assimilated by the body. Responsible for the chemical changes in food are the enzymes (en'zymz) present in the digestive secretions. **Digestive enzymes** are chemicals which change certain kinds of food into a form capable of being used by the body.

Intense emotions, excitement and fatigue, seriously disturb digestion. On the other hand, happiness and relaxation promote good digestion

REVIEW QUESTIONS

1. What two main types of glands are there in the human body?
2. Name the important organs of the excretory system.
3. Describe a respiratory cycle.
4. Name the important organs of the digestive system.

CHAPTER 29

ELECTRICITY AND LIGHT THERAPY

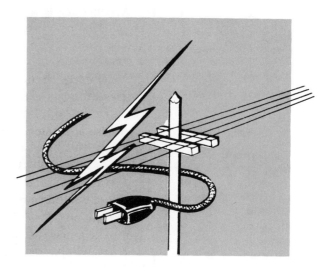

ELECTRICITY

The beneficial effects of electrical energy have long been recognized to be of value in the practice of cosmetology. Electricity can be a valuable tool, provided it is used intelligently and carefully. It can be used for the benefit of both the cosmetologist and the patron by supplying light, heat and the power to operate electrical appliances. As a result of the careful use of electric power, a considerable amount of time and energy can be saved, and the effectiveness of beauty treatments, considerably improved.

Although the exact nature of electricity is not yet completely understood, its generating sources and effects are known. It is generally believed that electricity is a form of energy which produces **magnetic, chemical** or **heating** effects.

A **current of electricity** is a stream of **electrons** (negatively charged particles) moving along a conductor.

An **electric wire** is composed of twisted fine metal threads (conductors) covered with rubber or silk (insulator or non-conductor).

A **conductor** is a substance which readily transmits an electric current. Most metals, carbon, the human body and watery solutions of acids and salts are good conductors of electricity.

Electrodes, special terminal devices, serve as points of contact when electricity is applied to the body.

A **non-conductor, or insulator,** is a substance that resists the passage of an electric current, such as rubber, silk, dry wood, glass, cement or asbestos.

FORMS OF ELECTRICITY

d.c.   +

a.c.

Two forms of electricity are employed, namely:

1. **Direct current (d.c.)** is a constant and even-flowing current, traveling in one direction.
2. **Alternating current (a.c.)** is a rapid and interrupted current, flowing first in one direction and then in the opposite direction.

A **converter** is an apparatus used to change a direct current into an alternating current. A **rectifier** is used to change an alternating current into a direct current. This is required to generate galvanism, a constant current of electricity, the action of which is chemical.

A **complete circuit of electricity** is the entire path traveled by the current from its generating source through various conductors (wire, electrode or body) and back to its original source.

A **fuse** is a safety device which prevents the overheating of electric wires. It will blow out when a line is overloaded (too many connections) or when a short circuit is present.

CAUTION: To reestablish the circuit, disconnect apparatus before inserting a new fuse.

Precaution—When replacing a blown fuse make sure to:

1. Use a new fuse with proper rating.
2. Stand on a dry surface.
3. Keep hands dry.

If an electrical appliance goes out of order while in operation, pull out plug and, if necessary, call an electrician.

ELECTRICAL MEASUREMENTS

Electrical measurements are expressed in terms of the following units:

The **volt** is a unit of electrical **pressure.**

The **ampere** is a unit of electrical **strength.**

The **ohm** is a unit of electrical **resistance.**

An electrical current flows through a conductor when the **pressure** is sufficiently great to overcome the resistance offered by the wire to the passage of the current.

Instead of the ampere, which is too strong, the **milliampere,** 1/1000th part of an ampere, is used for facial and scalp treatments. The **milliamperemeter** is an instrument for measuring the rate of flow of an electric current.

HIGH-FREQUENCY CURRENT

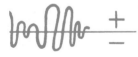

The high-frequency current is of primary interest to the cosmetologist since it is most commonly used in the beauty salon.

The high-frequency current is characterized by a high rate of vibration.

Of chief interest to the cosmetologist is the **Tesla current,** commonly called the "violet ray," used for both scalp and facial treatments.

The primary action of this current is thermal, or heat-producing. Because of its rapid vibrations, there are no muscular contractions. The physiological effects are either stimulating or soothing, depending on the method of application.

The electrodes for applying high-frequency are made of glass or metal. Their shapes vary, the facial electrode being flat and the scalp electrode being rake-shaped. As the current passes through the glass electrode, tiny violet sparks are emitted. All high-frequency treatments given should be started with a mild current and gradually increased to the required strength. The length of the treatment depends on the condition to be treated. For a general facial or scalp treatment, about five minutes should be allowed.

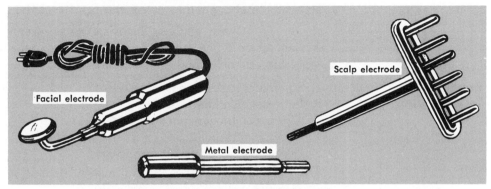

Facial electrode

Scalp electrode

Metal electrode

Methods Of Application

For proper use, follow the instructions provided by the manufacturer of Tesla equipment.

There are three methods of using the Tesla current:

Direct

1. **Direct surface application.** The cosmetologist holds the electrode and applies it over the patron's skin. In facial treatments, the electrode is applied directly over facial cream which has been previously applied.

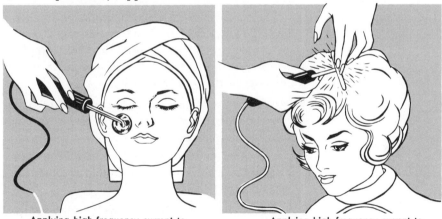

Applying high-frequency current to face using facial electrode

Applying high-frequency current to scalp using rake electrode

Indirect

2. **Indirect application.** The patron holds the metal or glass electrode, while the cosmetologist uses her fingers to massage the surface being treated. At no time is the electrode held by the cosmetologist. To prevent shock, the current is turned on after the patron has the electrode firmly in her hand; current is turned off before removing the electrode from the patron's hand.

CAUTION. Avoid contact by the patron with any metal, such as chair arms and stools. A burn may occur if such contact is made.

General Electrification

3. **General electrification.** By holding a metal electrode in her hand, the patron's body is charged with electricity without being touched by the cosmetologist.

Soothing And Stimulating Effects

To obtain sedative, calming or soothing effects with high-frequency current, the general electrification treatment is used, or the electrode is kept in close contact with the areas treated by the use of direct surface application.

To obtain a stimulating effect, lift the electrode slightly from the area to be treated and apply the current through the clothing or a towel.

CAUTION. When applying high-frequency current along with skin and scalp lotions **containing an alcoholic content,** you **must** apply the electricity **first,** and then the lotion.

Benefits Of Tesla High-Frequency

1. Stimulates circulation of the blood.
2. Increases glandular activity.
3. Aids in elimination and absorption.
4. Increases metabolism.
5. Germicidal action occurs during use.

The Tesla current may be used to treat falling hair, itchy scalp, tight scalp, excessively oily or dry skin and scalp.

ELECTRICAL EQUIPMENT

The **protection** and **safety** of the patron are the primary concern of the cosmetologist. All electrical equipment should be regularly inspected to determine whether they are in safe working condition. Carelessness in making electrical connections and in applying various types of currents may result in shock or burns. Observing safety precautions will help to eliminate accidents and assure greater satisfaction to the patrons.

The Vibrator

The vibrator is an electric appliance used in massage to produce a mechanical succession of manipulations. It has a stimulating effect on the muscular tissues, increases the blood supply to the areas treated, is soothing to the nerves, increases glandular activities, and stimulates the functions of the skin and scalp.

CAUTION. The vibrator should never be used when there is a pronounced weakness of the heart, or in cases of fever, abscesses or inflammation.

The vibrator may be used by attaching it to the back of the hand. The vibrations are thus transmitted through the hand or fingers to the areas being treated.

The vibrator is used over heavy muscular tissue, such as the scalp, shoulders and upper back. It is never used on a woman's face, but is used on a man's face.

Steamer Or Vaporizer

The steamer, or vaporizer, is electrical equipment that is applied over the head or face to produce a moist, uniform heat.

The **steamer** may be used instead of hot towels to cleanse and steam the face. The steam warms the skin, inducing the flow of both oil and sweat. It thus helps to cleanse the skin, clean out the pores, and soften any scaliness on the surface of the skin.

The **steamer** may also be used for scalp and hair reconditioning treatments. When fitted over the scalp, it produces controlled moist heat. Its action is to soften the scalp, increase the perspiration and promote the effectiveness of applied scalp cosmetics.

Another use for the steamer is to speed up the action of a lightener.

Thermal Curling Irons

Electrically heated curling irons come in various types and sizes. They have built-in heating elements and operate from electrical outlets. One type has perforations. Oil is injected into the barrel of the curling iron where it is vaporized. The vapor leaves the iron through small perforations to condition the hair as it curls.

Heating Cap

Heating caps are electrical devices, applied over the head, which provide a uniform source of heat. Their main use is as part of corrective treatments for the hair and scalp. When used for this purpose, they recondition dry, brittle and damaged hair, and also serve to activate a sluggish scalp.

Processing Machine

The accelerator machines, called by various names, have been designed as an aid to the professional hair colorist.

Their function is to reduce the processing time for lightening and tinting the hair. The processing time is reduced because the machine accelerates the molecular movement within the chemicals so that they work much faster.

Accelerating machines may be used efficiently and successfully for various hair coloring treatments, such as hair lightening, tinting, frosting, tipping, streaking and stripping. Accelerating machines must not be used over powdered lighteners.

Electric Hair Dryer

The electric hair dryer delivers hot, medium or cold air for the proper drying of the hair. It consists of an adjustable hood or helmet, with deflectors which distribute the air evenly, and is capable of drying heavy hair in a comparatively short time.

Electric Oil Heater

The small electric oil heater is used to heat oil and to keep the oil warm when giving an oil manicure.

SAFETY PRECAUTIONS

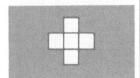

1. Disconnect appliances when finished using them.
2. Study instructions before using any electrical equipment.
3. Keep all wires, plugs, and equipment in a good condition.
4. Inspect all electrical equipment frequently.
5. Avoid wetting electric cords.
6. Sanitize all electrodes properly.
7. Protect the patron at all times.
8. Do not touch any metal while using any electrical apparatus.
9. Do not handle electric equipment with wet hands.
10. Do not allow patron to touch any metal surfaces when electric treatments are being given.
11. Do not leave room when patron is attached to any electric device.
12. Do not attempt to clean around an electric outlet when equipment is plugged in.
13. Do not touch two metallic objects at the same time while connected to an electric current.
14. Do not use any electric equipment without first obtaining full instruction for its care and use.

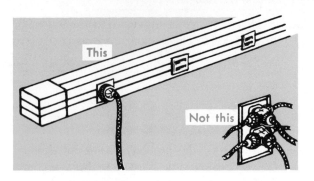

Use only one plug to each outlet. Overloading may cause fuse to blow out.

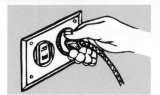

To disconnect current, remove plug without pulling cord. Never pull on cord, as the wires may become loosened and cause a short circuit.

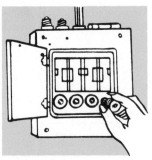

When replacing a blown-out fuse, make sure to:
1. Use new fuse with proper rating.
2. Stand on a dry surface.
3. Keep hands dry.

WARNING

Keep a flashlight at top of steps, so you won't stumble down a dark stairway. Using your flashlight, open fuse box and examine each fuse to locate "dead" one. When you replace a burned-out fuse, touch only its rim. Never put a coin in the fuse box instead of a fuse.

Be sure to have some good fuses on hand. To test a fuse, use a flashlight battery, and bulb (or the bulb assembly), and a piece of wire — as shown at right. If fuse is good, bulb will light.

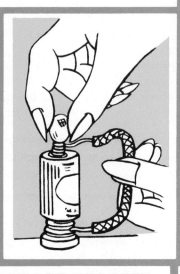

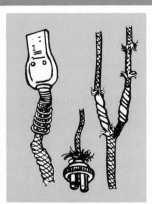

Examine cords regularly. Repair or replace worn cords to prevent short circuit, shock or fire.

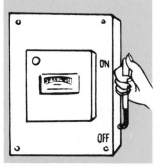

In an emergency, turn off main switch, as illustrated, to shut off electricity for entire salon or building.

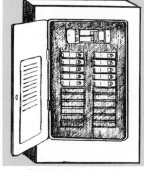

CIRCUIT-BREAKER

The circuit-breaker automatically disconnects any current with a defective appliance. It has the great advantage of restoring the current by a flick of the breaker switch to its "ON" position.

This is very important in the beauty salon by minimizing the possibility of long interruptions in the supply of electricity.

REVIEW QUESTIONS

Electricity

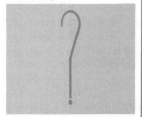

1. What is the nature of electricity?
2. What is a conductor?
3. What is a non-conductor or insulator? Give six examples.
4. What are electrodes?
5. What is a direct current (d.c.)?
6. What is an alternating current (a.c.)?
7. Which apparatus changes a direct current into an alternating current?
8. Which apparatus changes an alternating current to a direct current?
9. What is a volt?
10. What is an ampere?
11. What is an ohm?

High-Frequency Current

1. What is a high-frequency current?
2. Which type of high-frequency current is commonly used in the beauty salon?
3. What effects does the Tesla current produce on the body?
4. Name three kinds of electrodes used with high-frequency current.
5. Name three methods of applying the Tesla current.
6. Briefly describe how to use direct surface application.
7. Briefly describe how to use indirect application.
8. Briefly describe how to use general electrification.
9. Which method of application produces soothing results?
10. How are stimulating effects produced?
11. How long should a general facial or scalp treatment last?
12. What safety precaution should be observed in using hair tonics having a high alcoholic content?
13. List five benefits obtained by using the Tesla current.
14. List five scalp conditions which may be treated with the Tesla current.

Vibrator

1. What is a vibrator?
2. Under what conditions should a vibrator never be used?
3. Over which areas of the body is the vibrator used?

Steamer

1. How is a steamer, or vaporizer, used?
2. What are the effects produced by the steamer when used over the face?
3. What are the effects produced by the steamer when used over the scalp?

Thermal Curling Irons

1. What type of heating element does an electrically heated curling iron have?
2. How does vapor from a curling iron benefit the hair?

Heating Cap

1. What are heating caps?
2. What is their main use?
3. How do heating caps aid in corrective scalp and hair treatments?

Processing Machine

1. What is the function of a processing machine?
2. How does it reduce processing time?

LIGHT THERAPY

Light therapy (the′ra-pe) refers to treatment by means of light rays. Light or electrical waves travel at a tremendous speed — 186,000 miles per second.

There are many kinds of light rays, but in salon work we are concerned with only three — those producing heat, known as infra-red rays; those producing chemical and germicidal reaction, known as ultra-violet rays; and visible lights, all of which are contained within the spectrum of the sun.

If a ray of sunshine is passed through a glass prism (priz′m), it will appear in seven different colors, known as the **rainbow**, arrayed in the following manner: red, orange, yellow, green, blue, indigo and violet. These colors, which are visible to the eye, constitute the **visible rays**, comprising about 12% of sunshine.

Scientists have discovered that at either end of the visible spectrum are rays of the sun which are **invisible** to us. The rays beyond the violet are the **ultra-violet rays**, also known as **actinic** (ak-tin′ik) **rays**. These rays are the shortest and least penetrating rays of the spectrum, comprising about 8% of sunshine. The action of these rays is both chemical and germicidal (jur-mi-si′dal).

Beyond the red rays of the spectrum are the **infra-red rays**. These are pure heat rays, comprising about 80% of sunshine.

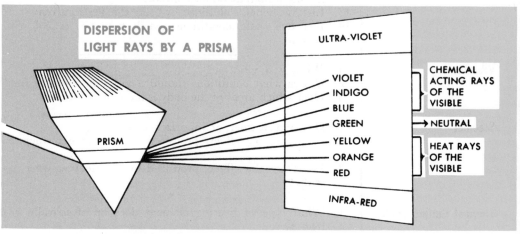

DISPERSION OF LIGHT RAYS BY A PRISM

Ultra-Violet Rays			Solar Spectrum	Infra-Red Rays
1847 AU to 3900 AU			3900 AU to 7700 AU	7700 AU to 14,000 AU
Far 1847-2200	Middle 2200-2900	Near 2900-3900	Violet Indigo Blue Green Yellow Orange Red	Penetrating
Germicidal	Therapeutic	Tonic		Analgesic
Cold Invisible Rays			Visible Rays	Invisible Heat Rays

NATURAL SUNSHINE IS COMPOSED OF:
   8% ultra-violet rays; 12% visible light rays; 80% infra-red rays.

PROPERTIES OF INFRA-RED RAYS:
   1. Long wave length
   2. Low frequency
   3. Deep penetrating power

PROPERTIES OF ULTRA-VIOLET RAYS:
   1. Short wave length
   2. High frequency
   3. Weak penetrating power

A **therapeutic lamp** (the-ra-pu′tik) is an electrical apparatus capable of producing certain light rays. There are separate lamps for infra-red and for ultra-violet rays.

Ultra-violet lamps (ul′trah-vi′o-let). There are three general types: The glass bulb, the hot quartz (kworts) and the cold quartz.

The **glass bulb lamp** is used mainly for cosmetic or tanning purposes.

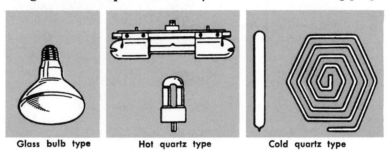

Glass bulb type   Hot quartz type   Cold quartz type

The **hot quartz lamp** is a general all-purpose lamp suitable for tanning, health, cosmetic or germicidal purposes.

The **cold quartz lamp** produces mostly short ultra-violet rays. It is used primarily in hospitals.

Infra-red (in′frah-red) **rays** give no light whatsoever, only a rosy glow when active. Special glass bulbs are also used to produce infra-red rays.

The **visible rays,** or **dermal lights**, are reproduced by carbon or tungsten filament in clear glass bulbs. They produce white light, or in colored bulbs, red or blue colors.

Protecting the eyes. The patron's eyes should always be protected with cotton pads, saturated with a boric acid or witch hazel solution, placed on the eyelids during light ray treatments. The cosmetologist and patron should always wear safety eye goggles when using ultra-violet rays.

ULTRA-VIOLET RAYS

Ultra-violet rays are invisible rays. Their action is both chemical and germicidal. Plant and animal life need ultra-violet rays for healthy growth. In the human body, these rays produce changes in the chemistry of the blood and also stimulate the activity of body cells.

Effects Of Rays

Ultra-violet rays increase resistance to disease by increasing the iron and vitamin D content and the number of red and white cells in the blood. They also increase elimination of waste products, restore nutrition where needed, stimulate the circulation, and improve the flow of blood and lymph (limf).

The slightest obstruction of any kind will hinder ultra-violet rays from reaching the skin. Consequently, the skin must be entirely cleansed before being subjected to ultra-violet rays.

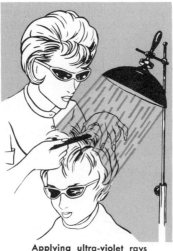

Applying ultra-violet rays to scalp

How applied. Ultra-violet rays are the shortest light rays of the spectrum. The farther they are from the visible light region, the shorter they become. The longer ultra-violet rays tend to increase the fixation of calcium in the blood. If the lamp is placed from 30 to 36 inches away, few of the shorter rays will reach the skin, so that the action is then limited to the effect of the longer rays.

The shorter rays are obtained when the lamp is within twelve inches from the skin. These rays are not only destructive to bacteria, but to tissue as well, if allowed to remain exposed for too long a period of time.

Average exposure may produce redness of the skin, and overdoses may cause blistering. It is well to start with a short exposure of two or three minutes, and gradually increase the time to seven or eight minutes. **The cosmetologist and patron must wear eye goggles to protect their eyes.**

Skin tanning is the result of exposure to ultra-violet rays, which stimulate the production of pigment, or coloring matter, in the skin.

Sunburn may be produced by ultra-violet rays in various degrees; however, for cosmetic purposes, a first degree sunburn only is given. This is manifested by a slight reddening, appearing several hours after application, showing no signs of itching, burning or peeling. Overexposure produces third and fourth degree burns, which are destructive to the tissues.

Skin and scalp disorders. Ultra-violet rays are used for acne, tinea, seborrhea and to combat dandruff. They also promote healing, as well as stimulate the growth of hair.

INFRA-RED RAYS

Generally speaking, infra-red rays produce a soothing and beneficial type of heat, which penetrates for some distance into the tissues of the body.

Use and effect of infra-red rays on exposed area:

1. Heats and relaxes the skin without increasing temperature of the body as a whole.
2. Dilates blood vessels in the skin, thereby increasing blood flow.
3. Increases metabolism and chemical changes within skin tissues.
4. Increases the production of perspiration and oil on the skin.
5. Relieves pain.

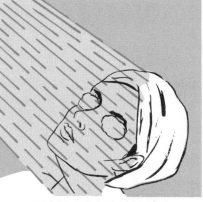

Applying infra-red rays to face

How To Apply Infra-Red Rays

The lamp is operated at an average distance of thirty inches. It is placed closer at the start, and to avoid the burning of the skin, it is then moved back gradually as the surface heat becomes more pronounced. **Always protect the eyes of the patron during exposure.** Place cotton pads saturated with boric acid or witch hazel solution over patron's eyelids.

> CAUTION. Do not permit the light rays to remain on body tissue more than a few seconds at a time. Move the hand back and forth across the ray's path to break constant exposure. Length of exposure should be about five minutes.

VISIBLE LIGHTS

The **lamp** used to reproduce visible lights is usually a dome-shaped reflector mounted on a pedestal with a flexible neck. The dome is finished with a highly polished metal lining capable of reflecting heat rays. The bulbs used with this lamp are available in white, red or blue.

Visible lights are used primarily in connection with facial and scalp treatments.

As with all other lamps, the patron's eyes must be protected from the glare and heat of the light. For proper eye protection, the patron's eyes are covered with cotton pads saturated with boric acid or witch hazel solution.

White Light

Use and effect of the white light:
1. Relieves pain, especially in congested areas; more particularly, around the nerve centers, such as the back of the neck and across the shoulders.

Blue Light

Use and effect of the blue light:
1. Has a tonic effect on the bare skin.
2. Is deficient in heat rays.
3. Has a soothing effect on the nerves.
4. To obtain the desired result, it is always used over the **bare skin.** Creams, oils, or powders must not be present on the skin.

Red Light

Use and effect of the red light:
1. Has strong heat rays.
2. Has a stimulating effect when used over the skin.
3. Penetrates more deeply than the blue light.
4. Heat rays aid the penetration of cosmetic creams into the skin.
5. Recommended for dry, scaly, and shriveled skin.
6. Used over creams and ointments to soften and relax tissue.

Light Therapy

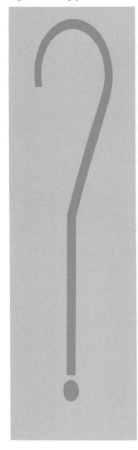

1. What is light therapy?
2. Which rays of the sun are invisible?
3. What is a therapeutic lamp?
4. Name three types of therapeutic lamps which produce ultra-violet rays.
5. Which ultra-violet lamps are desirable for the beauty salon?
6. Which four blood constituents are increased by exposure to ultra-violet rays?
7. What effects do ultra-violet rays have on the body functions?
8. Which skin and scalp disorders are helped by ultra-violet rays?
9. What benefit does the hair receive from ultra-violet rays?
10. What is the shortest distance the ultra-violet lamp should be kept from the skin?
11. Why should the eyes of both patron and cosmetologist be covered with goggles during exposure to ultra-violet rays?
12. How long should the skin be exposed for the first time?
13. To how many minutes can exposure be gradually increased?
14. Why should prolonged exposure be avoided?
15. What are the signs of first degree sunburn?
16. What causes the skin to tan?
17. Why should the skin be clean before exposure to ultra-violet rays?
18. Which types of therapeutic lamps produce infra-red rays?
19. How should the patron's eyes be protected during exposure?
20. How far should the infra-red lamp be kept from the skin?
21. Why should infra-red light rays be broken with a hand movement?
22. What are the five effects of infra-red rays on the body?
23. Which types of therapeutic lamps produce visible lights?
24. Why should the patron's eyes be protected during exposure?
25. What are the benefits of using a white light?
26. Which visible light lacks heat rays?
27. What are the benefits of using a blue light?
28. What are the three benefits of using a red light?

CHAPTER 30

CHEMISTRY

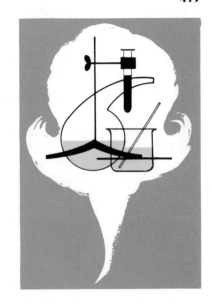

INTRODUCTION

The professional cosmetologist must be a many-sided individual. At various times she must act as a hairstylist, a psychologist, a business executive, an employee, a chemist, and an expert in all phases of cosmetology.

A basic knowledge of modern chemistry is an essential requirement for an intelligent understanding of the proper usage of the various chemicals and cosmetics in the beauty salon.

As a result of continuous study and research in chemistry, new products are constantly being developed for the benefit of both the cosmetologist and the patron. It is important that the professional cosmetologist understands these products and learns how to use them so that the patron will receive the maximum benefits.

CHEMISTRY DEFINITION

Chemistry is the science which deals with the composition, structure and properties of **matter,** and how matter changes under different chemical conditions.

In this chapter, the student will be introduced to some of the more fundamental aspects of chemistry. The subject will be presented in two forms: **organic** and **inorganic** chemistry. The student will also learn the nature of matter and its forms. This entire chapter will lay the foundation for a better understanding of the products with which cosmetologists work.

ORGANIC CHEMISTRY

Organic chemistry is the study of all substances in which **carbon** is present. Carbon can be found in all plants and animals, as well as in petroleum, soft coal, natural gas, and in many artificially prepared substances.

Most organic substances will burn. They are soluble in organic solvents, such as alcohol and benzene. They are not soluble in water.

Organic substances are slow in their chemical reactions. Examples of organic substances are grass, trees, gasoline, oil, soaps, detergents, plastics, antibiotics.

INORGANIC CHEMISTRY

Inorganic chemistry is the study of all substances that do **not** contain carbon, including all the elements.

Inorganic substances are soluble in water. Most of them will **not** burn.

Inorganic substances are quick in their chemical reactions. Examples of inorganic substances are water, air, iron, lead, iodine.

MATTER

Matter may be defined as anything that occupies space. It exists in three physical forms: solids, liquids and gases.

Look around the classroom and note what you see: hair, students, teachers, desks, chairs, walls. These items are matter in the solid state.

In the clinic area, you see water, shampoo, permanent waving lotion, setting lotion. These are matter in the liquid state.

Take a deep breath. The air you have just brought into your lungs is also matter. It is in its gaseous state.

STRUCTURE OF MATTER

Since it is not our purpose to graduate atomic physicists, but to help cosmetology students learn enough about matter to help them in their professional work, we will take just a quick look at the structure of matter.

Atoms

An atom is the smallest part of an element that possesses the characteristics of the **element.** Therefore, an atom of hydrogen has the properties of hydrogen. Should this atom be smashed, it would no longer possess the properties of hydrogen, nor would it resemble a hydrogen atom.

Molecules

A molecule is the smallest particle of an element or compound that possesses all the properties of the element or compound. If the molecule is of an element, the atoms are the same. If it is of a compound, the atoms are different. For example, a molecule of hydrogen contains two or more atoms of hydrogen, whereas a molecule of the compound of water is composed of two atoms of hydrogen and one atom of oxygen (H_2O).

Chemical Activities

In general, when we talk about the chemical activity of an element, we refer to the tendency of its atoms to combine with other elements. For example, hydrogen is a very active element and readily combines with other elements, while neon is completely inactive and does not combine with other elements.

TYPES OF MATTER

Matter exists in an almost infinite variety. This variety is made possible due to the atomic structure of matter, which permits the joining of a number of elements in countless combinations.

Matter exists in the form of elements, compounds and mixtures.

Elements

An element is the basic unit of all matter. It is a substance that **cannot** be made by the combination of simpler substances, and the element itself cannot be reduced to simpler substances. There are now 103 elements that are known, of which some of the more common are iron, sulphur, oxygen, zinc and silver.

Each element is given a letter symbol. Iron is Fe; sulphur, S; oxygen, O; zinc, Zn; and silver, Ag. All symbols can be obtained by referring to a chart of elements.

Compounds

When two or more elements unite chemically, they form a compound. Each element loses its characteristic properties and the new compound develops its own individual properties. For example, iron oxide (rust) has different properties from the two elements of which it is comprised—iron and oxygen. The new substance, which is a compound, cannot be altered by mechanical means, but only by chemical methods.

ELEMENTS AND COMPOUNDS

MATTER	TYPES AND DEFINITION	SMALLEST PARTICLE	ELEMENTS FOUND IN HAIR
	ELEMENTS SIMPLEST FORM OF MATTER	ATOM (Cannot be broken down by simple chemical reactions) About 100 different kinds	CARBON NITROGEN OXYGEN SULFUR HYDROGEN PHOSPHORUS
FORMS GASES LIQUIDS SOLIDS	COMPOUNDS FORMED BY COMBINATION OF ELEMENTS	MOLECULE (Consists of 2 or more atoms chemically combined) Unlimited kinds possible	COMPOUNDS USED ON HAIR WATER HYDROGEN PEROXIDE AMMONIUM THIOGLYCOLATE ANILINE DERIVATIVE TINTS AMMONIA ALCOHOL ACIDS ALKALIS

Oxides

Compounds are divided into four classes:

1. **Oxides** are compounds of any element combined with oxygen. For example, one part carbon and two parts oxygen equal **carbon dioxide,** which might be recognized as dry ice. Or, one part carbon and one part oxygen equal **monoxide,** better known as the poisonous exhaust of an automobile.

Acids

2. **Acids** are compounds of hydrogen, a non-metal, such as nitrogen and, sometimes, oxygen. For example, hydrogen + sulphur + oxygen = **sulphuric acid** (H_2SO_4). Acids turn **blue** litmus paper **red,** providing a quick way to test a compound.

Bases

3. **Bases,** also known as alkalies, are compounds of hydrogen, a metal and oxygen. For example, sodium + oxygen + hydrogen = **sodium hydroxide** (NaOH), which is used in the manufacture of soap. Bases will turn **red** litmus paper **blue.**

Salts

4. **Salts** are compounds that are formed by the reaction of acids and bases, with water also produced by the reaction. Two common salts and their formulas are sodium chloride (table salt) (NaCl), which contains sodium and chloride; and magnesium sulphate (Epsom salts) ($MgSo_4.7H_2O$), which contains magnesium, sulphur, hydrogen and oxygen.

Mixtures

A mixture is a substance that is made up of two elements, combined **physically** rather than chemically.

The ingredients in a mixture do not change their properties, as they do in a compound, but retain their individual characteristics. For example, concrete is composed of sand, gravel and cement. While concrete is a mixture having its own functions, its ingredients never lose their characteristics. Sand remains sand, gravel is still gravel, and cement, cement.

CHANGES IN MATTER

Matter may be changed in two ways, either through physical or chemical means.

Physical Changes

Physical change refers to an alteration of the properties without the formation of any new substance. For example, ice, a solid, melts at a certain temperature and becomes a liquid (water), and water, a liquid, freezes at a certain temperature and becomes a solid. There is no change in the inherent nature of the water, but merely a change in its form.

Chemical Changes

A **chemical change** is one in which a new substance or substances are formed, having properties different from the original substances. For example, soap is formed from the chemical reaction between an alkaline substance (potassium hydroxide) and an oil or fat. The soap resembles neither the alkaline substance nor the oil from which it is formed. Chemical reaction between the two forms a new substance, having its own characteristic properties.

PROPERTIES OF MATTER

When we talk about the properties of matter, we are talking about how we distinguish one form of matter from another.

Physical Properties

These refer to properties, such as **density, specific gravity, odor, color, taste.**

Density

1. **Density** of a substance refers to its weight divided by its volume. For example, the volume of one cubic foot of water weighs 62.4 lbs. Therefore, its density is (weight) 62.4 lbs. ÷ (volume) 1 cubic foot, or water has a density of 62.4 lbs. per cubic foot.

Specific Gravity

2. **Specific gravity** of a substance is also referred to as its relative density. This means that substances are referred to as either more or less dense than water. For example, copper is 8.9 times as dense as water; therefore, the specific gravity (or relative density) of copper is 8.9.

Odor

3. **Odor** of a substance helps us identify it in many instances. For example, the characteristic odor of ammonium thioglycolate, known as the "thio" odor, helps us identify this product.

Color

4. **Color** helps us identify many substances. For example, we recognize the color of gold, silver, copper, brass, coal.

Taste

5. **Taste** has helped us identify many substances. For example, oil of wintergreen can be identified by its peppermint-type taste.

Chemical Properties

The chemical properties of a substance refer to the ability of the substance to react, and the conditions under which it reacts. Two of the more widely known chemical properties a substance possesses are **combustibility** and ability to **support combustion**. For example:

Combustibility

1. **Phosphorus** is a highly combustible substance. For that reason, it is used on the tips of matches. The heat produced by rubbing the match tip against a surface is enough to cause it to burst into flames.

Combustion Supporting

2. One of the chemical properties of wood is its ability to support combustion. It is, therefore, used in the manufacture of matches. The phosphorous tip starts the fire and the wood supports the fire.

PROPERTIES OF COMMON ELEMENTS, COMPOUNDS AND MIXTURES

Knowledge about the properties of some of the most common elements, compounds and mixtures can be of help to the cosmetology student investigating the reasons why certain cosmetological reactions occur.

Oxygen

Oxygen (O) is the most abundant element, found both free and in compounds. It composes about half of the earth's crust, half of the rock, one-fifth of the air, and 90% of the water. It is a colorless, odorless, tasteless, gaseous substance, combining with most other elements to form an infinite variety of compounds, called **oxides.** One of the chief characteristics of this element is its ability to support combustion.

Hydrogen

Hydrogen (H) is a colorless, odorless, tasteless gas, and is the lightest element known. It is inflammable and explosive when mixed with air. It is found in chemical combination with oxygen in water, and with other elements in acids, bases and organic substances, such as wood, meat, fish, sugar and butter.

Air

Air is the gaseous mixture which makes up the earth's atmosphere. It is odorless, colorless, and generally consists of about one part by volume of oxygen and four parts of nitrogen. It also contains a small amount of carbon dioxide, ammonia, and organic matter, which are all essential to plant and animal life.

Hydrogen Peroxide

Hydrogen peroxide (H_2O_2) is a compound of hydrogen and oxygen. It is a colorless liquid with a characteristic odor and a slightly acid taste. Organic matter, such as silk, hair, feathers and nails, are lightened by hydrogen peroxide. The bleaching action takes place through the oxidizing property of hydrogen peroxide. A 20- to 40-volume hydrogen peroxide solution is used as a lightening agent for the hair. A 10-volume solution of hydrogen peroxide possesses antiseptic qualities.

Oxidizing Agents

Oxidizing agents are substances that will cause oxidation of other substances. Hydrogen peroxide is such a substance. It oxidizes the hair pigment to a colorless compound. During the action, the lightening agent is reduced and the pigment is oxidized. Oxidation is always accompanied by reduction.

Nitrogen

Nitrogen (N) is a colorless, gaseous element found free in the air. It constitutes part of the atmosphere, forming about four-fifths of the air, and is necessary to life because it dilutes the oxygen. It is found chiefly in the form of ammonia and nitrates.

ACIDITY AND ALKALINITY (PH SCALE)

The pH (potential hydrogen) of a liquid refers to its degree of acidity or alkalinity. Meters and indicators have been developed for the measurement of pH. Values are illustrated below.

The pH scale goes from 0 to 14. The neutral point is 7.

Cold wave solutions are alkaline up to 9.6.

Neutralizers are always acid.

Soaps up to 9.5 are satisfactory. Higher, unsatisfactory.

Shampoos are 6 to 10.0.

Depilatories, above 10.0.

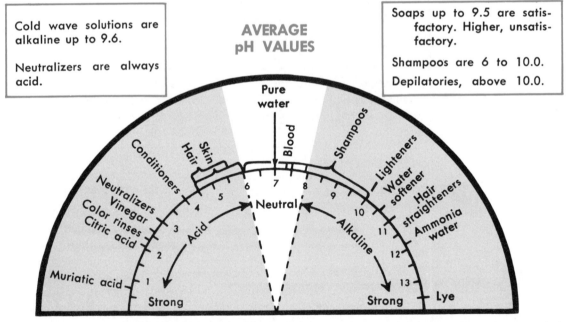

AVERAGE pH VALUES

Note: The cleansing action of soaps and shampoos depends upon their alkalinity and contact time with the skin, scalp or hair. Due to the short contact time, many alkaline products will achieve the desired results without damage to the skin, scalp or hair.

Acidity

Anything below 7 is acid. The lower the pH, the greater is the degree of acidity.

Alkalinity

Anything from 7 to 14 is alkaline. The higher the pH, the greater is the degree of alkalinity.

Since cosmetics vary in their pH values, be guided by your instructor.

CHEMISTRY OF WATER

Water (H$_2$O) is the most abundant of all substances, composing about 75% of the earth's surface, and about 65% of the human body. It is the universal solvent. De-mineralized or distilled water is used as a **non-conductor** of electricity. Water containing certain mineral substances is an excellent **conductor** of electricity.

Water serves many useful purposes in the beauty salon. Only water of known purity is fit for drinking purposes. Suspended or dissolved impurities in water render it unsatisfactory for cleaning objects and for use in beauty treatments.

Impurities can be removed from water by:

1. **Filtration:** passing water through a porous substance, such as filter paper or charcoal.
2. **Distillation:** heating water in a closed vessel arranged so that the resulting vapor passes off through a tube and is cooled and condensed to a liquid. This process purifies water used in the manufacture of cosmetics.

Boiling water at a temperature of 212° Farenheit will destroy most microbic life.

SOFT WATER

It is very important that **soft water** be used for shampooing, lightening or tinting the hair. **Rain water** is the softest water. **Hard water** contains mineral substances, such as the salts of calcium and magnesium, which curdle or precipitate soap instead of permitting a permanent lather to form. Hard water may be softened by **distillation,** or by use of **borax,** sodium carbonate (washing soda) or sodium phosphate. To soften hard water effectively in beauty salons, special equipment, such as zeolite tanks, are used.

Test For Soft Water

To **test for soft water,** use a soap solution made by dissolving three-quarters of an ounce of pure powdered castile soap in a pint of distilled water. Half fill a pint bottle with fresh water, and add 0.5 ml. (about 7 drops) of the soap solution. Shake the bottle vigorously. If a lather forms at once and persists, the water is very soft. If a lather does not appear at once, add another 0.5 ml. of soap solution and repeat the shaking. If more than 0.5 ml. of the soap solution is needed to produce a good lather, the water must be softened.

SHAMPOOING

All professional cosmetologists understand the importance of the shampoo and how the cleanliness of the hair affects other hair services. However, it is also important that they know how the shampoo cleanses the hair.

No discussion of the action of shampoos and how they function can be meaningful unless a study is made of the shampoo molecule.

SHAMPOO MOLECULES

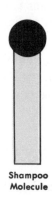

Shampoo Molecule

Shampoo molecules are large molecules which have been specially treated. They are composed of a **head** and **tail**, each with its own special function.

The **tail** of the shampoo molecule has an attraction for dirt, grease, debris and oil, but has no attraction for, or liking of, water.

The **head** of the shampoo molecule has a strong attraction for water, but does not like dirt.

Working as a team, both parts of the molecule do an effective job of cleansing the hair.

The shampoo is applied and thoroughly worked into the hair. The dirt, grease, debris and oil in the hair is attracted to the tails of the shampoo molecules and become firmly attached to them.

RINSING

During the rinsing step, as the stream of water is directed through the hair, the "water-loving" molecule heads attach themselves to the water molecules and are carried from the hair, taking with them the tails with the attached dirt.

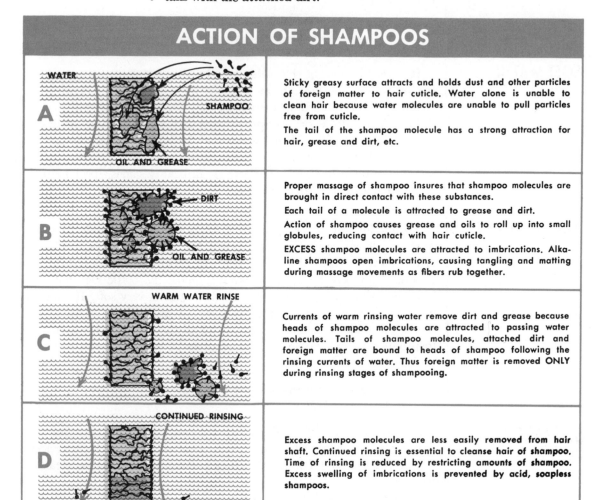

ACTION OF SHAMPOOS

A — Sticky greasy surface attracts and holds dust and other particles of foreign matter to hair cuticle. Water alone is unable to clean hair because water molecules are unable to pull particles free from cuticle.
The tail of the shampoo molecule has a strong attraction for hair, grease and dirt, etc.

B — Proper massage of shampoo insures that shampoo molecules are brought in direct contact with these substances.
Each tail of a molecule is attracted to grease and dirt.
Action of shampoo causes grease and oils to roll up into small globules, reducing contact with hair cuticle.
EXCESS shampoo molecules are attracted to imbrications. Alkaline shampoos open imbrications, causing tangling and matting during massage movements as fibers rub together.

C — Currents of warm rinsing water remove dirt and grease because heads of shampoo molecules are attracted to passing water molecules. Tails of shampoo molecules, attached dirt and foreign matter are bound to heads of shampoo following the rinsing currents of water. Thus foreign matter is removed ONLY during rinsing stages of shampooing.

D — Excess shampoo molecules are less easily removed from hair shaft. Continued rinsing is essential to cleanse hair of shampoo. Time of rinsing is reduced by restricting amounts of shampoo. Excess swelling of imbrications is prevented by acid, soapless shampoos.

CHEMISTRY OF SHAMPOOS

By combining an **alkali** with an oil or fat, shampoo soaps are formed. The oil used may be of vegetable origin, such as almond, peanut, coconut, olive, castor and palm-nut.

The fat used may be animal fat, lanolin, tallow and synthetic compounds.

Most shampoos contain varying amounts of the same fatty acids. Therefore, the shampoo soap formed varies with the substances used.

Shampoos with a high pH factor, which are highly alkaline, are especially damaging to all types of hair.

TYPES OF SHAMPOOS

The main purpose of a shampoo is to cleanse the scalp and hair. This may be accomplished by a wet or dry shampoo. Wet shampoos are watery solutions of soap and various cleansing agents. Dry shampoos do not use water, but contain either powdery substances or cosmetic products in liquid form.

Wet Shampoos

Wet shampoos, depending on their composition, are of three basic types:
1. Soap shampoos
2. Soapless shampoos (foaming or foamless)
3. Cream shampoos

Soap Shampoos

Soap shampoos are available in the form of cake, powder, jelly or liquid. The active cleansing agent is a soap made from olive oil, coconut oil or other oils. Liquid soap shampoos contain more than 50% water. When used on the hair, a soap shampoo will produce an alkaline reaction. With soft water, soap shampoos lather readily. When used with hard water, soap shampoos will not lather and tend to produce an insoluble soap residue on the hair.

Soapless Shampoos

Soapless shampoos come in the form of a powder, jelly, cream or liquid. They are effective cleansing agents. Their main ingredient is a sulfonated oil. Both the lathering and non-lathering types of soapless shampoos are available.

Soapless shampoos are just as effective in soft, hard, cold or hot water. They should be used with discretion, since frequent applications not only dry the scalp and hair, but render the hair more absorptive than usual.

Cream Or Paste Shampoos

Cream shampoos, or **pastes,** have a cleansing action due to soap, a synthetic detergent, or a combination of both. They may also contain a reconditioning agent for the hair. Cream shampoos, or pastes, without soap, are usually acid in reaction.

For other types of shampoos, see chapter on Shampooing and Rinsing.

PERMANENT WAVING

HAIR COMPOSITION

The Cortex

Peptide Bonds

Cross Bonds

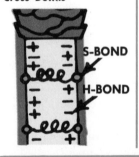

In order to understand the chemical actions of permanent waving, it is first necessary to understand the composition of the hair and hair bonds.

Hair is made of a hard protein called **keratin**. It has three layers: cuticle, cortex, medulla. Since permanent hair waving takes place in the cortical layer, special attention is given to a study of the cortex.

The cortex is composed of numerous parallel fibers of hard keratin, referred to as polypeptide chains. These parallel fibers are twisted around one another, something very much like heavy rope in appearance.

Each amino-acid is joined to another by peptide bonds (end bonds), forming a chain as long as the hair. They are the strongest bonds in the cortex, and most of the strength of hair is due to their properties.

Peptide bonds are chemical bonds, and if even a few are broken, the hair is weakened or damaged. If many of these bonds are broken, the hair will break off.

It is the presence of cross-bonds or links, however, that has given hair the ability to be permanently waved. There are two types of cross-bonds that are of major concern in hair work:

1. Sulphur bonds—(chemical)—called **S-bonds**
2. Hydrogen bonds—(physical)—called **H-bonds**

Hydrogen bonds are much more numerous than sulphur bonds, but they are much weaker and can be broken with water or chemicals.

Sulphur bonds are very strong and can only be broken by a strong chemical.

CHANGES IN HAIR CORTEX DURING PERMANENT WAVING

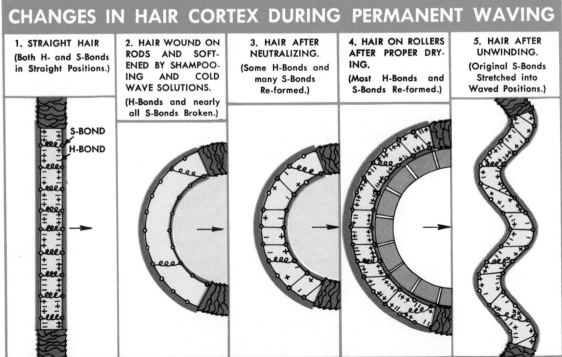

| 1. STRAIGHT HAIR (Both H- and S-Bonds in Straight Positions.) | 2. HAIR WOUND ON RODS AND SOFTENED BY SHAMPOOING AND COLD WAVE SOLUTIONS. (H-Bonds and nearly all S-Bonds Broken.) | 3. HAIR AFTER NEUTRALIZING. (Some H-Bonds and many S-Bonds Re-formed.) | 4. HAIR ON ROLLERS AFTER PROPER DRYING. (Most H-Bonds and S-Bonds Re-formed.) | 5. HAIR AFTER UNWINDING. (Original S-Bonds Stretched into Waved Positions.) |

Thio Solution

A thio solution (ammonium thioglycolate) with a pH of 9.4 to 9.6 causes the cuticle of the hair to swell and the imbrications to open, allowing the solution to penetrate into the cortex. The solution breaks down all the H-bonds and many of the S-bonds, permitting a "slippage" or alteration in the polypeptide chains. The chains assume the contour of the rods around which the hair is wound.

Neutralizer

When sufficient processing has taken place, the thio is rinsed from the hair and neutralizer is applied. The neutralizer is an acid solution with a pH of 3.0 to 4.0. This solution stops the action of the thio and re-hardens the hair by re-forming many of the S-bonds and some of the H-bonds. The rest of the H-bonds are re-formed during the drying of the hair. The S-bonds and H-bonds hold the polypeptide chains in their newly curled formation.

Caution

Caution must be exercised in the use of a thio solution. If it is permitted to remain in the hair for too long, it could weaken and break the polypeptide chains by destroying the end-bonds, thus causing hair breakage.

PROTEIN FILLERS

Protein fillers are used to recondition over-porous or damaged hair before a permanent waving lotion is applied.

The filler is a jelly-like, colorless substance, made of a mixture of protein and keratin. Some fillers also contain lanolin and cholesterol to protect the hair against the harshness of the permanent waving lotion.

The chemical properties of the filler are similar to those of the hair, so the filler is able to even out the hair's porosity along the entire hair shaft. This evening-out process takes place because the porous sections of the hair shaft absorb the filler more rapidly than do the less porous sections.

**WET WAVING
AND CURLING**

A temporary hair set is produced by **physical changes** which occur within the hair cortex. Because of the nature of these physical changes, hair can be set as frequently as desired. This is the basis of finger waving, pin curling, roller curling and all wet setting.

Water alone can be used because **it has the ability to break down the hydrogen bonds in the cortex.** These bonds, which occur between adjacent polypeptide chains, prevent them from moving. But, slippage of the chains must take place before a proper wave can be formed.

Stretching that part of each hair strand which is on the outside of the roller or curl must cause a temporary rearrangement of the chains. Water lubricates the chains so that they can move relative to one another. However, even though hydrogen bonds are broken, the total amount of movement is very small because the strong sulphur bonds are completely unaffected by the water and continue to restrict slippage of the polypeptide chains.

CHEMICAL HAIR RELAXING (STRAIGHT-ENING)

The procedure for chemical hair relaxing is very similar to the technique followed in permanent waving. However, since the objective to be attained is exactly the reverse of permanent waving, some of the techniques must also be reversed.

The cosmetologist starts with hair which is excessively curly, and her objective is to remove the curl permanently.

As in permanent waving, the process requires the breaking down of the S-bonds and the H-bonds in the cortex. The relaxing process, however, requires that the hair be held or directed in a straight position.

TYPES OF CHEMICAL RELAXERS

The two types of chemical hair relaxers that are in general use by professional cosmetologists are thio (thioglycolate), pH 9.4 to 9.6, and sodium hydroxide, pH 10 to 14. The over-all objective of both these products is exactly the same. Students must be cautioned, however, that sodium hydroxide is much stronger than thio, and, if not properly used, it can cause great damage to the patron's hair.

If left on the hair too long, it may change the hair color. If left on longer than 10 minutes, it may dissolve the hair.

FIXATIVE

The neutralizer, or fixative, employed is an acid solution with a pH of 3.0 to 4.0.

Before either of these products is employed, it is extremely important to read the chapter on Chemical Hair Relaxing for a detailed study of their application and the safety precautions required.

CHEMICAL HAIR STRAIGHTENING - SODIUM HYDROXIDE

1. CURLY HAIR
Both H- and S-Bonds holding polypeptide chains in position. chains in position.

2. HAIR BEING PROCESSED
All H-bonds broken, most S-bonds broken. Hand and comb manipulations starting to relax wave. (Polypeptide chains shift.)

3. HAIR BEING NEUTRALIZED
The neutralizer fixes polypeptide chains in a straight position after hair has been fully relaxed.

4. STRAIGHTENED HAIR . . .
after rinsing and proper drying. LANTHIONINE cross links now exist between polypeptide chains, keeping the hair in a permanently straight form. Drying re-forms the physical bonds.

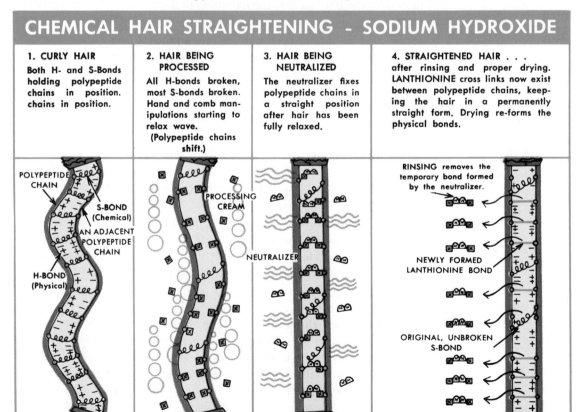

POLYPEPTIDE CHAIN

S-BOND (Chemical)

AN ADJACENT POLYPEPTIDE CHAIN

H-BOND (Physical)

PROCESSING CREAM

NEUTRALIZER

RINSING removes the temporary bond formed by the neutralizer.

NEWLY FORMED LANTHIONINE BOND

ORIGINAL, UNBROKEN S-BOND

HAIR COLORING

This presentation is limited to a discussion of the chemical composition, actions and reactions of the various types of hair colorings. See the chapter on **Hair Coloring** for information on techniques, application, and use of hair colorings.

Temporary Color

Temporary colorings for the hair come in various forms, such as color rinses, color sprays and color shampoos. They come in a wide range of colors and are easily applied. Temporary colors are washed out with the first shampoo. For these reasons, they are useful to a patron who is experimenting with new hair colors, or for a patron seeking a particular hair effect for a special occasion.

ACTION OF SIMPLE HAIR COLORINGS

Water or Color Rinses	SEMI PERMANENT RINSES		DRYING

Temporary colorings are harmless to the hair because they contain "true stains," which are colors accepted by the government for use in foods, drugs and cosmetics. They are also called "certified colors." Temporary colorings are composed of large molecules that are acid in chemical composition and unable to penetrate into the cortical layer. They shrink the cuticle scales, closing the imbrications and preventing the entrance of the large color molecules into the cortex. The coloring substance can only be trapped behind the imbrications of the cuticle.

Temporary coloring is easily washed from the hair because the shampoo is alkaline and opens the imbrications. The rinsing action of the shampoo then easily washes out the coloring substance.

Lightened hair is able to absorb more of the coloring substance because the lightener has already opened the cuticle, thus allowing more of the color to enter.

Semi-Permanent Tints

Semi-permanent colorings (tints) last from four to six weeks. They are aniline derivative tints, the same as permanent tints, but their molecules are larger than those of the permanent tints.

Semi-permanent tints offer patrons a number of benefits which are not found in other forms of hair coloring. Besides lasting from four to six shampoos, they have a very good range of colors. Semi-permanent tints are easily applied and do not require the use of hydrogen peroxide. They are effective in covering or blending partially grey hair without affecting the natural color. They also serve to highlight and bring out the natural color of the hair.

Semi-permanent tints are alkaline in chemical composition and cause an alkaline reaction on the hair. The alkali swells the cuticle, opening the imbrications and permitting the color molecules to enter the cortex. However, since semi-permanent tints are only mildly alkaline, the swelling of the cuticle and the opening of the imbrications are limited, permitting only a small number of the large molecules to enter into the cortex.

A neutral or slightly acid rinse is used to close the imbrications and trap the colored molecules inside the cortex. Gradually, the semi-permanent tints are washed out of the hair by alkaline shampoos, which open the cuticle imbrications, permitting the colored molecules to pass out of the cortex.

Permanent Color

Most patrons prefer their hair coloring to last much longer than a few shampoos. Originally, hair tints were intended solely to hide greying hair. Today, patrons of all ages choose to color their hair simply to enhance their appearance. Permanent hair tints may be found in a number of different types: aniline derivative tints, vegetable tints and metallic dyes.

Analine Derivative Tints

Aniline derivative tints, or oxidizing tints, are the primary tints used in professional services. They offer a number of distinct advantages over all other forms of coloring. They give a permanent color to the hair, requiring no further coloring treatment, except for new growth. A wide range of aniline derivative colors has been developed to meet every patron's desires. Of special interest is the fact that aniline derivative tints permit other services to be given to tinted hair.

ACTION OF HAIR TINTS

TINT BASE PLUS DEVELOPER ON HAIR	1. TINT MIXTURE ENTERS INTO CORTEX	2. TINT PIGMENTS FORMED	3. SHRINKING OF CUTICLE SCALES TO TRAP PIGMENT

CONDITIONER

DRYING AND CONDITIONING

These tints are composed of very small, colorless molecules which experience no difficulty in passing through the cuticle imbrications and penetrating into the cortex. A developer, usually hydrogen peroxide, is added to the tint immediately before application. Once inside the cortex, the developer combines the small, colorless molecules into giant, colored molecules. These large molecules cannot be shampooed from the hair because they are too large to pass out through the imbrications. In addition, they form bonds with the keratin chains in the cortex, and thus become firmly affixed. These bonds are acid, and, therefore, leave the H-bonds and the S-bonds free for other hair treatments.

Vegetable Tints (Henna)

Vegetable tints, usually henna, have a very limited usefulness in the professional practice of hair coloring. The tint is formed by mixing henna powder with water and a mild acid to form a paste. This henna paste is applied to the hair, where it coats the hair shaft, and some may penetrate into the cortex. It produces a lasting color effect, usually red or auburn. The color produced is usually harsh. Vegetable tints offer absolutely no range of colors.

Henna is very messy to work with and is of very little value for professional services.

Metallic Dyes

These hair dyes also have little purpose today. The metallic film on the hair cuticle, which gives the color, creates serious limitations. Some of the metallic salts enter the cortex and combine with the S-bonds. This interferes with permanent waving.

The metallic salts (lead, silver, copper) are very poisonous. They also cause a violent reaction with hydrogen peroxide on the hair.

Metallic dyes are no longer used professionally.

Compound Dyes

Compound dyes consist of a combination of vegetable dyes and metallic salts, to fix the color. These coloring agents are never used professionally, but are sometimes used at home. While they coat the hair shaft, some of the metallic salts may penetrate into the cuticle and combine with S-bonds. The action of compound dyes renders the hair unfit for permanent waving, tinting or lightening, chemical hair straightening.

Color Stripping

Color strippers are chemical agents which are designed to strip out color with the least risk of damage to the hair.

Tint (color) strippers are very strong oxidizing agents which reduce the giant color molecules in the cortex into small colorless particles. When these particles are small enough to pass through the imbrications of the cuticle, they may be easily rinsed from the hair.

Chemicals used in strippers may be inorganic sulfites or organic **reducing agents** with modifiers. Liquid 30 vol. hydrogen peroxide, with excess ammonia to pH 10.0-12.0, may also be used as an effective color stripper.

434

HAIR LIGHTENING

Hair lightening is the process which decreases or removes the natural color pigments in the hair.

Hair color pigments are:

Melanin—black to brown shades

Oxymelanin—red to yellow shades

Hair lightening occurs in two ways: through natural conditions or through artificial conditions.

Natural conditions: Color may be removed from the hair by the sun's rays, chlorinated water or other natural action.

Artificial conditions: This usually occurs through chemical means. Chemical hair lightening is a two-stage process. The first stage involves changing the melanin pigments into oxymelanin. The second stage, depending on the degree of lightening desired, involves the continued breaking down of the oxymelanin pigment until the desired effect is achieved.

CHEMICAL AGENTS

The chemical agent used for removing pigments from the hair shaft is a 6% (20-volume) solution of hydrogen peroxide.

The active ingredient of hydrogen peroxide is oxygen gas. To speed the liberation of oxygen gas, a small quantity of 28% ammonia water is added, which increases the pH to 10.0.

There are a number of commercial lighteners available to the cosmetologist. These products are:

1. Oil lighteners—mixtures of hydrogen peroxide and sulfonated oils
2. Cream lighteners, containing conditioning agents, bluing and thickener
3. Powder lighteners, containing an oxygen releasing booster and inert substances

The chemical action of all the commercial lighteners is basically the same as outlined above.

TONERS

Toners are permanent aniline derivative hair colorings. They consist primarily of pale, delicate colors requiring very careful application.

Since a toner is an aniline derivative tint, it must be handled exactly as other permanent aniline tints. The chemical actions are identical with those described for aniline derivative tints.

Toners are usually applied to lightened hair to add color and highlights to the hair.

COLOR FILLERS

Color fillers are employed to equalize the porosity of abused or damaged hair. They also deposit a base color prior to a tinting treatment.

The color filler is a jelly-like substance, usually a mixture of protein, keratin and certified color, which is applied directly to the cuticle.

Since the filler is composed of the same basic chemical properties as the hair itself, it evens out porosity along the entire hair shaft. Porosity is equalized because the very porous sections of the hair shaft absorb the filler more rapidly than do the less porous areas.

The use of color fillers helps to make hair coloring services easier and more successful.

CHEMISTRY AS APPLIED TO COSMETICS

Cosmetologists will be better equipped to serve the public if they have an understanding of the chemical composition, preparation and uses of cosmetics that are intended to cleanse and beautify the body.

Cosmetics may be classified according to their physical and chemical nature and the characteristics by which they are recognized. The object in classifying cosmetics is to assist in their study and identification.

PHYSICAL AND CHEMICAL CLASSIFICATIONS OF COSMETICS

1. Powders
2. Solutions
3. Suspensions
4. Emulsions
5. Ointments
6. Sticks
7. Pastes
8. Mucilages
9. Soaps

Powders

Powders are a uniform mixture of insoluble substances (inorganic, organic and colloidal) which have been properly blended, perfumed and/or tinted to produce a cosmetic which is free from coarse or gritty particles.

In the process of making powders, mixing and sifting processes are employed.

Solutions

A **solution** is a preparation made by dissolving a solid, liquid or gaseous substance in another substance, usually liquid.

Solute

A **solute** is a substance dissolved in a solution.

Solvent

A **solvent** is a liquid used to dissolve a solute.

Solutions are clear and permanent mixtures of solutes and solvents which do not separate on standing. Since a good solution is clear and transparent, filtration is often necessary, particularly if the solution is cloudy.

Solutions are easily prepared by dissolving and stirring a powdered solute in a warm solvent. The solute may be separated from the solvent by the application of heat which evaporates the solvent.

Water is a universal solvent. It is capable of dissolving more substances than any other solvent. Grain alcohol and glycerine are frequently used as solvents. Water, glycerine and alcohol readily mix with each other; therefore, they are **miscible.** On the other hand, water and oil do not mix with each other; hence they are **immiscible.**

The **solute** may be **either** a solid, liquid or gas. For example, **boric acid solution** is a mixture of a solid in a liquid; **glycerine and rose water** is a mixture of two miscible liquids; **ammonia water** is a mixture of a gas in water.

Solutions containing volatile substances, such as ammonia and alcohol, should be stored in a cool place; otherwise, the volatile substance will evaporate.

There are various kinds of solutions:

A **dilute solution** contains a small quantity of solute in proportion to the quantity of solvent.

A **concentrated solution** contains a large quantity of solute in proportion to the quantity of solvent.

A **saturated solution** will not dissolve or take up more of the solute than it already holds at a given temperature.

Suspensions

Suspensions are temporary mixtures of insoluble powders in liquid. Since the particles have a tendency to separate on standing, a thorough shaking is required before using. A suspension should not be filtered. Some skin lotions are actually suspensions. (Example: calamine lotion.)

Suspensions are made by first mixing the powders, then adding a small amount of liquid to form a smooth paste, and finally adding the balance of the liquid.

Emulsions

Emulsions (creams) are permanent mixtures of two or more immiscible substances (oil and water) which are united with the aid of a binder (gum), or an emulsifier (soap). Emulsions are usually milky white in appearance. If a suitable emulsifier and the proper technique are employed, the resultant emulsion will be stable. A stable emulsion can hold as much as 90% water. Depending on the amount of water and wax present, the cream may be either liquid or semi-solid in character. The amount of emulsifier used depends on its efficiency and the amount of water or oil to be emulsified.

Emulsions are prepared by hand or with the aid of a grinding and cutting machine, called a colloidal mill. In the process of preparing the emulsion, the emulsifier forms a protective film around the microscopic globules of either the oil or water. The smaller the globules, the thicker and more stable will be the emulsion.

Ointments

Ointments are semi-solid mixtures of organic substances (lard, petrolatum, wax) and medicinal agents. No water is present. For the ointment to soften, its melting point should be below that of the body temperature (98.6° Fahrenheit).

Ointments are prepared by melting the organic substances and mixing the medicinal agent into the mixture.

Sticks

Sticks are similar to ointments in that they are a mixture of organic substances (oils, waxes, petrolatum) which are poured into a mold to solidify. Sticks are a little harder than ointments. No water is present. Lipstick is an example of a cosmetic stick.

Pastes

Pastes are soft, moist cosmetics, having a thick consistency. They are bound together with the aid of gum, starch and water. If oils and fats are present, water is absent. The colloidal mill assists in the removal of grittiness from the paste.

Mucilages

Mucilages are thick liquids containing either natural gums (tragacanth or karaya) or synthetic gums, mixed with water. Since mucilages undergo decomposition, a preservative is required. Mucilages are used for hair setting lotions.

Soaps

Soaps are compounds formed in a chemical reaction between alkaline substances (potassium or sodium hydroxide) and the fatty acids in oil or fat. Besides soap, glycerine is also formed. Potassium hydroxide produces a **soft soap,** whereas sodium hydroxide forms a **hard soap.** A mixture of the two alkalies will yield a soap of intermediate consistency.

A **good soap** does not contain an excess of free alkali and is made from pure oils and fats.

U. S. P.

The cosmetologist should become familiar with the United States Pharmacopeia (U.S.P.), a book defining and standardizing drugs. The following are some of the terms of interest to cosmetologists:

Alcohol

Alcohol, also known as grain or ethyl alcohol, is a colorless liquid obtained by the fermentation of certain sugars. It is a powerful antiseptic and disinfectant; a 70% solution is usable for sanitizing instruments, and a 60% solution can be applied to the skin. It is widely used in perfumes, lotions and tonics.

Alum

Alum is an aluminum potassium or ammonium sulphate, supplied in the form of crystals or powder, which has a strong astringent taste and action. It is used in skin tonics and lotions. It is also used in powder form as a styptic, which is applied to small cuts.

Ammonia Water

Ammonia water, as commercially used, is a colorless liquid with a pungent, penetrating odor. It is a by-product of the manufacture of coal gas. As it readily dissolves grease, it is used as a cleansing agent, and is also used with hydrogen peroxide in lightening hair. A 28% solution of ammonia gas dissolved in water is available commercially.

Sodium Bicarbonate

Sodium bicarbonate (baking soda) is a precipitate made by passing carbon dioxide gas through a solution of **sodium carbonate.** It is a white powder adapted for uses such as a neutralizing agent.

Sodium Carbonate

Sodium carbonate (washing soda) is prepared by heating **sodium bicarbonate.** It is used for water softening and in bath salts. Sodium carbonate may also be used with boiling water in the sterilization of metallic instruments. A small quantity is added to the water to keep the instruments bright.

Bichloride Of Mercury

Bichloride of mercury is usually sold in tablet form of about $7\frac{1}{2}$ grains each. It is shaped peculiarly for ready identification. It is a very strong poison and should be used very sparingly in beauty salons.

Boric Acid

Boric acid, also called boracic acid, is a powder obtained from sodium borate, which is mined in the form of borax and crystallized with sulphuric acid. It is a mild healing and antiseptic agent. It is sometimes used as a dusting powder, and, in solution, as a cleansing lotion or eyewash.

Formaldehyde

Formaldehyde is a gas, but in water solution containing from 37% to 40% of the gas by weight, it is known as **formalin.** Formaldehyde has a very disagreeable, pungent odor. It is very irritating to the eyes, nose and mouth. Formalin may be used to sanitize instruments.

Glycerine

Glycerine is a sweet, colorless, odorless, syrupy liquid, formed by the decomposition of oils, fats or molasses. It is an excellent skin softener, and is an ingredient of cuticle oil, facial creams and lotions.

Tincture Of Iodine

Tincture of iodine is a 2% solution of iodine in alcohol. If the patron is not allergic to iodine, it can be safely used on the skin to treat minor cuts and bruises. Iodine stains are readily removed with alcohol. **Mercurochrome,** or a 3-5% peroxide solution, may also be used for cuts.

Phenol

Phenol, or **carbolic acid,** is not actually an acid, but is a coal tar derivative, appearing as a crystalline substance having a slightly acid reaction. Glycerine is added to make it more readily soluble in water. A 5% solution of phenol is used to sanitize metallic instruments.

Potassium Hydroxide

Potassium hydroxide (caustic potash) sticks are dissolved in distilled water to form an alkaline solution. When not in use, the sticks must be kept in sealed containers, as they tend to absorb moisture from the air and deteriorate. They are used in the making of soaps and cosmetic creams.

Zinc Oxide

Zinc oxide is a heavy white powder made by burning zinc carbonate with coal in a special furnace. It is used as a dusting powder and as an ointment for some skin conditions.

Witch Hazel

Witch hazel is a solution of alcohol and water, containing an astringent agent extracted from witch hazel bark.

Quarternary Ammonium Compounds

Quaternary ammonium compounds (Quats) are a group of effective disinfectants widely used as sanitizing agents in beauty salons.

REVIEW QUESTIONS

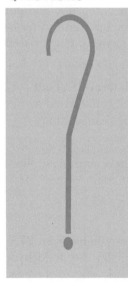

1. Why is a basic knowledge of chemistry important to cosmetologists?
2. What is the chemical symbol of a) water; and b) hydrogen peroxide?
3. Name two methods for removing impurities from water.
4. What type of water is best to use for shampooing?
5. What two parts make up a shampoo molecule?
6. a) What purpose does the tail of a shampoo molecule serve? b) The head?
7. What happens to the shampoo molecule during rinsing?
8. What part does the thio solution play in the permanent waving of hair?
9. What two types of chemical hair relaxers are in general use by professional cosmetologists?
10. What may happen to the hair if sodium hydroxide is left on the hair longer than 10 minutes?
11. Why do aniline derivative tints easily penetrate into the cortex?
12. What action takes place once the developer and tint are inside the cortex?
13. Why are aniline derivative tints permanent hair coloring?
14. What are "melanin" and "oxymelanin"?
15. What is the difference between a solute and a solvent?

COSMETICS
FOR BODY
CLEANLINESS

The chemistry of cosmetics embraces the study of products designed to cleanse and beautify the skin, hair and nails.

Cosmetics of this type are intended to cleanse the body by removing dirt, hair or foreign odors from the skin. This classification includes soaps, bath accessories, deodorants, anti-perspirants and depilatories.

KINDS OF SOAPS

Good toilet soaps should be made from purified fats which will not become rancid in the soap, and should not contain excessive free alkali. Soaps having a pH value above 9.5 tend to dry and roughen the skin. A pH value of about 8 is considered normal for the skin.

Kinds of Soaps		
Soaps	Common Ingredients	Uses
Castile soap (pure)	Olive oil and soda.	Best for the skin — produces little lather.
Castile soap (other kinds)	Synthetic detergents, olive or other oils.	Used for normal skin.
Green soap	Made from potash and olive or linseed oil and glycerine.	A medicinal liquid soap, used for oily skin.
Tincture of green soap	Mixture of green soap in about 35% alcohol and a small amount of perfume.	Used for correcting oily skin and scalp. Very drying, if used on normal or dry skin over a period of time.
Medicated soap	Contains a small percent of cresol, phenol or other antiseptics.	Used for acne conditions.
Shaving soap	Contains alkalies, coconut oil, vegetable and animal fats and a small amount of gum.	Used for shaving. The alkalinity softens the hair. The thick lather keeps the hair erect.
Shaving soap in pressure can	Shaving soap and gas under pressure.	Used the same as shaving soap.
Carbolic soap	A disinfectant soap containing 10% phenol.	Used for oily skin and acne infection.
Transparent soap	Contains glycerine, alcohol and sugar which render it transparent.	Used for normal skin.
Super-fatted soap	Contains a fatty substance, such as lanolin or cocoa butter.	Recommended for dry or sensitive skin. Keeps the skin soft after washing. Not suitable for hard water.
Naphtha soap	Contains naphtha, obtained from petroleum.	Do not use on face or scalp. Use mainly for laundry purposes.
Hard water soap	Contains coconut oil, varying amounts of washing soda or borax, sodium silicate and a phosphate.	Use only on oily skin. The alkaline substances will dry the skin.

BATH ACCESSORIES

Bath accessories include soaps, bath salts, bath oils, bath powders and body oils. Bath salts and oils are used during the bath, while bath powders and body oils are used after the bath.

Bath Accessories		
Kind	**Common Ingredients**	**Uses**
Bath salts	Carbonates or phosphates of sodium, color and perfume.	Soften and perfume the bath water.
Bath oils	Sulfonated oils (latherless) or sulfated fatty alcohols (produce lather), color and perfume.	Sulfonated oils are drying to the skin. If the body skin is dry, do not use them.
Bath dusting powders	Perfumed talc and other absorbent substances.	Impart a mild fragrance to the skin, and aid in drying body moisture.
Body oils	Vegetable and animal oils.	Replace natural oils removed by bathing.
Foam-bath salts	Sulfated compound related to coconut oil.	Drying to the skin.

DEODORANTS AND ANTI-PERSPIRANTS

Few preparations can be classified separately as deodorant or anti-perspirant products, since most combine the features of both. A **deodorant** is an agent which neutralizes or destroys disagreeable odors without suppressing the amount of perspiration. An **anti-perspirant** checks perspiration by its astringent action. The skin surrounding the pores swells, thereby temporarily closing the pores.

Deodorants and anti-perspirants are available in the form of creams, sticks, solutions and powders.

Deodorants and Anti-Perspirants		
Kind	**Common Ingredients**	**Uses**
Deodorant powders	Mixture of powder base, zinc compounds, boric acid, astringents, and antiseptics.	Destroy the odor of sweat without stopping perspiration.
Deodorant creams	Vanishing cream base, antiseptic and astringent.	Destroy the odor of sweat without stopping perspiration.
Deodorant solutions	Solution containing an antiseptic, an astringent, alcohol, glycerine and water.	Used to mask odor. The skin should be dry before wearing clothing. The acidity of the aluminum chloride will destroy clothing.
Deodorant sticks	Waxes and an astringent (zinc sulphocarbolate).	Easy to apply. Destroy odor without stopping perspiration.
Creams or liquids	Strong astringents, such as aluminum compounds.	Contract the sweat gland at the place of application. Prevent excessive sweating under the arms.

DEPILATORIES

Depilatories are preparations used for the temporary removal of superfluous hair in the armpits and on the legs. They consist of various alkali sulphides, calcium thioglycolate compounds, or resins and waxes. They are available in the form of a liquid, soft cream, paste, powder or hard cake.

Chemical Type

The chemical type of depilatory has the odor of spoiled eggs and is generally used over the legs and arms. It softens and dissolves the hair at the margin of the skin. To prevent irritation of the skin, use only as directed by the manufacturer.

Wax Type

The wax type of depilatory is odorless and is preferred for the face. After the melted wax hardens on the hairy surface, the patch is suddenly removed, and with it, the embedded hairs.

Before application, give a small patch test of the depilatory on the patron's skin. If skin redness or blisters do not develop, it is safe to use the depilatory over a larger skin surface.

For additional information, see chapter on Removal of Superfluous Hair.

COSMETICS FOR SKIN AND FACE

Grouped under this heading are all preparations designed to render the skin or face youthful and attractive in appearance. For this purpose, there are available creams, lotions, powders, makeup cosmetics and miscellaneous products.

Creams

Of all cosmetics used for the skin or face, creams comprise the largest and most varied group. Basically, creams are either stable emulsions of oily and watery substances, or an ointment base without water. Creams do not actually feed the tissues, but they do lubricate the skin.

Creams

Kind	Common Ingredients	Uses
Cold cream	Beeswax, vegetable or mineral oil, borax (1%), water and perfume.	Suitable for cleansing dry or normal skin.
Liquefying cleansing cream	Mineral oil, petrolatum, mineral wax, perfume, small amount of water.	May be used on oily skin. Melts quickly, does not penetrate the skin. Long use will dry the skin.
Vanishing cream	75% water, stearic acid, combined with a small amount of an alkali. Cocoa butter, lanolin, glycerine and alcohol are also used.	Used before makeup is applied, and as a hand cream. Leaves a protective film on the skin. Skin may become very dry from its use.
Emollient cream (Also called tissue cream and lubricating cream)	Waxes, lanolin, vegetable fats and oils, fatty acids, alcohols and some mineral oil products.	Slightly penetrate and soften the skin. Used for the lubrication of the skin during massage.
Hormone cream	Emollient cream base containing sex hormones.	For women of middle age. Prevents dryness and age lines.
Moisturizing cream	Emollient cream base containing moisturizing agents.	For dryness in aging skin due to lack of moisture and natural oil.

Creams (continued)		
Kind	**Common Ingredients**	**Uses**
Massage cream	Cold cream base, lanolin or casein (protein found in cheese).	For massage of normal or slightly dry skin.
Astringent cream	Mild ointment base containing zinc oxide and an astringent.	Recommended to correct excessive oiliness, and to close pores.
Acne cream	Boric acid, sulfur, zinc oxide, cade oil, camphor, benzoin and salicylic acids.	Helps clear the skin of simple acne and other minor lesions. Should be soft enough to spread easily without irritating the skin.
Foundation cream	Vanishing cream base is modified by increasing the glycerine content.	Applied to the face after cleansing, to provide a suitable base for makeup.
Eye cream and throat cream	Lanolin, vegetable oils, waxes and astringent substances.	Lubricate and soften fine lines. Make them less conspicuous.
Suntan cream	Contains a cream or ointment base and various color pigments.	Used to give the appearance of a darker skin color.

Lotions

Lotions are popular products used to a considerable extent in various kinds of cosmetic treatments. They are available as a clear solution or as a suspension, having an insoluble sediment at the bottom of the container.

Lotions		
Kind	**Common Ingredients**	**Uses**
Aromatic water	Essential oil (oil of rose, geranium, lavender, etc.) dissolved in distilled water with the aid of talc.	Imparts a cooling and fragrant effect to skin tonics and lotions.
Cleansing lotions	Alcohol or a sulfonated compound.	For oily skin.
Astringent lotions	Zinc, alum, boric or salicylic acid, in solution of water, glycerine and alcohol.	For oily skin and large pores.
Skin freshener lotions	Witch hazel, camphor, boric acid, mild organic acids, perfume and coloring.	Slightly astringent solution for dry skin.
Acne lotions	Precipitated sulfur, glycerine, spirits of camphor and distilled water.	Used to sponge the skin where simple acne exists.
Witch hazel	A solution of alcohol and water containing the astringent from witch hazel bark.	Used as an astringent and cooling lotion.
Eye lotions	Boric acid, bicarbonate of soda, zinc sulfate and glycerine, witch hazel, or other herbs.	Used to soothe, cleanse, and brighten the eyes.

Lotions (continued)		
Kind	**Common Ingredients**	**Uses**
Calamine lotion	Suspension of prepared calamine and zinc oxide in glycerine, bentonite and lime water.	Used as a soothing application to irritated surfaces of the skin and as a protective lotion.
Hardy's lotion	Corrosive sublimate, alcohol, zinc sulfate, lead acetate and water.	Recommended by a physician to remove freckles.
Medicated lotions	Antiseptics, sulfur compounds, or other medicinal agents.	Recommended by a physician for acne, or other skin eruptions.
Sunburn preventive lotion	Dilute solution of methyl salicylate in alcohol, glycerine and water.	Filters out most of the ultra-violet rays of the sun and produces a uniform tan.
Sunburn remedial lotion	Dilute solution of astringent or cooling agent (camphor) in alcohol, glycerine and water.	Helps to heal a first degree burn.

Powders

Next to creams, powders are widely used and constitute a profitable source of income. Since each kind of powder serves a particular purpose, the cosmetologist should be acquainted with the advantages of each powder used.

Face powder consists of a powder base, mixed with a coloring agent (pigment) and a suitable perfume. A good face powder for a normal skin should possess the following characteristics:

1. **Slip**—having a smooth feel to the skin. This quality is imparted by the talc or zinc stearate. The French or Italian talc, 200 mesh, is the best for face powders.

2. **Covering power**—having easy and even spread in order to cover skin shine, skin defects and enlarged pores. Zinc oxide, kaolin or titanium dioxide may be used.

3. **Adherency**—having the ability to remain on the skin. Zinc or magnesium stearate is used.

4. **Absorbency**—retaining the perfume, distributing the color, and absorbing perspiration and sebaceous secretions. Precipitated chalk and magnesium carbonate are employed for this purpose.

5. **Bloom**—imparting a velvet-like appearance to the skin. Chalk is used for this purpose.

6. **Color and perfume**—having a fragrant odor and uniform shade.

Toilet powder is used after bathing and shaving to relieve irritated surfaces. Talcum is the most satisfactory base for a toilet powder, as it is not absorbent and is not affected by moisture.

Cream powder is composed of a vanishing cream base, to which is added a face powder. Cream powder combines both the face powder and the vanishing cream in one application.

Cake powder has 3% tragacanth mucilage mixed with a face powder. The tragacanth mucilage binds the substances together in a compact form.

Liquid powder may contain an oil, zinc oxide, stearates, talc, perfume and coloring. It spreads quickly and uniformly over the skin, producing a non-drying thin film, or foundation, over which facial cosmetics can be applied.

COSMETICS FOR MAKEUP

The selection and application of proper makeup are the primary requisites for improving the complexion and beautifying the facial features. The introduction of a personalized makeup service in beauty salons has increased the demand and sale of these cosmetics.

Cheekcolor

Cheekcolor is available in the form of a compact powder, paste, cream and liquid.

Powder cheekcolor resembles the composition of a face powder except that a suitable color is added and the entire mixture is moistened and molded with aid of a binder. It is usually recommended for an oily skin.

Paste cheekcolor is composed of fats and waxes, having a red or brownish red color. It is recommended for a dry skin.

Liquid cheekcolor is composed of a dye dissolved in a solution of water, glycerine, alcohol and wax.

Creme cheekcolor usually has a petrolatum base and contains lanolin, fats and waxes. It is recommended for a dry skin.

Lipcolor comes in stick, cream or liquid form. Its three basic shades are blue-red, yellow-red and true red.

How to Select Cheekcolor

The blood, as seen through the skin, reveals the natural coloring in the cheeks. The color of blood is bright red. Depending on the nature of the skin, it may acquire a bluish, purplish or orange tone. The exact shade of rouge should match the natural skin color tone.

Rouge should always be selected to match the skin color tone rather than used as a color scheme to match a garment.

Lipcolor

How to Select Lipcolor

Lipcolor contains high melting ingredients to which is added either an insoluble pigment (delible) or a soluble bromoacid dye (indelible).

The color of the inner mucous membrane of the lower lip is a guide to color selection. If the lipstick blends with the color of this inner membrane, it will give the most natural effect.

Eye Makeup

How to Select Mascara

Eyebrow pencil consists of a wax base to which suitable coloring is added. An eyebrow pencil comes in various shades and may be used to darken the brows and lashes.

Mascara is sometimes used to darken the brows and the lashes. It is available in the form of cake, cream or liquid.

Cream mascara contains a pigment in a vanishing cream base.

Liquid mascara usually consists of an alcoholic solution of resin colored with a dyestuff. It is also available as a suspension of pigment in a mucilage. A brush is used for direct application.

The following is a general guide to the selection of mascara:

Color of Eyes and Eyelashes	Shade of Mascara
Black eyelashes, with dark brown or black eyes.	Black
Black eyelashes, with blue or grey eyes.	Blue or Black

Brown, golden or reddish eyelashes, with brown eyes.   Dark Brown

Blonde, reddish or light brown eyelashes, with green,

    grey or hazel eyes.   Brown or Green

How to Select Eyeshadow or Eyecolor

Eyeshadow or eyecolor is usually a suspension of pigments in a fatty base. It is colored black, brown, blue, green, bronze, silver and purple, and is carefully selected with regard to the color of the skin, hair and eyes, the time of day and the occasion.

Eyeshadow or eyecolor is used to emphasize the beauty of the eyes. Use sparingly and with good taste. The selected shade should blend with the tone of the natural shadow found between the inner corner of the eye and the root of the nose.

Color of Eyes	Eyecolor or Eyeshadow
Dark brown or black	Green, violet, brown
Blue	Blue, grey, violet
Green	Green, grey, brown
Hazel	Green, grey, brown
Grey	Grey, green, blue
Tawny	Brown, green

Miscellaneous Cosmetics

Grease paint is a mixture of fats, petrolatum and a coloring agent and is used for theatrical purposes.

Cake or pancake makeup is available in a compressed or compact form. It contains a dehydrated cream into which is blended a distinct color. It is removed from the container with a moist applicator and then spread over the face. As the water evaporates, a thin film of cream and color adhere to the face.

Muscle oil is an oil in which is dissolved either lecithin or cholesterol. It is used around the eyes and over the throat. It lubricates and softens the outer layer of the epidermis.

Beauty clay is composed of substances (kaolin, bentonite, fuller's earth or colloidal clay) to which is added honey, glycerine, zinc oxide, casein, oils, magnesium carbonate, starch, tragacanth gum powder, astringent, water or milk, depending on the nature of the pack or mask.

A beauty clay, or pack, can exert a cleansing, softening, astringent, refreshing, or stimulating action upon the skin.

Facial Packs and Masks are discussed in the chapter on Facial Treatments.

For more information, see section on Makeup in chapter on Facial Treatments.

Scalp Lotions And Ointments

Scalp lotions and ointments usually contain medicinal agents for the purpose of correcting a scalp condition and reconditioning the hair. The active ingredients of such preparations are irritants which stimulate the circulation of the scalp and hasten the shedding and renewal of epithelial tissue.

Scalp lotions contain such ingredients as lecithin, quinine, sulfur, salicylic acid, oils, resorcin, camphor and capsicum. Resorcin and quinine used over a period of time may discolor blonde hair.

Lotions for an **oily scalp** should contain a high percentage of alcohol and ingredients which possess astringent properties. On the other hand, lotions for a **dry scalp** should contain little or no alcohol or astringents. Instead, emulsified vegetable or animal oils should be the predominant ingredient.

Hair lotions or **tonics** are divided into groups according to the purpose for which they are used, some being used to regulate the activity of the oil glands of the scalp, others, to remove dandruff. They are found in liquid, oil or cream form.

For dry scalp, use olive oil, delicately perfumed.

For oily scalp, use sweet oil and alcohol.

Sulfur ointment contains precipitated sulfur in benzoated lard and is used in skin and scalp disorders.

Hair Dressings

Hair dressings are used to impart a gloss or fragrance to the hair and to keep unruly or curly hair in a fixed position.

Hair creams in both liquid and semi-solid form are used after a shampoo to give the hair gloss. They may be applied to either wet or dry hair. Such creams consist of lanolin, oil emulsions, fatty acids, waxes, mild alkalies and water. Hair creams are generally used on dry types of hair.

Other hair dressings which are used for oily types of hair and applied before the hair is set may contain resins, gums, starch, or other thickeners in water and alcohol. They hold the hair in place, leave a light film when dry, but give less gloss to the hair.

Hair Sprays

Styling trends led to a demand for a quick-drying preparation which would impart sufficient rigidity to the set to keep it in place, control loose ends and not detract from the natural sheen of the hair.

A new type of hair spray was developed with the production of plastics, such as polyvinylpyrrolidone (PVP). This hair spray gives a film with enough strength to control the hair, but with sufficient elasticity to allow combing without distorting the set. A product of this type can be used on wet hair as a setting lotion after the shampoo, thereby extending the duration of the set. The effect of this spray is better on weak, lightened, or over-processed hair.

CHAPTER 31

SALON MANAGEMENT

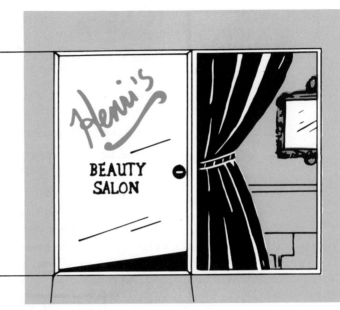

INTRODUCTION

Many opportunities exist in the field of cosmetology. Most cosmetologists want to advance themselves and eventually become owners or managers of beauty salons. Only those who are adequately prepared will be able to realize their ambitions.

The prospective owner or manager of a beauty salon should have a thorough training in cosmetology. In addition, she should have the experience of working in a number of different types of salons, of dealing with a variety of patrons, and of giving all kinds of cosmetic treatments. This background will be of great help in preparing a cosmetologist for her own business.

Going into your own business is a big responsibility. A self-inventory is necessary. A knowledge of business principles, bookkeeping, business laws, insurance, salesmanship and psychology are very helpful in conducting a beauty salon.

OPENING A BEAUTY SALON

When planning to open a beauty salon, careful consideration must be given to the selection of a location:

a) A good location is in an area large enough to support the beauty salon. It should be near other active business places which attract women, such as food, department stores, or super markets.

b) The salon should be clearly visible to women passing by.

c) Avoid too much competition in the immediate area.

d) Study the trading area for potential patrons. Find out about the size, income and buying habits of the area's population.

e) Sign a store lease for your protection.

A **store lease** guards against any increase in rent. The lease should refer to alterations and painting of the beauty salon. Before signing a lease, it is advisable that you ask your lawyer to help you in your negotiations.

REGULATIONS, BUSINESS LAWS AND INSURANCE

In conducting a business and employing help, it is necessary to comply with local, state and federal regulations and laws.

Local regulations may cover building and renovations (local building code).

Federal law covers social security, unemployment compensation or insurance, and cosmetics and luxury tax payments.

State laws cover sales taxes, licenses and workmen's compensation.

Income tax laws are covered by both the state and federal governments.

Insurance covers malpractice, premises liability, fire, burglary and theft, and use and occupancy policies.

PLANNING THE PHYSICAL LAYOUT

The layout of the beauty salon takes considerable amount of planning in order to achieve efficiency and economy.

"OPEN" STYLE OF OPERATION

The plan opposite shows a 4-operator salon, with 4 styling stations. Shampooing, hair drying, and manicuring are done in separate sections.

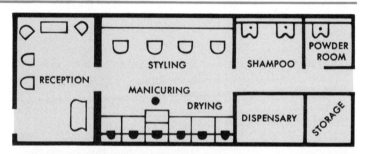

"CLOSED" STYLE OF OPERATION

Here 4 semi-private booths take care of all services, including hair coloring. Drying and manicuring are performed in a separate area.

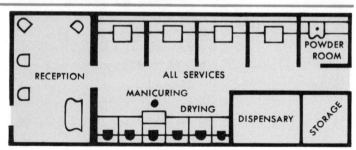

"COMBINATION" STYLE OF OPERATION

Here two open stations are utilized for styling, while two closed booths may be used for other services. Drying and manicuring are performed in a separate area.

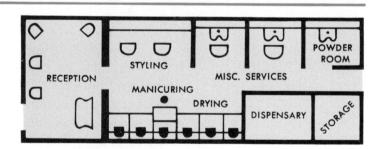

The beauty salon should have:
1. Maximum efficiency of operation.
2. Adequate aisle space.
3. The flow of operational services toward the reception room.
4. Enough space for each piece of equipment.

5. Furniture, fixtures and equipment chosen on the basis of cost, durability, utility and appearance. The purchase of standard and guaranteed equipment is a worthwhile investment.
6. A color scheme that is restful and flattering.
7. A dispensary; and plenty of storage space.
8. A clean rest room containing toilet and basin.
9. Good plumbing and sufficient lighting for satisfactory services.
10. Air conditioning, heating.

The reception area should not be overlooked when you plan the layout of your salon. This is the first contact a patron has with your establishment, and it sets the tone for the rest of the salon. An attractively decorated reception area can be one of your best promotional tools, as it immediately makes a patron comfortable, and gives her the impression that this is a salon that cares about the comfort of its patrons. It can also be an eye-catcher for passing women, who will find your salon invitingly pleasant and become prospects for your service.

ADVERTISING

Advertising includes all activities which attract attention to the salon and create a favorable impression in the public eye. Hence, the personality and ability of the manager and the staff, the quality of work performed, and the attractiveness of the salon are all natural advertising assets.

A pleased patron is the best form of advertising.

Advertising must attract and hold the reader's attention and create a desire for the beauty service or merchandise.

1. Plan an advertising budget of about 3% of the gross income.
2. Use newspaper advertising as the first medium.
3. Use direct mail to create a more intimate contact with the reader.
4. Classified advertising is comparatively inexpensive.
5. Radio advertising is more expensive, but is very effective.
6. TV is a dramatic but expensive medium of advertising.
7. A window display acts as a salesman to every passerby.
8. Personal public appearances are excellent advertising, especially at women's clubs, church functions, political gatherings, charitable affairs.

BUSINESS OPERATION AND PERSONNEL MANAGEMENT

Business problems are numerous, especially when you start a new salon. Contributing causes to beauty salon failures are:

1. Inexperience in dealing with the public and employees
2. Not enough capital to carry the business through until established, poor location, and too high overhead expenses
3. Lack of proper basic training in the beauty school
4. Business neglect and careless bookkeeping methods

The owner or manager must have business sense, knowledge, ability, good judgment and diplomacy.

Smooth beauty salon management depends on:

1. Sufficient investment capital
2. Efficiency of management
3. Cooperation between management and employees
4. Good business procedures
5. Trained and experienced personnel in the salon

**Be A Leader Of
Beauty Fashion**

There is no surer way of introducing the latest styles than by using them yourself. Your hair should always be becomingly styled; your nails manicured; and your face properly made up.

You can be your own best advertisement of the services you can perform. In addition, by looking good yourself, you can motivate your patrons to do the same.

Allocation Of Money

As part of your business operation, you must always know where your money is being spent. It is always a good idea to apportion your money so that maximum benefit is derived from it.

AVERAGE EXPENSES FOR BEAUTY SHOPS IN THE UNITED STATES (Based on total gross income)	
	Percent
Salaries and commissions (including payroll taxes)	53.5
Rent	13
Supplies	5
Advertising	3
Depreciation	3
Laundry	1
Cleaning	1
Light and power	1
Repairs	1.5
Insurance	.75
Telephone	.75
Miscellaneous expenses	1.5
Total expense	85
Net profit	15

The figures quoted above may be subject to variation in different localities. In large towns and cities items such as rent may run higher, while in small towns rent may be lower and utilities and telephone, higher. **The figures are suggested merely as a general guide.**

You will note that the largest items of expense are salaries, rent, supplies, and advertising. The first three merit your closest attention. The advertising item can be adjusted at your discretion.

When opening a beauty salon, provide for: plumbing, lighting, ventilation, electric outlets, air conditioning, heating, voltage, current (direct or indirect) carrying capacity of wires, and room size.

Booking Appointments

Booking appointments must be done with care, for booking can make the difference between success and failure. Services are sold in terms of time on the appointment page. Time, depending on how it is used, may spell either a gain or a loss.

**REVIEW
QUESTIONS**

**Opening A
Beauty Salon**

1. What constitutes a good location for a beauty salon?
2. What does a store lease guard against?
3. Why is the reception area of a beauty salon important?
4. What should advertising accomplish for a beauty salon?
5. What are four contributing causes of beauty salon failure?

TELEPHONE TECHNIQUES FOR THE BEAUTY SALON

INTRODUCTION

An important part of the beauty salon business is handled over the telephone. **Good telephone habits** and **techniques** make it possible for the salon owner and cosmetologist to increase business and win friends. With each call, you have a chance to build up the salon's reputation by rendering service of a high calibre.

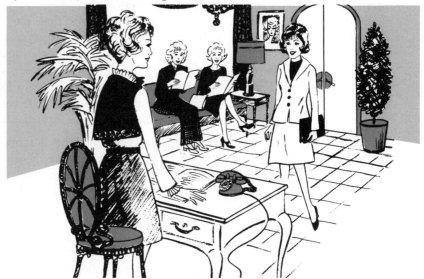

The telephone serves many useful purposes in the salon, such as:

1. To make or change appointments
2. To go after new business, or strayed or infrequent patrons
3. To remind patrons of needed services
4. To answer questions and render friendly service
5. To adjust complaints and satisfy patrons
6. To receive messages
7. To order equipment and supplies

Your success in using the phone depends to a large extent on the thoughtful effort exerted in observing certain fundamental principles. To the extent that these requirements are fulfilled, the telephone can be a very helpful aid to the success of the salon.

Business in the beauty salon can be effectively promoted over the phone, provided there is:

1. Good planning
2. Good telephone usage

GOOD PLANNING

Good planning consists mainly of assigning the **right person** and giving her the necessary information with which to do a good telephone job.

An understanding and capable cosmetologist, or receptionist, should be put in charge of telephone calls. She should be thoroughly familiar with the prices charged for the various beauty services, and be able to recommend appropriate services to **fit the needs of patrons.** In her absence, a reliable substitute should be trained to handle the salon's calls.

Next in importance is to have the phone located in a convenient and quiet place. A comfortable seat should be provided. Near the phone there should be readily accessible an appointment book, patrons' record cards, pencil or ball point pen and paper pad. To save time, have available an up-to-date list of telephone numbers commonly used, and a recent telephone directory.

Good business practice requires that the beauty salon's telephone number be freely and prominently displayed on stationery, advertising circulars, newspaper ads and appointment cards. Business cards should be readily available on the receptionist's desk, and in the reception area. They save patrons the trouble of having to look up the salon's phone number, making it easier for them to call your salon.

GOOD TELEPHONE USAGE

Good telephone usage can best be described as the golden rule of dealing with others as you would have them deal with you. The motto should be **"Phone as you would be phoned to."** When put into daily practice, it really means saying or doing the right thing, at the right time, and in the right manner.

Good telephone usage requires the application of a few basic principles which add up to **"common sense and common courtesy."**

Your Greetings

The first thing that the caller wants to know is the name of the speaker and the beauty salon she represents. The proper way to answer the phone is to say, "Good morning (afternoon or evening), Miss Jones of the Milady Beauty Salon speaking." Following this brief introduction, translate your greeting into such helpful expressions as "How are you?" "What can I do for you?" or "May I help you?".

The first few words you say over the phone immediately register your attractive personality and give prestige to the beauty salon. That is why it is so important to greet every caller with a **cordial welcome.** It shows that you are pleased to receive the call and want to be of service.

Basic Rules

Any receptionist, or cosmetologist, should be able to learn the following four basic rules and to follow them to improve her telephone conversations:

1. Display an interested, helpful attitude, as revealed by the tone of your voice and what you have to say.
2. Be prompt. Answer all calls as quickly as possible. Nothing irritates the caller more than waiting for you to answer.
3. Practice giving all necessary information to the caller. This means identifying yourself and your salon when making or receiving a call. If the requested information is not readily available, be courteous enough to say, "Will you please hold the line while I get the information for you?" Then put the caller on "hold."
4. Be tactful. Avoid saying or doing anything which may offend or irritate the caller. The tactful telephone user is careful:
   a) To inquire who is calling by saying, "May I ask who is calling, please?" Refrain from using such blunt questions as "Who's calling?"
   b) To address people by their last names. Make use of such expressions as "Thank you," "I'm sorry" or "I beg your

pardon." The caller appreciates such courtesy and consideration.

c) To avoid making side remarks during a call.

d) To let the caller end the conversation. Do not bang down the receiver at the end of a call.

Your Voice And Speech

Every time you telephone someone, you make a definite impression —good, bad or indifferent. Your voice, what you say, and how you say it are what reveal you to others.

If you want a **good telephone personality,** then be sure to acquire the habit of:

1. Clear speech
2. Correct speech
3. Pleasing tone of voice

In this way, the other person hearing your voice will readily understand what you are saying.

As a general rule, the most effective speech is that which is correct, and at the same time, natural. A cheerful, alert and enthusiastic voice most often comes from a person who has these desirable qualities as part of her personality.

To make a good impression over the phone, assume good posture; relax and draw a deep breath before answering the phone. Open the mouth, pronounce the words distinctly, use a low-pitched natural voice and speak at a moderate pace. Clear voices carry better than loud voices over the phone.

If your listeners sometimes break in with such remarks as "what was that?" or "I'm sorry, I didn't get that," it usually means that your voice is not doing its job well. In that event, you should try to find out what is wrong and have it corrected. The more common causes of this condition may be:

1. You are speaking too loudly or too softly.
2. Your lips are too close or too far away from the mouthpiece. They should be about the width of two fingers from the mouthpiece.
3. The pitch of your voice is too low or too high.
4. Your pronunciation is not precise.

PLANNING YOUR TELEPHONE CONVERSATION

Whether it be a friendly chat or a business conversation, list the main points on your pad so you will **know what to say.** In this way, you will project an image of someone who knows how to handle all types of situations in an efficient manner. The salon will benefit from this image as patrons will obtain a favorable impression of the people who are employed there.

If a patron is talking to you in a lengthy conversation, take notes of the main points of her conversation. When you answer her, you will be able to address yourself to the points in which she has expressed interest.

EFFECTIVE TELEPHONE TECHNIQUES

Regular observance of the simple requirements of good telephone practice will help you make friends, bring in more business, and create goodwill for the beauty salon.

To acquire skill in handling different situations and patrons, you should study and practice the following effective telephone techniques:

1. Booking appointments by phone
2. Adjusting complaints over the phone
3. Answering price objections over the phone

Booking Appointments By Phone

Whoever is assigned to handle salon appointments has an important responsibility. For this task, special qualifications and experience are required, such as:

1. Being familiar with all types of services and products available in the beauty salon, and the prices to be charged
2. Being familiar with the quality of work done by each cosmetologist
3. Using judgment in giving assignments and being equally fair with the cosmetologists in the salon
4. Being accurate in recording name, service, and time when making appointments
5. Spacing appointments uniformly to permit the efficient functioning of the beauty salon

How To Handle A Prospective Patron

The proper way to handle a prospective patron is illustrated in the following telephone conversation.

Receptionist (R): "Good afternoon. Miss Jones of the Milady Beauty Salon speaking. May I help you?"

Patron (P): "I am Mrs. Brown and would like to have a permanent."

R.: "At what time, please?"

P.: "Two o'clock on Wednesday."

R.: "I am sorry, Mrs. Brown. This time is already taken. We have a four o'clock opening. Would this time meet with your convenience?"

P.: "Yes, that's fine. But, I want that blond young girl."

R.: "Do you mean Miss Paul? She has no openings for Wednesday. But we have Miss Dell, a very capable hairstylist, who can take care of you at four o'clock."

P.: "I would really prefer Miss Paul."

R.: "I am sorry that we cannot accommodate you this time. Could you take another time instead? Perhaps, at your next appointment, if made early enough, we can arrange to have Miss Paul serve you."

P.: "All right, then. I will be in at four o'clock on Wednesday."

R.: "Very well, Mrs. Brown. Thank you. Good-bye."

How To Handle A Regular Patron

How to arrange a convenient appointment for the patron is illustrated by the following telephone conversation.

Patron (P): "This is Mrs. West. Can Stella give me a shampoo and set any time on Friday? I'd rather come in the afternoon."

Receptionist (R): "Just a moment, Mrs. West, I'll check. Stella is booked both Friday and Saturday. How about tomorrow?"

P.: "Tomorrow is rather inconvenient for me."

R.: "Then I would suggest an appointment with Mary on Friday afternoon. Mary is new with us, but she does very good work, and I'm sure you will be satisfied. Stella could take care of you tomorrow at one, or Mary on Friday, at three."

P.: "I do like to have Stella do my hair, but I simply can't come in then. I don't know what to do."

R.: "If any appointments are cancelled, I'll be glad to call you, Mrs. West. I have your number—536-4327. But in case there isn't a cancellation, should I give you the appointment on Friday at three with Mary? Stella could show Mary how you style your hair."

P.: "All right, I'll try Mary."

R.: "Friday at three, then, unless I call. Thank you, Mrs. West. Good-bye."

Adjusting Complaints By Phone

Some beauty salons resent complaints; they take it as a personal affront. Such an attitude only makes matters worse and frequently results in a loss of business. Instead, the patron's complaint should be given **careful consideration.** It affords an opportunity to improve service and retain the patron's goodwill.

Adjusting complaints, particularly over the phone, is a difficult task. Since the complainant is probably upset and short-tempered, try to use **self-control, tact** and **courtesy,** no matter how trying the circumstances may be. Only in this way will the complainant be made to feel that she has been fairly treated.

Remember that the tone of your voice must be sympathetic and reassuring. Your manner of speaking and the words you use should make the caller aware that you are really concerned about her complaint. Get her to tell you the whole story. **Avoid interrupting her.**

After hearing the complaint in full, your next move is to adjust it quickly and effectively. Any of the following techniques will accomplish good results.

1. Tell the unhappy patron that you are sorry for what happened and explain the reason for the difficulty. Inform her that it will not happen again.

2. Sympathize with the patron by telling her you understand how she feels and regret the inconvenience suffered. Express thanks for calling this matter to your attention.

3. Ask the caller how the beauty salon can remedy her complaint. If the request is fair and reasonable, agree and comply with it.

4. If the patron is dissatisfied with the results of the beauty service, try to correct the difficulty to her satisfaction. Pacify the patron by arranging for a corrective service free of charge.

How to adjust a complaint over the phone is illustrated by the following conversation:

R.: "Good morning, Miss Jones of the Milady Beauty Salon speaking."

P.: "May I speak to Mr. Charles?"

R.: "I'm sorry, but he can't come to the phone now. May I help you?"

P.: "Well . . . This is Mrs. Bell and I wanted to talk to Mr. Charles because I'm not satisfied with my permanent."

R.: "I'm sorry to hear that, Mrs. Bell. I'm sure Mr. Charles would want to talk with you himself. Would it be convenient for you to come to the salon so that he can see your hair? If you could do that sometime within the next few days, I'll be glad to make an appointment for a consultation."

P.: "I'm going to be near the shop tomorrow morning. Would 11 o'clock be all right?"

R.: "Yes, or it would be even better if you could see him a few minutes before eleven. Shall I tell him to expect you then?"

P.: "Yes, thank you."

R.: "Thank you, Mrs. Bell. I'm so glad you called."

Answering Price Objections

Suppose a patron phones in to ask for the price of a permanent wave. After being told what the cost is, the patron says, "I can get the same permanent wave around the corner for less." How are you going to answer this objection?

The best way to overcome such an objection is to build up more value in the patron's mind. You can appeal to her better judgment by presenting logical reasons. Try to show her how she will profit from the greater value and better service offered by your beauty salon.

In the telephone conversation, first get the patron to agree with you. You might say in a calm, assuring voice, "I quite agree, Mrs. Brown, but you can also get a pair of shoes for less. Yet, you prefer to pay more and get only the best for your feet. Why, Mrs. Brown? Because you know that although shoes may look the same, there may be a vast difference in the quality of the leather, the skill of the shoemaker, and the fit of the shoes. In the long run, the higher-priced shoe will give you better wear, and, therefore, cost less.

"By the same token, our permanent wave costs more because we use only the highest quality materials for your hair, and take great care to produce a natural-looking permanent. You can rest assured that the reason we charge more is to enable us to provide you with better service and a higher quality permanent."

RULES OF GOOD TELEPHONE USAGE

The telephone, when properly used, is a valuable aid for obtaining more business and for making appointments. Every time the telephone is used, it affords an opportunity to render service and spread goodwill for the beauty salon.

To get the most out of your telephone, observe the following rules at all times:

1. Be prompt. When the telephone rings, answer it immediately, after the first ring, if possible.

2. Be prepared. Know in advance what you intend to say. Be able to provide accurate information to any inquirer. Always keep a pencil, ball point pen and pad handy for messages.

3. Identify both yourself and your salon for every incoming and outgoing call.

4. Speak clearly into the phone. Don't mumble or shout. Use good English and avoid slang.

5. Be tactful and courteous when speaking over the phone. Refer to the caller by last name. Try to leave a good impression on your listener.

6. Be interested in and helpful to the people who call the beauty salon.

7. Avoid arguments and interruptions while on the phone.

REVIEW QUESTIONS

Telephone Techniques For The Beauty Salon

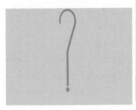

1. Name at least five uses a telephone has in a beauty salon.
2. Describe good telephone usage.
3. What are four basic rules to follow when using the telephone?
4. What three speech characteristics contribute to good telephone personality?
5. What should a cosmetologist do before undertaking a telephone conversation?
6. How will the use of good telephone techniques help a cosmetologist and a beauty salon?
7. How should a patron's complaint be handled?
8. How should a price objection be handled?

BEAUTY SALON SALESMAN- SHIP

INTRODUCTION

Selling is becoming an increasingly important responsibility of the cosmetologist as salons add wig and boutique departments to their beauty culture operations. The cosmetologist who is equally proficient as both a hairstylist and a salesman is most likely to be the one to succeed in business.

No attempt is made here to cover all aspects of selling, but if students use this material as a basis upon which to build, they will find that effective selling techniques will become part of their repertoire of skills.

Successful salesmanship requires ambition and determination. Effective salesmanship is a necessity in any business.

The first step in selling is to "Sell Yourself." Patrons must like and trust the cosmetologist in order for them to buy beauty services, cosmetics, wigs or other merchandise.

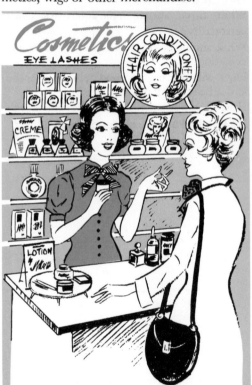

Every woman who enters a salon is a prospective purchaser of additional services or merchandise. The manner in which you greet her lays the foundation for suggestive selling. Greet her with a smile and say, "May I help you?" Be ready and eager to serve her. Recognizing the needs and preferences of patrons makes the intelligent use of suggestive selling possible.

SELLING PRINCIPLES

The cosmetologist who is to become a proficient salesperson must understand, and be able to apply, the following principles of selling:

1. Be familiar with the merits and benefits of each service and product.
2. Adapt the approach and selling method to the needs and psychology of each patron.
3. Be self-confident. It is essential to making selling agreeable and productive.
4. Stimulate attention, interest and desire which are the steps leading up to a sale.

5. Never misrepresent your service or product.

6. Use tact in handling a patron, without being rude or offensive.

7. Understand human nature so that you can apply appropriate sales technique.

8. Don't be negative.

9. To sell a product or service, deliver a sales talk in a relaxed, friendly manner and, if possible, demonstrate its use.

10. Recognize the right psychological moment to close any sale.

TYPES OF PATRONS AND WAYS OF HANDLING THEM

The cosmetologist who is most likely to be successful in selling additional services or merchandise to patrons is the one who can recognize the many different types of people and knows how to handle each type.

The following material describes seven of the most common types you are likely to come across and suggests ways on how each should be treated.

1. **Shy, Timid.** Make her feel at ease. Lead the conversation. Don't force her to talk. Cheer her up.

2. **Talkative Type.** Be a good, patient listener. Tactfully switch the conversation to her beauty needs.

3. **Nervous, Irritable Type.** Does not want much conversation. Wants simple, practical hairdo and fast operator. Get her started and finished as fast as possible.

4. **Inquisitive, Over-Cautious Type.** Explain everything in detail. Show her facts—sealed bottles, brand names. Ask her opinion.

5. **Conceited, "Know It All" Type.** Agree with her. Cater to her vanity. Suggest things in question form. Don't argue with her. Compliment her.

6. **Teenager.** Don't oversell her. Leave her hair longer. Give her special advice on hair care and proper makeup.

7. **Old Timer** (60 and over). Be extra courteous and solicitous of her comfort. Suggest permanent and hairstyle more becoming to a mature woman.

PERSONALITY IN SELLING

Greeting The Patron

Your selling power will increase progressively as you make patrons aware of your personal interest in their welfare. Treat patrons with friendliness and extend such little courtesies as a warm greeting and a pleasant smile. Take care of the patron's coat and do not let her wait too long for her treatment. Attention to these little details is greatly appreciated by patrons. The beauty service may be obtained elsewhere, but the personality and friendliness behind the service are what brings the patron back again to you.

Personal magnetism is a valuable asset in selling. Each person creates an atmosphere which may either attract or repel patrons. Since an attractive personality is conducive to making friends and increasing sales, the cosmetologist should develop the qualities which make for an outstanding personality.

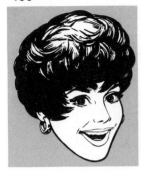

The following are positive qualities necessary for a successful selling career:

Optimism—the expectation that things will come out all right.

Acquisitiveness—the desire to acquire wealth and improve one's position in life.

Self assertiveness—the ability to face and to overcome problems and obstacles.

Initiative—the ability to do what is necessary without being told what or how to do it.

Cheerfulness—a congenial spirit which makes the work of selling agreeable both to the cosmetologist and the patron.

Tact—saying or doing the right thing, at the right time, in the right place, without any offense.

Sincerity—making your suggestions because you really believe the sale will be a good one for the patron.

Ability to smile—a smiling face tells the patron that you are pleased to be of service to her.

SALES PSYCHOLOGY

No matter how good a beauty service or product may be, unless there is a need for it, you will find it difficult to make a sale. Before attempting to sell anything, first determine whether the patron has a need for it. Every person who enters a salon is an individual with wants and needs different from anyone else. Determine how the patron can use a particular item before attempting to sell it to her.

Motives For Buying

What are the motives which prompt women to buy beauty services and merchandise? Women want to make the most of their natural endowments or substitute for what is lacking. A modern hairstyle, a youthful complexion, sparkling eyes, a tender skin, stylish clothes and correct makeup are among the most cherished desires of women. Personal influence and social prestige can be enhanced by a youthful appearance. Vanity or show, personal satisfaction and aesthetic gratification are other reasons why patrons desire beauty treatments. The buying motive which predominates and is the strongest is the one to which the cosmetologist should make her most successful appeal.

Help Patron Make Decision

If a patron is doubtful or undecided, help her to make a decision by giving honest and sincere advice. For instance, if a patron wants a permanent wave and you see that her hair is very dry, it is your responsibility to recommend the use of a conditioner and fully explain how it will help her hair.

In the beauty profession, you should instill ideas in conjunction with selling services and merchandise. Show the patron not only what the beauty service is, but also what it can mean to her in terms of results and benefits. Sell her the idea that a beauty treatment or product will improve her feminine attractiveness and personality. The selling of ideas along with beauty services gives greater value to the patron and more sales to the cosmetologist.

SALES TECHNIQUES

The best interests of the patron should be your first consideration. Under no circumstances should you approach a patron with the thought of the amount of money you can get from her. Sincerity and honesty are the foundation of good salesmanship.

Careful consideration on your part will acquaint you with the patron's needs, and those needs can be fulfilled to the complete satisfaction of the patron and to your financial advantage. Tact and diplomacy must be used, as well as courtesy.

Use Attractive Displays

To acquaint new and old patrons with the quality and cost of beauty services and merchandise, use attractive displays in the window, at the reception desk, cosmetic counter, service booth, and boutique area. Dress the windows so that they carry a definite message and appeal to the people passing the salon. Frequent rearrangement of case displays and changes in the featured service or merchandise will draw attention to new items. Price signs should accompany the placards. If the price is within reach of the patron, there will be no hesitation or embarrassment in obtaining more particulars about the advertisement.

An effective display can create interest in a particular service or product and help in its sale. Beauty products should make their appeal to the eye through color, and to the imagination through suggestion of feminine loveliness. Manufacturers and wholesale dealers will cooperate in arranging for well-lighted and attractive displays of their products.

Describe Benefits Of Beauty Service

Each beauty service requires a suitable sales technique, employing simple and suggestive language which will make the patron feel like buying. In creating interest and desire, use picture words and descriptive adjectives charged with feeling. Present to the patron a verbal picture of herself as a relaxed, refreshed and more charming individual after using the recommended beauty treatment.

Facial

Say to Mrs. Smith, "Our beauty facial invigorates the skin, making it radiant and lovely. A smooth and velvety skin will prompt others to remark 'what beautiful skin you have'." An emotional appeal is often more effective than the use of cold, reasoned facts.

For salesmanship to be successful, the language should be positive rather than negative. Refrain from using the word "don't" in selling language.

Hair Shaping

For example, a patron makes an appointment for a shampoo and set. Her hair needs shaping. (Use the term "shaping" instead of "cutting" because it sounds softer and is easier to sell.) The conversation might be as follows:

Cosmetologist: "Mrs. Jones, your hair is a little too long and not right for the style I'd like to give you. I would like to shape it a little so that it will conform to your head, and also frame your face. The set will last longer, your hair will be more manageable and it will dry in less time."

Mrs. Jones: "I didn't realize my hair was that long. Go ahead and shape it for I want my hairstyle to look as good as possible. Don't take off too much, please."

Cosmetologist: "Don't be concerned. I will take off only what is really necessary."

Don't Underestimate Patron

At no time should you underestimate either the patron's intelligence or ability to pay for what she actually wants or needs. Because a patron is simply dressed and makes no pretentious display of finances are no indications that the patron is not able to afford anything she wants. Regardless of financial status, each patron is entitled to courteous treatment and sincere consideration, whether her purchase is for a large or a small amount. When making a sale, you should refrain from mentioning price until the patron's interest is sufficiently aroused. Then it should be given in a casual manner, without attaching too much importance to it.

Selling Beauty Services And Accessories

Learn to identify patrons, not only by appearance, but also by name. Address the patron as "Miss Jones" or "Mrs. Smith" and not by "dearie" or "honey". Keep a reminder file of the patron's type of skin, hair and scalp; also include the type and price of service rendered and merchandise sold. When the patron calls again, you can refresh your memory as to previous work. Reminder forms help not only to sell more beauty treatments and products, but also assure the patron that you have a personal interest in her problems.

Another source of income is keeping up with the latest hairstyles. The progressive cosmetologist can create new coiffures whenever the occasion arises.

Every patron is a potential source of new customers and additional beauty treatments. A fashionable hairstyle will boost the reputation of the cosmetologist and, as a result, bring in new patrons. For complete grooming, beauty treatments should supplement one another. For example, reconditioning and corrective scalp treatments can be recommended between permanents. Explain to the patron that the hair will result in a much more satisfactory permanent wave, and the coiffure will be kept looking smarter and more vibrant, if dry and brittle hair is treated first. Encourage the patron to take a series of corrective treatments at a special price. For complete personal grooming, other services may be required, such as a facial, eyebrow shaping and a manicure.

In selling beauty services and merchandise, stress quality and other advantages over cheaper substitutes. The cosmetologist should have a ready answer for a price objection. She can say, "Although you are paying a higher price, you will be getting greater value and superior results from the money expended." The cosmetologist can also explain that the higher price is occasioned by the use of standard top quality materials and highly skilled cosmetologists.

Selling Supplies

Before the cosmetologist tries to sell accessory supplies, such as cosmetics, compacts, perfumes, atomizers, hair nets, wigs, jewelry, combs, brushes, she should have correct information concerning the following:

1. Location of the product
2. Name and brand of product
3. Contents and price of product
4. Comparative merits of similar products which differ in price

There should be a complete assortment of beauty accessories to meet the demand and to fit the pocketbook of the patrons. The range in shade and color of cosmetics should be large enough to suit all types of skin tones. The sale of one item leads to the sale of other items, if they are in stock. Reorder regularly, to assure a fresh and complete stock at all times.

Most women are anxious to know whether the color of powder, rouge and lipstick they are using is correct. A question of this nature may open the door to cosmetic sales. A complimentary skin analysis and makeup should be given to show the patron the cosmetics which are most suitable for her. Once the patron begins to buy her cosmetics through the beauty salon, she will establish the buying habit which will continue as long as high quality merchandise is sold.

The most effective way to convince women of the value of professional beauty services and accessories is to show them an actual treatment or application. Depend more on demonstrations than on spoken claims or promises.

REVIEW QUESTIONS

Beauty Salon Salesmanship

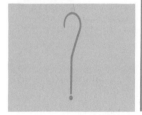

1. What are the ten principles of selling?
2. Name seven of the most common types of patron a cosmetologist is likely to come across.
3. Before attempting to sell a service or a product, what must a cosmetologist determine?
4. What is the foundation of good salesmanship?
5. What type of language is most suitable for selling?
6. How should beauty products make their appeal?
7. What potential does every patron have?
8. What is one of the most effective selling tools?
9. What is the best way of introducing the latest styles?
10. Why should the cosmetologist always look her best?

BUSINESS RECORDS AND SUPPLIES

Good business administration demands the keeping of a simple and efficient record system. Records are of value only if they are correct, concise and complete. Bookkeeping means keeping an accurate record of all income and expenses. Income is usually classified as income from services and income from retail sales. Expenses include rent, utilities, insurance, salaries, advertising, equipment and repairs. The assistance of an accountant will prove valuable. Retain check stubs, cancelled checks, receipts and invoices.

Proper business records are necessary to meet the requirements of local, state and federal laws regarding taxes and employees.

All business transactions must be recorded in order to maintain proper records. These are required by the owner, or manager, for the following reasons:

1. For efficient operation of the beauty salon
2. For determining income, expenses, profit and loss
3. For proving the value of the beauty salon to prospective buyer
4. For arranging a bank loan
5. For such reports as income tax, social security, unemployment and disability insurance, wage and hour law, accident compensation and labor tax.

Daily Records Important

Keeping daily records enables the owner, or manager, to know just how the business is progressing. A weekly or monthly summary helps to:

1. Make comparisons with other years.
2. Detect any changes in demands for different services.
3. Order necessary supplies.
4. Check on the use of materials according to the type of service rendered.
5. Control expenses and waste.

Each expense item bears on the total gross income. Accurate records show the cost of operation in relation to income.

Keep daily sales slips, appointment book and a petty cash book for at least six months. Payroll book, cancelled checks, monthly and yearly records are usually held for at least seven years. **Service** and **inventory** records are also important to keep. Sales records help to maintain a perpetual inventory. An organized **inventory** system can be used to:

1. Prevent overstocking.
2. Prevent running short of supplies needed for services.
3. Help in establishing the net worth at the end of the year.

Keep Service Records

A **service record** should be kept of treatments given and merchandise sold to each patron. Such information is the basis for timely suggestions and uniform services which result in increased sales. For this purpose, use card file system or memorandum book.

All service records should contain the name and address of the patron, date, amount charged, product used, and results obtained. Also, note the patron's preference and taste.

Keep a running inventory of all supplies. Classify them as to their use and retail value. Those to be used in the business are **consumption** supplies. Those to be sold are **retail** supplies. Consulting the inventory records indicates which merchandise is most popular, and prevents the running short of any item. In reordering, buy sufficient merchandise, so that it can be used or sold quickly, within a reasonable period of time. It is a better policy to have a slight excess of material rather than a deficiency in supplies.

Appointment Record

The use of a private appointment record divides the cosmetologist's working time to suit the patron's convenience. The appointment book accurately reflects what is taking place in the salon at a given time. The cosmetologist who makes advance preparation can render prompt and efficient service when the patron arrives. Besides, **waste in time and money** is prevented.

BUSINESS LAW FOR THE BEAUTY SALON

A beauty salon may be owned and operated by an **individual**, a **partnership**, or a **corporation**. Before deciding which type of ownership is most desirable, you should be acquainted with the relative merits of each.

Individual Ownership

1. The proprietor is boss and manager.
2. The proprietor can determine policies and make decisions.
3. The proprietor receives all profits and bears all losses.

Partnership

1. More capital is available for investment.
2. The combined ability and experience of each partner make it easier to share work and responsibilities, and to make decisions.
3. Profits are equally shared.
4. Each partner assumes each others unlimited liability for debts.

Corporation

1. A charter has to be obtained from the state.
2. A corporation is subject to taxation and regulation by the state.
3. The management is in the hands of a board of directors who determine policies and make decisions in accordance with the constitution of the charter.
4. The dividing of profits is proportionate to the number of shares possessed by each stockholder.
5. The stockholder is not legally responsible for losses.

Before Buying Or Selling A Beauty Salon

1. A written purchase and sale agreement should be formulated in order to avoid any misunderstandings between the contracting parties.
2. For safekeeping and enforcement, the written agreement should be placed in the hands of an impartial third person, who is to deliver the agreement to the grantee (one to whom the property is transferred upon the fulfillment of the specified contract).
3. The buyer or seller should take and sign a complete statement of inventory (goods, fixtures, etc.) and the value of each article.
4. If there is a transfer of chattel mortgage, notes, lease, and bill of sale, an investigation should be made to determine any default in the payment of debts.
5. Consult your lawyer for additional guidance.

**Agreement
To Buy Salon**

An agreement to buy an established salon should include the following:

1. Correct identity of owner.
2. True representations concerning the value and inducements offered to buy the beauty salon.
3. Use of salon's name and reputation for a definite period of time.
4. An understanding that the seller will not compete with the prospective owner within a reasonable distance from present location.

**Protection In Making
A Lease**

1. Secure exemption of fixtures or appliances which may be attached to the store or loft, so that they can be removed without violating the lease.
2. Insert into lease an agreement relative to necessary renovations and repairs, such as painting, plumbing, fixtures and electrical installation.
3. Secure option from landlord to assign lease to another person; in this way, the obligations for the payment of rental are kept separate from the responsibilities of operating the business.

**Protection Against Fire,
Theft And Lawsuits**

1. Employ honest and able employees, and keep premises securely locked.
2. Follow safety precautions to prevent fire, injury and lawsuits. Liability, fire, malpractice and burglary insurance should be obtained.
3. Do not violate the medical practice law of your state by attempting to diagnose, treat or cure a disease.
4. Become thoroughly familiar with the cosmetology law and the sanitary code of your city and state.
5. Keep accurate records of number of workers, salaries, length of employment, and social security numbers, for various state and federal laws that affect the social welfare of employees.

REMEMBER — **Ignorance of the law is no excuse for its violation**

WARNING

Do not have business transactions with a total stranger, and never pay a stranger cash. Never make out a check to an individual who is working for a firm; make check payable to the firm.

REVIEW QUESTIONS

**Business Records
And Supplies**

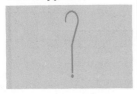

1. How should records be kept in order to be effective?
2. What purpose do accurate records serve?
3. How long should sales slips, appointment book and petty cash be kept?
4. How long should payroll book, cancelled checks, monthly and yearly records be kept?
5. What two types of supplies make up a beauty salon's inventory?
6. Under what three types of ownership may a beauty salon be operated?

THINGS TO CONSIDER WHEN GOING INTO BUSINESS

CAPITAL
  Amount available
  Amount required
ORGANIZATION
  Individual, partnership
  corporation
BANKING
  Opening a bank account
  Deposits, drawing checks
  Monthly statements
  Notes and drafts
SELECTING LOCATION
  Population
  Transportation facilities
  Transients
  Trade possibilities
  Space required
  Zoning ordinances
  Parking
DECORATING and
FLOOR PLAN
  Selection of furniture
  Floor covering
  Installing telephone
  Interior decorating
  Exterior decorating
    Window displays
    Electric signs
EQUIPMENT and SUPPLIES
  Selecting equipment
  Comparative values
  Installation
  Labor-saving steps
ADVERTISING
  Planning
  Direct mail
  Local house organs
  Newspaper
  Radio
  Television
LEGAL
  Lease, contracts
  Claims and lawsuits

BOOKKEEPING SYSTEM
  Installation
  Record of appointments
  Receipts and disbursements
  Petty cash
  Profit and loss
  Inventory
COST OF OPERATION
  Supplies, Depreciation,
  Rent, Light, Salaries,
  Telephone, Linen service,
  Sundries, Taxes
MANAGEMENT
  Methods of building goodwill
  Analysis of materials and labor
    in relation to service charges
  Greeting patrons
  Adjusting complaints
  Handling employees
  Selling merchandise
  Telephone techniques
OFFICE ADMINISTRATION
  Stationery and office supplies
  Inventory
INSURANCE
  Public liability and malpractice
  Compensation, unemployment
  Social Security
  Fire, theft and burglary
METHODS OF PAYMENT
  In advance
  C.O.D.
  Open account
  Time payments
COMPLIANCE WITH
LABOR LAWS
  Minimum wage law
  Hours of employment
  Minors
ETHICS
  Courtesy
  Observation of professional
    trade practices

COMPLIANCE WITH STATE COSMETOLOGY LAW governing salon physical layout and equipment
LICENSING of beauty salons, salon managers and cosmetologists

FIRST AID

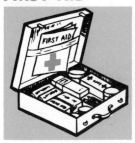

Emergencies arise in every line of business, and a knowledge of first aid measures is invaluable to the salon management and staff. Accidents arising in the beauty salon are mainly skin abrasions and burns.

A physician should be called as soon as possible after any accident has occurred, both as a courtesy to the patient and as a protection to the beauty salon. There are certain first aid treatments, however, which the layman can give while awaiting medical assistance. Use a standard first aid kit.

Abrasions

When the cuticle is cut with the nippers, or broken by carelessness in pushing, an antiseptic such as tincture of iodine, hydrogen peroxide, or mercurochrome should be applied.

Burns

Burns may be caused by electricity, hot irons, or flames, while scalds are usually due to exposure to hot liquids or live steam. Burns are classified as first degree, characterized by redness; second degree, having watery blisters; and third degree, involving deeper structures of the flesh with possible charring of tissues. First degree burns are treated by an application of cloths saturated with a solution of salt or baking soda. Apply a dry, sterile dressing.

Electric Shock

The clothing should be loosened and the patient removed to a cool place. The head should be raised, and the tongue drawn forward to prevent strangulation. Apply artificial respiration. Alcoholic stimulants should not be given.

Heat Exhaustion

Heat exhaustion is a general functional depression due to heat. It is characterized by a cool, moist skin, and collapse. Clothing should be loosened and the patient removed to a cool, dark, quiet place. She should be kept lying down for several hours, as rest and quiet will hasten recovery.

Nose Bleed

Nose bleed is a hemorrhage from the nose, and is treated by loosening the collar and applying pads saturated with cool water to the face and back of the neck.

For more information about emergency care, consult the latest edition of the First Aid Manual published by the American Red Cross.

Artificial Respiration

To deal with occurrences such as severe electric shock, protracted fainting, drowning, poisoning, and gas suffocation, there are three methods for giving artificial respiration: back pressure-arm lift method; prone pressure method; mouth-to-mouth breathing.

Back Pressure-Arm Lift Method

Place the patient in a face-down, prone position; bend her elbows; place her hands one upon the other and turn her face slightly to one side, resting the cheek upon her hands and allowing the free passage of air. Kneel at the head of the patient, facing her. Place your hands flat on patient's back with the tips of the thumbs just touching.

Prone Pressure Method

To force air out of the lungs, press downward on patient's back, keeping your elbows straight. Release the pressure by moving slowly backward. To expand the patient's chest, draw her arms upward and towards you, keeping the elbows straight. Finally, lower the patient's arms to the ground.

The above cycle should be repeated about twelve times a minute at a steady rate, and continued until natural breathing is restored.

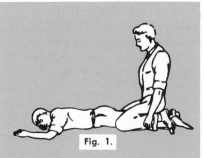

Fig. 1.

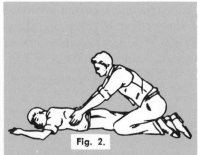

Fig. 2.

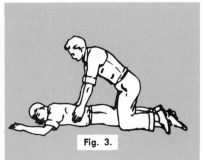

Fig. 3.

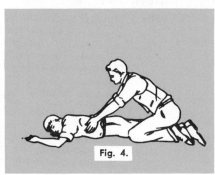

Fig. 4.

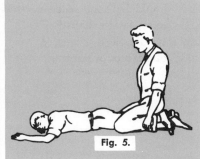

Fig. 5.

Fig. 1—Assume straddling position.
Fig. 2—Place hands.
Fig. 3—Swing forward.
Fig. 4—Sit back.
Fig. 5—And rest.

Mouth-to-Mouth Breathing

Mouth-to-mouth breathing can also be used for emergency first aid. First, remove any obstruction from the patient's air passage. Then, place patient on a flat surface with the head tilted backwards.

Open your mouth and place it tightly over the patient's mouth. At the same time, pinch the patient's nostrils and keep them closed. Blow into the patient's mouth. Remove your mouth and listen for the return flow of air from the patient's lungs. Continue this blowing and releasing movement.

Epileptic Fit

An epileptic fit is a nerve disorder, characterized by unconsciousness, convulsions, contortions of the face, foaming at the mouth, and rolling of the eyes.

Treatment consists of lying patient on the side and fixing a wad of cotton between her teeth to prevent biting the tongue. Mild stimulants may be administered in moderation after recovery. If the patient falls into a deep sleep after the attack, she should not be disturbed until she awakens naturally.

Fainting

Fainting is caused by a lack of blood flowing to the brain, bad air, indigestion, nervous condition, unpleasant odors, etc., and is characterized by pallor and loss of muscular control. There is a temporary suspension of respiration and circulation. If there is a sign of fainting and before it actually occurs, the patient should hold her head between her knees, as this action may check the faintness by causing the blood to flow quickly to the head. Treatment for fainting consists of loosening all tight clothing, changing the air in the room, and placing the patient in a reclining position with the head slightly lower than the body. If the patient is conscious, she should take aromatic spirits of ammonia and stimulants, such as hot coffee, tea or milk. If the patient is unconscious, cold applications to the face, chest, and over the heart are given, but cold water **should not** be dashed in the patient's face.

REVIEW QUESTIONS

First Aid

1. When an accident occurs, when should a physician be called?
2. What should be done when a cuticle is cut with a nippers?
3. What causes heat exhaustion?
4. How is a nose bleed treated?
5. Name four causes of fainting.

GLOSSARY

Compiled of words used in connection with beauty culture, defined in the sense of anatomical, medical, electrical and beauty culture relationship only. Key to pronunciation is as follows:

fāte, senāte, cåre, ăm, finâl,

ärm, ȧsk, sofǎ; ēve, ḗvent, ĕnd,

recênt, evẽr; īce, ĭll; ōld, ȯbey,

ôrb, ŏdd, cônnect, sǒft, fōod,

fo͝ot; ūse, u͝nite, ûrn, ŭp, circûs; those

abdomen (ăb-dō′měn): the belly; the cavity in the body between the thorax and the pelvis.

abducent nerve (ăb-dū′sênt): the sixth cranial nerve; a small motor nerve supplying the external rectus muscle of the eye.

abductor (ăb-dŭk′těr): a muscle that draws a part away from the median line (opp., adductor). i.e.: spreads the fingers.

abrasion (ă-brā′zhŭn): scraping of the skin; excoriation.

abscess (ăb′sĕs): a circumscribed cavity containing pus.

absorption (ăb-sôrp′shŭn): assimilation of one body by another; act of absorbing.

accessory nerve (ăk-sĕs′ô-rē nûrv): spinal accessory nerve; eleventh cranial nerve; affects the sternocleido-mastoid and trapezius muscles of the neck.

acetic (ă-sĕt′ĭk): pertaining to vinegar; sour.

acetone (ăs′ē-tōn): a colorless, inflammable liquid, miscible with water, alcohol, and ether, and having a sweetish, ethereal odor and a burning taste.

acid: a sour substance; any chemical compound having a sour taste.

acid rinse: a solution of water and lemon juice or vinegar.

acne (ăk′nē): inflammation of the sebaceous glands from retained secretion.

acoustic (ă-kōōs′tĭk): auditory; eighth cranial nerve; controlling the sense of hearing.

activator (ăk′tĭ-vā-têr): a substance employed to start the action of hair coloring products.

acute (ă-kūt′): attended with severe symptoms; having a short and relatively short course; not chronic; said of a disease.

additive: a substance which is to be added to another product.

adductor (ă-dŭk′těr): a muscle that draws a part toward the median line. i.e.: draws fingers together.

adipose tissue (ăd′ĭ-pōs): fatty tissue; areolar connective tissue containing fat cells; subcutaneous tissue.

adrenal (ăd-rē′nâl): an endocrine gland situated on the top of the kidneys.

adulterate (ă-dŭl′těr-āt): to falsify; to alter, make impure by combining other substances.

aeration (ā-ēr-ā′shŭn): airing; saturating a fluid with air, carbon dioxide or other gas; the change of venous into arterial blood in the lungs.

aerosol (â′rô-sōl): colloidal suspension of liquid or solid particles in a gas; aerosol container filled with liquified gas and dissolved or suspended ingredients which can be dispersed as a spray or aerosol.

afferent nerves (ăf′ēr-ênt): convey stimulus from the external organs to the brain.

agnail (ăg′nāl): hangnail.

affinity (ă-fĭn′ĭ-tē): 1) inherent likeness or relationship; 2) chemical attraction; the force that unites atoms into molecules.

albinism (ăl′bĭ-nĭz′m): congenital leucoderma or absence of pigment in the skin and its appendages; it may be partial or complete.

albino (ăl-bī′nō): a subject of albinism; a person with very little or no pigment in the skin, hair or iris.

albumin (ăl-bū′mĭn): a simple, naturally-occurring protein soluble in water, coagulated by heat; found, in egg white (ovalbumin), in blood (serum albumin), in milk (lactalbumin).

alcohol (ăl′kô-hôl): a readily evaporating colorless liquid with a pungent odor and burning taste; powerful stimulant and antiseptic.

alkali (ăl′kă-lī): an electropositive substance; capable of making soaps from fats; used to neutralize acids.

alkaline (ăl′kâ-līn): having the qualities of, or pertaining to, an alkali.

alkalinity (ăl-kâ-lĭn′ĭ-tē): the quality or state of being alkaline.

allergy (ăl′ēr-jē): a disorder due to extreme sensitivity to certain foods or chemicals.

alopecia (ăl-ô-pē′shē-â): deficiency of hair; baldness.

alopecia adnata (ăl-ô-pē′shē-â ăd-nă′tâ): baldness at birth.

alopecia areata (ăl-ô-pē′shē-â ā-rê-ă′tă): baldness in spots or patches.

alopecia prematura (ăl-ô-pē′shē-â): prē-mă-tū′ră): baldness beginning before middle age.

alopecia senilis (ăl-ô-pē′shē-â sĕ-nĭl′ĭs): baldness occurring in old age.

alum, alumen (ăl′ŭm, ă-lū′mên): sulphate of potassium and aluminum; an astringent; used as a styptic.

amino-acid (ăm′ĭ-nō): an important constituent of proteins.

amitosis (ăm-ĭ-tō′sĭs): cell multiplication by direct division of the nucleus in the cell.

ammonia (ă-mō′nē-ă): a colorless gas with a pungent odor; very soluble in water.

ammonium sulphide (ă-mō′nē-ŭm sŭl′fĭd): a combination of ammonia and sulphur.

ammonium thioglycolate (ă-mō′nē-ŭm thī-ô-glī′kô-lāt) (thio; thio relaxer): a chemical hair relaxer, similar in acid content to chemicals used in permanent waving and hair relaxing.

ampere (ăm-pâr′): the unit of measurement of strength of an electric current.

anabolism (ăn-ăb′ō-lĭz′m): constructive metabolism; the process of assimilation of nutritive matter and its conversion into living substance.

analysis, hair: an examination to determine the condition of the hair prior to a hair treatment.

anatomy (â-năt′ō-mē): the study of the gross structure of the body which can be seen with the naked eye.

angiology (ăn-jē-ŏl′ô-jē): the science of the blood vessels and lymphatics.

angular artery (ăng′û-lăr): supplies the lacrimal sac and the eye muscle.

anidrosis, anhidrosis (ăn-ĭ-drō′sĭs): a deficiency in perspiration.

aniline (ăn′ĭ-lĭn, -lēn): a product of coal tar used in the manufacture of artificial dyes.

antibody (ăn′tĭ-bŏd-ē): a substance in the blood which builds resistance to disease.

antidote (ăn′tĭ-dōt): an agent preventing or counteracting the action of a poison.

anti-perspirant (ăn-tĭ-pêr-spī′rânt): a strong astringent liquid or cream used to stop the flow of perspiration in the region of the armpits, hands or feet.

antiseptic (ăn-tĭ-sĕp′tĭk): a chemical agent that prevents the growth of bacteria.

antitoxin (ăn-tĭ-tŏk′sĭn): a substance in serum which binds and neutralizes toxin (poison).

aorta (ā-ôr′tă): the main arterial trunk leaving the heart, and carrying blood to the various arteries throughout the body.

aponeurosis (ăp-ô-nū-rō′sĭs): a broad, flat tendon; attachment of muscles.

appendage (â-pĕn′dĕj): that which is attached to an organ, and is a part of it.

aqueous (ā′kwē-ŭs): watery; pertaining to water.

aromatic (ăr-ô-măt′ĭk): pertaining to or containing aroma; fragrant.

arrector pili (ă-rĕk′tôr pī′lĭ): plural of arrectores pilorum.

arrectores pilorum (â-rĕk-tō′rēz pĭ-lôr′ûm): the minute involuntary muscle fibers in the skin inserted into the bases of the hair follicles.

artery: a vessel that conveys blood from the heart.

articulation (ăr-tĭk-û-lā′shŭn): joint; a connection between two or more bones, whether or not allowing any movement between them.

asepsis (ă-sĕp′sĭs): a condition in which pathogenic bacteria are absent.

aseptic (ă-sĕp′tĭk): free from pathogenic bacteria.

asteatosis (ăs-tē-ă-tō′sĭs): a deficiency or absence of the sebaceous secretions.

astringent (ăs-trĭn′jĕnt): a substance or medicine that causes contraction of the issues, and checks secretions.

athlete's foot: a fungus foot infection; epidermophytosis.

atom: the smallest quantity of an element that can exist and still retain the chemical properties of the element.

atrium (ăt′rē-ûm); pl., **atria** (-ă): the auricle of the heart.

atrophy (ăt′rô-fē): a wasting away of the tissues of a part of or of the entire body from lack of nutrition.

auditory (ô′dĭ-tô-rē): eighth cranial nerve; controlling the sense of hearing.

auricle (ô′rĭ-k′l): the external ear; one of the upper cavities of the heart.

auriculo-temporal (ô-rĭk′û-lô tĕm′pôr-âl): sensory nerve affecting the temple and pinna.

auricular (ô-rĭk′û-lâr): pertaining to the ear or cardiac auricle.

auricularis (ô-rĭk′û-lâr′ĭs): a muscle of the ear.

autonomic nervous system (ô-tô-nŏm′ĭk): the sympathetic nervous system; controls the involuntary muscles.

axon (ăk′sŏn): a long nerve fiber extending from the nerve cell.

B

bacillus (bă-sĭl′ûs); pl., **bacilli** (-ī): rod-like shaped bacterium.

back-combing: combing the short hair toward the scalp while the hair strand is held in a vertical position; also called teasing.

bacteria (băk-tē′rē-ă): microbes, or germs.

bactericide (băk-tē′rĭ-sīd): an agent that destroys bacteria.

bacteriology (băk-tē-rē-ŏl′ô-jē): the science which deals with bacteria.

bacterium (băk-tē′rē-ûm); pl., **bacteria** (-ă): unicellular vegetable micro-organism.

baldness: a deficiency of hair; hair loss.

bandeau hairpiece (băn-dō′): hairpiece sewn to a headband covering the hairline.

band wig (bănd): see bandeau hairpiece.

bang: the front hair cut so as to fall over the forehead; often used in the plural, as to wear bangs.

basal layer (bās′âl): the layer of cells at base of epidermis closest to the dermis.

base: the lower part or bottom; chief substance of a compound; an electropositive element that unites with an acid to form a salt.

base, protective (prô-tĕk′tĭv): the material to which the hair is attached in order to form a wig.

benign (bē-nīn′): mild in character.

benzine (bĕn′zēn): an inflammable liquid derived from petroleum and used as a cleansing fluid.

benzoin (bĕn′zō-ĭn, -zoin): a balsamic resin used as a stimulant, and also as a perfume.

bicarbonate of soda (bī-kär′bôn-ât): baking soda; relieves burns, itching, urticarial lesions and insect bites; is often used in bath powders as an aid to cleansing oily skin.

biceps (bī′sĕps): having two heads; a muscle producing the contour of the front and inner side of the upper arm.

bichloride (bī-klō′rĭd): a compound having two parts or equivalents of chlorine to one of the other element.

biology (bī-ŏl′ô-jē): the science of life and living things.

blackhead: a comedone; a plug of sebaceous matter.

bleach: see hair lightening.

bleb (blĕb): a blister of the skin filled with watery fluid.

blending (blĕnd′ĭng): the physical act of fusing the color of hair during tinting and lightening applications.

block: a head-shaped form upon which a wig is placed for a specific purpose.

blocking: the act of dividing the hair into practical working parts.

blonde; blond: a person of fair complexion, with light hair and eyes.

blood: the nutritive fluid circulating through the arteries and veins.

blood vascular system (văs′kû-lâr sĭs′tĕm): comprised of structures (the heart, arteries, veins and capillaries) which distribute blood throughout the body.

blood vessel: an artery, vein or capillary.

blue light: a therapeutic lamp used to soothe the nerves.

bluing rinse: a solution used to neutralize the unbecoming yellowish tinge on gray or white hair.

blunt cutting: cutting the hair straight off without thinning or slithering.

boil: a furuncle; a subcutaneous abscess. It is caused by bacteria which enter through the hair follicles.

boiling point: 212° F. or 100° C. The temperature at which a liquid begins to boil.

bond: 1) the linkage between different atoms or radicals of a chemical compound, usually effected by the transfer of one or more electrons from one atom to another; 2) it can be found represented by a dot or a line between atoms shown in various formulas.

booster (bōōs′tĕr): oxidizer added to hydrogen peroxide to increase its chemical action; such chemicals as ammonium persulfate or percarbonate are used.

borax (bō′răks): sodium tetraborate; a white powder used as an antiseptic and cleansing agent.

boric acid (bō′rĭk): acidum boricum; used as an antiseptic dusting powder; in liquid form, as an eye wash.

bouffant (bōō′fänt): the degree of height and fullness in a finished hairstyle.

brachial artery (brā′kĭ-âl): the main artery of the upper arm.

braid: to weave, interlace, or entwine together.

brain: that part of the central nervous sysem contained in the cranial cavity, and consisting of the cerebrum, the cerebellum, the pons, and the medulla oblongata.

brilliantine (brĭl-yân-tēn′): an oily composition that imparts luster to the hair.

bristle: the short, stiff hair of a brush; short, stiff hairs of an animal, used in brushes.

brittle: easily broken or shattered.

bromidrosis (brō-mĭ-drō′sĭs): perspiration which smells foul.

buccal nerve (bŭk′ăl): a motor nerve affecting the buccinator and the orbicularis oris muscle.

buccinator (bŭk′sĭ-nā-tẽr): a thin, flat muscle of the cheek, shaped like a trumpet.

bulbous (bŭl′bûs): pertaining to, or being like a bulb in shape or structure.

bulla (bōōl′ă): a large bleb or blister.

C

calamine lotion (kăl′ă-mīn; -mĭn): zinc carbonate in alcohol used for the treatment of dermatitis in its various forms.

calcium (kăl′sē-ŭm): a brilliant silvery-white metal; enters into the composition of bone.

callous, callus (kăl′ûs): skin which has become hardened; thick-skinned.

camphor (kăm′fẽr): a mild cutaneous stimulant; it produces redness and warmth, and has a slightly anaesthetic and cooling effect.

cancellous (kăn′sê-lûs): having a porous or spongy structure.

caninus (kā-nīn′ûs): the muscle which lifts the angle of the mouth.

canities (kā-nĭsh′ĭ-ēz): grayness or whiteness of the hair.

cap: the netting and binding of a wig which together form the base to which the hair is attached.

capillary (kăp′ĭ-lâ-rē): any one of the minute blood vessels which connect the arteries and veins; hair-like.

capitate (kăp′ĭ-tāt): the large bone of the wrist.

caput (kā′pût); poss., **capitis** (kăp′ĭ-tĭs): pertaining to the head.

carbohydrate (kär-bô-hī′drāt): a chemical containing carbon, hydrogen, and oxygen.

carbolic acid (kär-bŏl′ĭk): phenol made from coal tar; a caustic and corrosive poison; used in dilute solution as an antiseptic.

carbon: coal; an elementary substance in nature which predominates in all organic compounds and occurs in three distinct forms: black lead, charcoal, and lampblack.

carbon-arc lamp: an instrument which produces ultra-violet rays.

carbon dioxide (dī-ŏk′sīd): carbonic acid gas; product of the cumbustion of carbon with a free supply of air.

carbonic acid (kär-bŏn′ĭk): a weak, colorless acid, formed by the solution of carbon dioxide in water, and existing only in solution.

carbuncle (kär′bŭn-k′l): a large circumscribed inflammation of the subcutaneous tissue that is similar to a furuncle, but much more extensive.

cardiac (kär′dē-ăk): pertaining to the heart.

carotid (kă-rŏt′ĭd): the principal artery of the neck.

carpus (kär′pûs): the wrist; the eight bones of the wrist.

cartilage (kär′tĭ-lâj): gristle; a non-vascular connective tissue softer than bone.

catabolism (kā-tăb′ô-lĭz′m): chemical changes which involve the breaking down process within the cells.

catalyst (kăt′â-lĭst): a substance having the power to increase the velocity of a chemical reaction.

caustic (kôs′tĭk): an agent that burns and chars tissue.

caustic soda: sodium hydroxide.

cell: a minute mass of protoplasm forming the structural unit of every organized body.

cell division: the reproduction of cells by the process of each cell dividing in half and forming two cells.

cellular (sĕl′û-lăr): consisting of, or pertaining to, cells.

centrosome (sĕn′trô-sōm): a cellular body which controls the division of the cell.

cerebellum (sĕr-ê-bĕl′ûm): the posterior and lower part of the brain.

cerebral (sĕr′ê-brăl): pertaining to the cerebrum.

cerebrospinal system (sĕr-ê-brô-spī′nâl sĭs′tĕm): consists of the brain, spinal cord, spinal nerves and the cranial nerves.

cerebrum (sĕr′ê-brŭm): the superior and larger part of the brain.

certified color (sûr′tĭ-fīd): a commercial coloring product which temporarily coats the hair shaft.

chemical change: alteration in the chemical composition of a substance.

chemical dye remover: a dye remover containing a chemical solvent.

chemical hair relaxer (rē-lăks′ẽr): a chemical agent which is employed to straighten over-curly hair.

chemistry (kĕm′ĭs-trē): the science dealing with the composition of substances; the elements and their mutual reactions, and the phenomena resulting from the formation and decomposition of compounds.

chignon (shēn′yŏn): a knot or coil of hair worn at the crown or nape, created from natural hair or from a hairpiece.

chloasma (klô-ăz′mă): irregular large brown patches on the skin, such as liver spots.

chlorine (klō′rĭn, -rēn): greenish yellow gas, with a disagreeable suffocating odor; used in combined form as a disinfectant and a bleaching agent.

cholesterin; cholesterol (kô-lĕs′tẽr-ĭn; -ōl): a waxy alcohol found in animal tissues and their secretions; it is present in lanolin, and used as an emulsifier.

chronic (krŏn′ĭk): long-continued; the reverse of acute.

cicatrix (sĭ-kā′trĭks, sĭk′ă-trĭks); pl., **cicatrices** (sĭk-ă-trī′sēz): the skin or film which forms over a wound, later contracting to form a scar.

cilia (sĭl′ĭ-ă): the eyelashes; microscopic hair-like extensions which assist bacteria in locomotion.

circuit: the path of an electric current.

circulation: the passage of blood throughout the body.

citric acid (sĭt′rĭk): acid found in the lemon, orange, grapefruit; used for making a rinse.

clavicle (klăv′ĭ-k′l): collarbone, joining the sternum and scapula.

clipping (klĭp′ĭng): the act of cutting split hair ends with the shears or the scissors.

clockwise: the movement of hair, in shapings or curls, in the same direction as the hands of a clock.

coagulate (kô-ăg′û-lāt): to clot; to convert a fluid into a soft, jelly-like solid.

coccus (kŏk′ûs); pl., **cocci** (kŏk′sī): spherical cell bacterium.

coiffure (kwä-fūr′): an arrangement or dressing of the hair.

cold waving: a system of permanent waving involving the use of chemicals rather than heat.

collodion (kô-lō′dē-ôn): a thick liquid used to form an adhesive covering.

color blender: a preparation which cleanses, highlights and blends in gray hair.

color filler: a preparation used to recondition lightened, tinted or damaged hair.

color remover: a prepared commercial product which removes tint from the hair.

color rinse: a rinse which gives a temporary tint to the hair.

color shampoo: a preparation which colors the hair permanently without requiring presoftening treatment.

color test: a method of determining the action of a selected tint on a small strand of hair.

comedone (kŏm′ê-dōne): blackhead; a worm-like mass in an obstructed sebaceous duct.

comedone extractor (ĕks′trăk′tĕr): an instrument used for the removal of blackheads.

compact tissue (kŏm′păkt): a dense, hard type of bony tissue.

compound henna (kŏm′pound hĕn′ā): Egyptian henna to which has been added one or more metallic preparations.

compounds (kŏm′poundz): 1) made of two or more parts or ingredients; 2) in chemistry, a substance which consists of two or more chemical elements in union.

concentrated (kŏn′sên-trāt-ĕd): condensed; increasing the strength by diminishing the bulk.

conditioning (kŏn-dĭ′shŭn-ĭng): the application of special chemical agents to the hair, to help restore its strength, and give it body in order to protect it against possible breakage.

conducting cords (kŏn-dŭckt′ĭng): insulated copper wires which convey the current from the wall plate to the patron and operator.

conductor: any substance which will attract or allow a current to flow through it easily.

configuration (kŏn-fĭg′ū-rā′shŭn): the arrangement and spacing of the atoms of a molecule.

congeal (kŏn-jēl′): to change from a fluid to a solid state.

congenital (kŏn-jĕn′ĭ-tâl): existing at birth; born with.

congestion (kŏn-jĕs′chŭn): overfullness of the capillary and other blood vessels in any locality or organ; local hyperemia.

connecting cords: the insulated strands of copper wires which join together the apparatus and the commercial electric current.

constitutional (kŏn-stĭ-tū′shŭn-âl): belonging to or affecting the physical or vital powers of an individual.

contagion (kŏn-tā′jûn): transmission of specific diseases by contact.

contraction (kŏn-trăk′shŭn): the act of shrinking, drawing together.

converter (kŏn-vûr′tĕr): an apparatus used to convert the direct current to alternating current.

corium (kō′rē-ûm): the derma or true skin.

cornification (kôr-nĭ-fĭ-kā′shŭn): the process of becoming a horny substance or tissue; a callosity.

corpuscles, red (kôr′pŭs′lz): cells in blood, whose function is to carry oxygen to the cells.

corpuscles, white: cells in the blood whose function is to destroy disease germs.

corrosive (kô-rō′sĭv): something causing corrosion.

corrugations (kŏr-ŭ-gā′shŭns): alternate ridges and furrows; wrinkles.

corrugator supercilli (kŏr′ŭ-gā-tĕr sū-pĕr-sĭl′ē-ī): draws eyebrows inward and downward, thus causing vertical wrinkles at the root of the nose.

cortex (kôr′tĕks): the second layer of the hair.

cortical (kôr′tĭ-kâl): pertaining to the cortex.

cosmetic dermatology (kŏz-mĕt′ĭk dûr-mă-tŏl′ô-jē): a branch of dermatology devoted to improving the health and beauty of the skin and its appendages.

cosmetology (kŏz-mĕ-tŏl′ô-jē): the science of beautifying and improving the complexion, skin, hair and nails.

counterclockwise: the movement of hair, in shapings or curls, in the opposite direction to the hands of a clock.

cowlick: a tuft of hair standing up.

cranium (krā′nē′ûm): the bones of the head excluding bones of the face; bony case for the brain.

crayon: a temporary hair coloring, massaged or brushed on with a lipstick-like applicator.

cream: a semi-solid cosmetic.

crepe wool (krāp wōōl): a sheep wool substance used as tissue strips, headbands, fillers or for confining hair ends in winding.

cresol (krē′sōl): a colorless, oily liquid or solid derived from coal tar and wood tar and used as a disinfectant.

crest: a ridge, line or thin mark made by folding or doubling, as a crest between two waves.

croquignole (krō′kĭ-nōl): winding of the hair under from ends to the scalp.

cross bonds: the bonds holding together the long chains of amino-acids, which compose hair; the bonds holding together the parallel chains of amino-acids to form hair.

crown: the top part of the head.

crust (krŭst): a scab.

curd (kûrd): soap residue found on the hair after an unsatisfactory shampoo.

curl: a circle, or circles, within a circle.

curl, base: the stationary or immovable foundation of the curl, which is attached to the scalp.

curl, cascade (kăs′kād): a "stand-up" curl which is wound from the hair ends to the scalp.

curl direction: see direction, curl.

curl, Maypole (Mā′pōl): see curl, overlapping.

curl, overlapping: a strand of wet hair wound around the finger with the hair ends on the outside.

curl, pin: a strand of hair which is combed smooth and ribbon-like and wound into a circle with the ends on the inside; sometimes called a flat curl —sculpture curl.

curl, ridge: a curl placed behind and close to the ridge of a finger wave, and pinned across its stem.

curl, roller: a curl formed over a specially made roller.

curl, sculpture (skŭlp′tyûr): same as pin curl.

curl, stand-up: see curl, cascade.

curl stem: that part of the pin curl between the base and the first arc of the circle.

curl, thermal (thûr′mâl): a curl formed with thermal irons.

current, alternating; A.C. (kŭr′ênt, ôl′tĕr-nāt-ĭng): a rapid and interrupted current, flowing first in one direction and then in the opposite direction.

current, direct; D.C. (dī′rĕkt): a constant and even flowing current, travelling in one direction.

current, high-frequency (hī-frē′kwên-sē): an electric current characterized by a high rate of vibration.

cutaneous (kû-tā′nē-ûs): pertaining to the skin.

cuticle (kū′tĭ-k′l): the outer layer of the skin or hair.

cutis (kū′tĭs): the deeper layer of the skin (dermis).

cyst (sĭst): a closed, abnormally developed sac containing fluid, semi-fluid or morbid matter.

cysteine (sĭs′tĭ-ēn): an amino-acid produced by digestion; it is easily **oxidized** to cystine; obtained by reduction of cystine.

cystine (sĭs'tĭn): a sulphur containing amino-acid found in hair and nails.

cytoplasm (sī'tô-plăz'm): the protoplasm of the cell body, exclusive of the nucleus.

D

dandricide (dăn'drĭ-sīd): a chemical substance; counteracts the effects of dandruff.

dandruff (dăn'drŭf): pityriasis; scurf or scales formed in excess upon the scalp.

decolorize: see hair lightening.

deltoid (dĕl'toid): a muscle of the shoulder.

demarcation (dē-mär-kā'shûn): a line setting bounds or limits.

dendrite (dĕn'drīt): a tree-like branching of nerve fibers extending from a nerve cell.

deodorant (dē-ō'dĕr-ânt): a substance that removes or conceals offensive odors.

depilatory (dĕ-pĭl'ă-tô-rē): a substance, usually a caustic alkali, used to destroy the hair; having the power to remove hair.

depressor (dē-prĕs'ĕr): that which presses or draws down; a muscle that depresses.

dermatitis (dûr-mă-tī'tĭs): inflammation of the skin.

dermatitis, contact: an inflammation of the skin caused by coming in contact with chemicals, dyes, etc., to which the individual may be allergic.

dermatitis, cosmetic: an inflammation of the skin caused by coming in contact with some cosmetic product to which the individual may be allergic.

dermatitis, occupational (ŏk-û-pā'shûn-âl): an inflammation of the skin caused by the kind of employment in which the individual is engaged.

dermatology (dûr-mă-tŏl'ô-jē): the science which treats of the skin and its diseases.

dermis, derma (dûr'mĭs, dûr'mă): the layer below the epidermis; the corium or true skin.

detergent (dē-tûr'jênt): an agent that cleanses.

developer: an oxidizing agent, such as 20-volume hydrogen peroxide solution; when mixed with an aniline derivative tint it supplies the necessary oxygen gas.

diagnosis (dī-ăg-nō'sĭs): the recognition of a disease from its symptoms.

dialysis (dī-ăl'ĭ-sĭs): the process of separating different substances in solution by diffusion through a moist membrane or septum; separation.

diathermy (dī'ă-thûr-mē): a method of raising the temperature in the deep tissues, using high-frequency current.

diffusion (dĭ-fū'zhûn): a spreading out; dialysis.

digits (dĭj'ĭts): fingers or toes.

dilator (dī-lā'tĕr; dĭ-): that which expands or enlarges.

dilute (dĭ-lūt'; dĭ-): to make thinner by mixing, especially with water.

diplococcus (dī-plô-kŏk'ŭs): bacteria exhibiting pairs.

direction, curl: the movement of hair in order to form a particular pattern or style. Forward: toward the face. Backward (reverse): away from the face.

direction, stem: the direction in which the stem moves from the base to the first arc.

disease: a pathologic condition of any part or organ of the body, or of the mind.

disease carrier: a healthy person capable of transmitting disease germs to another person.

disinfectant (dĭs-ĭn-fĕk'tânt): an agent used for destroying germs.

dispensary (dĭs-pĕn'sà-rē): a place where medicines or other supplies are prepared and dispensed.

dispersion (dĭs-pûr'shôn): 1) the act of scattering or separating; 2) the incorporation of the particles of one substance into the body of another, comprising solutions, suspensions and colloid solutions.

distill (dĭs-tĭl'): to extract the essence or active principle of a substance.

disulfide (dī-sŭl'fīd): (sulphur): a chemical compound in which two sulphur atoms are united with a single atom of an element; i.e., carbon.

dormant (dôr'mânt): inactive; asleep.

double application tints: products requiring two separate applications; also called two process tints or two step tints.

duct: a passage or canal for fluids.

dye remover: see color remover.

E

eczema (ĕk'zĕ-mă): an inflammatory itching disease of the skin.

efferent (ĕf'ĕr-ênt): motor nerves conveying impulses away from the central nervous system.

effilate (ĕf'ĭ-lāt): to cut the hair strand by a sliding movement of the scissors.

effleurage (ĕ-flū-razh'): a stroking movement in massage.

Egyptian henna (ē-jĭp'shân hĕn'ă): a pure vegetable hair dye.

elasticity (ē-lăs'tĭs'ĭ-tē): the property that allows a thing to be stretched, and to return to its former shape.

electricity: a form of energy, which, when in motion, exhibits magnetic, chemical or thermal effects.

electrode (ē-lĕk'trōd): a pole of an electric cell; an applicator for directing the use of electricity on a patron.

electrolysis (ē-lĕk-trŏl'ĭ-sĭs): decomposition of a chemical compound or body tissues by means of electricity.

electron (ē-lĕk'trŏn): an extremely minute corpuscle or charge of negative electricity, the smallest known to exist.

electropositive (ē-lĕk'trō-pŏz'ĭ-tĭv): relating to or charged with positive electricity.

electro-static (ē-lĕk'trō-stăt'ĭk): pertaining to static electricity.

element (ĕl'ê-mĕnt): 1) a simple substance which cannot be decomposed by chemical means, and which is made up of atoms which are alike in their peripheral electronic configurations and in their chemical properties; 2) any one of the 103 ultimate chemical entities of which matter is believed to be composed.

emollient (ē-mŏl'yênt): an agent that softens or soothes the surface of the skin.

emulsifier (ē-mŭl'sĭ-fī-ĕr): a substance, as gelatin, gum, etc., for emulsifying a fixed oil.

emulsion (ē-mŭl'shûn): a product consisting of minute globules of one liquid dispersed throughout the body of a second liquid.

end bonds (peptide bonds) (pĕp'tīd): the chemical bonds which join together the amino-acids to form the long chains which are characteristic of all proteins.

endocrine (ĕn'dô-krĭn): any internal secretion or hormone.

enzyme (ĕn'zīm): a substance which induces a chemical change in other substances, without undergoing any change itself.

epicranius (ĕp-ĭ-krā'nē-ûs): the occipito-frontalis; the scalp muscle.

epidemic (ĕp-ĭ-dĕm′ĭk): common to many people; a prevailing disease.

epidermis (ĕp-ĭ-dûr′mĭs): the outer layer of the skin.

epilation (ĕp-ĭ-lā′shŭn): the removal of hair by the roots.

epithelium (ĕp-ĭ-thē′lē-ŭm): a cellular tissue or membrane, with little intercellular substance, covering a free surface or lining a cavity.

eponychium (ĕp-ō-nĭk′ē-ŭm): the extension of cuticle at base of nail-body.

erythrocyte (ĕ-rĭth′rō-sīt): a red blood cell; red corpuscle.

esophagus; oesophagus (ĕ-sŏf′ă-gŭs): the canal leading from the pharynx to the stomach.

ester (ĕs′tĕr): an organic compound formed by the reaction of an acid and an alcohol.

esthetic (ĕs-thĕt′ĭk): sensitive to art and beauty; showing good taste; artistic.

ethics: principles of good character and proper conduct.

ethmoid (ĕth′moid): resembling a sieve; a bone forming part of the walls of the nasal cavity.

etiology (ĕ-tē-ŏl′ō-jē): the science of the causes of disease.

evaporation: change from liquid to vapor form.

excoriation (ĕks-kō-rē-ā′shŭn): act of stripping or wearing off the skin; an abrasion.

excrete (ĕks-krēt′): to separate (waste matter) from the blood or tissue and eliminate from the body as through the kidneys or sweat glands.

excretion (ĕks-krē′shŭn): that which is thrown off or eliminated from the body.

exhalation (ĕks-hà-lā′shŭn): the act of breathing outward.

extensibility (ĕks-tĕn-sĭ-bil′ĭ-tē): capable of being extended or stretched.

extensor (ĕks-tĕn′sôr): a muscle which serves to extend or straighten out a limb or part.

extremity (ĕks-trĕm′ĭ-tē): the distant end or part of any organ; a hand and foot.

exudation (ĕks-û-dā′shŭn): act of discharging from the body through pores as sweat, moisture or other liquid.

eye-shadow: a cosmetic applied on the eyelids to accentuate their brilliance.

F

facial (fā′shâl): pertaining to the face; the seventh cranial nerve.

Fahrenheit (fä′rên-hīt): pertaining to the Fahrenheit thermometer or scale; water freezes at 32° F. and boils at 212° F.

fall: an artificial section of hair running across the back of the head.

fascia (făsh′ē-ă): a sheet of connective tissue covering, supporting, or binding together internal parts of the body.

felon (fĕl′ŭn): paronychia of the nail.

fermentation (fûr-mĕn-tā′shŭn): a chemical decomposition of organic compounds into more simple compounds, brought about by the action of an enzyme.

fetid (fĕt′ĭd): having a foul smell; stinking.

fever blister: an acute skin disease characterized by the presence of vesicles over an inflammatory base; herpes simplex.

fiber: a slender, threadlike structure that combines with others to form animal or vegetable tissue.

fibrin (fī′brĭn): the active agent in coagulation of the blood.

filler: a commercial product used to provide fill for porous spots in the hair during tinting, lightening and permanent waving.

finger test: a test given to determine the degree of porosity in the hair.

fission (fĭsh′ŭn): reproduction of bacteria by cellular division; any splitting or cleaving; **atomic f.:** the splitting of the neutrons of an atom in two main fragments.

fissure (fĭsh′ûr): a narrow opening made by separation of parts; a furrow; a slit.

fixative (fĭk′să-tĭv): a chemical agent capable of stopping the processing of the permanent wave solution or the chemical hair relaxer and hardening the hair in its new form; neutralizer; stabilizer.

flagella (flă-jĕl′ă): slender whip-like processes which permit locomotion in certain bacteria.

flexor (flĕk′sôr): a muscle that bends or flexes a part or a joint.

fluorescent (floo′ôr-ĕs′n′t): an ability to emit light after exposure to light, the wave length of the emitted light being longer than that of the light absorbed.

"fly away": an excessive electrostatic condition of hair which causes individual hair strands to repel one another and stand away from the head.

foamer (fō′mĕr): a substance which creates an excessive amount of foam.

follicle (fŏl′ĭ-k'l): the depression in the skin containing the hair root.

formaldehyde (fôr-măl′dĕ-hīd): a pungent gas possessing powerful disinfectant properties.

Formalin (fôr′mă-lĭn): a 37% to 40% solution of formaldehyde.

formula (fôr′mû-lă): a prescribed method or rule; a recipe or prescription.

fragilitas crinium (fră-jĭl′ĭ-tăs krĭ′nē-ŭm): brittleness of the hair.

freckle: a yellow or brown spot on the skin; lentigo.

free edge: part of the nail body extending over the fingertip.

French lacing: see teasing.

frequency (frē′kwên-sē): the number of complete cycles per second of current produced by an alternating current generator. Standard frequencies are 25 and 60 cycles per second.

friction: the resistance encountered in rubbing one body on another.

frizz: hair having too much of a curl.

frontal: in front; relating to the forehead; the bone of the forehead.

frontalis (frŏn-tā′lĭs): anterior portion of the muscle of the scalp.

frosting (frŏst′ĭng): to lighten or darken small selected strands of hair over the entire head to blend with the rest of the hair.

fulling (fool′ĭng): a massage movement in which the limb is rolled back and forth between the hands.

fumigate (fū′mĭ-gāt): disinfect by the action of fumes.

fungus (fŭn′gŭs): a vegetable parasite; a spongy growth of diseased tissue on the body.

furuncle (fū-rŭn′k'l): a small skin abscess (boil).

fuse: to liquefy by heat; a special device which prevents excessive current from passing through a circuit.

fusion (fū′zhŭn): the act of uniting or cohering.

G

ganglion (găn′glē-ŏn); pl., **ganglia** (-ă): bundles of nerve cells in the brain, in organs of special sense, or forming units of the sympathetic nervous system.

gastric juice (găs′trĭk): the digestive fluid secreted by the glands of the stomach.

gauze: a thin, open-meshed cloth used for dressings.

gel: comprised of a solid and a liquid which exist as a solid or semi-solid mass.

gelatine: the tasteless, odorless, brittle substance extracted by boiling bones, hoofs and animal tissues used in various foods, medicines, etc.

gene: the ultimate unit in the transmission of hereditary characteristics.

genetic (jĕ-nĕt′ĭk): the genesis or origin of something.

gentian violet jelly: (jĕn′shăn): an antiseptic used in the first aid treatment of a scalp burn.

germ: a bacillus; a microbe; an embryo in its early stages.

germicide (jûr′mĭ-sīd): any chemical, especially a solution that will destroy germs.

germinative layer (jûr-mĭ-nā′tĭv): stratum germinativum; the deepest layer of the epidermis resting on the corium.

gland: a secretory organ of the body.

globule (glŏb′ūl): a small, spherical droplet of fluid or semi-fluid material.

glossopharyngeal (glŏs-ô-fâ-rĭn′jĕ-āl): pertaining to the tongue and pharynx; the ninth cranial nerve.

glycerin; glycerine (glĭs′ĕr-ĭn): sweet, oily fluid, used as an application for roughened and chapped skin; also used as a solvent.

granules (grăn′ūlz): small grains; small pills.

granulosum (grăn-û-lōs′ûm): granular layer of the epidermis.

great auricular (grāt ô-rĭk′û-lär): a nerve affecting the face, ear, neck and parotid gland.

greater occipital (ŏk-sĭp′ĭ-tâl): sensory and motor nerve affecting the back part of the scalp.

gristle (grĭs″l): cartilage.

grooming (grōōm′ĭng): to make neat or tidy.

ground wire (ground wīr): a wire which connects an electric current to a ground (waterpipe or radiator).

H

hacking (hăk′ĭng): a chopping stroke made with the edge of the hand in massage.

hair: pilus; a slender threadlike outgrowth on the body.

hair bulb: the lower extremity of the hair.

hair clipping: removing the hair by the use of hair clippers; removing split hair ends of the hair with the scissors.

hair coloring: artificially changing the color of the hair.

haircutting: shortening and thinning of the hair, and molding the hair into a becoming style; hair shaping.

hair density: the number of hairs per square inch on the scalp.

hair dressing: the art of arranging the hair into various becoming shapes or styles.

hair follicle (fŏl′ĭ-k'l): the depression of the skin containing the root of the hair.

hair lightener: a chemical substance used to remove the natural color pigment from the hair.

hair lightening: the removal of natural pigment or artificial color from the hair.

hair papilla (hâr pă-pĭl′ă): a small, cone-shaped elevation at the bottom of the hair follicle.

hairpiece: an artificial section of woven hair used in place of or in conjunction with the natural hair.

hair pressing: a method of straightening curly or kinky hair by means of heated irons or a pressing comb.

hair pressing oil: an oily or waxy mixture used in hair pressing.

hair relaxing, chemical: a permanent method of straightening over-curly hair.

hair restorer: a preparation containing a metallic dye (not used professionally).

hair root: that part of the hair contained within the follicle.

hair shaft: the portion of the hair which projects beyond the skin.

hair shaping: the art of haircutting.

hair straightener: a physical or chemical agent used in straightening kinky or over-curly hair.

hair stream: the natural direction in which the hair grows after leaving the follicle.

hair, superfluous (sŭ-pûr′flōō-ûs): unwanted or excess hair, usually found on the faces of women. See: hirsuties.

hair test: a sampling of how the hair will react to a particular treatment.

hair texture (tĕks′tŭr): the general quality of hair, as to coarse, medium or fine; the feel of the hair.

hair tinting: the physical act of adding color pigment to either virgin or tinted hair.

halitosis (hăl-ĭ-tō′sĭs): offensive odor from the mouth; foul breath.

hangnail (hăng′nāl): a tearing up of a strip of epidermis at the side of the nail; agnail.

H-bond: see hydrogen bond.

heating cap: an electrical device, applied over the head, to provide a uniform source of heat.

heating coil: an electric coil which heats the air in a hair dryer.

helix (hē′lĭks; hĕl′ĭks): the fleshy tip of the ear (ear lobe).

hematocyte (hĕ′mă-tô-sīt): a blood corpuscle.

hemoglobin; haemoglobin (hē-mô-glō′bĭn): the coloring matter of the blood.

hemorrhage (hĕm′ô-râj): bleeding; a flow of blood, especially when profuse.

henna (hĕn′ă): the leaves of an Asiatic thorny tree or shrub used as a dye, imparting a reddish tint; it is also used as a cosmetic.

henna, compound (kŏm′pound): Egyptian henna to which has been added one or more metallic preparations.

heredity (hĕ-rĕd′ĭ-tē): the inborn capacity of the organism to develop ancestral characteristics.

herpes (hûr′pēz): an inflammatory disease of the skin having small vesicles in clusters.

herpes simplex (sĭm′plĕks): fever blister; cold sore.

hexachlorophenol (hĕks-ă-klō-rŏ-fē′nŏl): white, free flowing powder, essentially odorless; used as a bactericidal agent in antiseptic soaps, deodorant products, including soaps and various cosmetics.

high-frequency (hī-frē′kwĕn-sē): violet ray; an electric current of medium voltage and medium amperage.

highlighting shampoo tint: a preparation used with shampoo when a very slight change in hair shade is desired.

hirsute (hûr′sūt, hēr-sūt′): hairy; having coarse, long hair; shaggy.

hirsuties (hûr-sū′shĭ-ēz): hypertrichosis; growth of an unusual amount of hair in unusual locations, as on the faces of women or the backs of men; hairy; superfluous hair.

histology (hĭs-tŏl′ō-jē): the science of the minute structure of organic tissues; microscopic anatomy.

hives: urticaria; a skin eruption.

homogeneous (hō-mŏj′ê-nūs): having the same nature or quality; a uniform character in all parts.

homogenizer (hō-mŏj′ê-nīz-êr): serving to produce a uniform suspension of emulsions from two or more normally immiscible substances.

hormone (hôr′mōn): a chemical substance formed in one organ or part of the body and carried in the blood to another organ or part which it stimulates to functional activity or secretion.

humerus (hū′mêr-ûs): the bone of the upper part of the arm.

humidity: moisture; dampness.

hydro (hī′drō): a prefix denoting water; hydrogen.

hydro carbon: any compound composed only of hydrogen and carbon.

hydrogen: the lightest element; it is an odorless, tasteless, colorless gas found in water and all organic compounds. **h. acceptor:** a substance which, on reduction, accepts hydrogen atoms from another substance called a hydrogen donor.

hydrogen bond (physical bond): that bond formed between two molecules when the nucleus of a hydrogen atom, originally attached to a florine, nitrogen or oxygen atom of a molecule, is attracted to the florine, nitrogen or oxygen atom of a second molecule of the same or different substance.

hydrogen peroxide: a powerful oxidizing agent; in liquid form it is used as an antiseptic and for the activation of lighteners and hair tints.

hydrophilic (hī-drō-fīl′ĭk): capable of combining with or attracting water.

hygiene: the science of preserving health.

hygroscopic (hī-grō′skŏp′ĭk): readily absorbing and retaining moisture.

hyoid (hī′oid): the "u" shaped bone at the base of the tongue.

hyperhidrosis, hyperidrosis (h-′pĕr-ĭ-drō′sĭs): excessive sweating.

hypertrophy (hī′pĕr-trō′fē): abnormal increase in the size of a part or an organ; overgrowth.

hypoglossal (h:′pō-glŏ′sâl): the twelfth cranial nerve; motor nerve to base of tongue.

hyponychium (hī-pō-nĭk′ē-ûm): the portion of the epidermis upon which the nail-body rests under the free edge.

I

imbrications (ĭm-brĭ-kā′shŭnz): cells arranged in layers overlapping one another; found in cuticle layer of hair.

immerse (ĭ-mûrs′): to plunge into; dip; submerge in a liquid.

immersion (ĭ-mûr′chŭn): plunging or dipping into a liquid, especially so as to cover completely.

immunity (ĭ-mūn′ĭ-tē): freedom from, or resistant to disease.

incubation (ĭn-kû-bā′shŭn): the period of a disease between the implanting of the contagion and the development of the symptoms.

index: the forefinger; the pointing finger.

infection (ĭn-fĕk′shŭn): the invasion of the body tissues by disease germs.

infection, general: the result of the disease germs gaining entrance into the blood stream and thereby circulating throughout the entire body.

infection, local: confined to only certain portions of the body, such as an abscess.

infectious (ĭn-fĕk′shŭs): capable of spreading infection.

inflammation (ĭn-flâ-mā′shŭn): the reaction of the body to irritation with accompanying redness, pain, heat, and swelling.

infra-orbital (ĭn-frâ ôr′bĭ-tâl): below the orbit; a sensory and motor nerve affecting the cheek muscles, nose, and upper lip.

infra-red: rays pertaining to that part of the spectrum lying outside of the visible spectrum and below the red rays.

infra-trochlear (trŏk′lē-âr): sensory nerve affecting the skin of the nose and the inner muscle of the eye.

ingredient: any one of the things of which a mixture is made up.

ingrown hair: a wild hair that has grown underneath the skin, which may cause an infection.

ingrown nail: the growth of the nail into the flesh instead of toward the tip of the finger or toe, which may cause an infection.

inhalation (ĭn-hǎ-lā′shŭn): the inbreathing of air or other vapors.

inoculation (ĭn-ŏk-û-lā′shŭn): the process by which protective agents are introduced into the body.

inorganic (ĭn-ôr-gǎn′ĭk): composed of matter not relating to living organisms.

insanitary; unsanitary: not sanitary or healthful; injurious to health; unclean.

insoluble (ĭn-sŏl′û-b′l): incapable of being dissolved or very difficult to dissolve.

insulator (ĭn′sû-lā-tĕr): a non-conducting material or substance; materials used to cover electric wires.

intensity (ĭn-tĕn′sĭ-tē): the amount of force or energy of heat, light, sound, electric current, etc., per unit area; the quality of being intense.

intercellular (ĭn-tĕr-sĕl′û-lär): between or among cells.

intestine (ĭn-tĕs′tĭn): the digestive tube from the stomach to the anus.

involuntary muscles (ĭn-vŏl′ûn-tâ-rē): function without the action of the will.

iodine: a non-metallic element used as an antiseptic for cuts, bruises, etc.

ion: an atom or group of atoms carrying an electric charge.

ionization (ī-ŏn-ĭ-zā′shŭn): the separating of a substance into ions.

iris: the colored, muscular, disk-like diaphragm of the eye which regulates the pupil or opening in the center.

irradiation (ĭ-rā′dē-ā′shŭn): the process of exposing an object to the natural or artificial sunlight.

irreversible (ĭr-ê-vĕr′sĭ-b′l): not capable of being reversed.

irritability (ĭr-ĭ-tà-bĭl′ĭ-tē): readily excited or stimulated.

J

joint: a connection between two or more bones.

jowl: the hanging part of a double chin.

jugular (jōō′gû-lâr): pertaining to the neck or throat; the large vein in the neck.

K

keratin (kĕr′ă-tĭn): a fiber protein characteristic of horny tissues: hair, nails, feathers, etc.; it is insoluble in protein solvents and has a high sulfur content.

keratinization (kĕr′ă-tĭn-ĭ-zā′shŭn): the process of being keratinized.

keratoma (kĕr-ă-tō′mă): a callosity: a horny tumor; an acquired thickened patch of the epidermis.

kidney: a glandular organ which excretes urine.

kilowatt (kĭl′ō-wŏt): one thousand watts of electricity.

knead (nēd): to work and press with the hands as in massage.

L

labii (lā′bē-ī): of or pertaining to the lip.

labium (lā′bē-ŭm); pl., **labia** (-ă): lip.

laceration (lăs′ĕr-ā′shŭn): a tear of the skin or tissues.

lachrymal; lacrimal (lăk′rĭ-mâl): pertaining to tears or weeping; bone at the front of the orbits.

lacquer, nail (lăk′ĕr): a thick liquid which forms a glossy film on the nail.

lanolin (lăn′ō-lĭn): purified wool fat.

lanugo (lă-nū′gō): the fine hair which covers most of the body.

larynx (lăr′ĭnks): the upper part of the trachea or wind pipe; the organ of voice production.

lather: froth made by mixing soap and water.

latissimus dorsi (lă-tĭs′ĭ-mŭs dôr′sī): a broad, flat superficial muscle of the back.

lecithin (lĕs′ĭ-thĭn): a colorless crystalline compound, soluble in alcohol; it is found in animal tissues, especially nerve tissue, and the yolk of egg.

lemon rinse: a product containing lemon juice or citric acid; used to eliminate soap curds.

lentigo (lĕn-tĭ′gō); pl., **lentigines** (lĕn-tĭ-jĭ′nēz): a freckle; circumscribed spot or pigmentation in the skin.

lesion (lē′zhŭn): a structural tissue change caused by injury or disease.

lesser occipital (lĕs′ĕr ŏk-sĭp′ĭ-tâl): the nerve supplying muscles at the back of the ear.

leucocyte (lū′kō-sīt): a white corpuscle; white blood cell.

leucoderma (lū-kō-dûr′mă): abnormal white patches on the skin; absence of pigment in the skin.

leuconychia (lū-kō-nĭk′ē-ă): a whitish discoloration of nails; white spots.

ligament (lĭg′ă-mênt): a tough band of fibrous tissue, serving to connect bones, or to hold an organ in place.

lightener (bleach): the chemical employed to remove color from hair.

lightening (bleaching): see: hair lightening.

light therapy: the application of light rays for treatment of disorders.

lipophilic (lĭp-ō-fĭl′ĭk): having an affinity or attraction to fat and oil.

liquefy (lĭk′wĕ-fī): to reduce to the liquid state; said of both solids and gases.

liquor cresolis compound (lĭk′ĕr krē-sōl′ĭs kŏm′-pound): a powerful germicide.

litmus paper (lĭt′mŭs): a blue coloring matter that is reddened by acids and turned blue again by alkalies.

liver spots: the discolorations of chloasma.

lobe: a branch extending from a body; ear lobe.

lock-jaw: tetanus; specifically trismus; a firm closing of the jaw due to tonic spasm of the muscles of mastication.

lotion: a liquid solution used for bathing the skin.

louse; pl., **lice:** pediculus; an animal parasite infesting the hairs of the head.

lubricant: anything that makes things smooth and slippery, such as oil.

lucidum (lū′sĭ-dŭm): the clear layer of the epidermis.

lung: one of the two organs of respiration.

lunula (lū′nŭ-lă): the half-moon shaped area at the base of the nail.

lymph (lĭmf): a clear yellowish or light straw colored fluid, which circulates in the lymph spaces, or lymphatics of the body.

lymphatic system (lĭm-făt′ĭk): consists of lymph flowing through the lymph spaces, lymph vessels, lacteals, and lymph nodes or glands.

Lysol (lī′sōl): a trade name; a disinfectant and antiseptic; a mixture of soaps and phenols.

M

macroscopic (măk-rō-skŏp′ĭk): visible to the unaided eye.

macula (măk′ū-lă); pl., **maculae** (-lē): a spot or discoloration level with skin; a freckle; macule.

magnetism (măg′nĕ-tĭz′m): the power possessed by a magnet to attract or repel other masses.

malar (mā′lăr): of or pertaining to the cheek; the cheek bone.

malformation (măl-fôr-mā′shŭn): an abnormal shape or structure; badly formed.

malignant (mă-lĭg′nănt): resistant to treatment; growing worse; occurring in severe form; a tumor recurring after removal.

malpighian (măl-pĭg′ē-ân): stratum mucosum; the deeper portion of the epidermis.

mandible (măn′dĭ-b′l): the lower jaw bone.

mandibular nerve (măn-dĭb′ŭ-lăr): the fifth cranial nerve which supplies the muscles and skin of the lower part of the face.

manganese (măn′gă-nēs): a grayish-white, metallic chemical element which rusts like iron, but is not magnetic.

manicure: the artful care of the hands and nails.

manipulation (mă-nĭp-û-lā′shŭn): act or process of treating, working or operating with the hands or by mechanical means, especially with skill.

marcel: a series of even waves or tiers put in the hair with the aid of a heated iron.

marrow: a soft, fatty substance filling the cavities of bone.

mascara (măs-kă′ră): a preparation used to darken the eyelashes.

mask: a special cosmetic formula used to beautify the face.

massage (mă-säzh′): manipulation of the body by rubbing, pinching, kneading, tapping, etc., to increase metabolism, promote absorption, relieve pain, etc.

matting (măt′ĭng): tangling together into a thick mass.

matrix (mā′trĭks): the formative portion of a nail.

maxilla (măk-sĭl′ă): upper jaw bone.

medulla (mĕ-dŭl′ă): the marrow in the various bone cavities; the pith of the hair.

melanin (mĕl′ă-nĭn): the dark or black pigment in the epidermis and hair, and in the choroid or coat of the eye.

melanophore (mĕl-ân′ō-fôr): a pigment cell containing melanin.

membrane (mĕm′brăn): a thin sheet or layer of pliable tissue, serving as a covering.

mental nerve: a nerve which supplies the skin of the lower lip and chin.

mentalis (měn-tā'lĭs): the muscle that elevates the lower lip, and raises and wrinkles the skin of the chin.

metabolism (mě-tăb'ŏ-lĭz'm): the constructive and destructive life process of the cell.

metacarpus (mět-ă-kär'pŭs): the bones of the palm of the hand.

metatarsus (mět-ă-tär'sŭs): the bones which comprise the instep of the foot.

metallic salts: a compound of a base and an acid.

meta-toluene-diamine (mět'ă-tŏl'ū-ēn-dī-ăm'ĭn): the name given to an oxidation dye used to provide lighter shades of red and blonde; it is an aniline derivative type.

meter: an instrument used for measuring.

microbe: a micro-organism; a minute one-celled animal or vegetable bacterium.

micrococcus (mī-krŏ-kŏk'ŭs): a minute bacterial cell having a spherical shape.

micro-organism (mī'krŏ-ôr'găn-ĭz'm): microscopic plant or animal cell; a bacterium.

microscope (mī'krŏ-skōp): an instrument for making enlarged views of minute objects.

miliaria rubra (mĭl-ē-ā'rē-ă rōōb'ră): prickly heat; burning and itching usually caused by exposure to excessive heat.

milium (mĭl'ē-ûm); pl., **milia** (-ă): a small whitish pearl-like mass due to a retention of sebum beneath the epidermis; a whitehead.

mineral salts: salts derived from an inorganic chemical compound.

miscible (mĭs'ĭ-b'l): the property of certain liquids to mix with each other in equal proportions.

mixture: a preparation made by incorporating an insoluble ingredient in a liquid vehicle; sometimes used to identify an aqueous solution containing two or more solutes.

modifier (mŏd'ĭ-fī-ēr): anything that will change the form or characteristics of an object or substance.

mole: a small brownish spot on the skin.

molecule (mŏl'ê-kūl): the smallest unit of any substance having all the properties of the substance.

monilethrix (mŏ-nĭl'ê-thrĭks): beaded hair; a condition in which the hairs show a series of constrictions, giving the appearance of a string of fusiform beads.

mordant (môr'dânt): a substance, such as alum, phenol, aniline oil, which fixes the dye used in coloring.

motor nerves: carry impulses from nerve centers to muscles for certain motions.

mould: to form or to shape into a definite pattern.

mucous membrane (mū'kûs měm'brān): a membrane secreting mucus which lines passages and cavities communicating with the exterior.

muscle: the contractile tissue of the body by which movement is accomplished.

muscle tone: the normal degree of tension in a healthy muscle.

myology (mī-ŏl'ŏ-jē): the science of the function, structure, and diseases of muscles.

N

naevus; nevus (nē'vûs); pl., **naevi; nevi** (-vī): a birthmark; a congenital skin blemish.

nail: unguis; the horny protective plate located at the end of the finger or toe.

nail-bed: that portion of the skin on which the body of the nail rests.

nail-body: the horny nail blade resting upon the nail-bed.

nail-grooves: the furrows on the sides of the nail upon which the nail moves as it grows.

nail lacquer: a thick liquid which forms a glossy film on the nail.

mantle: the fold of the skin into which the nail root is lodged.

nail matrix (mā'trĭks): the portion of the nail-bed extending beneath the nail-root.

nail-root: located at the base of the nail, imbedded underneath the skin.

nail-wall: folds of skin overlapping sides and base of the nail-body.

nape: the back of the neck.

naris (nā'rĭs); pl., **nares** (-rēz): a nostril

nasalis (nâ-zā'lĭs): a muscle of the nose.

neck line: in haircutting, where the hair growth of the head ends and the neck begins; hairline.

nerve: a whitish cord, made up of bundles of nerve fibers, through which impulses are transmitted.

neuritis (nû-rī'tĭs): inflammation of nerves, marked by neuralgia.

neurology (nû-rŏl'ŏ-jē): the science of the structure, function and pathology of the nervous system.

neuron (nū'rŏn): the unit of the nervous system, consisting of the nerve cell and its various processes.

neutral: exhibiting no positive properties; indifferent; in chemistry, neither acid nor alkaline.

neutralization (nū-trăl-ĭ-zā'shûn): a chemical reaction between an acid and a base; rehardening the hair in cold waving or in chemical hair relaxing.

neutralizer (nū'trăl-īz-ēr): an agent capable of neutralizing another substance. (See fixative.)

nit: the egg of a louse, usually attached to a hair.

nitrate (nī'trāte): an oxidizing agent.

nitrite (nī'trīte): a reducing agent; sodium nitrite is used as a sanitizing agent and acts as an anti-rusting agent.

nitric acid (nī'trĭk): concentrated acid employed as a caustic.

nitro-cellulose (nī-trŏ-sĕl'û-lōs): used in nail polishes.

nitrogen (nī'trŏ-jĕn): a colorless, gaseous element, tasteless and odorless, found in air and living tissue.

nodule (nŏd'yūle): a small, circumscribed, solid elevation that usually extends into the deeper layers of the skin.

non-conductor (kŏn-dŭk'tĕr): any substance that resists the passage of electricity, light or heat towards or through it.

non-pathogenic (păth-ŏ-jĕn'ĭk): non-disease producing; growth promoting.

non-striated (strī'āt-ĕd): involuntary, smooth muscle which functions without the action of the will.

nucleus (nū'klê-ûs); pl., **nuclei** (-ī): the active center of cells.

nutrition (nû-trĭsh'ûn): the process of nourishment.

O

oblique (ŏb-lēk'; lĭk'); **obliquus** (-ûs): slanting, or inclined.

obsolete (ŏb-sŏ-lēt'): old; gone out of date.

occipital (ŏk-sĭp'ĭ-tâl): the bone which forms the back and lower part of the head.

occipito-frontalis (ŏk-sĭp'ĭ-tō-frŏn-tā'lĭs): epicranius; the scalp muscle.

occupational disease (ŏk-ū-pā'shŭn-ăl): due to certain kinds of employment, in which contact with chemicals, dyes is involved.

oculist (ŏk'ū-lĭst): a specialist in diseases of the eyes.

oculomotor (ŏk'ū-lō-mō'tĕr): third cranial nerve; controlling the motion of the eye.

oculus (ŏk'ū-lŭs); pl., oculi (-lī): the eye.

ohm (ōm): a unit of measurement used to denote the amount of resistance in an electrical system or device.

Ohm's law (ōmz lô): the simple statement that the current in an electric circuit is equal to the pressure divided by the resistance.

ointment: a fatty, medicated mixture used externally.

oleic acid (ō-lē'ĭk): an oily acid used in making soap and ointments.

olfactory (ŏl-făk'tō-rē): relating to the sense of smell; first cranial nerve, the special nerve of smell.

onychatrophia (ŏn-ĭ-kă-trō'fē-ă): atrophy of the nails.

onychauxis (ŏn-ĭ-kôk'sĭs): enlargement of the nails.

onychia (ō-nĭk'ē-ă): inflammation of the matrix of the nail with pus formation and shedding of the nail.

onychoclasis (ŏn-ĭ-kō-klā'sĭs): breaking of the nail.

onychocryptosis (ŏn-ĭ-kō-krĭp-tō'sĭs): ingrowing nail.

onychogryposis (ŏn-ĭ-kō-grĭ-pō'sĭs): denotes enlargement with increased curvature of the nail.

onycholysis (ŏn-ĭ-kŏl'ĭ-sĭs): loosening of the nail without shedding.

onychomycosis (ŏn-ĭ-kō-mī-kō'sĭs): refers to any parasitic disease of the nails.

onychophagy (ŏn-ĭ-kŏf'ă-jē): the morbid habit of eating or biting the nails.

onychophosis (ŏn-ĭ-kŏf-ō'sĭs): growth of horny epithelium in the nail-bed.

onychophyma (ŏn-ĭ-kŏf-ī'mă): a morbid degeneration of the nail.

onychoptosis (ŏn-ĭ-kŏp-tō'sĭs): falling off of the nails.

onychorrhexis (ŏn-ĭ-kō-rĕk'sĭs): abnormal brittleness of the nails with splitting of free edge.

onychosis; onychonosus (ŏn-ĭ-kō'sĭs; ŏn-ĭ-kō-nō'sûs): any disease of the nails.

onyx (ŏ'nĭks): a nail of the fingers or toes.

opaque (ō-pāk'): impervious to light rays; neither transparent nor translucent.

optic (ŏp'tĭk): second cranial nerve; the nerve of sight; pertaining to the eye, or to vision.

orangewood stick: a stick made of orangewood used in manicuring the nails.

orbicularis oculi (ôr-bĭk-û-lā'rĭs ŏk'û-lī): orbicularis palpebrarum; the ring muscle of the eye.

orbicularis oris (ō'rĭs): orbicular muscle; muscle of the mouth.

orbit: the bony cavity of the eyeball; the eye-socket.

organic (ôr-găn'ĭk): relating to an organ; pertaining to substances derived from living organisms.

organism (ôr'găn-ĭz'm): any living being, either animal or vegetable.

origin: the beginning; the starting point of a nerve; the place of attachment of a muscle to a bone.

oris (ō'rĭs): peraining to the mouth; an opening.

os (ŏs): a bone.

oscillation (ŏs-ĭ-lā'shŭn): movement like a pendulum; a swinging or vibration.

osmidrosis (ŏs-mĭ-drō'sĭs; ŏz-): bromidrosis; foul smelling perspiration.

osmosis (ŏs-mō'sĭs; ŏz-): the passage of fluids and solutions through a membrane or other porous substance.

osseous; osseus (ŏs'ê-ûs): bony.

osteology (ŏs-tê-ŏl'ō-jē): science of the anatomy, structure, and function of bones.

ovary (ō'vă-rē): one of the two reproductive glands in the female, containing the ova or germ cells.

oxidation (ŏk-sĭ-dā'shŭn): the act of combining oxygen with another substance.

oxygen: a gaseous element, essential to animal and plant life.

oxygenation (ŏk'sĭ-jê-nā'shŭn): saturation with oxygen, noting especially the aeration of the blood in the lungs.

oxymelanin (ŏk'sĭ-mĕl'ă-nĭn): a compound formed by a combination of an oxidizing agent with the dark melanin (color) pigments in the hair; (generally found in the red to yellow shades).

P

pack: a special cosmetic formula used to beautify the face.

palatine bones (păl'ă-tĭn): situated at the back part of the nasal depression.

palmar (păl'măr): referring to the palm of the hand.

papilla, hair (pă-pĭl'ă): a small cone-shaped elevation at the bottom of the hair follicle in the dermis.

papillary layer (păp'ĭ-lă-rē): the outer layer of the dermis.

papule (păp'ūl): a pimple; a small, circumscribed elevation on the skin containing no fluid.

para (păr'ă): see para-phenylene-diamine.

para-phenylene-diamine (păr-ă-fēn'ĭ-lēn-dĭ-ăm'ĭn; dĭ'ă-mēn): an aniline derivative used in hair tinting.

parasite (păr'ă-sīt): a vegetable or animal organism which lives on or in another organism, and draws its nourishment therefrom.

parasiticide (păr-ă-sĭt'ĭ-sīd): a substance that destroys parasites.

para tint: a tint made from an aniline derivative.

para toluene diamine (păr'ă tŏl'ū-ēn dī-ăm'ĭn): a variety of aniline derivative dyes commonly used in preparations compounded to provide red and blonde tones. (meta: prefix meaning higher, or change relating to the position of the amine free arm on the toluene ring.)

parietal (pă-rī'ê-tăl): pertaining to the wall of a cavity; a bone at the side of the head.

paronychia (păr-ô-nĭk'ē-ă): felon; an inflammation of the tissues surrounding the nail.

parotid (pă-rŏt'ĭd): near the ear; a gland near the ear.

patch test: see predisposition test.

pathogenic (păth-ô-jĕn'ĭk): causing disease; disease producing.

pathology (păth-ŏl'ô-jē): the science of the nature of disease.

pectoralis (pĕk-tô-rā'lĭs): a muscle of the breast.

pediculosis capitis (pê-dĭk'û-lō'sĭs kăp'ĭ-tĭs): lousiness of the hair of the head.

pedicure (pĕd'ĭ-kūr): care of feet and toe nails.

penetration (pĕn-ē-trā'shŭn): act or power of penetrating.

peptide (pĕp'tĭd): a compound of two or more amino-acids containing one or more peptide groups; continuous filaments in the case of fiber protein or keratin.

peptide bonds: see end bonds.

percarbonate (pĕr-kär'bô-nāt): quantity of salts or esters of carbonic acid.

percussion (pĕr-kŭsh'ŭn): a form of massage consisting of repeated light blows or taps of varying force.

pericardium (pĕr-ĭ-kär'dē-ŭm): the membranous sac around the heart.

peripheral nervous system (pê-rĭf'ĕr-ăl): consists of the nerve endings in the skin and sense organs.

permanent wave, cold: a system of permanent waving employing chemicals rather than heat.

permanent wave, heat: accomplished by changing the hair structure from an ordinary and natural straightness to one of permanent curliness or waviness.

permeable (pûr'mê-ă-b'l): permitting the passage of liquids.

peroxide of hydrogen: a powerful oxidizing agent; in liquid solution it is used as an antiseptic; used in tinting and lightening treatments.

perspiration (pûr'spĭ-rā'shŭn): sweat; the fluid excreted from the sweat glands of the skin.

persulfate (pĕr-sŭl'fāt): a sulfate which contains more sulfuric acid than the ordinary sulfide.

petrissage (pĕt-rĭ-säj): the kneading movement in massage.

petrolatum (pĕt-rô-lā'tŭm): petroleum jelly; Vaseline; a purified, yellow mixture of semi-solid hydrocarbons obtained from petroleum.

petroleum (pê-trô'lê-ŭm): an oily liquid coming from the earth and consisting of a mixture of hydrocarbons.

pH: symbol for potential hydrogen concentration; the relative degree of acidity or alkalinity.

pH number: a measure of the degree of acidity or alkalinity of a solution.

phalanx (fā'lănks); pl., **phalanges** (fă-lăn'jēz): the long bone of the finger or toe.

pharynx (făr'ĭnks): the upper portion of the digestive tube, behind the nose and mouth.

phenol (fē'nŏl): carbolic acid; caustic poison; in dilute solution is used as an antiseptic and disinfectant.

phyma (fī'mă); pl., **phymata** (fī'mă-tă): a circumscribed swelling on the skin, larger than a tubercle.

physics (fĭz'ĭks): the branch of science that deals with matter, motion, light, heat, electricity, sound and mechanics.

physiology (fĭz-ē-ŏl'ô-jē): the science of the functions of living things.

pigment (pĭg'mĕnt): any organic coloring matter, as that of the red blood cells, the hair, skin, iris, etc.

pigmentation (pĭg-mĕn-tā'shŭn): the deposition of pigment in the skin or tissues.

pilus (pī'lŭs); pl., **pili** (-lī): hair.

pimple: any small, pointed elevation of the skin; a papule or small pustule.

pituitary (pĭ-tū'ĭ-târ-ē): a ductless gland located at the base of the brain.

pityriasis (pĭt-ĭ-rī'ă-sĭs): dandruff; an inflammation of the skin characterized by the formation and flaking of fine branny scales.

pityriasis capitis simplex (kăp'ĭ-tĭs sĭm'plĕks): a scalp inflammation marked by dry dandruff or branny scales.

pivot, hair shaping: the exact point from which the hair is directed in forming a curvature or shaping.

plasma (plăz'mă): the fluid part of the blood and lymph.

platelets (plāt'lĕts): blood cells which aid in the forming of clots.

platysma (plă-tĭz'mă): a broad, thin muscle of the neck.

pledget (plĕj'ĕt): a compress or small, flat mass of lint, absorbent cotton, or the like.

plexus (plĕk'sŭs): a network of nerves or veins.

pliability (plī-ă-bĭl'ĭ-tē): flexibility.

pneumogastric nerve (nū-mô-găs'trĭk nûrv): vagus nerve; tenth cranial nerve.

polypeptide (pŏl-ē-pĕp'tĭd): strings of amino-acids joined together by peptide bonds, the prefix "poly" meaning many.

pollex (pŏl'ĕks): the thumb.

pomade (pô-mād'): a medicated ointment for the hair.

pore: a small opening of the sweat glands of the skin.

porosity (pô-rŏs'ĭ-tē): ability of the hair to absorb moisture.

porous: full of pores.

positive: affirmative; not negative; the presence of abnormal condition; having a relatively high potential in electricity.

posterior (pŏs-tē'rē-ĕr): situated behind; coming after or behind.

posterior auricular (ô-rĭk'û-lăr): a nerve which supplies muscles in the posterior surface of the ear.

postiche (pôs-tēsh'): artificial hairpiece; curls, braids, or other extra hairpiece used in creating coiffures.

potassium hydroxide (pô-tăs'ē-ŭm hī-drŏk'sīd): a powerful alkali, used in the manufacture of soft soaps.

potassium permanganate (pĕr-măn'gâ-nāt): a salt of permanganate acid; used as an antiseptic and deodorant.

precipitate (prē-sĭp'ĭ-tāt): to cause a substance in solution to settle down in solid particles; to decrease solubility.

predisposition (prē-dĭs-pô-zĭsh'ŭn): a condition of special susceptibility to disease; allergy.

predisposition test: a skin test designed to determine an individual's over-sensitivity to certain chemicals (patch test, allergy test, skin test).

pressing: a method of straightening over-curly or kinky hair with a heated comb or iron.

primary colors: pigments or colors that are, or thought to be, fundamental; red, yellow and blue are the primary colors in pigments.

primary hair: the baby fine hair that is present over almost the entire smooth skin of the body.

prism (prĭz'm): a transparent solid with triangular ends and two converging sides; it breaks up white light into its component colors.

procerus (prô-sē'rŭs): muscle that covers bridge of the nose.

processing (prŏs'ĕs-ĭng): the action of a chemical in softening and reforming the structure of the hair. (In permanent waving and hair relaxing.)

processing machine: an apparatus employed to hasten the action of the chemical in hair tinting or lightening.

prognosis (prŏg-nō'sĭs): the foretelling of the probable course of a disease.

progressive tints (prô-grĕs'ĭv): hair restorers requiring time to oxidize; color develops gradually.

prong: the round rod of the thermal (marcel) iron.

properties (prŏp'ĕr-tēz): the identifying characteristics of a substance which are observable; a peculiar quality of anything; i.e., color, taste, smell, etc.

prophylaxis (prô-fĭ-lăk'sĭs): prevention of disease.

protective base (prô-tĕk'tĭv): a petroleum base, applied to the entire scalp in order to protect it from the active agents contained in the chemical hair relaxer.

protein: a complex organic substance present in all living tissues, such as skin, hair and nails; necessary in the daily diet; also present in skin and hair conditioners.

protoplasm (prō'tō-plăz'm): the material basis of life; a substance found in all living things.

protozoa (prō-tō-zō'ä): subkingdom of animals, including all the unicellular animal organisms.

psoriasis (sō-rī'ä-sĭs): a skin disease with circumscribed red patches, covered with adherent white silver scales.

puberty (pū'bĕr-tē): the period of life in which the organs of reproduction are developed.

pull burn: scalp irritation resulting from uneven winding of the hair during permanent waving.

pull test: a test to determine the degree of elasticity of the hair.

pulmonary (pŭl'mō-nȧ-rē): relating to the lungs.

pumice (pŭm'ĭs): hardened volcanic substance, white or gray in color, used for buffing in manicuring; also called pumice stone.

purification (pū-rĭ-fĭ-kā'shŭn): the act of cleaning or removing foreign matter.

pus: a fluid product of inflammation, consisting of a liquid containing leucocytes and the debris of dead cells and tissue elements.

pusher: a steel instrument used to loosen the cuticle from the nail.

pustule (pŭs'tūl): an inflamed pimple containing pus.

Q

quadratus labii superioris (kwŏd-rā'tŭs lā'bē-ī sû-pē'rē-ŏr'ĭs): a muscle of the upper lip.

quarantine (kwŏr'ȧn-tēn): the isolation of a person to prevent spread of a contagious disease.

quinine (kwī'nīn): enters into the composition of many hair lotions in small quantities; its effect is slightly antiseptic.

R

radial nerve (rā'dè-ăl): a nerve which affects the arm and hand.

radiation (rā-dè-ā'shŭn): the process of giving off light or heat rays.

radius (rā'dè-ûs): the outer and smaller bone of the forearm.

rash: a skin eruption having little or no elevation.

ratting: see teasing.

reconditioning (rē-kŏn-dĭ'shŭn-ĭng): the application of a special substance to the hair in order to improve its condition.

rectifier (rĕk'tĭ-fĭ-ēr): an apparatus to change an alternating current of electricity into a direct current.

rectus (rĕk'tûs): in a straight line; the name of small muscles of the eye.

reddish cast: a tinge of red.

reducing agent: a substance capable of adding hydrogen; in cosmetology, a cold wave solution would be a reducing agent.

reflex: an involuntary nerve reaction.

relaxer (rē-lăk'sēr): a chemical applied to the hair to remove the natural curl.

relaxer testing: checking the action of the relaxer in order to determine the speed at which the natural curl is being removed.

reproductive (rē-prō-dŭk'tĭv): pertaining to reproduction or the process by which plants and animals give rise to offspring.

resilient (rĕ-zĭl'ĭ-ĕnt): elastic.

resistance (rē-zĭst'ȧns): the difficulty of moisture or chemical solutions to penetrate the hair shaft.

respiration (rĕs-pĭ-rā'shŭn): the act of breathing; the process of inhaling air into the lungs and expelling it.

respiratory system (rĕ-spīr'ȧ-tō-rē): consists of the nose, pharynx, larynx, trachea, bronchi and lungs which assist in breathing.

rete (rē'tē): any interlacing of either blood vessels or nerves.

reticular layer (rĕ-tĭk'û-lâr): the inner layer of the corium.

retina (rĕt'ĭ-nȧ): the sensitive membrane of the eye which receives the image formed by the lens.

retouch: application of hair color, lightener or chemical hair relaxer to new growth of hair.

reversible (rē-vērs'ĭ-b'l): capable of going through a series of changes in either direction, forward or backward, as a reversible chemical reaction.

rhagades (răg'ȧ-dēz): cracks, fissures or chaps on the skin.

rickettsia (rĭk-ĕt'sē-ä): a type of pathogenic microorganism, capable of producing disease.

ringed hair: a variety of canities in which the hair appears white or colored in rings.

ringworm: a vegetable parasitic disease of the skin and its appendages which appears in circular lesions and is contagious.

rinse: to cleanse with a second or repeated application of water after washing; a prepared rinse water.

risorius (rĭ-zôr'ē-ûs): muscle at the side of the mouth.

rolling: a massage movement in which the tissues are pressed and twisted.

root: in anatomy, the base; the foundation or beginning of any part.

rotary (rō'tȧ-rē): circular motion of the fingers as in massage.

ruffing (rŭf'ĭng): back combing; teasing of the hair.

S

saccular (săk'û-lâr): consisting of little sacs, such as oil glands.

sachet (sȧ-shā'): a perfumed bag or pad.

saline (sā'līn): salty; containing salt.

saliva (sȧ-lī'vȧ): the secretion of the salivary glands; spittle.

salt: in chemistry, the union of a base with an acid.

sanitary (săn'ĭ-tȧ-rē): pertaining to cleanliness in relation to health; tending to promote health.

sanitation (săn-ĭ-tā'shŭn): the use of methods to bring about favorable conditions of health.

sanitize: to make sanitary.

saprophyte (săp'rō-fīt): a micro-organism which grows normally on dead matter, as distinguished from a parasite.

S-bonds: see: sulphur bonds.

scab: a crust formed on the surface of a sore.

scabies (skā'bĭ-ēz): a skin disease caused by an animal parasite, attended with intense itching; the itch.

scale: any thin plate of horny epidermis; regular markings used as a standard in measuring and weighing.

scalp: the skin covering of the cranium.

scapula (skăp'û-lä): the shoulder blade; a large, flat, triangular bone of the shoulder.

scar: a mark remaining after a wound has healed.

scarf skin: epidermis.

science: knowledge duly arranged and systematized.

scurf (skûrf): thin, dry scales or scabs on the body, especially on the scalp; dandruff.

sebaceous cyst (sē-bā'shŭs sĭst): a distended, oily or fatty follicle or sac.

sebaceous glands: oil glands of the skin.

seborrhea (sĕb-ô-rē'ă): an oily condition caused by the over-action of the sebaceous glands.

seborrhea capitis (kăp'ĭ-tĭs): seborrhea of the scalp, commonly called dandruff; pityriasis.

seborrhea oleosa (ō-lē-ō'să): excessive oiliness of the skin, particularly of the forehead and nose.

seborrhea sicca (sĭk'ă): an accumulation on the scalp, of greasy scales or crusts, due to over-action of the sebaceous glands; dandruff or pityriasis.

seborrheic (sĕb-ô-rē'ĭk): seborrheal; pertaining to the over-action of the sebaceous glands.

sebum (sē'bŭm): the fatty or oily secretions of the sebaceous glands.

secondary hair: the stiff, short, coarse hair found on the eyelashes, eyebrows and within the openings or passages of the nose and ears.

secretion (sē-krē'shŭn): a product manufactured by a gland for a special purpose.

sectioning (sĕk'shŭn-ĭng): dividing the hair into separate parts.

senility (sē-nĭl'ĭ-tē): quality or state of being old.

sensation (sĕn-sā'shŭn): a feeling or impression arising as the result of the stimulation of an afferent nerve.

sensitivity (sĕn-sĭ-tĭv'ĭ-tē): the state of being easily affected by certain chemicals or external conditions.

sensory nerve: afferent nerve; a nerve carrying sensations.

sepsis (sĕp'sĭs): the presence of various pus-forming and other pathogenic organisms, or their toxins, in the blood or tissues; septicemia.

septic (sĕp'tĭk): relating to or caused by sepsis.

septum (sĕp'tŭm): a dividing wall; a partition.

serratus anterior (sĕ-rā'tŭs ăn-tē'rĕ-ôr): a muscle of the chest assisting in breathing and in raising the arm.

shaft: slender, stem-like structure; the long, slender part of the hair above the scalp.

shampoo: to subject the scalp and hair to washing and massaging with some cleansing agent, such as soap and water.

shaping, haircutting: the process of shortening and thinning the hair to a particular style or to the contour of the head.

shaping, hairstyling: the formation of uniform arcs or curves in wet hair, thus providing a base for finger waves, pin curls or various patterns in hairstyling.

sheath: a covering enclosing or surrounding some organ.

shingling: cutting the hair close to the nape of the neck and gradually longer toward the crown.

shortwave: a form of high-frequency current used in permanent hair removal.

singeing: process of lightly burning hair ends with a lighted wax taper.

single application tints: products which lighten and add color to the hair in a single application; also called one process or one step tints.

sinus (sī'nŭs): a cavity or depression; a hollow in bone or other tissue.

skeletal muscles (skĕl'ĕ-tăl): muscles connected to the skeleton.

skeleton: the bony framework of the body.

skin: the external covering of the body.

skin texture: the general feel and appearance of the skin.

skull: the bony case or the framework of the head.

slicing: carefully removing a section of hair from a shaping in preparation for making a pin curl.

slip: a smooth and slippery feeling imparted by talc to face powder.

slippage: the shifting and changing of position of the sulphur bonds.

slithering (slĭth'ẽr-ĭng): tapering the hair to graduated lengths with scissors.

smaller occipital (ŏk-sĭp'ĭ-tăl): sensory nerve affecting skin behind the ear.

soap cap: a solution of equal parts of shampoo, hydrogen peroxide and tint; employed when a slight change in color is desired.

soapless shampoo: a shampoo made with sulfonated oil, alcohol, mineral oil and water; this type of shampoo does not foam, and is usually alkaline in reaction.

sodium (sō'dē-ûm): a metallic element of the alkaline group.

sodium bicarbonate (bī-kär'bŏn-ât): baking soda; it relieves burns, bites; is often used in bath powders as an aid to cleansing oily skin.

sodium carbonate (kär'bŏn-ât): washing soda; used to prevent corrosion of metallic instruments when added to boiling water.

sodium hydroxide (hī-drŏk'sīd): a powerful alkaline product used in some chemical hair relaxers; caustic soda.

sodium lauryl sulfite (lô'rêl sûl'fīt): a metallic element of the alkaline group, in white or light yellow crystals; used in detergents.

sodium perborate (pẽr'bŏ-rāt): a compound, formed by treating sodium peroxide with boric acid; on dissolving the substance in water, peroxide of hydrogen is generated; used as an antiseptic.

sodium sulphite (sûl'fīt): a soft, white metallic salt of sulphurous acid.

softening: the application of a chemical product to hair in order to make it more receptive to hair coloring or permanent waving.

solar (sō'lär): pertaining to the sun.

solarium (sō-lä'rē-ûm): a sun parlor.

solubility (sŏl-û-bĭl'ĭ-tē): the extent to which a substance (solute) dissolves in a liquid (solvent) to produce a homogeneous system (solution).

solute (sŏl'ūt): the dissolved substance in a solution.

solution: the act or process by which a substance is absorbed into a liquid.

solvent (sŏl'vĕnt): an agent capable of dissolving substances.

spatula (spăt'û-lă): a flexible, knife-like implement for handling creams and pomades, etc.

spectrum (spĕk'trŭm): the band of rainbow colors produced by decomposing light by means of a prism.

sphenoid (sfē'noid): wedge-shaped; a bone in the cranium.

spinal accessory (spī'nâl ăk-sĕs'ô-rē): eleventh cranial nerve.

spinal column: the backbone or vertebral column.

spinal cord: the portion of the central nervous system contained within the spinal, or vertebral canal.

spinal nerves: the nerves arising from the spinal cord.

spine: a short process of bone; the backbone.

spiral: coil; winding around a center, like a watch spring.

spirillum (spī-rĭl'ûm); pl., **spirilla** (-ă): curved bacterium.

splash neutralizer: a chemical agent capable of stopping the action of the cold waving solution and setting or hardening the hair in its new form.

spore (spôr): a tiny bacterial body having a protective wall to withstand unfavorable conditions.

spray gum: a sticky juice applied as a liquid going through the air in small drops.

squama (skwā′mă): an epidermic scale made up of thin, flat cells.

stabilized: made stable or firm, preventing changes.

stabilizer: see fixative.

stable: in a balanced condition; not readily destroyed or decomposed; resisting molecular change.

stain: an abnormal skin discoloration.

staphylococcus (stăf-ĭ-lō-kŏk′ŭs): cocci which are grouped in clusters like a bunch of grapes; found in pustules and boils.

static electricity: a form of electricity generated by friction.

steamer, facial: an apparatus, used in place of hot towels, for steaming the scalp or face.

stearic acid (stē-ăr′ĭk): a white, fatty acid, occuring in solid animal fats and in some of the vegetable fats.

steatoma (stē-ă-tō′mă): a sebaceous cyst; a fatty tumor.

steatosis (stē-ă-tō′sĭs): fatty degeneration; adiposis.

stem direction: the direction in which the stem moves from the base to the first arc.

stem, pin curl: that part of the pin curl between the base and the first arc of the circle.

sterilization: the process of making sterile; the destruction of germs.

sterno-cleido-mastoideus (stûr′nō-klī′dō-măs-toid′ē-ŭs): a muscle of the neck which depresses and rotates the head.

stimulation (stĭm-û-lā′shŭn) the act arousing increased functional activity.

stomach: the dilated portion of the alimentary canal, in which the first process of digestion takes place.

strand test: a preliminary test given before a tint or lightening application to determine the required development time; a test to determine the degree of porosity and elasticity of the hair, as well as the ability of the hair to withstand the effects of chemicals.

stratum (strā′tŭm); pl., **strata** (-ă): layer of tissue.

stratum corneum (kôr′nē-ŭm): horny layer of the skin.

stratum germinativum (jûr-mĭ-nā′tĭv-ŭm): the deepest layer of the epidermis resting on the corneum.

stratum granulosum (grăn-û-lō′sŭm): granular layer of the skin.

stratum lucidum (lū′sĭ-dŭm): clear layer of the skin.

stratum mucosum (mū-kō′sŭm): mucous or malpighian layer of the skin.

streaking (strēk′ĭng): lightening broad sections of hair attractively placed around the face.

streptococcus (strĕp-tō-kŏk′ŭs): pus-forming bacteria that arrange in curved lines resembling a string of beads; found in erysipelas and blood poisoning.

striated (strī′āt-ĕd): marked with parallel lines or bands; striped; voluntary muscle.

stripping: the removal of color from the hair shaft; lightening. Strong shampoos or soap removing some of the color from the hair is also known as stripping.

stroking: a gliding movement over a surface; to pass the fingers or any instrument gently over a surface; effleurage.

strontium sulphide (strŏn′shē-ŭm sŭl′fīd): a light gray powder capable of liberating hydrogen sulphide in the presence of water; used as a depilatory.

styptic (stĭp′tĭk): an agent causing contraction of living tissue; used to stop bleeding; an astringent.

subcutaneous (sŭb-kū-tā′nē-ŭs): under the skin.

subcutis (sŭb-kū′tĭs): subdermis; subcutaneous tissue; under or beneath the corium or dermis, the true skin.

subdermis (sŭb-dûr′mĭs): subcutis or subcutaneous tissue of the skin.

submental artery (sŭb-mĕn′tâl är′tĕr-ē): supplies blood to the chin and lower lip.

sudamen (sû-dā′mĕn); pl., **sudamina** (sû-dăm′ĭ-nă): a disorder of the sweat glands with obstruction of their ducts.

sudoriferous glands (sū-dôr-ĭf′ĕr-ŭs glăndz): sweat glands of the skin.

sulfite (sŭl′fīt): any salt or sulfurous acid.

sulfonated oil (sŭl′fôn-āt-êd): an organic substance prepared by reacting oils with sulphuric acid; has an alkaline reaction and is miscible with water; used as a base in soapless shampoos.

sulphide (sŭl′fīd): a compound of sulphur with another element or base.

sulphur (sŭl′fûr): a chemical element whose compounds are used in lightening, in hair preparations and in medicine.

sulphur bonds: sulphur cross bonds in the hair, which hold the chains of amino-acids together in order to form a hair strand.

supercilium (sū-pĕr-sĭl′ē-ûm); pl., **supercilia** (-ă): the eyebrow.

suppuration (sŭp-û-rā′shûn): the formation of pus.

supraorbital (sū-pră-ôr′bĭ-tâl): above the orbit or eye.

supra-trochlear (sū-pră-trŏk′lē-âr): above the trochlea or pulley of the superior oblique muscle.

surface tension: the tension or resistance to rupture possessed by the surface film of a liquid.

susceptible (sū-sĕp′tĭ-b′l): capable of being influenced or easily acted on.

suspension (sû-spĕn′shûn): a mixture of a liquid and insoluble particles which have a tendency to settle on standing.

swirl: formation of a wave in a diagonal direction from back to side of head.

switch: long wefts of hair, tail-like in formation, mounted with a loop at the end.

sympathetic nervous system (sĭm-pă-thĕt′ĭk): controls the involuntary muscles which affect respiration, circulation and digestion.

symptom, objective (sĭmp′tôm, ŏb-jĕk′tĭv): that which can be seen, as in pimples, pustules, etc.

symptom, subjective (sŭb-jĕk′tĭv): can be felt, as in itching.

system: a group of organs which especially contribute toward one of the more important vital functions.

systematic: proceeding according to system or regular method.

systemic (sĭs-tĕm′ĭk): pertaining to a system or to the body as a whole.

T

tactile corpuscle (tăk′tĭl kôr′pŭs-′l): touch nerve endings found within the skin.

tannic acid (tăn′ĭk): a plant extract used as an astringent.

tapotement (tà-pôt-män′): a massage movement using a short, quick slapping or tapping movement.

tapping: a massage movement; striking lightly with partly flexed fingers.

tartaric acid (tär'tâ-rĭk): a colorless crystalline acid compound.

teasing: combing small sections of hair from the ends toward the scalp, causing the shorter hair to mat at the scalp, forming a cushion or base. Also known as ratting, French lacing or ruffing.

temple: the flattened space on the side of the forehead.

temporal bone (těm'pô-rål): the bone at the side and base of the skull.

temporalis (těm-pô-rā'lĭs): the temporal muscle.

tendon: fibrous cord or band connecting muscle with bone.

tensile (těn'sĭl): capable of being stretched.

tension: stress caused by stretching or pulling.

terminology (těr-mĭ-nŏl'ô-jē): the special words or terms used in science, art or business.

tertiary (terminal) hair (těr'shĕ-â-rē hâr): the long, soft hair found on the scalp.

test curls: a method to determine how the patron's hair will react to permanent waving solution and neutralizer.

test, hair tint: a test made upon the scalp, behind the ear, or in the bend of the arm, for predisposition to the agent used; a test to determine the reaction of the color upon the sample strand, regarding both color and breakage.

tetanus (tět'â-nŭs): a disease with spasmodic and continuous contraction of the muscles; lockjaw.

textometer (těks-tŏm'ĕ-těr): a device used to measure the elasticity and reaction of the hair to alkaline solutions.

texture of hair: the general quality as to coarse, medium or fine; feel of the hair.

texture of skin: the general feel and appearance of the skin.

thallium (thǎ'lĭ-ŭm): a bluish-white metallic element, the salts of which have been used for epilation; thallium is highly toxic to humans.

therapeutic lamp (thěr-ă-pū'tĭk): an electrical apparatus producing any of the various rays of the spectrum; used for skin and scalp treatments.

therapy (thěr'ă-pē): the science and art of healing.

thermal (thûr'mål): relating to heat.

thermal curling: the process of forming curls with thermal irons.

thermal hair straightening: straightening over-curly hair with heated thermal irons.

thermal irons: an implement used to curl, wave or straighten hair by the application of heat.

thermal waving: forming waves in the hair with heated thermal iron.

thermostat (thûr'mô-stǎt): an automatic device for regulating temperature.

thinning, hair: decreasing the thickness of the hair where it is too heavy.

thio (thī'ō): see ammonium thioglycolate.

thioglycolic acid (thī-ō-glī'kô-lĭk): a colorless liquid or white crystals with a strong unpleasant odor, miscible with water, alcohol or ether; (used in permanent wave solutions, hair relaxers and depilatories.)

thorax (thō'rǎks): the part of the body between the neck and the abdomen; the chest.

thrombocyte (thrŏm'bō-sīt): a blood platelet which aids in clotting.

thyroid gland (thī'roid): a large, ductless gland situated in the neck.

tincture (tĭnk'tûr): an alcoholic solution of a medicinal substance.

tinea (tĭn'ē-ă): a skin disease, especially ringworm.

tint: to give a coloring to; as used in cosmetology, pertaining to hair tinting; to color the hair by means of a hair tint or color rinse.

tinting: the process of adding artificial color to hair.

tipping: similar to frosting, but the darkening or lightening is confined to small strands of hair at the front of the head.

tissue: a collection of similar cells which perform a particular function.

tissue, connective (kŏ-něk'tĭv): binding and supporting tissue.

toluene diamine (tŏl'ū-ēn dī-ăm'ĭn): a colorless liquid, obtained from a coal tar product, used as a solvent and also in a drug designed to increase the amount of bile secreted.

tone: healthy functioning of the body or its parts.

toner: an aniline derivative tint applied to highly lightened hair to achieve a pale, delicate color.

tonic: increasing the strength or tone of the system.

toupee (tōō-pē'): a small wig used to cover the top or crown of a man's head.

toxemia (tŏk-sē'mē-ă): form of blood poisoning.

toxin; toxine (tŏk'sĭn; -sēn): a poisonous substance of undetermined chemical nature, elaborated during the growth of pathogenic micro-organisms.

tracheo (trā'kē-ă; trǎ-kē'ă): wind pipe.

translucent (trăns-lū'sênt): somewhat transparent.

transformation (trăns-fôr-mā'shŭn): an artificial band of hair worn over a person's own hair.

transformer (trăns-fôr'mēr): used for the purpose of increasing or decreasing the voltage of the current used; it can only be used on an alternating current.

transverse facial (trăns-vûrs'): an artery supplying the skin, the parotid gland and the masseter muscle.

trapezius (tră-pē'zē-ŭs): muscle that draws the head backward and sideways.

triangularis (trī-ăn-gû-lā'rĭs): a muscle that pulls down the corner of the mouth.

triceps (trī'sěps): three-headed.

trichology (trī-kŏl'ō-jē): the science of the care of the hair.

trichonosus (trĭk-ô-nō'sûs): any disease of the hair.

trichophytosis (trĭ-kŏf-ĭ-tō'sĭs): ringworm of the skin and scalp, due to growth of a fungus parasite.

trichoptilosis (trĭ-kŏp-tĭ-lō'sĭs): a splitting of the hair ends, giving them a feathery appearance.

trichorrhexis (trĭk-ô-rěk'sĭs): brittleness of the hair.

trichosis (trĭ-kō-sĭs): abnormal growth of hair.

trifacial: the fifth cranial nerve; also known as the triceminal nerve.

trigeminal (trī-jěm'ĭ-nâl): relating to the fifth cranial or trigeminus nerve.

true skin: the corium.

trypsin (trĭp'sĭn): an enzyme in the digestive juice secreted by the pancreas; trypsin changes proteins into peptones.

tubercle (tū'běr-k'l): a rounded, solid elevation on the skin or membrane.

tumor: a swelling; an abnormal enlargement.

turbinal; turbinate (tûr'bĭ-nâl; -nāt): a bone in the nose; turbinated body.

tweezers: a pair of small forceps to remove or extract hair.

tyrosine (tī-rō'sĭn): an amino-acid widely distributed in proteins, particularly in casein.

U

ulcer (ŭl'sēr): an open sore not caused by a wound.

ulna (ŭl'nă): the inner and larger bone of the forearm.

ultra-violet: invisible rays of the spectrum which are beyond the violet rays.

unadulterated (ŭn-ă-dŭl'tēr-āt-ĕd): pure.

undulation (ŭn-dû-lā'shŭn): a wave-like movement or shape.

unguentum (ŭn-gwĕn'tûm); pl., **unguenta** (-ă): a salve or ointment.

unguis (ŭn'gwĭs)); pl., **ungues** (-gwēz): the nail of a finger or toe.

unguium, tinea (ŭn'gwē-ŭm, tĭn'ê-ă): ringworm of the nails.

unit: a single thing or value.

United States Pharmacopeia (U.S.P.) (fär-mà-kô-pē'yà): an official book of drug and medicinal standards.

unstable: liable to fade.

urea (ū-rē'à): a diuretic; also employed externally in treating infected wounds; occurs as colorless to white crystals or powder; soluble in water.

urea peroxide: a combination of urea and peroxide in the form of a cream developer or activator; employed in hair tinting.

V

vaccination (văk-sĭ-nā'shŭn): inoculation with the virus of cowpox, or vaccina, as a means of producing immunity against small pox.

vaccine (văk'sĭn; -sēn): any substance used for preventive inoculation.

vacuum (văk'û-ûm): a space from which most of the air has been exhausted.

vagus (vā'gûs): pneumogastric nerve; tenth cranial nerve.

vapor: the gaseous state of a liquid or solid.

varicose veins (văr'ĭ-kōs): swollen or knotted veins.

vascular (văs'kû-làr): supplied with small blood vessels; pertaining to a vessel for the conveyance of a fluid as blood or lymph.

Vaseline (văs'ê-lĭn; ēn): a tradename; petrolatum; a semi-solid greasy or oily mixture of hydrocarbons obtained from petroleum.

vein; vena (vē'nà): a blood vessel carrying blood toward the heart.

vena cava (kā'vă): one of the large veins which carries the blood to the right auricle of the heart.

ventilate: to renew the air in a place.

ventricle (vĕn'trĭ-k'l): a small cavity; particularly in the heart.

vermin (vûr'mĭn): parasitic insects, as lice and bedbugs.

verruca (vĕ-rōō'kă): a wart; a growth of the papillae and epidermis.

vertebra (vûr'tê-bră); pl., **vertebrae** (-brē): a bony segment of the spinal column.

vesicle (vĕs'ĭ-k'l): a small blister or sac; a small elevation on the skin.

vibrator (vī'bră-tēr): an electrically driven massage apparatus causing a swinging, shaking sensation on the body, producing stimulation.

violet-ray: high-frequency; Tesla; an electric current of medium voltage and medium amperage.

virgin hair: normal hair which has had no previous lightening or tinting treatments.

virus (vī'rûs): poison; the specific poison of an infectious disease.

viscid (vĭs'ĭd): sticky or adhesive.

viscosity (vĭs-kōs'ĭ-tê): 1) resistance to change of form; 2) a resistance to flow that a liquid exhibits; 3) the degree of density, thickness, stickiness and adhesiveness of a substance.

viscous (vĭs'kûs): sticky or gummy.

visible rays: light rays which can be seen; are visible to the eye.

vitiligo (vĭt-ĭ-lī'gō): milky-white spots of the skin.

volatile (vŏl'à-tĭl): easily evaporating; diffusing freely; not permanent.

volt: the fractional unit of electromotive force.

voltage: electrical potential difference expressed in volts.

voluntary: under the control of the will.

vomer (vō'mēr): the thin plate of bone between the nostrils.

W

wart (wôrt): verruca.

water, hard: water containing certain minerals; does not lather with soap.

water, soft: water which readily lathers with soap; relatively free of minerals.

water softener: certain chemicals, such as the carbonate or phosphate of sodium, used to soften hard water to permit the lathering of soap.

wattage (wŏt'àj): amount of electric power expressed in watts.

wave, cold: a method of permanent waving requiring the use of certain chemicals rather than heat.

wave, finger: arranging waves into the hair, which has been wet with fingers and comb.

wave, marcel: thermal wave produced by means of heated thermal irons.

wave, permanent: a wave given to the hair which is of permanent duration.

wave, pin curl: alternating the direction of rows of pin curls in order to form a wave pattern.

wave, shadow: a wave with low ridges and shallow waves.

wave, skip: a pattern formed by a combination of alternating ridges and curls.

weft (wĕft): an artificial section of woven hair used for practice work or as a substitute for natural hair.

wen (wĕn): a sebaceous cyst, usually on the scalp.

wetting agent: a substance that causes a liquid to spread more readily on a solid surface, chiefly through a reduction of surface tension.

wheal (whēl): a raised ridge on the skin, usually caused by a blow, a bite of an insect, urticaria, or sting of a nettle.

whitehead (whīt'hĕd): milium.

whorl (whûrl; whôrl): a spiral turn, in general; a hair whorl or cowlick; a spiral turn causing a tuft of hair which goes contrary to the usual growth of the hair.

wig: an artificial covering for the head consisting of a network of interwoven hair.

wiglet: a hairpiece with a flat base which is used in special areas of the head.

winding, croquignole (krō'kwĭ-nōl): winding under the hair, from the hair ends towards the scalp.

winding, spiral (spī'rál): winding the hair from the scalp to the ends.

wind pipe: trachea.

wrapping: winding hair on rollers or rods in order to form curls.

wrinkle: a small ridge or a furrow.

Z

zinc sulphate (sŭl'fāt): a salt often employed as an astringent, both in lotions and creams.

zinc sulphocarbonate (zĭnk sŭl-fô-kär'bôn-āt): a fine white powder having the odor of carbolic acid; used as an antiseptic and astringent in deodorant preparations.

zygomatic (zī-gô-măt'ĭk): pertaining to the malar or cheek bone.

zygomaticus (zī-gô-măt'ĭ-kûs): a muscle that draws the upper lip upward and outward.

ANSWERS TO REVIEW QUESTIONS

CHAPTER 1

HYGIENE AND GOOD GROOMING

(Answers to Questions on Page 4)

1. The science of healthful living.
2. The care given by the individual to preserve his or her health.
3. Sanitary measures taken by the government to promote public health.
4. Cleanliness, oral hygiene, good posture, exercise, relaxation, adequate sleep, balanced diet and wholesome thoughts.
5. Providing pure air, pure food, pure water, adequate sewerage, control of disease, adequate medical facilities.
6. Cheerfulness, courage and hope.
7. Worry and fear.
8. Clean.
9. Deodorant.
10. Antiseptic.
11. Contagious.
12. Oral hygiene means keeping teeth and gums in good condition by brushing at least twice a day with a good dentifrice.

CHAPTER 2

VISUAL POISE

(Answers to Questions on Page 10)

1. (a) Improved personal appearance. (b) Preventing body fatigue. (c) Permitting of graceful movements.
2. 45.
3. Up; floor; up; flat.
4. Together.
5. Floor.
6. Chair.
7. Low-heeled.
8. Exercise keeps the muscles of the body in good condition.
9. They give the body support and balance, and help maintain good posture.
10. Healthy feet are necessary in order to maintain good posture and perform good work.
11. A correct sitting position will help to eliminate general fatigue and back strain.
12. Sit with the lower back against the chair. Rest the body weight upon the full length of the thighs.

CHAPTER 3

PERSONALITY DEVELOPMENT

(Answers to Questions on Page 16)

1. Personality is the outward reflection of the inner being.
2. Personalities are developed according to the way everyday problems are managed and solved.
3. The English a person speaks is a reflection of his or her background and culture.
4. A pleasing personality can help a student to become successful.
5. Personality analysis is necessary for self-improvement.
6. Temper, envy, jealousy, self-pity, hate and cruelty are some enemies of a good personality.
7. The foundation of politeness is thoughtfulness of others.
8. (a) A smile of greeting. (b) A word of welcome.
9. Success.
10. Success.
11. Liveliness.
12. Grammar.
13. Ideas.
14. Fashion, personal grooming, education and literature.
15. Manners.

CHAPTER 4

PROFESSIONAL ETHICS

(Answers to Questions on Page 20)

1. Ethics deal with proper conduct and business dealings in relation to employer, patrons and co-workers.
2. Courtesy, honesty, obeying the cosmetology law, and keeping your word.
3. Bad breath and body odor offend the patron and co-workers.
4. Repeating gossip will cause loss of confidence.
5. The use of profane language denotes lack of culture.
6. State Board members are acting in line of duty and contribute to the higher standards of cosmetology.
7. By complying with the cosmetology laws, the cosmetologist is contributing to the public health, welfare and safety of the community.
8. By obeying the rules and regulations of the school, the student develops habits of good citizenship and self-discipline.

CHAPTER 5

BACTERIOLOGY

(Answers to Questions on Page 26)

1. Bacteriology is the science or study of bacteria.
2. These measures protect the student, the cosmetologist and the patron against pathogenic bacteria.
3. Bacteria are minute, one-celled vegetable microorganisms found nearly everywhere.
4. Microorganisms, germs and microbes.
5. They are very minute; fifteen hundred rod-shaped bacteria barely reach across a pinhead.
6. Non-pathogenic bacteria: non-disease producing, beneficial or harmless type. Pathogenic bacteria: disease producing and harmful type.
7. (a) Parasites are bacteria that live on living matter. (b) Saprophytes are bacteria that live on dead organic matter.
8. (a) Coccus — round shape. (b) Bacillus — rod shape. (c) Spirillum — corkscrew shape.
9. Staphylococci; streptococci.

10. Each organism divides in the middle, forming two daughter cells which grow to full size and then reproduce again.

11. A local infection, such as a boil, is confined to a small part of the body. A general infection, such as blood poisoning, results when bacteria or their poisons enter the bloodstream.

12. An infection is caused by an invasion of the body tissues by disease producing bacteria.

13. Staphylococcus and streptococcus.

14. Tuberculosis, virus infections, ringworm and head lice.

15. (a) Certain bacteria, when adverse conditions arise, are capable of surrounding themselves with a tough, resistant covering; they then become spores. (b) Anthrax and tetanus.

16. One that may be transmitted from one person to another.

17. By the practice of personal hygiene, cleanliness and sanitation at all times.

18. Through the mouth, nose, eyes and breaks or wounds in the skin.

19. (a) Unbroken skin; (b) body secretions, such as perspiration; (c) white blood cells; (d) antitoxins.

20. The ability of the body to fight and overcome certain diseases caused by germs and their poisons.

21. Natural immunity means natural resistance to disease. Acquired immunity is secured after the body has by itself overcome certain diseases, or by injections of serum.

22. A human disease carrier is a person who, although immune to the disease himself, can infect other persons with the germs of the disease. Two examples are diphtheria and typhoid fever.

23. Disinfectants, intense heat and ultra-violet rays.

CHAPTER 6

STERILIZATION AND SANITATION

(Answers to Questions on Page 35)

Sterilization

1. Sterilization is the process of completely destroying all kinds of bacteria, whether harmful or beneficial.

2. Chemical.

3. Ultra-violet rays and chemical vapors keep objects clean after they have been sanitized.

4. Pathogenic bacteria.

5. Infectious diseases may be spread from one person to another.

6. Asepsis—free from disease germs. Sterile—free from all germs. Sepsis—poisoning due to germs.

7. Quats.

8. Formalin.

9. A chemical agent which may kill or prevent the growth of bacteria.

10. A chemical agent which destroys bacteria.

11. A chemical vapor used to keep sanitized objects in a sanitary condition until ready for use.

12. (a) Quats—1 to 5 minutes; (b) 25% Formalin—10 minutes; (c) 10% Formalin—20 minutes.

13. A wet sanitizer is a receptacle containing a disinfectant solution. It is best used by immersing clean implements into it for required time.

14. Clean each object with soap and water and place it into a suitable disinfectant solution for required time.

15. (a) Convenient to prepare; (b) quick acting; (c) non-corrosive; (d) non-irritating to skin.

16. Rinse implements in clean water; dry them with a clean towel, and place them in a cabinet sanitizer until ready to be used.

17. Wrap them in an individual paper envelope and place them in a dust-proof cabinet, or place them in a cabinet sanitizer until ready for use.

18. A closed, airtight cabinet containing an active fumigant (formaldehyde gas).

19. Place one tablespoon of borax and one tablespoon of Formalin solution on a small tray or blotter on the bottom of a cabinet sanitizer.

20. Formalin is a 37% to 40% solution of formaldehyde gas dissolved in water.

21. Rub the surface and sharp edges with a cotton pad dampened with 70% alcohol.

22. Gently rub surface of electrodes with a cotton pad dampened with 70% alcohol.

23. Infections.

24. 25% Formalin.

25. Short disinfection time, odorless, non-toxic and stable.

26. 1:1000 solution.

27. (a) Purchase chemicals in small quantities. (b) Store in cool, dry place. (c) Measure carefully. (d) Label all containers. (e) Keep under lock and key. (f) Avoid spilling.

28. No. All have the power to destroy bacteria, both harmful and harmless.

Sanitation

1. Sanitation refers to the employment of measures designed to promote public health and prevent disease.

2. State Board of Cosmetology and the Health Department.

3. The responsibility for sanitation rests with each student.

4. Sanitizing all equipment, implements and linen, and washing the hands before and after serving each patron.

5. Keep loose hair and waste material in covered receptacles, and remove them regularly.

6. Before and after giving a beauty service, and after using the toilet.

7. To prevent disease.

8. It is one of the most common means of transmitting disease.

9. Remove creams from containers with a clean spatula or wooden tongue blade.

10. They should be kept in dustproof containers and applied to the face with cotton pledgets.

11. Wet and dry sanitizers, disinfectant and antiseptic solutions, towel cabinet, and hot and cold running water.

12. All towels must be laundered after use on each patron, and then placed in an airtight, dustproof cabinet until used again.

13. It should be sanitized before being used on a patron.

CHAPTER 7

SHAMPOOING AND RINSING

(Answers to Questions on Page 50)

Shampooing

1. Shampoos are preparations for cleansing the scalp and hair.

2. As often as necessary, depending upon how quickly the hair and scalp become soiled.

3. Select and arrange required materials; prepare patron properly; examine hair and scalp; brush hair.

4. Wet the hair with warm water; work liquid shampoo into the hair to form a thick lather; massage entire scalp; rinse hair thoroughly; repeat shampoo and rinse; dry hair.

5. Discard used materials; sanitize soiled items; place unused supplies in their proper place.

6. Before and after the shampoo.

7. To prevent oils and perspiration from mixing with scales and dirt and forming a breeding place for bacteria.

8. (a) Prior to a lightener; (b) prior to a tint; (c) prior to a permanent wave; (d) prior to chemical hair relaxer; (e) if scalp is irritated.

9. A shampoo with a high alkaline content.

10. When the hair has been tinted or toned, or if the hair is in a damaged condition.

11. When the patron is prevented by illness from having a wet shampoo.

RINSING

1. A hair rinse consists of water alone, or a mixture of water with a mild acid, coloring agent, or special ingredients.

2. (a) To add temporary color to the hair. (b) To dissolve soap curds from the hair. (c) To give hair a soft, lustrous appearance. (d) To neutralize the yellowish tinge of white or grey hair. (e) To seal in tint or toner after a color treatment.

3. (a) Lemon rinse separates the hair strands, making the hair easier to comb. The lemon rinse has a slight lightening effect. (b) Vinegar rinse separates the hair strands, making the hair easier to comb.

4. A prepared rinse containing a blue base color.

5. It softens the hair, adds luster, and prevents the hair from tangling, making it easier to comb.

6. Color rinses are used to highlight or add temporary color to the hair.

7. Color rinses usually last from one shampoo to the next.

8. As a final rinse after a soap shampoo, acid rinse (vinegar, lemon or citric acid), and bluing rinse.

9. It is a rinse formulated to prevent the stripping of color after a tint or toner treatment.

10. A vinegar rinse may be used.

CHAPTER 8

SCALP AND HAIR TREATMENTS

(Answers to Questions on Page 58)

1. To preserve the health, cleanliness, and beauty of the hair and scalp.

2. They increase the blood circulation to the scalp, soothe the nerves, stimulate the muscles and activity of the glands, render the scalp more flexible, and increase the growth and health of the hair.

3. Thorough brushing, vigorous hand manipulations, and through the use of electrical currents.

4. The condition of the hair, whether dry or oily; any abnormal condition, such as abrasions, loss of hair, scaling of scalp, scalp disease; not to give scalp treatment prior to tinting, lightening, permanent waving, or chemical hair straightening.

5. A series of treatments, once a week for normal scalp, and more frequent for scalp disorders.

6. It removes dust and dirt, gives the hair added luster, and also stimulates the blood circulation to the scalp.

7. To keep the scalp and hair in a clean, healthy condition, and also to prevent baldness.

8. Dandruff, dry scalp, oily scalp and excessive hair loss.

9. Poor blood circulation to the scalp, improper diet and uncleanliness.

10. (a) If a scalp disorder or abrasions are present. (b) Prior to a permanent wave, lightener, tint, or chemical hair relaxer treatment.

11. When hair tonics or lotions with alcoholic content are used in connection with high-frequency, they should be applied after using the current, never before.

CHAPTER 9

HAIR SHAPING

(Answers to Questions on Page 74)

1. Hair shaping is the process of thinning, tapering and shortening the hair to mold it into a becoming shape.

2. Haircutting scissors, thinning shears, straight razor, razor with safety guard, and combs.

3. (a) To prepare the hair for easier curling and waving. (b) To accentuate a particular hairstyle. (c) To shape thick, unruly hair, to achieve a more lasting hairstyle. (d) To secure better results before giving a permanent wave.

4. Slithering is the process of thinning, or thinning and tapering, the hair by using regular haircutting scissors.

5. Combing the short hair of the strand toward the scalp.

6. The hair in these areas is usually thin and sparse and does not require thinning.

7. The cut ends would be seen in the finished hairstyle.

8. It is impossible to correct a haircut when too much hair has been removed during the thinning process.

9. (a) Fine hair: from one-half to one inch from scalp. (b) Medium hair: from one to one and one-half inches from scalp. (c) Coarse hair: from one and one-half to two inches from scalp.

10. If coarse hair is thinned too close to the scalp, the short, stubby hair ends will protrude through the top layer; fine hair, on the other hand, being softer and more pliable, will lay flatter on the head.

11. Sectioning the hair prior to hair shaping enables one to shape the hair systematically, and the final results would be a uniformly shaped hairstyle.

12. The hair must be damp in order to avoid being pulled, and to prevent the razor from being dulled.

13. A "stair-step" appearance results from the hair not being cut uniformly with scissors held over the comb.

14. (a) Protect the tips of scissor blades with fingertips of the left hand or with a comb. (b) Avoid nipping the skin with the points of the scissors. (c) Avoid giving high necklines.

CHAPTER 10

FINGER WAVING

(Answers to Questions on Page 80)

1. It is a wave that is made in wet hair, with the use of the fingers and a comb.
2. By properly draping the patron with a clean towel and shampoo cape.
3. By placing a net over the hair.
4. Because finger waving is the foundation of all modern hairstyling.
5. Naturally wavy hair and permanently waved hair.
6. The evenness of the waves and a suitable style to fit the individual.
7. They do not contain harmful ingredients.
8. Waving lotion helps to keep the hair in place while waves are being formed.
9. To protect the patron from excessive heat of the hair dryer.

CHAPTER 11

HAIRSTYLING

(Answers to Questions on Page 118)

1. A cosmetologist must have a knowledge of basic hairstyling in order to keep up with the ever-changing trends of hair fashion.
2. This personal consideration will probably result in a hairstyle more suitable to the patron.
3. A correct hair shaping supplies the foundation upon which a well-designed hairstyle may be created.
4. Hair shaping, permanent waving, and curl placement.
5. The hair should be in good, healthy condition.
6. Removing tangles in a systemic manner prevents hair damage.
7. Hair should be combed straight back.
8. Sculpture curls.
9. The hair must first be conditioned, properly tapered, wound uniformly, and each curl placed correctly either on base, on one-half off base, or completely off base.
10. Naturally or permanently waved hair.
11. Base, stem and circle.
12. The base is the stationary or immovable foundation of the curl which is attached to the scalp.
13. The stem is that part of a pin curl between the base and the first arc of the circle.
14. The stem gives the circle its direction, action and mobility.
15. The pin curl circle governs the width and strength of the wave.
16. The stem.
17. No-stem, half-stem and full-stem.
18. A no-stem curl is used for strength when a stationary line is desired.
19. It gives the base of the curl a firm, immovable position, permitting only the circle or curl to move.
20. The half-stem curl is used when the hairstyle requires some freedom of movement.
21. Movement occurs because the half-stem allows the circle to move away from its base.
22. The full-stem curl is used when the hairstyle requires a great deal of movement.

23. Square, triangular, rectangular and arc (half moon or "C" shape).
24. The shape of the base has no effect upon the resulting curl.
25. By using a full-stem curl.
26. The size of the curl determines the size of the wave.
27. To obtain an even, smooth wave and a uniform end curl.
28. For fine hair, when a fluffy comb-out is desired.
29. Forward curl — toward the face; reverse curl — away from the face.
30. The way the hair is directed (shaped) to create a guideline for a curl or wave pattern.
31. Forward and reverse.
32. The hair is directed in a circular motion, following the side hair part, downward and towards the face.
33. To prevent splits or breaks from occurring in the finished hairstyle.
34. Square-base pin curls are recommended when an even construction is desired.
35. The arc or half-moon base is used.
36. By stretching the strand during the making of the curl.
37. So that the curl holds firmly as placed.
38. Slide the clip or clippie through part of the base and/or stem at an angle and across the ends of the curl.
39. In the direction in which they are intended to be combed.
40. Give the hair a reverse shaping; then set vertical pin curls in three rows: the first row is set with reverse pin curls; the second row, forward pin curls; the third row, reverse pin curls.
41. Ridge curls are pin curls placed behind the ridge line of a shaping or finger wave.
42. The skip wave is formed by the use of a combination finger wave and pin curl pattern, with the pin curls placed in alternate finger wave formations.
43. Skip waves are recommended when wide, smooth-flowing vertical waves are desired, usually at the sides of the head.
44. The hair should be 3 to 5 inches in length.
45. Stand-up curl.
46. The cascade curl may be used to create a lift to the hairstyle.
47. Roller curls are used to create volume and/or indentation wherever needed in a hairstyle.
48. Stand-up curls are formed one at a time, while rollers can accommodate, at one time, the equivalent of from two to four stand-up curls.
49. Make the base a quarter of an inch shorter than the roller.
50. The hair is first sectioned into panels; then, it is subdivided into roller bases.
51. End papers permit control of the hair ends during winding.
52. It is used when there is not enough room to place a roller.
53. It is made in a similar way as a stand-up curl, having a flat base and containing more hair.
54. Volume means lift in a hairstyle.
55. Indentation means hollowness in a hairstyle.

56. Full volume is created by directing the hair up from the head, rolling the ends under and then rolling the hair down to the scalp onto its base.

57. Indentation is created by keeping hair at scalp level and rolling the hair over to one-half off its base.

58. Six of the following: balance point, swing point, terminal point, pivot point, pendulum point, radial point, fulcrum point, radiation point, rotary point, spotmatic.

59. Cylinder roller.

60. The texture of the hair.

61. The facial type, natural parting and the desired hairstyle.

62. A diagonal part is often used for a round or square facial type face, to create the illusion of height.

63. For hairstyles directed to one side, creating the illusion of decreasing the width of the forehead.

64. They form a cushion for the top covering hair in order to achieve a desired hairstyle.

65. Teasing, ratting, matting, French lacing.

66. Ruffing.

67. (a) Brush out curls. (b) Place general wave. (c) Accentuate and develop lines and style. (d) Finish.

68. To hold the hair in place.

69. (a) Shape of the entire head; (b) characteristics of features; (c) body structure and posture.

70. The oval facial type.

71. To create the illusion of length.

72. Style the hair to create the illusion of width at the forehead and to minimize the width at the jawline.

73. Style the hair to create the illusion of width at the jawline and to minimize the width at the forehead.

74. At the back of the head, a smooth head-hugging hairstyle, and dress the hair close to the sides.

75. Cover the neck with soft waves or curls.

76. (a) Curl: a circle or circles within a circle.
    (b) Strand: a lock or section of hair.
    (c) Slicing: carefully removing a section of hair from a shaping in preparation for making a pin curl.

CHAPTER 12

THE CARE AND STYLING OF WIGS

(Answers to Questions on Page 156)

1. (a) Fashion; (b) necessity; (c) quick changes.

2. (a) How wigs can improve the patron's appearance. (b) How wigs are made and fitted. (c) How to select and style wigs to patron's best advantage. (d) How to clean and service wigs.

3. (a) The kind of hair it contains. (b) The way it is constructed. (c) How it is fitted to the patron's measurements.

4. (a) Human hair; (b) synthetic or man-made hair; (c) animal hair; (d) a blend of synthetic, animal and human hair.

5. Cut a small piece of hair from the back area of the wig. Burn this hair and observe — human hair burns slowly and gives off a strong odor; synthetic hair burns more quickly and gives off little or no odor and tiny, hard beads can be felt in the burnt ash.

6. So that the wig will fit the patron's head correctly.

7. (a) Custom made wigs are hand knotted into a fine mesh foundation. (b) With weft wigs, the hair is machine sewn into a net cap in circular rows.

8. Brush the hair down smoothly and pin it as flat and tight as possible. Keeping close to the head, and without pressure, take flat measurements with a tape.

9. Wet the net foundation with warm water; pin it on a block of the desired size, and allow it to dry and shrink naturally.

10. Reconditioning treatments.

11. Depending on how often it is worn, usually every two to four weeks.

12. Long wefts of hair mounted with a loop at the end.

13. A hairpiece with a flat base which is used on special areas of the head.

14. A hairpiece which is sewn to a headband covering the hairline.

15. If properly handled, the style can last indefinitely.

16. On the contrary, if properly worn and cared for, a synthetic wig will protect the wearer's natural hair.

17. Modacrylic fibers.

18. The sunlight will have no effect upon it.

19. Modacrylic fiber is much lighter than human hair.

20. a) Arranging hair fibers so that all root ends are together. b) Using a hackle to mix or blend hair.

CHAPTER 13

BLOW WAVING AND CURLING

(Answers to Questions on Page 164)

1. Because it helps to create free and natural effects, and is timesaving.

2. The proper use of combs, brushes and blowers.

3. Hair that has a natural wave.

4. They concentrate the heat on the hair where it is most needed.

5. They cannot withstand the intense heat coming out of the blower.

CHAPTER 14

PERMANENT WAVING

(Answers to Questions on Page 195)

1. A method of waving the hair involving physical and chemical action.

2. Curling rods.

3. Neutralizer.

4. A waving solution and a neutralizer or fixative.

5. It softens the hair to the shape of the curling rods.

6. It stops the action of the waving lotion and re-hardens the hair into a new position.

7. A correct analysis of the patron's scalp and hair condition.

8. (a) Scalp condition; (b) hair porosity; (c) hair texture; (d) hair elasticity; (e) hair density; (f) hair length.

9. The texture and porosity of the hair.

10. Without elasticity, the hair will not hold the curl.

11. The student should follow the teacher's instructions or the manufacturer's directions.

12. The size of the rod, the blocking (sub-sectioning), and the hair texture.
13. The elasticity and texture of the hair.
14. Wrapping the hair smoothly and without tension permits better saturation and action of the waving lotion and neutralizer.
15. To avoid hair breakage, as the hair swells after absorbing waving lotion.
16. (a) Size of rod and density, and texture of the hair. (b) The length of the blockings.
17. When the waving lotion remains on the skin or scalp too long.
18. To determine in advance how the patron's hair will react to the permanent waving process.
19. Hair porosity and texture.
20. To protect dry, brittle and damaged hair.
21. (a) Immediately after the last rod is secured. (b) Following the rewet application of lotion. (c) Every 30 seconds thereafter.
22. To protect the patron.
23. Blot with a piece of cotton saturated with cold water. Do not rub. Apply neutralizer, if necessary.
24. When the wave forms a firm letter "S".
25. Weak or fine hair.
26. It is very curly when wet, frizzy when dry, and difficult to comb into a wave pattern.
27. It softens the hair and causes it to expand.
28. If a tint is given first, the waving lotion will lighten the hair and may cause an uneven color; if the permanent wave is given first, the tint may distort and weaken the wave pattern.
29. Both the method used for application and the chemicals in the rinse may disturb the wave pattern.
30. Apply a milder waving solution to those hair sections that are too curly. Retain it on the hair until the curl has relaxed sufficiently. Then thoroughly neutralize the hair.
31. A mild or very mild waving lotion.
32. By containing all essential information, a permanent wave record eliminates guesswork.
33. It relieves the salon owner, to some extent, of the responsibility for accidents or damage to patron's hair.

CHAPTER 15

HAIR COLORING AND LIGHTENING

(Answers to Questions on Page 233)

HAIR COLORING

1. The application of an artificial color preparation to the hair.
2. (a) To change grey hair to an attractive color. (b) To change natural shade of hair to a more attractive color. (c) To restore hair to its natural color.
3. Structure of the hair and scalp; proper selection of chemical agents; correct method of application; chemical reaction of solutions following application.
4. Temporary, semi-permanent and permanent.
5. One which has had no previous lightening or tinting treatment.
6. Color rinses contain certified color and remain on the hair until the next shampoo.
7. A semi-permanent hair coloring is a tint formulated to last from four to six weeks.

8. Aniline derivative tints.
9. Pure vegetable tints, metallic dyes and compound dyes.
10. The metallic and compound dyes.
11. Hair colorings having a base derived from aniline, a coal tar product.
12. When mixed with peroxide, they penetrate the cuticle layer of the hair shaft, and deposit the coloring in the cortical layer of the hair.
13. (a) A skin test is required by Federal law. (b) To determine if the patron is allergic to the tint.
14. Behind the ear or in the bend of the arm.
15. The patron's age and skin tone.
16. To determine the patron's hair condition and color results.
17. (a) Signs of a positive skin test. (b) Scalp sores or eruptions. (c) Contagious scalp disease. (d) Presence of metallic dye or compound dye.
18. Bristles of the brush may contribute to scalp irritation.
19. A single application tint.
20. One-process and one-step tints.
21. To the new growth of the hair.
22. When the hair is resistant to color.
23. (a) When the patron desires a drastic change in her color. (b) When a toner shade is desired.
24. Two-process and two-step tints.
25. To cleanse the hair and to highlight its natural color.
26. (a) Check the natural color of the hair at the scalp area. (b) Make two or more strand tests. (c) Select the appropriate color filler shade.
27. (a) Lightener application method. (b) Dye solvent application method.
28. Each patron's hair problem should be handled on an individual basis.
29. By working in a circular motion with a pledget of cotton dipped in leftover tint, commercial tint remover, cream or peroxide.
30. A color filler.
31. A color filler is recommended for discolored and damaged hair, in order to achieve a uniform porosity and shade prior to the application of the tint.
32. They recondition lightened, tinted, permanently waved and damaged hair.
33. A dye which accumulates on the outside of the hair shaft. Metallic and compound dyes.
34. A method of removing dye from the hair by means of dye solvent, commercial products or lightening treatment.
35. An aniline derivative tint.

HAIR LIGHTENING

1. Hair lightening is a partial or total removal of natural pigment or artificial color from the hair.
2. Hair tinting or toner application.
3. Applicator bottles and brushes.
4. (a) Oil lighteners; (b) cream lighteners; (c) powder lighteners.
5. (a) Frosting: strands of hair are lightened over various parts of the head. (b) Tipping: wisps of hair are lightened in various areas. (c) Streaking: a strand is lightened, usually at the front hairline.
6. The ultimate effect desired on the patron's hair.
7. 20 volume strength.
8. To hasten the lightening action.

9. Over-porous and other types of damaged hair.

10. Toners are aniline derivative tints having a pale and delicate color.

11. To the new growth of hair.

12. (a) Use of a strong lightening formula; (b) over-lapping; (c) retaining the lightener on the hair too long.

13. It makes the hair porous and lighter in color.

14. To prevent hair breakage.

15. It softens the outer cuticle of the hair, and makes it more receptive to the penetrating action of the aniline derivative tint.

16. To make it porous enough to receive the delicate color.

17. To prevent hair breakage or scalp irritation.

CHAPTER 16

CHEMICAL HAIR RELAXING

(Answers to Questions on Page 245)

1. Chemical hair relaxing is the process of straightening over-curly hair by the use of chemical agents.

2. It is a softening and swelling action on the hair.

3. To determine the true condition of the patron's hair, so that a correct hair relaxing treatment can be given.

4. Porosity, texture, elasticity and any possible hair damage.

5. (a) The Thio Method. (b) The Sodium Hydroxide Method.

6. The stabilizer.

7. Stabilizer or fixative.

8. Hair strand test.

9. To determine the degree of porosity, to determine the elasticity, and to determine the results to be expected.

10. Because the chemical hair relaxer may cause serious infection if any scalp eruptions or abrasions are present.

11. It serves as a record guide for future services.

12. To protect against lawsuits.

13. Hair which has previously been hot comb straightened, damaged by tinting or lightening, or treated with metallic dyes.

14. Hair having good porosity requires less processing time because the chemical is readily absorbed and the hair softens and relaxes quicker.

15. To protect the scalp and skin from possible burns or irritation caused by the sodium hydroxide chemical hair relaxer.

16. The sodium hydroxide in the hair relaxer can be very harmful to the cosmetologist's hands.

17. To help stop the action of the chemical relaxer by removing most of it from the hair.

18. To brush hair before the relaxer is applied may cause scalp irritation.

19. The ingredients in the cream shampoo will readily stick to the hair and help prevent tangling.

20. The hair is still soft, due to the action of the relaxer, and combing out tangles may cause breakage.

21. In order to remove all chemicals from the hair. Any chemical left in the hair will cause continuous processing and breakage.

22. It stops the action of the chemical relaxer, and at the same time, reforms the cystine (sulfur) cross bonds in their new position.

23. The hair is ready for combing when the neutralizer has rehardened the hair.

24. The conditioner is applied to offset the harshness of the relaxer and to help restore some of the natural oils to the scalp and hair.

25. Since the hair is in a fragile or weakened condition, the hair is wound on rollers without tension.

26. Because the hot comb treatments could cause chemical reactions which would result in hair breakage and loss of hair.

27. The same as the regular chemical relaxer treatment, except that the relaxer is applied to the new growth only.

28. (a) No. (b) Yes.

29. (a) Rinse out about one-half of the cream with warm water. (b) Comb the hair smooth and straight, with the remainder of the relaxer left in the hair for about five minutes. (c) Rinse balance of cream from the hair.

CHAPTER 17

THERMAL HAIR STRAIGHTENING

(Answers to Questions on Page 254)

1. Over-curly hair is temporarily straightened.

2. A soft press is accomplished with a pressing comb.

3. A hard press is accomplished with thermal irons over the comb press. It may also be accomplished with a double comb press.

4. Cuticle, cortex and medulla.

5. Most resistant: wiry, curly hair.

6. Hair that has been abused by lightening and tinting treatments.

7. The length, texture, shade and condition of the hair; the normalcy, tightness or flexibility of the scalp; abrasions and disease.

8. If the patron has a scalp injury, or a contagious hair or scalp condition.

9. Application of special scalp and hair preparations, massage, hair brushing, and exposure of scalp and hair to therapeutic light.

10. Keep the teeth of the comb facing upward, while the handle is kept away from the flame.

11. Pressing comb, heater, pressing oil, hair brush and comb, brilliantine or pomade.

12. Divide hair into small sections; apply pressing oil to hair; test temperature of heated comb; press hair with pressing comb.

13. Apply brilliantine or pomade to the scalp hair and brush it through the hair; comb and style the patron's hair. Place supplies in their proper places.

14. Burning of the hair, skin or scalp; hair breakage and skin irritation.

15. Immediately apply 1% gentian violet jelly to the burn.

CHAPTER 18

THERMAL CURLING AND WAVING

(Answers to Questions on Page 268)

THERMAL CURLING

1. Thermal curling is the art of creating curls in the hair with the aid of thermal irons and a comb.

2. Hard rubber combs.

3. Volume in a curl is the degree of lift or fullness desired in a hairstyle.
4. When fullness or maximum lift is desired in the hairstyle.
5. It is placed off base.
6. Failure to catch all the hair ends in the irons when the hair ends are being curled.
7. Nothing. The patron must wait until the hair grows out again.
8. The hair would revert back to its original over-curly state.
9. Heated thermal irons may cause damage to the hair.

THERMAL WAVING

1. Thermal waving is the art of imparting waves into the hair with the aid of heated thermal irons and a comb.
2. The temperature of heated irons is adjusted to the texture and condition of the patron's hair.
3. Each section of waved hair is made to fit perfectly into another.
4. Use a small section of waved hair as a guide for waving the rest of the hair.
5. Shadow thermal waves are shallow waves with ridges that are not too sharp.

CHAPTER 19

MANICURING

(Answers to Questions on Page 291)

MANICURING

1. Manicuring is the artful care of the hands and nails.
2. She selects and arranges sanitized implements, cosmetics and materials in an orderly manner.
3. Before and after each manicure.
4. Used manicuring implements are sanitized after each manicure.
5. Nail file, emery boards, cuticle pusher, orange-wood sticks, cuticle nippers.
6. Nail polish remover, cuticle solvent, cuticle oil, cuticle cream, nail polish, base coat and top coat.
7. Remove old polish; shape the nails; soften cuticle; apply cuticle solvent; loosen and push back cuticle; trim dead cuticle; remove soil beneath free edges; scrub nails; apply base coat, nail polish and top coat.
8. At least once a week.
9. Nails are filed with the growth of the nails to avoid splitting.
10. Apply an approved antiseptic to prevent infection.
11. To stop bleeding from a small cut.
12. It softens the cuticle.
13. It softens cuticle and removes dead cuticle.
14. A base coat serves as an adhesive base for liquid nail polish.
15. The top coat or sealer protects the nails from chipping.
16. Oil manicures are recommended for brittle nails and dry cuticles.
17. (a) Capping of fragile tips. (b) Repairing of partially broken or split nails. (c) Reattaching broken off tips.
18. For women whose hands are on display, such as models, actresses, saleswomen, and for women who may want to wear press-on artificial nails for special occasions.
19. Not more than 48 hours.
20. The massage keeps the patron's hands flexible and well-groomed, and the skin smooth.
21. To prevent accidents and injury to the patron and manicurist.
22. (a) Wash her hands before and after each manicure. (b) Sanitize all used implements after each manicure. (c) Use a clean towel for each patron.

PEDICURING

1. Pedicuring is the professional care of the feet, legs and toenails.
2. Corns, callouses, ingrown nails, foot infections, and ringworm of the feet (athlete's foot).
3. Watery blisters and thick, white skin between the toes.
4. It is an infectious condition which can be spread from one person to another.
5. File the toenails, rounding them slightly to conform to shape of toes. To avoid ingrown nails, do not file or clip into corners of nails.
6. A weekly pedicure gives the toes a well-groomed appearance. Foot bath prevents rough, harsh heels, and foot and leg massage increases circulation and keeps the skin smooth and soft.

CHAPTER 20

THE NAIL AND DISORDERS OF THE NAIL

(Answers to Questions on Page 296)

THE NAIL

1. Nails are the horny protective coverings at the tips of the fingers and toes.
2. It is firm and flexible, and exhibits a slightly pinkish color. Its surface should be smooth, curved and unspotted, without any hollows or wavy ridges.
3. It is composed mainly of keratin, a protein substance.
4. Onyx.
5. To protect the tips of the fingers and toes.
6. Keratin.
7. (a) The nail root is at the base of the nail, underneath the skin. (b) The nail body is the visible portion of the nail resting upon the nail bed. (c) The free edge is that portion of the nail which extends over the fingertip. (d) The nail bed is the part of the skin upon which the nail rests.
8. The lanula is the whitish half-moon area at the base of the nail body.
9. Nutrition and general good health.
10. General poor health, disease of the nails, and injury to the matrix.
11. The matrix.
12. In the matrix.
13. The light color of the lunula may be due to the reflection of light where the matrix and the connective tissue of the nail bed join.
14. (a) The cuticle is the overlapping epidermis around the nail. (b) The mantle is the deep fold of skin in which the nail root is imbedded. (c) The nail grooves are slits, or tracks, on the sides of the nail upon which the nail moves as it grows.
15. It is that portion of the epidermis under the free edge of the nail.
16. It is the extension of the cuticle at the base of the nail which partly overlaps the lunula.

17. The perionychium is that portion of the cuticle surrounding the entire nail border.

18. From the matrix which contains nerves, lymph and blood vessels.

19. The cells of the matrix undergo a reproducing and hardening process to produce the nail.

20. About one eighth of an inch per month.

21. It will be replaced if the matrix is in good condition.

DISORDERS OF THE NAIL
(Questions on Page 300)

1. No, the patron should be referred to a doctor.

2. Hangnail is a condition in which the cuticle splits around the nail. Dryness of the cuticle, cutting off too much cuticle, or carelessness in removing the cuticle may cause hangnail.

3. Proper nail care, such as oil treatments, will help the condition.

4. Illness.

5. a—4. b—5. c—3. d—2. e—1.

6. An antiseptic is applied immediately.

7. Corrugations, furrows, white spots, hypertrophy, atrophy, pterygium, bitten nails, brittle nails, hangnail, eggshell nails, blue nails, bruised nails.

8. Onychorrhexis.

9. Oil manicures.

10. Any nail disease.

11. Onychocryptosis.

12. Bacterial infection.

13. It is an inflammation of the nail matrix, accompanied by pus formation.

14. A vegetable parasite.

15. A vegetable parasite.

16. a—3. b—1. c—2.

17. Athlete's foot.

18. Deep, itchy, colorless vesicles appear.

19. It is contagious.

CHAPTER 21
THEORY OF MASSAGE

(Answers to Questions on Page 304)

1. Massage is the application of external manipulations to the face, or any part of the body, by hand, mechanical or electrical devices.

2. For reasons of health and beauty.

3. (a) Strong, flexible hands; (b) a quiet temperament; (c) self-control; (d) the use of psychology.

4. (a) Skin abrasions; (b) skin diseases; (c) broken capillaries.

5. (a) Effleurage—stroking. (b) Petrissage—kneading. (c) Friction—deep rubbing. (d) Percussion or tapotement—tapping, slapping and hacking. (e) Vibration—shaking.

6. The skin is nourished and rendered soft and pliable. Skin glands are stimulated.

7. (a) Muscle fibers are stimulated and strengthened. (b) Fat cells are reduced. (c) Blood circulation is increased. (d) Nerves are soothed and rested. (e) Pain is sometimes relieved.

8. (a) Therapeutic lamps, high-frequency current, and facial steamers. (b) Therapeutic lamps, high-frequency current, scalp steamers, heating caps, and vibrators.

9. Soft, light, slow and rhythmical movements.

10. Massage movements of moderate pressure, speed and time.

11. Firm, kneading—or fast, firm (but light) slapping massage movements.

CHAPTER 22
FACIAL TREATMENTS

(Answers to Questions on Page 320)

FACIAL TREATMENTS

1. a, b, d, e.

2. a, b, c, f, g.

3. About once a week.

4. To determine the condition of the patron's skin, in order to give her the facial most suitable for her skin.

5. If the skin is dry, oily or normal; if comedones, milia or acne are present; if broken capillaries are visible; if the skin is soft, harsh or rough; its color and fine lines.

6. Relaxed.

7. Cold.

8. Dry.

9. Oily.

10. An insufficient flow of sebum from the oil glands.

11. Excessive secretions of the oil glands.

12. Comedone.

13. Clean.

MASKS AND PACKS

1. When a cleansing, softening, smoothing, stimulating and refreshing effect is desired.

2. Clean.

3. For normal or oily skin.

4. Dry skin and skin inclined to wrinkle.

5. For normal or oily type skin.

6. To reduce the visibility of freckles.

CHAPTER 23
FACIAL MAKEUP

(Answers to Questions on Page 336)

FACIAL MAKEUP

1. Makeup is applied to the face for the purpose of improving its appearance. It is also used to emphasize good points and minimize facial defects, making them less conspicuous.

2. Cream, liquid, cake.

3. It creates a pleasing contour of the face, provides a uniform shade of color, conceals blemishes, and protects the skin against dirt and weather.

4. (a) Eyeshadow: to upper lids. (b) Mascara: to eyelashes and eyebrows. (c) Eyebrow pencil: to eyebrows.

5. (a) Eyecolor complements the eyes by making them look brighter and more expressive. (b) Mascara makes the eyelashes appear fuller and longer. (c) Eyebrow pencil darkens and fills in the eyebrows.

6. Liquid, cream, dry (cake) and brush-on.

7. (a) Cream rouge is applied before the face powder. (b) Dry rouge is applied after the face powder.

8. (a) Oily skin: cake foundation. (b) Dry skin: cream foundation.

9. It is unsanitary to use the same lipcolor applicator on more than one patron.

10. The oval face is generally accepted as the perfect face.

11. By the use of shading foundation cream.

12. By applying a lighter foundation cream to the forehead.

13. To minimize a bulging forehead, a darker foundation should be applied to the prominent part of the forehead and blended downward on the temples.

14. A highlight is produced by using a shade lighter than the original foundation on a particular part of the face.

15. To bring out the parts of the facial features to be emphasized.

16. A shadow is formed by using a foundation darker than the original.

17. To minimize or subdue prominent features, and to make them less noticeable.

18. Color harmony can be achieved when the makeup tones flatter the color combination of the eyes, hair and skin.

EYEBROW ARCHING
(Questions on Page 340)

1. The correct shaping of the eyebrow has a marked effect on the beauty and contour of the face.

2. To soften the brows and open the pores, making tweezing less painful.

3. Pull out the hair, in the direction in which it grows out of the follicle, with a quick, jerking motion.

4. To avoid an infection.

5. To contract the brows and surrounding skin.

6. The eyes can be made to appear closer together by extending the eyebrow line to the inside corner of the eyes.

7. To make the eyes appear farther apart, space brows farther apart by widening the distance between them; also slightly extend the brows outward.

8. The illusion of a shorter face can be created by making the eyebrows almost straight, and not extending the eyebrow line beyond the outer corners of the eyes.

9. The eyebrow arch is slightly elevated to detract from a high forehead.

10. The face will appear less round and more narrow if there is a high arch (or slight lift) on the outer ends of the eyebrows.

CHAPTER 24

ELECTROLYSIS — SUPERFLUOUS HAIR REMOVAL

(Answers to Questions on Page 345)

ELECTROLYSIS

1. Hypertrichosis.

2. Heredity, glandular disturbances, and unique racial characteristics.

3. The only method of permanent hair removal.

4. Galvanic and the shortwave methods.

5. The galvanic method destroys the papilla by causing decomposition. The shortwave method destroys the papilla by means of coagulation caused by heat.

6. Thermolysis, diathermy, high-frequency.

7. Shortwave method.

8. Because of greater speed, safety and less sensation to patron.

9. Yes. If the papilla has not been reached due to either distorted hair follicles or due to a poor insertion of the needle.

10. All areas, except the inner nostrils, eyelids and areas where the skin shows signs of inflammation or eruption.

11. No.

TEMPORARY REMOVAL OF SUPERFLUOUS HAIR
(Questions on Page 348)

1. Shaving, tweezing and depilatories.

2. Under the armpits and on the legs.

3. Around the eyebrows, mouth and chin.

4. Oil bleach mixed with two parts of peroxide.

5. Cream, paste, powder.

6. Some persons are allergic to chemical depilatories.

7. The hair will be sufficiently dissolved in ten minutes. If left on longer, it may cause skin irritation.

8. A chemical depilatory may be used on a healthy skin, preferably of the thicker type. Thin skin is usually quite sensitive.

9. (a) It is simple to use. (b) It is painless. (c) It leaves skin soft and smooth.

10. (a) It requires a skin test. (b) Some patrons may be allergic to chemical depilatories.

11. (a) Avoid applying wax that is too hot. (b) Apply it in strips. (c) Apply an emollient cream or an antiseptic lotion immediately after removal of the wax.

12. If wax is applied over warts, moles, growths or abrasions, serious infection may occur.

13. To prevent skin burns.

14. As the hair grows out, repeated treatments at regular intervals are necessary.

CHAPTER 25

CELLS

(Answers to Questions on Page 352)

1. A cell is the basic unit of all living things, including humans.

2. They differ as to size, shape, structure and function.

3. Protoplasm.

4. Nucleus, cytoplasm.

5. (a) The nucleus plays an important part in the reproduction of the cell. (b) Cytoplasm supplies the food materials necessary for growth and reproduction.

6. Reproduction takes place by indirect division.

7. It is a complex chemical process whereby body cells are nourished and supplied with energy to carry on their many activities.

8. Anabolism and catabolism.

9. The cell takes in whatever food, water and oxygen it needs.

10. The cell uses up whatever it has taken in.

11. They are groups of the same kind of cells, all performing the same function.

12. (a) Connective tissue; (b) muscular tissue; (c) nerve tissue; (d) epithelial tissue; (d) liquid tissue.

13. It is a structure containing two or more different tissues, combining to accomplish a definite function.

14. The heart.

15. The lungs.
16. They are groups of organs which work together in performing body functions.
17. Skeletal, muscular, nervous, circulatory, endocrine, excretory, respiratory, digestive and reproductive systems.
18. The nervous system.
19. The skeletal system.
20. The muscular system.
21. The circulatory system.

CHAPTER 26
THE SKIN AND DISORDERS OF THE SKIN
(Answers to Questions on Page 359)

THE SKIN

1. The skin is a slightly moist, soft, strong, flexible covering of the body, and it is acidic.
2. A fine texture, healthy color and free of blemishes.
3. The epidermis and dermis.
4. It is the outermost layer of the skin and the outer protective covering of the body.
5. (a) Stratum corneum (horny layer); (b) stratum lucidum (clear layer); (c) stratum granulosum (granular layer); (d) stratum germinativum.
6. Stratum corneum.
7. Stratum lucidum.
8. Stratum granulosum.
9. Stratum germinativum.
10. The dermis is a highly sensitive and vascular layer of connective tissue. Within its structure are numerous blood vessels, lymph vessels, nerves, sweat glands, oil glands, hair follicles, arrector pili muscles and papillae.
11. Papillary and reticular layers.
12. Papillae, melanin.
13. Fat cells, blood vessels, lymph vessels, oil glands, sweat glands, hair follicles, arrector pili muscles.
14. It gives smoothness to the body, contains fat for use as energy, and is a protective cushion for the outer skin.
15. ½ to ⅔ of the entire blood supply in the body is distributed to the skin.
16. Blood and lymph nourish the skin.
17. Motor, sensory and secretory nerve fibers.
18. The fingertips.
19. To arrector pili muscles attached to hair follicles.
20. The elastic fibers in the dermis.
21. In the deepest layer of the stratum germinativum of the epidermis, and in the papillary layer of the dermis.
22. They react to heat, cold, touch, pressure and pain.
23. They regulate the excretion of perspiration from sweat glands, and control the flow of sebum to the surface of the skin.
24. After the skin is stretched, it regains its former shape almost immediately.
25. Loss of elasticity.
26. The coloring matter melanin, and the blood supply.
27. Protection sensation, heat regulation, secretion, excretion, and absorption.
28. Blood circulation through the skin, and evaporation of sweat.
29. 98.6 degrees Fahrenheit.

30. Hormone creams.
31. Hair, nails, sweat glands, oil glands.

SWEAT AND OIL GLANDS

1. Sudoriferous or sweat glands, sebaceous or oil glands.
2. They consist of a coiled base and a tube-like duct, which form a pore at the surface of the skin.
3. Over the entire area of the skin, more numerous on the palms, soles, forehead and armpits.
4. They help to eliminate waste products in the form of sweat.
5. Heat, exercise, mental excitement and certain drugs.
6. They consist of small sacs whose ducts open into the neck of the hair follicle.
7. Sebum, an oily substance.
8. It lubricates the skin and hair, keeping them soft and pliable.
9. Oil glands are found in all parts of the body, with the exception of the palms and soles.

DISORDERS OF THE SKIN
(Questions on Page 367)

1. To prevent their spread, and to avoid more serious conditions.
2. To help prevent the spread of infection to others.
3. To safeguard her own and the public's health.
4. Dermatology is the study of the skin, its nature, structure, functions, diseases and treatment.
5. A skin specialist.
6. A structural change in the tissues caused by injury or disease.
7. An objective lesion can be seen. (Pimples). A subjective lesion can be felt. (Itching).
8. Macule, papule, wheal, tubercle, tumor, vesicle, bulla and pustule.
9. Scale, crust, excoriation, fissure, ulcer, scar and skin stain.
10. Any departure from a normal state of health.
11. (a) Blackheads; (b) whiteheads.
12. A worm-like mass of hardened sebum obstructing the duct of the oil glands.
13. Acne is a chronic inflammatory disorder of the sebaceous (oil) glands.
14. Milia, acne, comedones and seborrhea.
15. Bromidrosis—foul smelling perspiration. Anidrosis —lack of perspiration. Hyperidrosis—excessive perspiration. Miliaria rubra—prickly heat.
16. Dermatitis is a term used to denote an inflammatory condition of the skin.
17. An inflammation of the skin of acute or chronic nature. Its cause is unknown.
18. The lesions are round, dry patches covered with coarse, silvery scales.
19. On the scalp, elbows, knees, chest and lower back.
20. It is a virus infection. Fever blister.
21. Lips, nostrils or other parts of the face.
22. Eruptive skin infections. Aniline derivative tinting and cold waving.
23. Small yellowish to brownish colored spots, caused by sunlight and air.
24. Moth patches or liver spots.
25. Birthmark.
26. Abnormal white patches of skin due to genetic defect; an acquired condition of leucoderma, affecting the skin or the hair.

27. A congenital absence of pigment in the body, including the skin, hair and eyes.
28. Keratoma.
29. A small brownish spot or blemish of the skin.
30. Verruca.

CHAPTER 27

HAIR AND DISORDERS OF THE HAIR

(Answers to Questions on Page 378)

1. A slender, thread-like outgrowth of the skin and scalp of the human body.
2. Trichology.
3. It gives the cosmetologist an understanding of proper hair care and treatment that is beneficial to patrons.
4. The hair serves as an adornment, but it also protects the head from heat, cold and injury.
5. Harmful cosmetic applications or faulty hair treatments.
6. Keratin.
7. The hair root and hair shaft.
8. Strongly alkaline solutions cause intense swelling of the hair and breakage of the bonds.
9. It is that portion of the hair beneath the surface of the skin.
10. It is that portion of the hair which extends beyond the skin.
11. It is a tube-like depression or pocket in the skin.
12. The direction of the natural flow of hair on the scalp.
13. A club-shaped structure forming the lower part of the hair root. It fits over and covers the papilla.
14. A small cone-shaped elevation at the bottom of the hair follicle that fits into the hair bulb.
15. Arrector pili muscle and sebaceous gland.
16. From the small blood vessels in the papilla.
17. The papilla produces hair cells during hair growth.
18. Germs and dirt.
19. Fear or cold, which causes the arrector pili muscles to contract.
20. They secrete sebum, an oily substance, which keeps the hair and scalp in a soft and pliable condition.
21. (a) Diet; (b) blood circulation; (c) emotional disturbances; (d) stimulation of endocrine glands; (e) drugs.
22. The shape and size of the hair follicle.
23. (a) Straight hair is usually round. (b) Wavy hair is usually oval. (c) Curly hair is almost flat.
24. Cuticle, cortex and medulla.
25. The cuticle.
26. The cortex.
27. The medulla.
28. Palms of the hands, soles of the feet, lips and eyelids.
29. Lanugo hair is fine, soft and downy, and is usually found on all areas of the body.
30. It helps in the evaporation of perspiration.
31. Growth, fall, and replacement of the hair.

32. The new hair is formed by cell division, which occurs at the root of the hair around the papilla.
33. About one-half inch per month.
34. (a) Light blonde—140,000. (b) Black—108,000. (c) Brown—110,000.
35. (a) Moisture in the air deepens the natural wave. (b) Cold air will cause hair to contract. (c) Heat will cause hair to expand and absorb moisture.
36. About 120 square inches.
37. The coloring matter in hair.
38. Between 50 and 80.
39. From 2 to 4 years.
40. The loss of natural pigment, and the presence of air spaces in the hair.
41. (a) A cowlick is a tuft of hair standing up. (b) A whorl is an area of the scalp where the hair forms in a swirl effect, such as in the crown area.
42. A person who is born with white hair and without pigment coloring in the skin or iris of the eyes.
43. Sight, touch, hearing and smell.
44. Texture, porosity, elasticity, and condition of the hair.
45. Touch and sight.
46. Degree of coarseness or fineness of the hair.
47. Ability of hair to absorb moisture.
48. Ability of hair to stretch and return to its original form without breakage.
49. (a) Normal dry hair can be stretched about one-fifth of its length. (b) When wet, it can be stretched from 40-50% of its length.

DISORDERS OF THE HAIR
(Questions on Page 383)

1. Dandruff is recognized as being the small, white scales that appear on the scalp and hair.
2. A direct cause of dandruff is the excessive shedding of the epithelial cells.
3. (a) Poor circulation; (b) infection; (c) injury; (d) lack of nerve stimulation; (e) improper diet; (f) uncleanliness.
4. (a) Pityriasis; (b) pityriasis capitis simplex; (c) pityriasis steatoides.
5. Alopecia is the technical term for any form of hair loss.
6. No. When hair has grown to its full length, it comes out by itself and is replaced by new hair.
7. It is a form of baldness occurring in old age.
8. It is a form of baldness beginning any time before middle age by a slow thinning process.
9. The natural shedding of hair occurs most frequently in spring and fall.
10. It is the sudden falling out of hair in round patches, or baldness in spots.
11. Ringworm is the common term for tinea.
12. It is caused by vegetable parasites.
13. Ringworm starts with a small, reddened patch of little blisters which spread outward and heal in the middle with scaling. Several such patches may be present.
14. Head lice. No.
15. Boil.
16. Canities.

17. Worry, anxiety, nervous strain, prolonged illness, heredity.

18. (a) It is the technical name for split hair ends. (b) Superfluous hair.

19. Alternate bands of gray and dark hair.

20. Hirsuties.

21. (a) Trichorrhexis nodosa; (b) monilethrix.

22. It is the technical term for brittle hair.

CHAPTER 28

ANATOMY

(Answers to Questions on Page 388)

BONES OF THE SKULL

1. Bone is the hardest structure of the body.

2. (a) Give shape and strength to the body. (b) Protect the organs from injury. (c) Serve as an attachment for muscles. (d) Act as levers for all bodily movements.

3. The skull is the skeleton of the head.

4. It is divided into two parts: the cranium and the skeleton of the face.

5. Eight bones.

6. (a) Occipital; (b) two parietal; (c) frontal; (d) two temporal.

7. Back and lower part of the cranium.

8. The sides and top of head.

9. The frontal bone.

10. Temporal bones.

11. Sphenoid bone.

12. Fourteen bones.

13. (a) Two nasal bones; (b) two zygomatic bones; (c) two maxillae bones; (d) mandible bone.

14. The whole upper jaw.

15. The lower jaw.

16. Zygomatic bones.

17. In the front part of the throat.

18. It forms the top part of the spinal column, and is located in the neck region.

19. Thorax.

SHOULDER, ARM AND HAND BONES

1. Clavicle and scapula.

2. (a) Upper arm—humerus; (b) Forearm—ulna and radius.

3. (a) Wrist—eight; (b) Palm—five; (c) Fingers—fourteen.

4. Carpal bones.

5. Metacarpal bones.

6. Digits.

7. Phalanges are the three bones that make up each finger and two in the thumb.

MUSCLE (Questions on Page 392)

1. Muscle is a contractile, elastic, fibrous tissue by which movements of the body are produced.

2. Muscles cover, shape and support the skeleton, and effect all body movements.

3. (a) Voluntary or striated muscle; (b) involuntary or non-striated muscle; (c) cardiac or heart muscle.

4. Voluntary muscles, such as those of the face, arms and legs, are controlled by the will. Involuntary muscles, such as those of the stomach and intestines, are not controlled by the will.

5. The skeletal and nervous systems.

6. (a) Origin of a muscle refers to its more fixed attachment. (b) Insertion of a muscle refers to its more movable attachment.

7. Chemicals, massage, electric current, light rays, heat rays, moist heat, nerve impulses.

MUSCLES OF THE HEAD, FACE, NECK AND BACK

1. The epicranius covers the entire top of the scalp, from the base of the skull to the eyebrows. The occipitalis is the back portion; the frontalis is the front portion.

2. It raises the eyebrow and draws the scalp forward, causing transverse wrinkles across the forehead.

3. The orbicularis oculi.

4. Corrugator.

5. Orbicularis oris.

6. Procerus.

7. Trapezius.

8. Platysma.

9. Trapezius.

MUSCLES OF THE ARM AND HAND

1. Deltoid, biceps and triceps.

2. Pronators, supinators, flexors and extensors.

3. The pronators turn the palm downward. The supinators turn the palm upward.

4. The flexor muscles bend the wrist, draw the hand up, and close the fingers toward the forearm. The extensor muscles straighten out the hand and fingers.

THE NERVOUS SYSTEM (Questions on Page 398)

1. (a) To understand how to administer scalp and facial treatments for the patron's benefit. (b) To understand what effects these treatments have on the nerves in the skin and on the body as a whole.

2. The brain, spinal cord and their nerves.

3. The cerebro-spinal, the peripheral and the sympathetic nervous systems.

4. Controls consciousness, voluntary functions of the five senses, and voluntary muscle actions.

5. The peripheral system consists of sensory and motor nerve fibers which carry messages to and from the cerebro-spinal nervous system.

6. The functions of the sympathetic nervous system are independent of the will. This system controls involuntary body functions, such as breathing, circulation, digestion and glandular activity.

7. A neuron is the structural unit of the nervous system.

8. It is composed of a cell body, and long and short fibers called cell processes.

9. Nerves are long white cords made up of fibers, which carry messages to and from various parts of the body.

10. Sensory and motor nerves.

11. Sensory nerves carry messages regarding touch, heat, cold, sight, hearing, smell, taste and pain to the nerve centers in the brain.

12. (a) Sensory nerves—afferent nerves. (b) Motor nerves—efferent nerves.

13. Motor nerves carry messages from the brain to the muscles, which produce movements of the body.

14. A quick removal of the hand away from a hot object.

15. Worry, excessive mental work, excessive muscular activity.

16. Chemicals, massage, electrical currents, light rays, heat rays, moist heat.

17. There are twelve pairs of cranial nerves. Thirty-one pairs of spinal nerves.

18. The fifth or trigeminal nerve, the seventh or facial nerve, the eleventh or accessory nerve.

19. The fifth cranial nerve.

20. It is the chief sensory nerve of the face, and the motor nerve of the muscles of mastication.

21. The seventh cranial nerve.

22. (a) The optic nerve; (b) the olfactory nerve; (c) the acoustic (auditory) nerve.

23. The scalp at the back part of the head, as far up as the top of the head.

24. The spinal portion of the eleventh cranial nerve.

25. (a) Supra-orbital. (b) Nasal. (c) Infra-orbital. (d) Mental. (e) Auriculo-temporal. (f) Zygomatic.

26. a) Temporal. (b) Mandibular. (c) Cervical. (d) Posterior auricular. (d) Buccal. (f) Zygomatic.

Nerves of the Arm and Hand

1. The ulnar nerve supplies the little finger side of the arm and palm of the hand. The radial nerve supplies the thumb side of the arm and back of the hand.

2. The digital nerve supplies the fingers.

The Circulatory System (Questions on Page 403)

1. The circulatory system supplies nourishment to the entire body as well as to the skin, hair and nails.

2. (a) Carries water, oxygen, food and secretions to all cells of the body. (b) Carries away carbon dioxide and waste products for elimination. (c) Helps to equalize the body temperature. (d) Aids in protecting the body from harmful bacteria and infections through action of the white blood cells. (e) Clots the blood.

3. It keeps the blood moving within the circulatory system.

4. Arteries, veins, capillaries.

5. The arteries.

6. The capillaries.

7. They carry impure blood from all parts of the body back to the heart.

8. (a) The pulmonary system; (b) the general or systemic system.

9. The blood consists of blood plasma, red and white corpuscles and blood platelets.

10. 98.6 degrees Fahrenheit.

11. Blood plasma is composed of about 9/10th's water, and carries food elements, waste products and other substances.

12. Red blood cells carry oxygen to the cells of the body.

13. White blood cells protect the body against disease.

14. Lymph is a colorless, watery fluid, circulating through the lymph-vascular system.

15. (a) Supplies parts of the body not reached by the blood. (b) Carries nourishment from the blood to the body cells. (c) Removes waste material from the body cells. (d) Carries on an interchange with the blood. (e) Fights infection.

16. Lymph is derived from the blood plasma.

Blood Vessels of the Head, Face and Neck
(Questions on Page 404)

1. Common carotid arteries.

2. Internal common carotid artery; external common carotid artery.

3. Internal branches of the common carotid arteries.

4. External branches of the common carotid arteries.

5. Facial artery.

6. Submental artery.

7. Frontal artery.

8. The back of the head, up to the crown.

9. (a) Superior labial artery; (b) inferior labial artery.

10. Parietal artery—the crown and side of the head. Frontal artery—forehead.

11. Frontal and parietal arteries.

12. Posterior auricular artery.

13. The infra-orbital artery.

14. Internal jugular and external jugular.

Blood Circulation of Arms and Hands

1. The ulnar and radial arteries.

2. The ulnar artery.

3. The radial artery.

Endocrine, Excretory, Respiratory and Digestive Systems (Questions on Page 406)

1. The duct glands and the ductless glands.

2. The kidneys, liver, skin, large intestine, lungs.

3. With each cycle an exchange of gases takes place. During inhalation, oxygen is absorbed into the blood, while carbon dioxide is expelled during exhalation.

4. Mouth, pharynx, esophagus, stomach, small intestine.

CHAPTER 29

ELECTRICITY AND LIGHT THERAPY

(Answers to Questions on Page 413)

Electricity

1. Electricity is a form of energy which produces magnetic, chemical or heating effects.

2. A conductor is a substance which readily transmits an electric current.

3. A non-conductor or insulator is a substance that resists the passage of an electrict current. Rubber, silk, dry wood, glass, cement, and asbestos are examples of non-conductors.

4. Electrodes are special terminal devices which serve as points of contact when applying electricity to the body.

5. Direct current (d.c.) is a constant and even-flowing current, traveling in one direction.

6. Alternating current (a.c.) is a rapid and interrupted current, flowing first in one direction and then in the opposite direction.

7. A converter.

8. A rectifier.

9. A volt is a unit of electrical pressure.

10. An ampere is a unit of electrical strength.

11. An ohm is a unit of electrical resistance.

High-Frequency Current

1. A high-frequency current is characterized by a high rate of vibration.

2. Tesla current, commonly called the "violet ray."

3. The primary action of this current is heat-producing, which is either stimulating or soothing, depending on the method of application.

4. (a) Facial electrode; (b) scalp electrode; (c) metal electrode.

5. (a) Direct surface application; (b) indirect application; (c) general electrification.
6. The cosmetologist holds the electrode and applies it over the patron's skin.
7. The patron holds the metal or glass electrode while the cosmetologist uses her fingers to massage the surface being treated. At no time does the cosmetologist hold the electrode.
8. The patron holds the metal electrode in her hand; her body is charged with electricity without being touched by the cosmetologist.
9. General electrification.
10. The cosmetologist lifts the electrode slightly from the area to be treated and applies the current through the clothing or a towel.
11. Approximately five minutes.
12. The high-frequency must be applied first and then the lotion.
13. (a) Stimulates circulation of the blood. (b) Increases glandular activity. (c) Aids in elimination and absorption. (d) Increases metabolism. (e) Germicidal action occurs during use.
14. (a) Falling hair; (b) itchy scalp; (c) tight scalp; (d) excessively oily scalp; (e) excessively dry scalp.

VIBRATOR

1. A vibrator is an electric appliance used in massage to produce a mechanical succession of manipulations.
2. The vibrator should never be used when there is a pronounced weakness of the heart, or in cases of fever, abscesses or inflammation.
3. The vibrator is used over heavy muscular tissue, such as the scalp, shoulders and upper back.

STEAMER

1. The steamer or vaporizer is applied over the head or face to produce a moist, uniform heat.
2. It helps to cleanse the skin, clean out the pores, and soften any scaliness on the surface of the skin.
3. It softens the scalp, increases perspiration, and promotes the effectiveness of applied scalp cosmetics.

THERMAL CURLING IRON

1. Built in heating element.
2. The vapor leaves the iron through small perforations and conditions the hair as it curls.

HEATING CAP

1. Heating caps are electrical devices, applied over the head, which provide a uniform source of heat.
2. Their main use is as part of corrective treatments for the hair and scalp.
3. Heating caps help to recondition dry, brittle and damaged hair, and also serve to activate a sluggish scalp.

PROCESSING MACHINE

1. To reduce the processing time for lightening and tinting the hair.
2. The machine accelerates the molecular movement within the chemicals of the product so that they work faster.

ELECTRICITY AND LIGHT THERAPY
(Questions on Page 418)

1. Treatment by means of light rays.
2. Ultra-violet rays and infra-red rays.
3. An electrical apparatus used in producing various rays of the sun.

4. Glass bulb lamp, hot quartz lamp, and cold quartz lamp.
5. Glass bulb lamp and hot quartz lamp.
6. Iron, vitamin D, red and white blood cells.
7. They increase the blood and lymph flow, restore nutrition and increase the elimination of waste products.
8. Acne, tinea, seborrhea and dandruff.
9. They stimulate the growth of hair.
10. About twelve inches.
11. To prevent irritation and injury to the eyes.
12. About two to three minutes.
13. Seven or eight minutes.
14. Prolonged exposure may cause severe sunburn and blisters.
15. Slight reddening of the skin, appearing several hours after application, without any signs of itching, peeling or burning.
16. The ultra-violet rays stimulate the production of pigment or coloring matter in the skin.
17. The slightest covering on the skin prevents these ultra-violet rays from reaching the skin.
18. Special glass bulbs.
19. The eyes should be covered with pads dipped in boric acid or witch hazel solution.
20. About thirty inches from the skin.
21. To prevent constant exposure on the tissues.
22. (a) Heat and relax the skin. (b) Dilate blood vessels in the skin, thereby increasing blood flow. (c) Increace metabolism and chemical changes within skin tissues. (d) Increase the production of perspiration on the skin. (e) Relieve pain.
23. Dermal lights, having a tungsten or carbon filament in clear or colored bulbs.
24. To protect the eyes from the heat and glare of the light.
25. The heat relieves pain in congested areas.
26. Blue light.
27. It has a tonic effect on the bare skin, and soothes the nerves.
28. (a) The heat penetrates the skin. (b) It has a stimulating effect on the skin. (c) It aids penetration of creams and ointments.

CHAPTER 30

CHEMISTRY

(Answers to Questions on Page 438)

1. It gives them the ability to understand the proper usage of the various chemicals and cosmetics used in the beauty salon.
2. (a) H_2O; (b) H_2O_2.
3. Filtration and distillation.
4. Soft water.
5. A head and a tail.
6. (a) The tail attracts dirt, grease, debris and oil, but has no attraction for water. (b) The head attracts water, but does not attract dirt.
7. As the stream of water goes through the hair, the molecule heads of the shampoo attach themselves to the water molecules and are carried from the hair, taking with them the attached dirt.

8. The thio solution penetrates the cuticle and softens the cortex by breaking down all the H-bonds and many of the S-bonds. This permits slippage of the polypeptide chains to take place and assume the contour of the rods.

9. Thioglycolate and sodium hydroxide.

10. The hair may be dissolved.

11. These tints are composed of very small, colorless molecules that easily pass through the cuticle imbrications.

12. The developer combines the small, colorless molecules into giant colored molecules.

13. The large colored molecules that are developed inside the cortex cannot be shampooed from the hair because they are too large to pass out through the imbrications.

14. Melanin is the name given to black to brown hair color pigments. Oxymelanin are the red to yellow hair pigments.

15. A solute is a substance dissolved in a solution. A solvent is a liquid used to dissolve a solute.

CHAPTER 31
SALON MANAGEMENT
(Answers to Questions on Page 450)

OPENING A BEAUTY SALON

1. A good location should be in a large enough area to support the salon. It should be near other active business places which attract women.

2. A store lease guards against an increase in rent.

3. The reception area is the first contact the patron has with the salon, and it sets the tone for the rest of the salon.

4. Advertising should attract the reader's attention, and create a desire for the service advertised.

5. (a) Inexperience in dealing with the public and employees. (b) Not enough capital. (c) Lack of proper basic training in the beauty school. (d) Business neglect.

TELEPHONE TECHNIQUES FOR THE BEAUTY SALON
(Questions on Page 457)

1. (a) To make or change appointments. (b) To go after new business, or strayed or infrequent patrons. (c) To remind patrons of needed services. (d) To answer questions and render friendly service. (e) To adjust complaints and satisfy patrons. (f) To receive messages. (g) To order equipment and supplies.

2. "Phone as you would be phoned to."

3. (a) Display an interested, helpful attitude. (b) Be prompt in answering the phone. (c) Give all necessary information to the caller. (d) Be tactful.

4. (a) Clear speech; (b) correct speech; (c) pleasing tone of voice.

5. List the main points on a pad so she will know what to say.

6. The use of good telephone techniques helps make friends, brings in more business, and creates goodwill for the beauty salon.

7. A cosmetologist should give a patron's complaint careful consideration by using self-control, tact and courtesy.

8. The best way to overcome a price objection is to build up the value of your services in the patron's mind.

BEAUTY SALON SALESMANSHIP
(Questions on Page 463)

1. (a) Be familiar with the product or service. (b) Adapt the selling approach to each patron. (c) Be self-confident. (d) Stimulate attention, interest and desire. (e) Never misrepresent your product or service. (f) Use tact in handling a patron. (g) Understand human nature. (h) Don't be negative. (i) Deliver a sales talk in a relaxed, friendly manner. (j) Recognize the right psychological moment to close the sale.

2. (a) Shy, timid; (b) talkative; (c) nervous, irritable; (d) inquisitive, over-cautious; (e) conceited, "Know It All"; ((f) teenager; (g) old-timer.

3. First determine whether the patron has a need for it.

4. Sincerity and honesty are the foundation of good salesmanship.

5. Simple and suggestive language will tend to make the patron feel like buying.

6. The use of picture words and descriptive adjectives charged with feeling.

7. Every patron is a potential source of new customers and additional beauty treatments.

8. Demonstrating a product or service is one of the most effective selling tools.

9. By the salon's cosmetologists wearing the latest hairstyles themselves.

10. She is a walking advertisement of the services rendered in her salon.

BUSINESS RECORDS AND SUPPLIES
(Questions on Page 466)

1. Records should be kept correct, concise and complete.

2. (a) They contribute to the efficient operation of the beauty salon. (b) Determine income, expense, profit and loss. (c) Prove the value of the beauty salon to a prospective buyer. (d) Helpful in arranging for a bank loan. (e) Needed for government reports.

3. At least six months.

4. At least seven years.

5. Consumption and retail supplies.

6. Individual, partnership, corporation.

FIRST AID (Questions on Page 470)

1. A physician should be called as soon as possible after any accident has occurred.

2. An antiseptic, such as tincture of iodine, should be applied.

3. Heat exhaustion is a general functional depression due to heat.

4. A nose bleed is treated by loosening the collar and applying pads saturated with cool water to the face and back of the neck.

5. Lack of blood flowing to the brain, bad air, indigestion, nervous condition, unpleasant odors.

CROSS INDEX

BIBLIOGRAPHY

In the revision of this textbook, the following basic references and authorities were consulted. The books herein listed can be purchased directly from the Milady Publishing Corp., 3839 White Plains Road, Bronx, New York 10467.

Basic References:

Air Jet Hairstyling—Michael D. Morro
A Man's Guide to Business and Social Success—Ruth Tolman
Beautician's Guide to Beauty, Charm and Poise—Ruth Tolman
Chemistry in Your Beauty Shop—Arnold Lowman, Ph.D.
Common Skin Diseases—H. Goodman, M.D.
Curling Iron Techniques with Directional Design—Mary Lou Augustine
Electricity and Light—Noble M. Eberhart, M.D.
Electrolysis, Thermolysis and the Blend—Arthur R. Hinkel
Essentials of Histology—Gerrit Bevelander, Ph.D.
Gray's Anatomy—Warren H. Lewis
Hair Structure and Chemistry Simplified—A. H. Powitt
Harry's Cosmetology—Ralph G. Harry
Human Anatomy and Physiology—Dr. King and Dr. Showers
New Gould's Medical Dictionary—G. M. Gould, A.M., M.D.
Principles and Practices of Beauty Culture—Florence E. Wall, A.M., F.A.I.C.
Salesmanship in the Beauty Salon—Margaret B. Fleck
Standard Textbook of Cosmetology—Constance V. Kibbe
Stedman's Practical Medical Dictionary—Norman B. Taylor, M.D.
Synopsis of Diseases of the Skin—Sutton and Sutton
The Complete Guide to Wigs and Hairpieces—Rebecca Hyman
The Make-Up Artist in the Beauty Salon—Vincent J-R Kehoe
The Scalp in Health and Disease—Howard T. Behrman, A.B., M.D.
Your Skin and Its Care—Dr. Behrman and Dr. Levin

Trade Periodicals:

National Beauty School Journal
Modern Beauty Shop
American Hairdresser/Salon Owner

Authorities Consulted:

Illustrations by Warren Meek
Garo Artinian in the revision of the chapter on electrolysis
Milady Textbook Educational Board

The publisher expresses sincere thanks to those manufacturers who so willingly cooperated in the revision of this text.